Oncologic Thermoradiotherapy: Need for Evidence, Harmonisation, and Innovation

Oncologic Thermoradiotherapy: Need for Evidence, Harmonisation, and Innovation

Editors

Stephan Bodis
Pirus Ghadjar
Gerard C. Van Rhoon

MDPI • Basel • Beijing • Wuhan • Barcelona • Belgrade • Manchester • Tokyo • Cluj • Tianjin

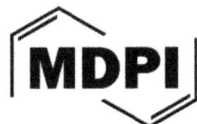

Editors

Stephan Bodis
Radiation Oncology
Department ITIS Foundation
University and University
Hospital Zurich
Zurich
Switzerland

Pirus Ghadjar
Radiation Oncology
Charite Berlin
Berlin
Germany

Gerard C. Van Rhoon
Radiation Oncology - Unit of
Hyperthermia
Erasmus University
Rotterdam
Netherlands

Editorial Office
MDPI
St. Alban-Anlage 66
4052 Basel, Switzerland

This is a reprint of articles from the Special Issue published online in the open access journal *Cancers* (ISSN 2072-6694) (available at: www.mdpi.com/journal/cancers/special_issues/thermoradiotherapy_oncology).

For citation purposes, cite each article independently as indicated on the article page online and as indicated below:

LastName, A.A.; LastName, B.B.; LastName, C.C. Article Title. *Journal Name* **Year**, *Volume Number*, Page Range.

ISBN 978-3-0365-4532-5 (Hbk)
ISBN 978-3-0365-4531-8 (PDF)

© 2022 by the authors. Articles in this book are Open Access and distributed under the Creative Commons Attribution (CC BY) license, which allows users to download, copy and build upon published articles, as long as the author and publisher are properly credited, which ensures maximum dissemination and a wider impact of our publications.

The book as a whole is distributed by MDPI under the terms and conditions of the Creative Commons license CC BY-NC-ND.

Contents

About the Editors . . . . **vii**

Preface to "Oncologic Thermoradiotherapy: Need for Evidence, Harmonisation, and Innovation" . . . . **ix**

Stephan Bodis, Pirus Ghadjar and Gerard van Rhoon
Oncologic Thermoradiotherapy: Need for Evidence, Harmonisation, and Innovation
Reprinted from: *Cancers* **2022**, *14*, 2418, doi:10.3390/cancers14102418 . . . . **1**

Baard-Christian Schem, Frank Pfeffer, Martin Anton Ott, Johan N. Wiig, Nils Sletteskog and Torbjørn Frøystein et al.
Long-Term Outcome in a Phase II Study of Regional Hyperthermia Added to Preoperative Radiochemotherapy in Locally Advanced and Recurrent Rectal Adenocarcinomas
Reprinted from: *Cancers* **2022**, *14*, 705, doi:10.3390/cancers14030705 . . . . **5**

Sota Nakahara, Takayuki Ohguri, Sho Kakinouchi, Hirohide Itamura, Takahiro Morisaki and Subaru Tani et al.
Intensity-Modulated Radiotherapy with Regional Hyperthermia for High-Risk Localized Prostate Carcinoma
Reprinted from: *Cancers* **2022**, *14*, 400, doi:10.3390/cancers14020400 . . . . **21**

Carrie Anne Minnaar, Innocent Maposa, Jeffrey Allan Kotzen and Ans Baeyens
Effects of Modulated Electro-Hyperthermia (mEHT) on Two and Three Year Survival of Locally Advanced Cervical Cancer Patients
Reprinted from: *Cancers* **2022**, *14*, 656, doi:10.3390/cancers14030656 . . . . **35**

Yohan Lee, Sunghyun Kim, Hyejung Cha, Jae Hun Han, Hyun Joon Choi and Eun Go et al.
Long-Term Feasibility of 13.56 MHz Modulated Electro-Hyperthermia-Based Preoperative Thermoradiochemotherapy in Locally Advanced Rectal Cancer
Reprinted from: *Cancers* **2022**, *14*, 1271, doi:10.3390/cancers14051271 . . . . **55**

Andras Szasz
Heterogeneous Heat Absorption Is Complementary to Radiotherapy
Reprinted from: *Cancers* **2022**, *14*, 901, doi:10.3390/cancers14040901 . . . . **71**

Mark W. Dewhirst, James R. Oleson, John Kirkpatrick and Timothy W. Secomb
Accurate Three-Dimensional Thermal Dosimetry and Assessment of Physiologic Response Are Essential for Optimizing Thermoradiotherapy
Reprinted from: *Cancers* **2022**, *14*, 1701, doi:10.3390/cancers14071701 . . . . **113**

Azzaya Sengedorj, Michael Hader, Lukas Heger, Benjamin Frey, Diana Dudziak and Rainer Fietkau et al.
The Effect of Hyperthermia and Radiotherapy Sequence on Cancer Cell Death and the Immune Phenotype of Breast Cancer Cells
Reprinted from: *Cancers* **2022**, *14*, 2050, doi:10.3390/cancers14092050 . . . . **137**

Niloy R. Datta, Bharati M. Jain, Zatin Mathi, Sneha Datta, Satyendra Johari and Ashok R. Singh et al.
Hyperthermia: A Potential Game-Changer in the Management of Cancers in Low-Middle-Income Group Countries
Reprinted from: *Cancers* **2022**, *14*, 315, doi:10.3390/cancers14020315 . . . . **159**

Adela Ademaj, Danai P. Veltsista, Pirus Ghadjar, Dietmar Marder, Eva Oberacker and Oliver J. Ott et al.
Clinical Evidence for Thermometric Parameters to Guide Hyperthermia Treatment
Reprinted from: *Cancers* 2022, 14, 625, doi:10.3390/cancers14030625 171

Emanuel Stutz, Emsad Puric, Adela Ademaj, Arnaud Künzi, Reinhardt Krcek and Olaf Timm et al.
Present Practice of Radiative Deep Hyperthermia in Combination with Radiotherapy in Switzerland
Reprinted from: *Cancers* 2022, 14, 1175, doi:10.3390/cancers14051175 229

Michiel Kroesen, Netteke van Holthe, Kemal Sumser, Dana Chitu, Rene Vernhout and Gerda Verduijn et al.
Feasibility, SAR Distribution, and Clinical Outcome upon Reirradiation and Deep Hyperthermia Using the Hypercollar3D in Head and Neck Cancer Patients
Reprinted from: *Cancers* 2021, 13, 6149, doi:10.3390/cancers13236149 247

Redi Poni, Esra Neufeld, Myles Capstick, Stephan Bodis, Theodoros Samaras and Niels Kuster
Feasibility of Temperature Control by Electrical Impedance Tomography in Hyperthermia
Reprinted from: *Cancers* 2021, 13, 3297, doi:10.3390/cancers13133297 261

Ioannis Androulakis, Rob M. C. Mestrom, Miranda E. M. C. Christianen, Inger-Karine K. Kolkman-Deurloo and Gerard C. van Rhoon
A Novel Framework for the Optimization of Simultaneous ThermoBrachyTherapy
Reprinted from: *Cancers* 2022, 14, 1425, doi:10.3390/cancers14061425 285

Stephan Scheidegger, Sergio Mingo Barba and Udo S. Gaipl
Theoretical Evaluation of the Impact of Hyperthermia in Combination with Radiation Therapy in an Artificial Immune—Tumor-Ecosystem
Reprinted from: *Cancers* 2021, 13, 5764, doi:10.3390/cancers13225764 301

H. Petra Kok and Johannes Crezee
Fast Adaptive Temperature-Based Re-Optimization Strategies for On-Line Hot Spot Suppression during Locoregional Hyperthermia
Reprinted from: *Cancers* 2021, 14, 133, doi:10.3390/cancers14010133 317

About the Editors

Stephan Bodis

Stephan Bodis is a Swiss and US Board Certified Radiation Oncologist. Residency and fellowships in oncology and radiation oncology at University Hospital Zurich, Institut Gustave Roussy Paris, Harvard Medical School Teaching Hospitals and the Massachusetts Institute of Technology in Boston and Cambridge. Head of Radiation Oncology Departments Kantonsspitäler Aarau and Baden in Switzerland for 18 years. Currently Associate Professor at University Hospital and University Zurich, President IT'IS Foundation Board Zurich, Member of Zurich Ethics Committee. Research focus in clinical (radiation) oncology, oncologic thermotherapy/hyperthermia, infrastructural need for radiation oncology care in LMIC. Author of >100 peer-reviewed papers. Community contributions in national and international meetings, organisations with focus on health care, cancer research, and oncologic thermotherapy. Pivotal input to integrate oncologic hyperthermia in Swiss Health Care.

Pirus Ghadjar

Medical school and oncology residency at Charite University Berlin, residency in radiation oncology and urology at Bern University Hospital. Clinical research fellowship in radiation oncology at the prestigious Memorial-Sloan Kettering Cancer Center in New York. Currently holds a Professorship at Charite University Medecine Berlin and is the Head of the Charite Hyperthermia Center. He has over 150 peer-reviews publications. Pirus Ghadjar is member/board member of numerous national and international organisations dedicated to cancer care, hyperthermia/thermotherapy and palliative care. As head of the Charite Hyperthermia Center he managed to expand the equipment pool through constructive and innovative research cooperations with the industry. His research areas in hyperthermia/thermotherapy are in basic science, high-frequency electromagnetic field modelling, phantom construction, QA and development of hardware and software components in this field.

Gerard C. Van Rhoon

Gerard van Rhoon, Ph.D. 1994 Delft University of Technology. Professor in Physical Aspects of Electromagnetic Fields and Health at the Erasmus MC Cancer Institute. In 2019, co-appointed at Delft University of Technology. He made pivotal contributions to integrate hyperthermia as regular health care in The Netherlands. From the first hour of his career involved in clinical applications of hyperthermia in cancer. His research involves design of technology to apply well-controlled localised heating of tumors at all body sites. He authored >190 peer-reviewed publications. Awards: 1987 Lund Science Award, 2008 Dr. BB Singh Award and ESHO Award, 2012 Dr. Sugahara Award, 2017 Robinson STM Award. Community contributions: Executive Committee Intl. J. of Hyperthermia, Auditor Physics in Medicine and Biology, President of the European Society for Hyperthermic Oncology ESHO, 2001-2006 Health Council of The Netherlands of Committee 673 EMF in society.

Preface to "Oncologic Thermoradiotherapy: Need for Evidence, Harmonisation, and Innovation"

The road of acceptance of oncologic thermotherapy/hyperthermia as a synergistic modality in combination with standard oncologic therapies is still bumpy. This is partially due to the lack of level I evidence from international, multicentric, randomized clinical trials, including large patient numbers and a long term follow-up. Therefore, we need more level I EVIDENCE from clinical trials, we need HARMONISATION and global acceptance for existing technologies and a common language understood by all stakeholders and we need INNOVATION in the fields of biology, clinics, and technology in order to move thermotherapy/hyperthermia forward. This is the main focus of this book.

Acknowledgements: To all authors who contributed to this Special Issue, to Cosmina Vircan for her editorial assistance.

Stephan Bodis, Pirus Ghadjar, and Gerard C. Van Rhoon
Editors

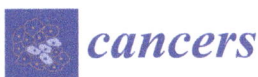

Editorial

Oncologic Thermoradiotherapy: Need for Evidence, Harmonisation, and Innovation

Stephan Bodis [1,2,*], Pirus Ghadjar [3] and Gerard van Rhoon [4]

1. Foundation for Research on Information Technologies in Society (IT'IS), 8004 Zürich, Switzerland
2. Department of Radiation Oncology, University Hospital Zurich, 8032 Zürich, Switzerland
3. Department Radiation Oncology, Charité–Universitätsmedizin Berlin, Corporate Member of Freie Universität Berlin and Humboldt-Universität zu Berlin, Augustenburger Platz 1, 13353 Berlin, Germany; pirus.ghadjar@charite.de
4. Department of Radiotherapy, Erasmus MC Cancer Institute, University Medical Center, 3015 GD Rotterdam, The Netherlands; g.c.vanrhoon@erasmusmc.nl
* Correspondence: s.bodis@bluewin.ch

Evidence, Harmonisation and Innovation

The road of acceptance of oncologic thermotherapy/hyperthermia as a synergistic modality in combination with standard oncologic therapies is still bumpy. This is partially due to lack of evidence from international, multicentric, randomized clinical trials combined with biologic/pharmacologic systemic therapy and/or radiotherapy and/or surgery including a long term follow up.

Despite valid data and numerous publications over many decades, the lack of level I evidence for clinical trials, the lack of a thermotherapy/hyperthermia glossaries understood by all stakeholders with defined technical terms, and a widening technology gap between available and desirable hard-software components created a lukewarm climate for acceptance and reimbursement of thermotherapy/hyperthermia by most national health authorities and national health care insurances. Due to recently published randomized studies, a series of published meta-analysis and the first draft of a thermotherapy/hyperthermia glossary this field is moving forward.

Novel international research networks jointly by academia and industry (e.g., HYPERBOOST (https://www.hyperboost.eu/, last accessed on 2 May 2022); an EU horizon 2020 multimillion educational grant for PhDs) in the areas of AI/IT, biology, physics and technology are strengthening this joint effort substantially. We do hope that this special edition of Cancers can support these running, joint efforts.

Evidence

In this special issue new evidence is presented. In a long term retrospective study of preoperative chemoradiation plus deep hyperthermia Schemm et al. [1]. reports an encouraging level in five-year survival with better RFS for patients reaching T50 temperatures above 39.9 °C. The impact of a high thermal dose was also found in the retrospective study on RT+HT for prostate cancer by Nakahare et al. [2]: CEM43T90 > 7 min. predicted improved biochemical disease-free survival. The paper by Minnaar et al. [3] performed a two- to three-year follow-up on the results of the South African Phase III Trial comparing chemoradiotherapy with and without modulated Electro-Hyperthermia (mEHT) and found a beneficial effect on the two- to three-year survival survival for patients with locally advanced cervical cancer treated by chemoradiation plus mEHT. The retrospective study by Lee et al. [4] evaluated the results of neoadjuvant 40 Gy plus mEHT followed by surgery in patients with advanced rectal cancer and observed an indication for longer survival in patients treated with mEHT energy above 3800 kJ.

The review by Szasz [5] discusses whether heterogenous heating is beneficial over homogenous heating. On the other hand, the review by Dewhirst et al. [6] emphasizes the importance of hyperthermia to improve perfusion and long duration reoxygenation (i.e., 24–48 h post hyperthermia).

For sure integration of mechanistic and pre-clinical immunology research data will further strengthen insights into biological mechanisms, increase understanding of the different patterns of in vivo tumor responses, and promote clinical trials integrating immunology in the field of oncologic thermotherapy. In this issue Sengedorj et al. [7] demonstrate that HT combined with RT changes the immunophenotype of breast cancer cells and upregulates immune suppressive immune checkpoint molecules. Therefore, adding an immune checkpoint inhibitor to combined HT-RT should be further explored as another potential clinical benefit.

Harmonization

This issue contributes to further define the role of thermoradiotherapy. For instance, the review by Datta et al. [8] discusses the potential role of hyperthermia as a potential game-changer in the management of cancer in low-middle-income group countries. It reflects on different hyperthermia technologies that are available including annular-phased array systems for regional hyperthermia as well as capacitive hyperthermia systems without and with the use of amplitude modulation [1–4]. As each technology involves advantages and disadvantages, it is most important to consciously use it for appropriate clinical indications, preferably within prospective clinical trials. It is not primarily the choice of technology but rather the commonly observed unreasonable and mostly undocumented use of the method as explained by Ademaj et al. [9], that has dragged the collective success of thermoradiotherapy. An excellent example on how to introduce hyperthermia in a harmonized way at a national level is presented by Stutz et al. [10]. By introducing the Swiss Hyperthermia Network (https://www.ksa.ch/zentren-kliniken/radio-onkologie/leistungsangebot/swiss-hyperthermia-network, last accessed on 2 May 2022), hyperthermia treatment has been made available at a national level for all Swiss inhabitants enabling at the same time a platform to discuss with the Swiss Federal Office of Public Health (https://www.bag.admin.ch/bag/en/home.html, last accessed on 2 May 2022) proper implementation of reimbursement for hyperthermia treatment of selected evidence-based indications. The data provided in this issue support the use of different hyperthermia technologies for different well described clinical scenarios and will therefore improve the overall clinical acceptance of thermoradiotherapy in oncology.

Innovation

This special issue is a scholarly example of innovation (i.e., defined as the successive introduction of new ideas, devices, and methods to generate improved output and value). The various contributions provide numerous suggestions to innovate thermotherapy, aiming at improved efficiency of combined thermoradiotherapy. The papers by Schemm et al. [1] and Nakahara et al. [2] are new support of the existence of a thermal dose effect relationship and is another confirmation for the need to always strive for the highest quality assurance and control for optimal treatment outcome. As reported by various papers improved efficiency can be achieved by innovating the heating and improved patient selection to fit with the correct level (complexity) of technology (Kroesen et al. [11], Poni et al. [12], Androulakis et al. [13]) enhanced understanding of the biological principles, either by experimental or clinical research (Dewhirst et al. [6], Sengedorj et al. [7]) or through building new more advanced biological models (Scheidegger et al. [14]) and supported by adequate computer modelling to predict the temperature distribution in the tissue (Kok et al. [15]). At the same time the contribution of Ademaj et al. [9] makes it crystal clear that to better understand which mechanisms are dominant to maximize treatment outcome during the clinical application of thermoradiotherapy, we still have a world to gain in accurate and complete documentation of the quality of the thermal therapy delivered to the patient. Improved documentation will open the gate way for further exploitation of thermal therapy using new technology to guide treatment quality and hence making thermal therapy more effective and efficient. Both items are crucial to increase the wider acceptance of thermal therapy by the oncological community and ultimately to bring the benefits of thermal therapy to the patients in all countries.

In this issue we find contributions from Africa, America, Asia, and Europe. Beside local, regional and national efforts we also need to strengthen international platforms and networks of oncologic thermorediotherapy. This is a must for a better global exchange of knowledge and information transfer. These oncologic thermo-therapy networks will further stimulate innovations, both for HI and LMI countries, strengthen harmonization including a well understood and accepted "vocabulary for thermotherapy", improve acceptance of health care authorities and the public opinion, regulatory processes and QA. And, last but not least, all of these efforts must always be based on evidence.

Funding: This research received no external funding.

Conflicts of Interest: The authors declare no conflict of interest.

References

1. Schem, B.-C.; Pfeffer, F.; Ott, M.A.; Wiig, J.N.; Sletteskog, N.; Frøystein, T.; Myklebust, M.P.; Leh, S.; Dahl, O.; Mella, O. Long-Term Outcome in a Phase II Study of Regional Hyperthermia Added to Preoperative Radiochemotherapy in Locally Advanced and Recurrent Rectal Adenocarcinomas. *Cancers* **2022**, *14*, 705. [CrossRef] [PubMed]
2. Nakahara, S.; Ohguri, T.; Kakinouchi, S.; Itamura, H.; Morisaki, T.; Tani, S.; Yahara, K.; Fujimoto, N. Intensity-Modulated Radiotherapy with Regional Hyperthermia for High-Risk Localized Prostate Carcinoma. *Cancers* **2022**, *14*, 400. [CrossRef] [PubMed]
3. Minnaar, C.A.; Maposa, I.; Kotzen, J.A.; Baeyens, A. Effects of Modulated Electro-Hyperthermia (mEHT) on Two and Three Year Survival of Locally Advanced Cervical Cancer Patients. *Cancers* **2022**, *14*, 656. [CrossRef] [PubMed]
4. Lee, Y.; Kim, S.; Cha, H.; Han, J.H.; Choi, H.J.; Go, E.; You, S.H. Long-Term Feasibility of 13.56 MHz Modulated Electro-Hyperthermia-Based Preoperative Thermoradiochemotherapy in Locally Advanced Rectal Cancer. *Cancers* **2022**, *14*, 1271. [CrossRef] [PubMed]
5. Szasz, A. Heterogeneous Heat Absorption Is Complementary to Radiotherapy. *Cancers* **2022**, *14*, 901. [CrossRef] [PubMed]
6. Dewhirst, M.W.; Oleson, J.R.; Kirkpatrick, J.; Secomb, T.W. Accurate Three-Dimensional Thermal Dosimetry and Assessment of Physiologic Response Are Essential for Optimizing Thermoradiotherapy. *Cancers* **2022**, *14*, 1701. [CrossRef] [PubMed]
7. Sengedorj, A.; Hader, M.; Heger, L.; Frey, B.; Dudziak, D.; Fietkau, R.; Ott, O.J.; Scheidegger, S.; Barba, S.M.; Gaipl, U.S.; et al. The Effect of Hyperthermia and Radiotherapy Sequence on Cancer Cell Death and the Immune Phenotype of Breast Cancer Cells. *Cancers* **2022**, *14*, 2050. [CrossRef]
8. Datta, N.R.; Jain, B.M.; Mathi, Z.; Datta, S.; Johari, S.; Singh, A.R.; Kalbande, P.; Kale, P.; Shivkumar, V.; Bodis, S. Hyperthermia: A Potential Game-Changer in the Management of Cancers in Low-Middle-Income Group Countries. *Cancers* **2022**, *14*, 315. [CrossRef] [PubMed]
9. Ademaj, A.; Veltsista, D.P.; Ghadjar, P.; Marder, D.; Oberacker, E.; Ott, O.J.; Wust, P.; Puric, E.; Hälg, R.A.; Rogers, S.; et al. Clinical Evidence for Thermometric Parameters to Guide Hyperthermia Treatment. *Cancers* **2022**, *14*, 625. [CrossRef] [PubMed]
10. Stutz, E.; Puric, E.; Ademaj, A.; Künzi, A.; Krcek, R.; Timm, O.; Marder, D.; Notter, M.; Rogers, S.; Bodis, S.; et al. Present Practice of Radiative Deep Hyperthermia in Combination with Radiotherapy in Switzerland. *Cancers* **2022**, *14*, 1175. [CrossRef] [PubMed]
11. Kroesen, M.; van Holthe, N.; Sumser, K.; Chitu, D.; Vernhout, R.; Verduijn, G.; Franckena, M.; Hardillo, J.; van Rhoon, G.; Paulides, M. Feasibility, SAR Distribution, and Clinical Outcome upon Reirradiation and Deep Hyperthermia Using the Hypercollar3D in Head and Neck Cancer Patients. *Cancers* **2021**, *13*, 6149. [CrossRef] [PubMed]
12. Poni, R.; Neufeld, E.; Capstick, M.; Bodis, S.; Samaras, T.; Kuster, N. Feasibility of Temperature Control by Electrical Impedance Tomography in Hyperthermia. *Cancers* **2021**, *13*, 3297. [CrossRef] [PubMed]
13. Androulakis, I.; Mestrom, R.M.C.; Christianen, M.E.M.C.; Kolkman-Deurloo, I.-K.K.; van Rhoon, G.C. A Novel Framework for the Optimization of Simultaneous ThermoBrachyTherapy. *Cancers* **2022**, *14*, 1425. [CrossRef] [PubMed]
14. Scheidegger, S.; Mingo Barba, S.; Gaipl, U.S. Theoretical Evaluation of the Impact of Hyperthermia in Combination with Radiation Therapy in an Artificial Immune—Tumor-Ecosystem. *Cancers* **2021**, *13*, 5764. [CrossRef] [PubMed]
15. Kok, H.P.; Crezee, J. Fast Adaptive Temperature-Based Re-Optimization Strategies for On-Line Hot Spot Suppression during Locoregional Hyperthermia. *Cancers* **2022**, *14*, 133. [CrossRef] [PubMed]

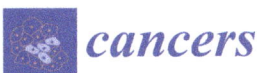

Article

Long-Term Outcome in a Phase II Study of Regional Hyperthermia Added to Preoperative Radiochemotherapy in Locally Advanced and Recurrent Rectal Adenocarcinomas

Baard-Christian Schem [1], Frank Pfeffer [2], Martin Anton Ott [3], Johan N. Wiig [4], Nils Sletteskog [5], Torbjørn Frøystein [6], Mette Pernille Myklebust [6], Sabine Leh [7], Olav Dahl [6,8,*] and Olav Mella [6,8]

1 The Western Norway Regional Health Authority, 4034 Stavanger, Norway; trazom@online.no
2 Department of Gastrointestinal Surgery, Haukeland University Hospital and Institute of Clinical Medicine, Medical Faculty, University of Bergen, 5021 Bergen, Norway; frank.pfeffer@uib.no
3 Department of Surgery, Haugesund Hospital, Helse Fonna, 5504 Haugesund, Norway; martin.anton.ott@helse-fonna.no
4 Department of Gastroenterological Surgery, Section of Surgical Oncology, Norwegian Radium Hospital, Oslo University Hospital HF, 0424 Oslo, Norway; joniwii@online.no
5 Department of Surgery, Førde Central Hospital, 6807 Førde, Norway; nils.sletteskog@helse-forde.no
6 Department of Oncology and Medical Physics, Haukeland University Hospital, 5021 Bergen, Norway; torbjorn.froystein@helse-bergen.no (T.F.); mette.pernille.myklebust@helse-bergen.no (M.P.M.); olav.mella@helse-bergen.no (O.M.)
7 Department of Pathology, Haukeland University Hospital and Institute of Clinical Medicine, Medical Faculty, University of Bergen, 5021 Bergen, Norway; sabine.leh@helse-bergen.no
8 Medical Faculty, Institute of Clinical Science, University of Bergen, 5021 Bergen, Norway
* Correspondence: olav.dahl@helse-bergen.no

Simple Summary: Regional hyperthermia added to standard preoperative chemoradiotherapy for locally advanced and recurrent rectal cancer gives a high complete response rate and an improved long-term recurrence free survival.

Abstract: Hyperthermia was added to standard preoperative chemoradiation for rectal adenocarcinomas in a phase II study. Patients with T3-4 N0-2 M0 rectal cancer or local recurrences were included. Radiation dose was 54 Gy combined with capecitabine 825 mg/m^2 × 2 daily and once weekly oxaliplatin 55 mg/m^2. Regional hyperthermia aimed at 41.5–42.5 °C for 60 min combined with oxaliplatin infusion. Radical surgery with total or extended TME technique, was scheduled at 6–8 weeks after radiation. From April 2003 to April 2008, a total of 49 eligible patients were recruited. Median number of hyperthermia sessions were 5.4. A total of 47 out of 49 patients (96%) had the scheduled surgery, which was clinically radical in 44 patients. Complete tumour regression occurred in 29.8% of the patients who also exhibited statistically significantly better RFS and CSS. Rate of local recurrence alone at 10 years was 9.1%, distant metastases alone occurred in 25.6%, including local recurrences 40.4%. RFS for all patients was 54.8% after 5 years and CSS was 73.5%. Patients with T50 temperatures in tumours above median 39.9 °C had better RFS, 66.7% vs. 31.3%, $p = 0.047$, indicating a role of hyperthermia. Toxicity was acceptable.

Keywords: rectal cancer; hyperthermia; chemoradiotherapy; tumour control

1. Introduction

Patients presenting locally advanced rectal cancer (LARC) or primarily non-resectable rectal cancer have a dire prognosis [1]. Locally recurrent rectal cancer is difficult to control [2,3]. Preoperative radiation for advanced rectal cancer [4–6] and palliative radiotherapy for metastasized or irresectable rectal cancer [7–9] is well established.

The clinical benefit of superficial hyperthermia for malignant melanomas and deep pelvic hyperthermia as an adjuvant to radiotherapy for cervical cancer has been documented [10–13]. Additive effect of some chemotherapeutic drugs, including cisplatin have been shown experimentally [14]. It was therefore of interest to explore whether a preoperative combination of radiation, chemotherapy and hyperthermia could improve the results of surgery for rectal cancer. At the time the study was initiated, few clinical studies had treated primary rectal cancer by radiation combined with deep hyperthermia [13,15–17]. The combination of radiation with capecitabine was also new [18], as were the combination of hyperthermia and oxaliplatin in rectal recurrences [19] and experimental cell cultures [20,21]. Whole body hyperthermia and oxaliplatin in colorectal cancer patients was an experimental option not in general use [22]. We therefore first performed a phase I study to assess the feasibility of a combination of radiation, 5-day continuously administered 5-fluorouracil (5-FU), and weekly hyperthermia and oxaliplatin before surgery for rectal cancer [23]. Excellent local control was achieved, but acute diarrhoea was a frequent side effect. As the continuous administration of 5-FU via a central venous line was cumbersome in an outpatient setting, we replaced 5-FU with oral capecitabine in the current new phase II study. As various heating techniques had been used in earlier studies [17,24], we decided to explore the use of regional hyperthermia following the European quality assurance guidelines [25]. During the follow up of our patients, promising results have been published for LARC patients [26,27].

The present phase II study was open for patients with LARC without distant metastases and patients with local recurrences considered to be surgically curable, some with sufficient tumour shrinkage after preoperative treatment. During and after the inclusion and follow up of the study, the standard treatment has changed regarding radiation dose and inclusion of chemotherapy. We therefore waited with publication until long-term results were available. The present series of advanced and recurrent rectal cancer patients with good local control warrant consideration among the new therapeutic options. The secondary aim is the presentation of treatment-related toxicity.

2. Materials and Methods

From April 2003 to April 2008, 50 patients with histologically verified rectal adenocarcinomas were recruited. By a mistake, one patient with locally advanced tumour was examined with abdominal computed tomography (CT) the day after first treatment, which revealed multiple liver metastases, and this patient was therefore excluded due to major protocol violation.

2.1. The Inclusion Criteria

The inclusion criteria were patients with LARC (defined as T3 and T4 tumours with distance to the mesorectal facia less than 3 mm on magnetic resonance imaging (MRI), within 15 cm from the anal verge by proctoscopy) or recurrence after surgery alone. Age was below 76 years. The patients should not have evidence of distant metastases, and performance status should be 0–2. The patients should not have hypertension, cardiac failure or myocardial infarction in the previous 6 months. No chronic pulmonary or renal disease. No prior radiation or cancers, except basal cell carcinomas or stage 0 cervical cancer. Haematological tests should demonstrate Hgb > 10 g/dL, leucocytes > 3×10^9/L or thrombocytes > 100×10^9/L, and creatinine clearance > 30 mL/min. Due to the hyperthermia applicator size, maximal pelvic diameter should be less than 49 cm, and the patient should have no pacemaker or other metallic implanted object. Diagnostic procedures included clinical examination, rigid rectoscopy by a senior surgeon, biopsy confirming adenocarcinoma, CT of the pelvic area and abdomen with contrast in the rectum, and MRI of the pelvic area. Endorectal ultrasound was optional, and cystoscopy was performed if any invasion of the bladder was suspected. Blood counts included Hgb, leucocytes with differential counts, thrombocytes, analysis of Na, K, Cl, Ca, Mg and creatinine, bilirubin, ASAT, ALAT, ϒ-GT, LDH and creatinine kinase.

The primary tumours were classified according to TNM 4th edition [28]. Indications for preoperative radiotherapy of LARC was based on the MRI examination showing a threatened circumferential resection margin with less than 3 mm from the mesorectal fascia (MRF) according to Norwegian national guidelines, or tumour deposits outside the MRF.

2.2. Statistics and Ethics

The outcomes were defined as local control, relapse-free survival included any local or distant recurrence with secondary colorectal cancer censored (RFS), cancer recti-specific survival (CSS) and overall survival (OS) as defined by Punt [29]. Toxicity was graded according to Common Terminology Criteria for Adverse Events v3.0 (CTCAE), Publish Date: 9 August 2003 (https://ctep.cancer.gov/protocoldevelopment/electronic_applications/docs/ctcaev3.pdf, accessed on 8 September 2020) [30].

Survival was assessed by Kaplan-Meier estimates with 95% confidence intervals (95% CI), and differences assessed by the log-rank test. Differences with a two-tailed p-value less than 0.05 were considered statistically significant. IBM SPSS version 26 (IBM Corp, Armonk, NY, USA) and R (version 4.0.3, R Foundation for Statistical Computing, Vienna, Austria) were used for analyses and creating survival curves.

After oral and written information on the experimental nature of the study, all patients signed a written informed consent form. The study was conducted according to the guidelines of the Declaration of Helsinki. It was approved by the Regional Ethics Committee, Health Region West (REK III nr. 159.01) and thereby in accordance with Norwegian law and regulations.

3. Treatment

Radiation therapy was based on 3D dose planning, mostly a three-field technique with one backfield and two side fields. Tumour with regional glands received 2 Gy × 23 with a boost of 2 Gy × 4–5 against primary tumour and mesorectum or metastatic lymph nodes. Total tumour dose was therefore 54–56 Gy based on tumour size and bowel volume to be included in the boost volume, as well as comorbidity, age and acute side effects. The treatment was administered once daily, 5 days weekly. Pauses except Saturdays and Sundays were compensated for by a 6th fraction the following week(s).

Chemotherapy was administered as peroral capecitabine 825 mg/m^2 5 days a week, concomitant with radiation (See Figure 1). Maximal dose was 1650 mg/day, administered in one dose the evening before radiation and the other half in the morning before radiation. Oxaliplatin was administered at a dose of 55 mg/m^2 each week, with a maximal dose 100 mg. Oxaliplatin was given as infusion during the hyperthermia session; at least five infusions, and if possible six infusions were administered. The drug was infused in 5% glucose, administered as a 2 h peripheral vein infusion, which started 1 h before planned start of hyperthermia.

Regional hyperthermia was administered by a BSD 2000 machine (Pyrexar Medical, Salt Lake City, UT, USA), using the Sigma-Eye applicator or the Sigma-60 applicator for patients with the highest pelvic diameters [17]. Hyperthermia was administered once a week from the first or second day of radiation, each treatment given as soon as possible after receiving the radiation fraction. Prior to radiation, catheters for Bowman temperature probes were inserted into tumour tissues using local anesthetics, and in women also in the vagina. Usually, a single catheter was inserted into the tumour, but for large tumours two catheters were used to optimize monitoring of the tumour heating. With problems of insertion of catheters or shrinkage of tumours, the probe measured rectal luminal temperature. One catheter was inserted in the urinary bladder. The positions of the catheters were verified by CT before the radiation. The treatment time was 60 min, calculated from the time the temperature probe in the tumour (or in rectal lumen if no probe was inserted in the tumour) reached 41.0 °C or started 30 min after initiation of the hyperthermia session. Normal tissues should be kept below 43.0 °C. The focus of heating was controlled by phase and amplitude steering [31]. If the awake patient reported discomfort or pain repeated doses of fentanyl up to 0.10 mg was given intravenously. With continuous bladder temperatures > 42.5 °C, the bladder was irrigated by 10–30 mL of isotone saline holding room temperature for cooling. Bladder installations were kept at a minimum to avoid cooling of possible tumour near the bladder. Only tumour-tissue temperature-probe data are used for quality assessment of the hyperthermia given. The T20, T50 and T90 are defined as the temperature equal to or exceeded by 20%, 50% and 90% of the measured temperatures, respectively [32], and were calculated using the RhyThM software [33].

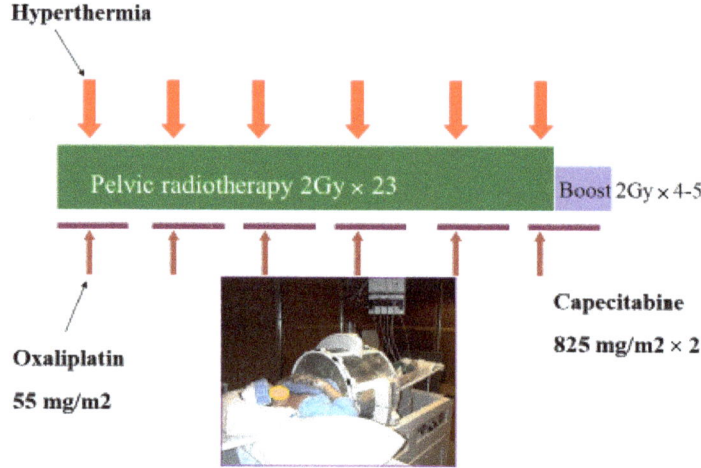

Figure 1. Treatment schedule for preoperative combination treatment by radiation, chemotherapy and hyperthermia for rectal adenocarcinoma.

Surgery. Rectal resections were performed according to total mesorectal excision (TME) principles. A partial, total or extended TME was carried out depending on the location. With invasion of neighbouring organs in locally advanced or recurrent tumours, a total pelvic exenteration procedures was performed. Totally 25 patients had a permanent colostomy. The resection margins were classified by the pathologists as R0 resection with a margin > 1 mm, R1 with a margin < 1 mm, and R2 in case of involved margins. The tumour regression grade (TRG) was classified by the Dworak criteria [34]. Follow up after surgery for at least 5 years followed the Norwegian national guidelines.

4. Results

In total 43 patients with LARC and 6 patients with recurrent rectal tumours without previous preoperative radio (chemo)therapy, 32 male and 17 female, were included. The characteristics for the patients are shown in Table 1. Fourteen tumours were locally advanced rectal adenocarcinomas, with growth into or beyond the MRF (two patients with T3N1 tumours had only 3 and 2 mm to the MRF) and were considered moderate-risk patients, while 29 patients had high-risk tumours.

Table 1. Patient characteristics for patients included and treated according to the study protocol.

Category	Total	Male	Female
Included	49	32	17
Age (years)	59.1 (range 21.0–75.6)	60.3 (range 21.0–75.6)	56.9 (range 39.4–74.7)
Locally advanced	43	27	16
Level 0–5 cm	19	15	4
Level 6–10 cm	21	11	10
Level 11–15 cm	3	1	2
Mean height cm	6.7	6.1	7.4
T3	19	11	8
T4	24	16	8
N0	3	3	0
N1	17	11	1
N2	21	12	9
Nx	2	1	1
Moderate	14	7	7
High risk	29	20	9
Local recurrence	6	5	1

The median radiation dose was 54.0 Gy (range 50–56, of these, seven received 56 Gy). The median number of hyperthermia sessions was 5.4 (range 1–6) and 92% of the patients had at least four hyperthermia sessions. The temperature data measured in the tumours (n = 152 catheters) was mean (T-mean) 39.92 °C (95%CI 38.22–41.62), T-min 39.14 °C (95%CI 37.6–40.68), T-max 40.61 °C (95%CI 39.56–41.66), T20 was 40.29 °C (39.32–41.26), T50 39.91 °C (95%CI 39.06–40.76), and T90 was 39.36 °C (95%CI 38.58–40.14). There were no significant relation between T-stage, primary tumours versus recurrences or T size and median T50.

All patients had at least one oxaliplatin dose, 94% had four and more doses, and 71% had all six scheduled courses. One patient had only three weeks with capecitabine, two only four weeks, while 94% had the scheduled 5–6 weeks of oral chemotherapy together with radiation.

A total of 41 of the 43 patients with locally advanced tumours had the scheduled surgery at a median time of 84 days (range 69–216) after the start of radiation. The longest delay was for a very advanced tumour, which first had an exploratory laparotomy finding that the tumour was irresectable, and a new attempt later with the successful removal of a seemingly large tumour, however showing no vital tumour cells when examined by microscopy. Two patients were not operated as planned preoperative examinations revealed distant metastases. All six patients with local recurrences were operated as scheduled. The resections were recorded as R0 in 41 (87%) of the operated patients, R1 in 3 (6%) and R2 in 3 (6%) patients. The pathological assessment of TRG showed no malignant cells, complete regression (TRG4, pCR) in 14 (29.8%) of the specimens, 22 (46.9%) with TRG 3, 7 (14.9%) with moderate response, TRG 2, and only 4 (8.5%) with minimal regression, TRG 1.

The rate of local recurrence alone at 5 and 10 years was 9.1% (95%CI 4.4–13.8) and at 15 years the local recurrence rate was 12.3% (95%CI 0.8–23.8) for all included patients. Distant metastases only occurred in 25.6% (95%CI 12.3–38.9) of the patients after 5 years, 40.4% (95%CI 26.4–54.4) including concurrent local recurrences. For all patients, 5-year RFS was 54.8% (95%CI 40.8–68.8), Figure 2. There was no difference in RFS according to presentation as locally advanced tumours or recurrences. CSS for all patients at 5 years was 73.5% (95%CI 61.2–85.8) and at 10 years 62.5% (95%CI 48.9–76.2), Figure 3. CSS was similar for LARC patients and patients with recurrence. OS was 73.5% (95%CI 61.2–85.8) at 5 years, and dropped to 55.1% (95%CI 41.3–68.9) after 10 years (Figure A1).

Classification of tumour response as TRG 4 (pCR) among the 47 operated patients yielded better RFS compared with the other groups ($p = 0.032$), see Figure 4. For patients with TRG 4 the 5-year CSS was 92.9% (95%CI 79.4–100.0) versus 72.7% (95%CI 57.5–87.9) for patients with residual tumour cells, and 10-year CSS 83.6 % (95%CI 62.5–100) versus 57.4% (95%CI 40.0–74.8), ($p = 0.063$), respectively. Thus the CSS differences were not statistically significant.

When evaluating outcome in relation to the thermometry data, we were only able to retrieve the original disk recordings for 39 patients, thus data were unavailable for 10 patients. It was found that the RFS was significantly better, 66.7% (95%CI 40.6–86.7) for patients with recordings above 39.9 °C (T50, median of all recordings) versus 31.3% (95%CI 9.3–53.3), $p = 0.047$, in the lower group, see Figure 5.

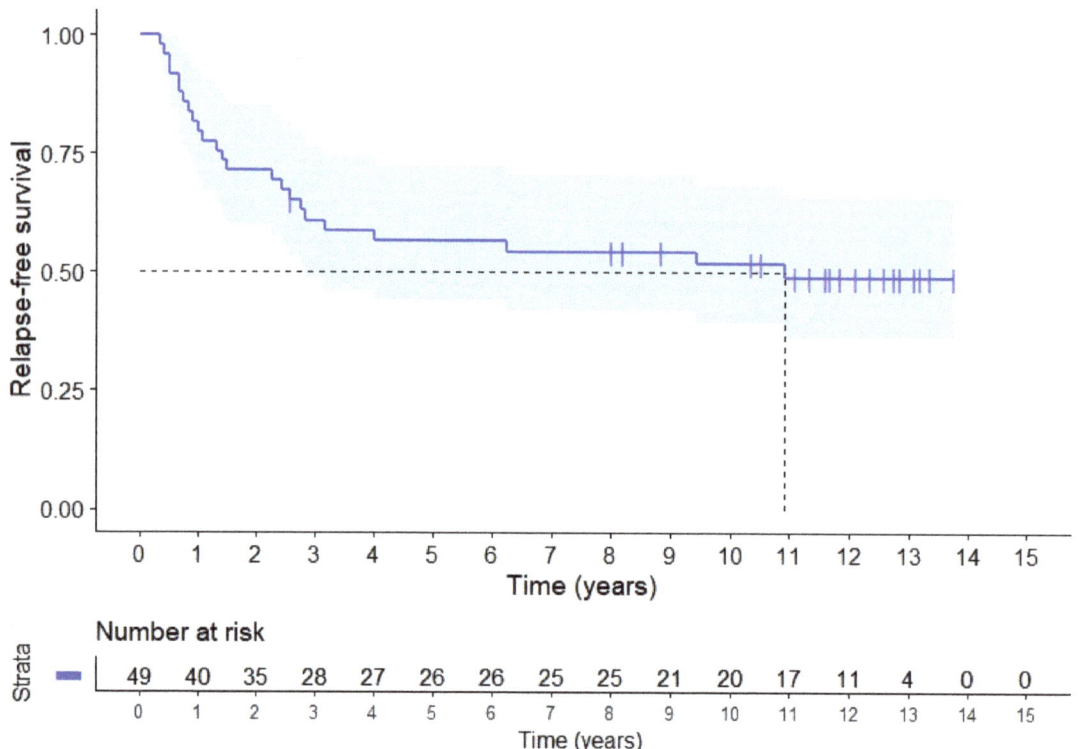

Figure 2. Relapse-free survival (RFS) for 49 rectal cancer patients with locally advanced or recurrent rectal adenocarcinoma.

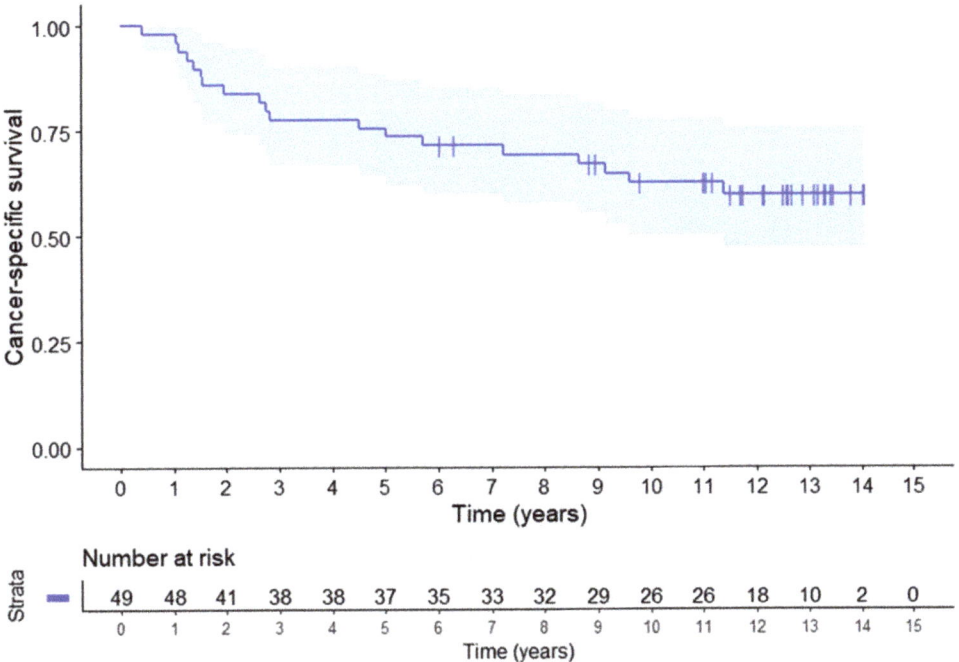

Figure 3. Cancer specific survival (CSS) for 49 patients, 43 with locally advanced and 6 patients with local recurrences of rectal adenocarcinomas.

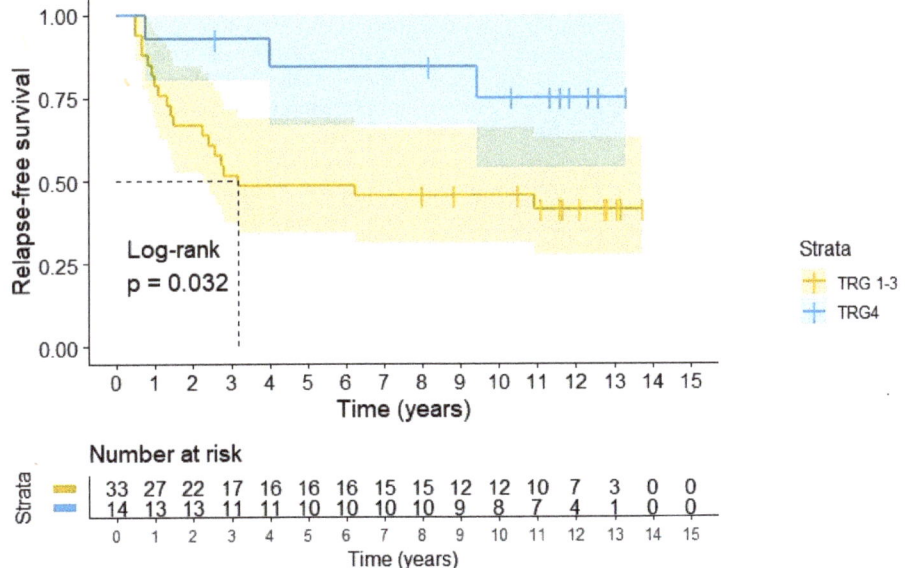

Figure 4. RFS according to histopathology classification according to Dworak's TRG grades for 47 patients operated for rectal adenocarcinomas after preoperative radiochemotherapy with hyperthermia. TRG4 means pCR.

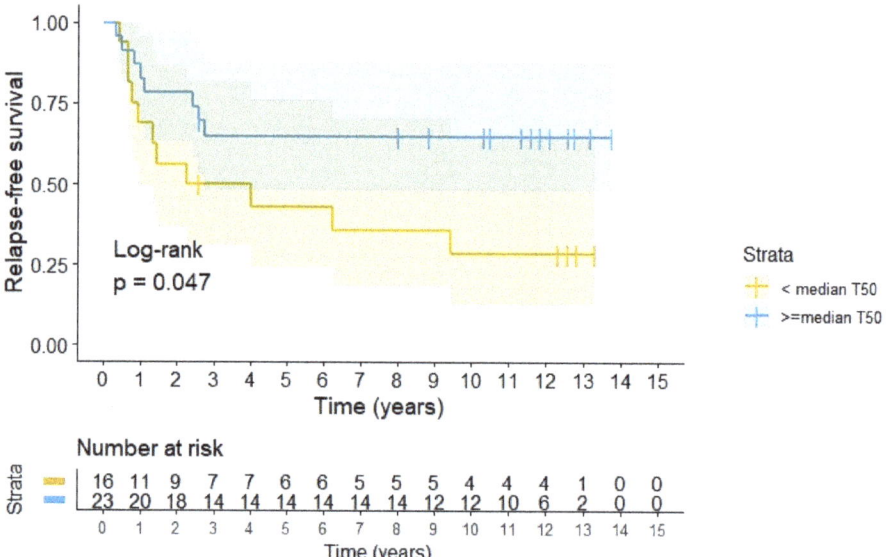

Figure 5. RFS according to quality of heating divided above or below 39.91 °C, the median of the T50 measured in the tumours during all heating sessions among 39 patients.

Toxicity. Table 2 shows that most patients who had the scheduled treatment including surgery, had some acute side effects: 23% had grade 1, 34% had grade 2, 40% had grade 3, and only one (2%) recorded as grade 4 due to reduced general condition caused by several side effects. The most frequent side effects were diarrhoea due to chemotherapy and radiation, skin toxicity due to radiation and nausea related to chemotherapy. Fever reaction without infection after oxaliplatin was recorded in 40% of the patients. Twenty-seven patients (57%) experienced no long-term toxicity. Grade 1 occurred in two patients (4%, subileus and an accidentally fixed urether catheter), grade 2 in four patients (8%, one slight vaginal athresia and one abdominal pain possibly related to the oncological treatment, one patient had surgery for a ventral hernia, and one patient was not operated on due to liver metastases presented a Guillain Barre syndrome, probably unrelated to the treatment). Grade 3 was recorded in six patients (12%), two patients with bladder symptoms (irritation and paresis), one hip arthrosis and one subileus after several years, and one stoma surgery due to local pain. Grade 4 was observed in five patients (10%): two with stenotic ureters, two patients had ileus, one of them also hip surgery and one pelvic pain. One Grade 5 patient died 2 weeks after surgery due to sepsis and adult respiratory distress syndrome, considered a complication after major surgery. In summary the side effects were as expected for the present cohort of locally advanced tumours with some elderly patients, and no obvious unexpected toxicity related to the hyperthermia treatment was observed.

Table 2. Acute toxicity observed during preoperative therapy and first month after surgery in 47 patients.

Grade	Maximal Acute Toxicity	Skin Toxicity	Diarrhoea	General Condition	Urinary	Nausea	Oxaliplatin Fever	Other
1	11	5	17	2	4	8	11	5
2	16	4	13	7	3	4	1	9
3	19	3	7	3	0	0	2	9
4	1	0	0	1	0	0	0	0
No surgery	2							

5. Discussion

Since this study was done, the surgical techniques used in combination with radiation and delivery of radiation have evolved and have reduced the local recurrence rate to about 5% for operable rectal cancer [35,36]. We therefore were initially not too enthusiastic of our achievement with the use of hyperthermia. However, most of the patients could be resected 12 weeks after the preoperative treatment in our series. We obtained a R0 resection rate of 87%, which seems better than 61% in a previous national study including locally advanced T4 rectal cancer patients [37]. Pathological assessment of the operation specimens revealed no residual tumour cells (TRG 4) in 29.8% of the patients, which is higher than the standard 10–20% pCR as reported after preoperative radiochemotherapy for rectal cancer [38–42], but some report even higher percentages [39,43,44]. In general the TRG4 rate is influenced by the initial tumour stage, the given treatment, as well as the timing between preoperative treatment and surgery. The high TRG4 rate in the present cohort of advanced rectal cancers is very promising. The most important aspect of the TRG4 is that no viable tumour cells after preoperative treatment is a predictor of higher RFS as demonstrated in Figure 4 in accordance with the findings in other series [40,45–48]. In the pCR group, 11 of 14 patients had no recurrence versus 14 of 33 in the other categories ($p < 0.05$). In our cohort the 5-year CSS was 92.9% for patients with pCR versus 72.7% with residual tumour cells, but this did not reach statistical significance, possibly due to the small sample size.

The isolated local recurrence rate at 5 years was 9% in this series of locally advanced rectal cancer patients. This is the same as observed in 2005 in a series of 3388 Norwegian patients with operable rectal cancer treated for cure by surgery alone including 5% pre-operative and 5% postoperative radiation [48]. In a previous Norwegian series of LARC patients defined as T4 tumours, the local recurrence rates at 5 years were 18% (95%CI 14–23) for patients with a R0-resection and 40% (95%CI 26–52) if the procedure was classified as R1 [35]. We observed two local recurrences after about 10 years. Whether these recurrences are true local recurrences or de novo development of new primary tumours cannot be determined, and we have therefore recorded them as local recurrences. Habr-Gama has reported adenomas after pCR for rectal cancer [49]. Thus, new primary cancer at the tumour bed may develop from such residual adenomas.

For comparison, the 5-year relative survival rate for all operated rectal cancers in Norway was 79% in 2004-06 [35]. The overall survival at 5 years in our series was 73.5%, clearly improved from 29% in the previous Norwegian series where 5-year survival was 49% after R0 resection and 20% after a R1 resection. In a more recent randomized trial, the 5-year overall survival for locally advanced rectal cancer was 66% after preoperative radiochemotherapy and 53% after preoperative radiation alone [1]. However, after 10-years there was no significant difference between radiation alone or radiochemotherapy in this trial [49].

The current study was designed to assess a possible role of hyperthermia. When 86 rectal cancer patients, treated with preoperative radiotherapy followed by surgical resection and adjuvant 5-FU and hyperthermia once or twice a week, were compared with predicted outcomes from a nomogram based on randomised European trials without hyperthermia, the observed OS (87.3%) versus predicted OS (75.5%), distant metastasis free survival (87.3%) vs. predicted (75.5%), and local control (95.8% vs. 95.8%, respectively), was better after hyperthermia [50]. Recently a series of 112 patients with locally advanced and recurrent rectal cancer had preoperative radiation (55.8–59.4 Gy) and regional hyperthermia with 5FU or capecitabine and oxaliplatin in locally advanced patients [51]. They reported a local recurrence rate of 2.3% with hyperthermia vs. 21.3% without hyperthermia and DFS of 89.1% vs. 70.4%, respectively. In another study including 78 LARC patients also using a similar regimen as our study with radiation 50.4 Gy combined with 5-FU and hyperthermia twice per week, pCR was seen in 14% with combined TRG 4 and TRG 3 in 50% of the patients [52]. DFS and OS were also in accord with our data. They also report that those patients achieving best quality hyperthermia had best tumour response. These studies therefore also support a role of hyperthermia in rectal cancer. Currently there has not been published a prospectively randomized study demonstrating the effect of deep hyperthermia added to preoperative treatment in rectal cancer patients.

It proved difficult to achieve the temperature aim stated in our protocol in most patients, mainly due to local pain and discomfort limiting power output, despite the use of fentanyl. However, achieving a temperature above median of T50 for the patients where temperature was recorded in tumours, resulted in a significant better RFS. Our findings support general reviews demonstrating that hyperthermia in addition to its own effect, is a sensitizer for radiation [27,53–55] as well as a chemosensitizer [53]. For further details on mechanism of action of hyperthermia, see references [12,53,56]. In addition, hyperthermia may also have positive immunological effects [57,58].

The role of oxaliplatin in the preoperative treatment of rectal cancer is controversial. Some authors report only increased toxicity (diarrhoea) [59], while others showed improved pCR, local control and distant metastases, but no effect on OS [60]. Other authors have reported improved outcomes in patients treated with oxaliplatin [61–63]. Avoiding the last scheduled dose of oxaliplatin significantly reduced pathological response in a recent study [64]. We cannot assess the contribution of oxaliplatin in our cohort, but we notice that oxaliplatin is part of current total neoadjuvant therapy for rectal cancer where induction chemotherapy is used before radiation [65–68]. Giving more chemotherapy before surgery was recently documented in two large randomized studies and several phase II studies, yielding pCR rates around 30% for total neoadjuvant therapy versus 14% for standard radiochemotherapy in a meta-analysis [69–71]. Although the disease free survival (DFS) at 3 years seems promising [71], the 4.6 year local recurrence rate was 8.3% in the experimental arm versus 6% after standard radiochemotherapy in the Rapido trial [69]. It should be noted that the time from diagnosis to surgery was 10 weeks longer in the experimental arm, which may have favoured this group. Distant metastases were recorded for 20.0% in the experimental group compared with 26.8% in the standard group in this trial, and disease-related treatment failure was 23.7% in the experimental group versus 30.4% ($p = 0.019$) in the standard of care group, but there was no difference in OS. Therefore, the effect of this more intense preoperative chemotherapy treatment on reduction of distant metastases must be further validation in new studies to assess the impact of more intense chemotherapy over longer time. Preoperative chemotherapy with mFOLFIRINOX may be an alternative option as pCR was 27.5% after chemotherapy alone versus 11.7% after standard preoperative chemoradiation followed by adjuvant chemotherapy, and 3-year DFS was 75.7% and 68.5%, respectively [72].

Surgery alone or after preoperative radiation has been the traditional treatment of local recurrences of rectal cancer [73,74]. Radiotherapy alone yields poor local control after surgery for rectal cancer [2], while radiochemotherapy followed by surgery seems better [49]. Currently carbon-ion radiotherapy seems to offer even better local control, but distant failures remain a problem [75,76]. Our data and the recent phase II studies imply a role of hyperthermia in recurrent rectal cancer [51,52].

In the present study, there was no unexpected long-term toxicity associated with addition of hyperthermia and the overall acute and long-term toxicity seems to be in line with current use of preoperative radiochemotherapy for rectal cancer [1,77,78]. No negative effects on quality of life with addition of hyperthermia to neoadjuvant radiochemotherapy was reported in this setting [79]. We must however admit that side effects recorded in the patient's journal and retrospectively collected as done in our study, are a weakness of our study.

6. Conclusions

This study of radiochemotherapy combined with deep regional hyperthermia showed, after long follow-up, good local control and survival, and no indications of increased treatment-related long-term side effects. The achieved temperatures during hyperthermia were relatively low, indicating a possibility for even better tumour effects with improvement of heating technology.

Author Contributions: Conceptualization, B.-C.S., O.M. and O.D.; methodology, B.-C.S., O.M., T.F., F.P., J.N.W., M.A.O. and N.S.; software, O.D.; validation, S.L.; formal analysis, O.D.; resources, O.M.; data curation, O.D. and M.P.M.; writing—original draft preparation, O.D.; writing—review and editing, all authors; visualization, B.-C.S., M.P.M. and O.D.; supervision, O.M.; project administration, O.M.; funding acquisition, O.D. All authors have read and agreed to the published version of the manuscript.

Funding: This research was supported by an unrestricted grant from the Trond Mohn Foundsation, earlier Bergen Research Foundation, BFS2015PAR02, and the Norwegian Cancer Society (Hyperthermia equipment). The sponsors had no influense on the study design.

Institutional Review Board Statement: The study was conducted according to the guidelines of the Declaration of Helsinki, and approved by the Regional Ethics Committee of Western Norway, protocol code REK III nr. 159.01, date of approval 7 November 2001.

Informed Consent Statement: Informed consent was obtained from all subjects involved in the study.

Data Availability Statement: Anonymous data may be disclosed upon any reasonable relevant request according to EU General Data Protection Regulation (GDPR) and Norwegian legislation.

Acknowledgments: The study were supported by an unrestricted grant from Trond Mohn Foundation and the Norwegian Cancer Society.

Conflicts of Interest: The authors declare no conflict of interest.

Appendix A

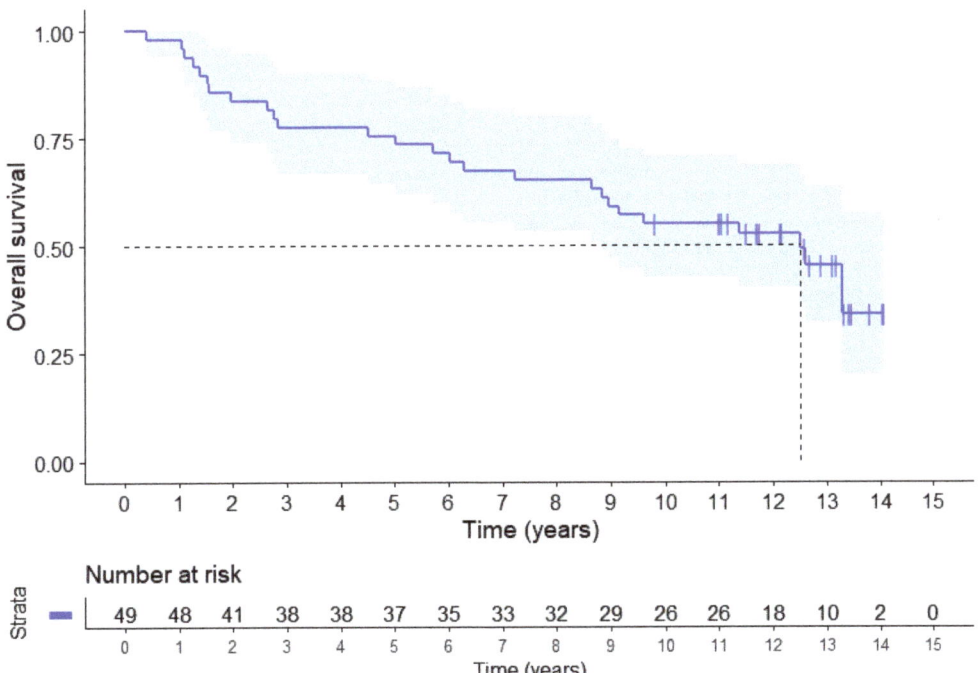

Figure A1. Overall survival for 49 rectal cancer patients, 43 with locally advanced and 6 with recurrent adenocarcinomas.

References

1. Braendengen, M.; Tveit, K.M.; Berglund, Å.; Birkemeyer, E.; Frykholm, G.; Påhlman, L.; Wiig, J.N.; Byström, P.; Bujko, K.; Glimelius, B. Randomized phase III study comparing preoperative radiotherapy with chemoradiotherapy in nonresectable rectal cancer. *J. Clin. Oncol.* **2008**, *26*, 3687–3694. [CrossRef] [PubMed]
2. Tanaka, H.; Yamaguchi, T.; Hachiya, K.; Okada, S.; Kitahara, M.; Matsuyama, K.; Matsuo, M. Radiotherapy for locally recurrent rectal cancer treated with surgery alone as the initial treatment. *Radiat. Oncol. J.* **2017**, *35*, 71–77. [CrossRef] [PubMed]
3. Temple, W.J.; Saettler, E.B. Locally recurrent rectal cancer: Role of composite resection of extensive pelvic tumors with strategies for minimizing risk of recurrence. *J. Surg. Oncol.* **2000**, *73*, 47–58. [CrossRef]
4. Dahl, O.; Horn, A.; Morild, I.; Halvorsen, J.F.; Odland, G.; Reinertsen, S.; Reisæter, A.; Kavli, H.; Thunold, J. Low-dose preoperative radiation postpones recurrences in operable rectal cancer. Results of a randomized multicenter trial in western Norway. *Cancer* **1990**, *66*, 2286–2294. [CrossRef]
5. Colorectal Cancer Collaborative Group. Adjuvant radiotherapy for rectal cancer: A systematic overview of 8507 patients from 22 randomized trials. *Lancet* **2001**, *358*, 1291–1304. [CrossRef]
6. Krook, J.E.; Moertel, C.G.; Gunderson, L.L.; Wieand, H.S.; Collins, R.T.; Beart, R.W.; Kubista, T.P.; Poon, M.A.; Meyers, W.C.; Mailliard, J.A.; et al. Effective surgical adjuvant therapy for high-risk rectal carcinoma. *N. Engl. J. Med.* **1991**, *324*, 709–715. [CrossRef]
7. Bjerkeset, T.; Dahl, O. Irradiation and surgery of primarily inoperable rectal adenocarcinoma. *Dis. Colon Rectum* **1980**, *23*, 298–303. [CrossRef]
8. Mella, O.; Dahl, O.; Horn, A.; Morild, I.; Odland, G. Radiotherapy and resection for apparently inoperable rectal adenocarcinoma. *Dis. Colon. Rectum* **1984**, *27*, 663–668. [CrossRef]
9. Reerink, O.; Verschueren, R.; Szabo, B.; Hospers, G.; Mulder, N. A favourable pathological stage after neoadjuvant radiochemotherapy in patients with initially irresectable rectal cancer correlates with a favourable prognosis. *Eur. J. Cancer* **2003**, *39*, 192–195. [CrossRef]
10. Dahl, O.; Dalene, R.; Schem, B.C.; Mella, O. Status of clinical hyperthermia. *Acta Oncol.* **1999**, *38*, 863–873. [CrossRef]
11. Harima, Y.; Nagata, K.; Harima, K.; Ostapenko, V.V.; Tanaka, Y.; Sawada, S. A randomized clinical trial of radiation therapy versus thermoradiotherapy in stage IIIB cervical carcinoma. *Int. J. Hyperth.* **2001**, *17*, 97–105. [CrossRef] [PubMed]
12. Overgaard, J.; Gonzalez Gonzalez, D.; Hulshof, M.C.; Arcangeli, G.; Dahl, O.; Mella, O.; Bentzen, S.M. Randomised trial of hyperthermia as adjuvant to radiotherapy for recurrent or metastatic malignant melanoma. European Society for Hyperthermic Oncology. *Lancet* **1995**, *345*, 540–543. [CrossRef]
13. Van der Zee, J.; González, D.; van Rhoon, G.C.; van Dijk, J.D.; van Putten, W.L.; Hart, A.A. Comparison of radiotherapy alone with radiotherapy plus hyperthermia in locally advanced pelvic tumours: A prospective, randomised, multicentre trial. Dutch Deep Hyperthermia Group. *Lancet* **2000**, *355*, 1119–1125. [CrossRef]
14. Schem, B.C.; Mella, O.; Dahl, O. Thermochemotherapy with cisplatin or carboplatin in the BT4 rat glioma in vitro and in vivo. *Int. J. Radiat. Oncol. Biol. Phys.* **1992**, *23*, 109–114. [CrossRef]
15. Korenaga, D.; Matsushima, T.; Adachi, Y.; Mori, M.; Matsuda, H.; Kuwano, H.; Sugimachi, K. Preoperative hyperthermia combined with chemotherapy and radiotherapy for patients with rectal carcinoma may prevent early local pelvic recurrence. *Int. J. Colorectal Dis.* **1992**, *7*, 206–209. [CrossRef]
16. Rau, B.; Wust, P.; Hohenberger, P.; Löffel, J.; Hünerbein, M.; Below, C.; Gellermann, J.; Speidel, A.; Vogl, T.; Riess, H.; et al. Preoperative hyperthermia combined with radiochemotherapy in locally advanced rectal cancer: A phase II clinical trial. *Ann. Surg.* **1998**, *227*, 380–389. [CrossRef]
17. Wust, P.; Hildebrandt, B.; Sreenivasa, G.; Rau, B.; Gellermann, J.; Riess, H.; Felix, R.; Schlag, P.M. Hyperthermia in combined treatment of cancer. *Lancet Oncol.* **2002**, *3*, 487–497. [CrossRef]
18. Dunst, J.; Reese, T.; Sutter, T.; Zühlke, H.; Hinke, A.; Kölling-Schlebusch, K.; Frings, S. Phase I trial evaluating the concurrent combination of radiotherapy and capecitabine in rectal cancer. *J. Clin. Oncol.* **2002**, *20*, 3983–3991. [CrossRef]
19. Hildebrandt, B.; Wust, P.; Dräger, J.; Lüdemann, L.; Sreenivasa, G.; Tullius, S.G.; Amthauer, H.; Neuhaus, P.; Felix, R.; Riess, H. Regional pelvic hyperthermia as an adjunct to chemotherapy (oxaliplatin, folinic acid, 5-fluorouracil) in pre-irradiated patients with locally recurrent rectal cancer: A pilot study. *Int. J. Hyperth.* **2004**, *20*, 359–369. [CrossRef]
20. Rietbroek, R.C.; van de Vaart, P.J.M.; Haveman, J.; Blommaert, F.A.; Geerdink, A.; Bakker, P.J.M.; Veenhof, C.H.N. Hyperthermia enhances the cytotoxicity and platinum-DNA adduct formation of lobaplatin and oxaliplatin in cultured SW 1573 cells. *J. Cancer Res. Clin. Oncol.* **1997**, *123*, 6–12. [CrossRef]
21. Urano, M.; Ling, C.C. Thermal enhancement of melphalan and oxaliplatin cytotoxicity in vitro. *Int. J. Hyperth.* **2002**, *18*, 307–315. [CrossRef] [PubMed]
22. Hegewisch-Becker, S.; Gruber, Y.; Corovic, A.; Pichlmeier, U.; Atanackovic, D.; Nierhaus, A.; Hossfeld, D.K. Whole-body hyperthermia (41.8 degrees C) combined with bimonthly oxaliplatin, high-dose leucovorin and 5-fluorouracil 48-hour continuous infusion in pretreated metastatic colorectal cancer: A phase II study. *Ann. Oncol.* **2002**, *13*, 1197–1204. [CrossRef] [PubMed]
23. Schem, B.C.; Froystein, T.; Hjertaker, B.T.; Larsen, A.; Mella, O. Trimodality treatmenet with regional hyperthermia (HT), radiotherapy (RT) and chemotherapy in primary inoperable or recurrent rectal carcinoma. In Proceedings of the International Conference of Hyperthermic Oncology—ICHO, St. Louis, MO, USA, 20–24 April 2004; pp. 88–89.

24. Ohno, S.; Sumiyoshi, Y.; Mori, M.; Sugimachi, K. Hyperthermia for rectal cancer. *Surgery* **2002**, *131*, S121–S127. [CrossRef] [PubMed]
25. Lagendijk, J.J.W.; Van Rhoon, G.C.; Hornsleth, S.N.; Wust, P.; De Leeuw, A.C.C.; Schneider, C.J.; Van Ddk, J.D.P.; Van Der Zee, J.; Van Heek-Romanowski, R.; Rahman, S.A.; et al. ESHO quality assurance guidelines for regional hyperthermia. *Int. J. Hyperth.* **1998**, *14*, 125–133. [CrossRef]
26. Gani, C.; Schroeder, C.; Heinrich, V.; Spillner, P.; Lamprecht, U.; Berger, B.; Zips, D. Long-term local control and survival after preoperative radiochemotherapy in combination with deep regional hyperthermia in locally advanced rectal cancer. *Int. J. Hyperth.* **2016**, *32*, 187–192. [CrossRef]
27. Peeken, J.C.; Vaupel, P.; Combs, S.E. Integrating Hyperthermia into Modern Radiation Oncology: What Evidence Is Necessary? *Front. Oncol.* **2017**, *7*, 132. [CrossRef]
28. Hermanek, P.; Hutter, R.V.; Sobin, L.H.; Wagner, G.; Wittekind, C. *TNM Atlas: Illustrated Guide to TNM/pTNM Classification of Malignant Tumours*, 4th ed.; Union Internationale Contre le Cancer—UICC: Geneva, Switzerland, 1997.
29. Punt, C.J.A.; Buyse, M.; Köhne, C.-H.; Hohenberger, P.; Labianca, R.; Schmoll, H.J.; Påhlman, L.; Sobrero, A.; Douillard, J.-Y. Endpoints in adjuvant treatment trials: A systematic review of the literature in colon cancer and proposed definitions for future trials. *J. Natl. Cancer Inst.* **2007**, *99*, 998–1003. [CrossRef]
30. Trotti, A.; Colevas, A.; Setser, A.; Rusch, V.; Jaques, D.; Budach, V.; Langer, C.; Murphy, B.; Cumberlin, R.; Coleman, C. CTCAE v3.0: Development of a comprehensive grading system for the adverse effects of cancer treatment. *Semin. Radiat. Oncol.* **2003**, *13*, 176–181. [CrossRef]
31. Hornsleth, S.N.; Frydendal, L.; Mella, O.; Dahl, O.; Raskmark, P. Quality assurance for radiofrequency regional hyperthermia. *Int. J. Hyperth.* **1997**, *13*, 169–185. [CrossRef]
32. Oleson, J.R.; Samulski, T.V.; Leopold, K.A.; Clegg, S.T.; Dewhirst, M.W.; Dodge, R.K.; George, S.L. Sensitivity of hyperthermia trial outcomes to temperature and time: Implications for thermal goals of treatment. *Int. J. Radiat. Oncol. Biol. Phys.* **1993**, *25*, 289–297. [CrossRef]
33. Fatehi, D.; de Bruijne, M.; van der Zee, J.; van Rhoon, G.C. RHyThM, a tool for analysis of PDOS formatted hyperthermia treatment data generated by the BSD2000/3D system. *Int. J. Hyperth.* **2006**, *22*, 173–184. [CrossRef] [PubMed]
34. Dworak, O.; Keilholz, L.; Hoffmann, A. Pathological features of rectal cancer after preoperative radiochemotherapy. *Int. J. Colorectal Dis.* **1997**, *12*, 19–23. [CrossRef] [PubMed]
35. Guren, M.G.; Kørner, H.; Pfeffer, F.; Myklebust, T.Å.; Eriksen, M.T.; Edna, T.-H.; Larsen, S.G.; Knudsen, K.O.; Nesbakken, A.; Wasmuth, H.H.; et al. Nationwide improvement in rectal cancer treatment outcomes in Norway, 1993–2010. *Acta Oncol.* **2015**, *54*, 1714–1722. [CrossRef]
36. Kapiteijn, E.; Marijnen, C.A.; Nagtegaal, I.D.; Putter, H.; Steup, W.H.; Wiggers, T.; Rutten, H.J.; Pahlman, L.; Glimelius, B.; Van Krieken, J.H.; et al. Preoperative radiotherapy combined with total mesorectal excision for resectable rectal cancer: 12-year follow-up of the multicentre, randomised controlled TME trial. *Lancet Oncol.* **2011**, *12*, 575–582.
37. Eriksen, M.; Norwegian Gastrointestinal Cancer Group; Wibe, A.; Hestvik, U.; Haffner, J.; Wiig, J.; Norwegian Rectal Cancer Group. Surgical treatment of primary locally advanced rectal cancer in Norway. *Eur. J. Surg. Oncol.* **2006**, *32*, 174–180. [CrossRef]
38. 2017 European Society of Coloproctology (ESCP) Collaborating Group; Battersby, N.; Glasbey, J.C.; Neary, P.; Negoi, I.; Kamarajah, S.; Sgro, A.; Bhangu, A.; Pinkney, T.; Frasson, M.; et al. Evaluating the incidence of pathological complete response in current international rectal cancer practice; the barriers to widespread safe deferral of surgery. *Colorectal Dis.* **2018**, *20*, 58–68.
39. Hartley, A.; Ho, K.F.; McConkey, C.; Geh, J.I. Pathological complete response following pre-operative chemoradiotherapy in rectal cancer: Analysis of phase II/III trials. *Br. J. Radiol.* **2005**, *78*, 934–938. [CrossRef]
40. Maas, M.; Nelemans, P.J.; Valentini, V.; Das, P.; Rödel, C.; Kuo, L.-J.; A Calvo, F.; García-Aguilar, J.; Glynne-Jones, R.; Haustermans, K.; et al. Long-term outcome in patients with a pathological complete response after chemoradiation for rectal cancer: A pooled analysis of individual patient data. *Lancet Oncol.* **2010**, *11*, 835–844. [CrossRef]
41. Tan, Y.; Fu, D.; Li, D.; Kong, X.; Jiang, K.; Chen, L.; Yuan, Y.; Ding, K. Predictors and Risk Factors of Pathologic Complete Response Following Neoadjuvant Chemoradiotherapy for Rectal Cancer: A Population-Based Analysis. *Front. Oncol.* **2019**, *9*, 497. [CrossRef]
42. Teo, M.T.W.; McParland, L.; Appelt, A.L.; Sebag-Montefiore, D. Phase 2 Neoadjuvant Treatment Intensification Trials in Rectal Cancer: A Systematic Review. *Int. J. Radiat. Oncol. Biol. Phys.* **2018**, *100*, 146–158. [CrossRef]
43. Li, J.; Ji, J.; Cai, Y.; Li, X.-F.; Li, Y.-H.; Wu, H.; Xu, B.; Dou, F.-Y.; Li, Z.-Y.; Bu, Z.-D.; et al. Preoperative concomitant boost intensity-modulated radiotherapy with oral capecitabine in locally advanced mid-low rectal cancer: A phase II trial. *Radiother. Oncol.* **2012**, *102*, 4–9. [CrossRef] [PubMed]
44. Petrelli, F.; Trevisan, F.; Cabiddu, M.; Sgroi, G.; Bruschieri, L.; Rausa, E.; Ghidini, M.; Turati, L. Total Neoadjuvant Therapy in Rectal Cancer: A Systematic Review and Meta-analysis of Treatment Outcomes. *Ann. Surg.* **2020**, *271*, 440–448. [CrossRef] [PubMed]
45. Bujko, K.; Kolodziejczyk, M.; Nasierowska-Guttmejer, A.; Michalski, W.; Kepka, L.; Chmielik, E.; Wojnar, A.; Chwalinski, M. Tumour regression grading in patients with residual rectal cancer after preoperative chemoradiation. *Radiother. Oncol.* **2010**, *95*, 298–302. [CrossRef] [PubMed]

46. Kong, J.C.; Guerra, G.R.; Warrier, S.K.; Lynch, A.C.; Michael, M.; Ngan, S.Y.; Phillips, W.; Ramsay, G.; Heriot, A.G. Prognostic value of tumour regression grade in locally advanced rectal cancer: A systematic review and meta-analysis. *Colorectal Dis.* 2018, *20*, 574–585. [CrossRef] [PubMed]
47. Rödel, C.; Martus, P.; Papadoupolos, T.; Füzesi, L.; Klimpfinger, M.; Fietkau, R.; Liersch, T.; Hohenberger, W.; Raab, R.; Sauer, R.; et al. Prognostic significance of tumor regression after preoperative chemoradiotherapy for rectal cancer. *J. Clin. Oncol.* 2005, *23*, 8688–8696. [CrossRef]
48. Wiig, J.N.; Larsen, S.G.; Dueland, S.; Giercksky, K.E. Clinical outcome in patients with complete pathologic response (pT0) to preoperative irradiation/chemo-irradiation operated for locally advanced or locally recurrent rectal cancer. *J. Surg. Oncol.* 2005, *92*, 70–75. [CrossRef]
49. Braendengen, M.; Glimelius, B. Preoperative radiotherapy or chemoradiotherapy in rectal cancer—Is survival improved? An update of the "Nordic" LARC study in non-resectable cancers. *Radiother. Oncol.* 2018, *127*, 392–395. [CrossRef]
50. Zwirner, K.; Bonomo, P.; Lamprecht, U.; Zips, D.; Gani, C. External validation of a rectal cancer outcome prediction model with a cohort of patients treated with preoperative radiochemotherapy and deep regional hyperthermia. *Int. J. Hyperth.* 2018, *34*, 455–460. [CrossRef]
51. Ott, O.; Gani, C.; Lindner, L.; Schmidt, M.; Lamprecht, U.; Abdel-Rahman, S.; Hinke, A.; Weissmann, T.; Hartmann, A.; Issels, R.; et al. Neoadjuvant Chemoradiation Combined with Regional Hyperthermia in Locally Advanced or Recurrent Rectal Cancer. *Cancers* 2021, *13*, 1279. [CrossRef]
52. Gani, C.; Lamprecht, U.; Ziegler, A.; Moll, M.; Gellermann, J.; Heinrich, V.; Wenz, S.; Fend, F.; Königsrainer, A.; Bitzer, M.; et al. Deep regional hyperthermia with preoperative radiochemotherapy in locally advanced rectal cancer, a prospective phase II trial. *Radiother. Oncol.* 2021, *159*, 155–160. [CrossRef]
53. Datta, N.R.; Kok, H.P.; Crezee, H.; Gaipl, U.S.; Bodis, S. Integrating Loco-Regional Hyperthermia Into the Current Oncology Practice: SWOT and TOWS Analyses. *Front. Oncol.* 2020, *10*, 819. [CrossRef] [PubMed]
54. De Haas-Kock, D.F.; Buijsen, J.; Pijls-Johannesma, M.; Lutgens, L.; Lammering, G.; van Mastrigt, G.A.; De Ruysscher, D.K.; Lambin, P.; van der Zee, J. Concomitant hyperthermia and radiation therapy for treating locally advanced rectal cancer. *Cochrane Database Syst. Rev.* 2009, CD006269. [CrossRef] [PubMed]
55. Horsman, M.R.; Overgaard, J. Hyperthermia: A potent enhancer of radiotherapy. *Clin. Oncol. (R Coll. Radiol.)* 2007, *19*, 418–426. [CrossRef]
56. Elming, P.B.; Sørensen, B.S.; Oei, A.L.; Franken, N.A.P.; Crezee, J.; Overgaard, J.; Horsman, M.R. Hyperthermia: The Optimal Treatment to Overcome Radiation Resistant Hypoxia. *Cancers* 2019, *11*, 60. [CrossRef]
57. Hader, M.; Frey, B.; Fietkau, R.; Hecht, M.; Gaipl, U.S. Immune biological rationales for the design of combined radio- and immunotherapies. *Cancer Immunol. Immunother.* 2020, *69*, 293–306. [CrossRef]
58. Hader, M.; Savcigil, D.P.; Rosin, A.; Ponfick, P.; Gekle, S.; Wadepohl, M.; Bekeschus, S.; Fietkau, R.; Frey, B.; Schlücker, E.; et al. Differences of the Immune Phenotype of Breast Cancer Cells after Ex Vivo Hyperthermia by Warm-Water or Microwave Radiation in a Closed-Loop System Alone or in Combination with Radiotherapy. *Cancers* 2020, *12*, 1082. [CrossRef]
59. Allegra, C.J.; Yothers, G.; O'Connell, M.J.; Beart, R.W.; Wozniak, T.F.; Pitot, H.C.; Shields, A.F.; Landry, J.C.; Ryan, D.P.; Arora, A.; et al. Neoadjuvant 5-FU or Capecitabine Plus Radiation With or Without Oxaliplatin in Rectal Cancer Patients: A Phase III Randomized Clinical Trial. *J. Natl. Cancer Inst.* 2015, *107*, djv248. [CrossRef]
60. Thavaneswaran, S.; Kok, P.S.; Price, T. Evaluating the addition of oxaliplatin to single agent fluoropyrimidine in the treatment of locally advanced rectal cancer: A systematic review and meta-analysis. *Expert Rev. Anticancer. Ther.* 2017, *17*, 965–979. [CrossRef]
61. Dueland, S.; Ree, A.; Grøholt, K.; Saelen, M.; Folkvord, S.; Hole, K.; Seierstad, T.; Larsen, S.; Giercksky, K.; Wiig, J.; et al. Oxaliplatin-containing Preoperative Therapy in Locally Advanced Rectal Cancer: Local Response, Toxicity and Long-term Outcome. *Clin. Oncol. (R Coll. Radiol.)* 2016, *28*, 532–539. [CrossRef]
62. Martijnse, I.S.; Dudink, R.L.; Kusters, M.; Vermeer, T.A.; West, N.P.; Nieuwenhuijzen, G.A.; Van Lijnschoten, I.; Martijn, H.; Creemers, G.-J.; Lemmens, V.E.; et al. T3+ and T4 rectal cancer patients seem to benefit from the addition of oxaliplatin to the neoadjuvant chemoradiation regimen. *Ann. Surg. Oncol.* 2012, *19*, 392–401. [CrossRef]
63. Rödel, C.; Graeven, U.; Fietkau, R.; Hohenberger, W.; Hothorn, T.; Arnold, D.; Hofheinz, R.-D.; Ghadimi, M.; Wolff, H.A.; Lang-Welzenbach, M.; et al. Oxaliplatin added to fluorouracil-based preoperative chemoradiotherapy and postoperative chemotherapy of locally advanced rectal cancer (the German CAO/ARO/AIO-04 study): Final results of the multicentre, open-label, randomised, phase 3 trial. *Lancet Oncol.* 2015, *16*, 979–989. [CrossRef]
64. Broggi, S.; Passoni, P.; Gumina, C.; Palmisano, A.; Bresolin, A.; Burgio, V.; Di Chiara, A.; Elmore, U.; Mori, M.; Slim, N.; et al. Predicting pathological response after radio-chemotherapy for rectal cancer: Impact of late oxaliplatin administration. *Radiother. Oncol.* 2020, *149*, 174–180. [CrossRef] [PubMed]
65. Fernández-Martos, C.; Pericay, C.; Aparicio, J.; Salud, A.; Safont, M.; Massuti, B.; Vera, R.; Escudero, P.; Maurel, J.; Marcuello, E.; et al. Phase II, randomized study of concomitant chemoradiotherapy followed by surgery and adjuvant capecitabine plus oxaliplatin (CAPOX) compared with induction CAPOX followed by concomitant chemoradiotherapy and surgery in magnetic resonance imaging-defined, locally advanced rectal cancer: Grupo cancer de recto 3 study. *J. Clin. Oncol.* 2010, *28*, 859–865. [PubMed]
66. Ludmir, E.B.; Palta, M.; Willett, C.G.; Czito, B.G. Total neoadjuvant therapy for rectal cancer: An emerging option. *Cancer* 2017, *123*, 1497–1506. [CrossRef] [PubMed]

67. Masi, G.; Vivaldi, C.; Fornaro, L.; Lonardi, S.; Buccianti, P.; Sainato, A.; Marcucci, L.; Martignetti, A.; Urso, E.D.L.; Castagna, M.; et al. Total neoadjuvant approach with FOLFOXIRI plus bevacizumab followed by chemoradiotherapy plus bevacizumab in locally advanced rectal cancer: The TRUST trial. *Eur. J. Cancer* 2019, *110*, 32–41. [CrossRef] [PubMed]
68. Schrag, D.; Weiser, M.R.; Goodman, K.A.; Gönen, M.; Hollywood, E.; Cercek, A.; Reidy-Lagunes, D.L.; Gollub, M.J.; Shia, J.; Guillem, J.G.; et al. Neoadjuvant chemotherapy without routine use of radiation therapy for patients with locally advanced rectal cancer: A pilot trial. *J. Clin. Oncol.* 2014, *32*, 513–518. [CrossRef]
69. Bahadoer, R.R.; A Dijkstra, E.; van Etten, B.; Marijnen, C.A.M.; Putter, H.; Kranenbarg, E.M.-K.; Roodvoets, A.G.H.; Nagtegaal, I.D.; Beets-Tan, R.G.H.; Blomqvist, L.K.; et al. Short-course radiotherapy followed by chemotherapy before total mesorectal excision (TME) versus preoperative chemoradiotherapy, TME, and optional adjuvant chemotherapy in locally advanced rectal cancer (RAPIDO): A randomised, open-label, phase 3 trial. *Lancet. Oncol.* 2021, *22*, 29–42. [CrossRef]
70. Cercek, A.; Roxburgh, C.S.; Strombom, P.; Smith, J.J.; Temple, L.K.; Nash, G.M.; Guillem, J.G.; Paty, P.B.; Yaeger, R.; Stadler, Z.K.; et al. Adoption of Total Neoadjuvant Therapy for Locally Advanced Rectal Cancer. *JAMA Oncol.* 2018, *4*, e180071. [CrossRef]
71. Kasi, A.; Abbasi, S.; Handa, S.; Al-Rajabi, R.; Saeed, A.; Baranda, J.; Sun, W. Total Neoadjuvant Therapy vs Standard Therapy in Locally Advanced Rectal Cancer: A Systematic Review and Meta-analysis. *JAMA Netw. Open* 2020, *3*, e2030097. [CrossRef]
72. Conroy, T.; Lamfichekh, N.; Etienne, P.L.; Rio, E.; Francois, E.; Mesgouez-Nebout, N.; Vendrely, V.; Artignan, X.; Bouché, O.; Gargot, D.; et al. Total neoadjuvant therapy with mFOLFIRINOX versus preoperative chemoradiation in patieents with locally advanced rectal cancer: Final results of PRODIGE 23 phase III trial, a UNICANCER GI trial. *J. Clin. Oncol.* 2020, *38*, 4007. [CrossRef]
73. Iversen, H.; Martling, A.; Johansson, H.; Nilsson, P.; Holm, T. Pelvic local recurrence from colorectal cancer: Surgical challenge with changing preconditions. *Colorectal Dis.* 2018, *20*, 399–406. [CrossRef] [PubMed]
74. Lee, D.J.; Sagar, P.M.; Sadadcharam, G.; Tan, K.Y. Advances in surgical management for locally recurrent rectal cancer: How far have we come? *World J. Gastroenterol.* 2017, *23*, 4170–4180. [CrossRef] [PubMed]
75. Shinoto, M.; Yamada, S.; Okamoto, M.; Shioyama, Y.; Ohno, T.; Nakano, T.; Nemoto, K.; Isozaki, Y.; Kawashiro, S.; Tsuji, H.; et al. Carbon-ion radiotherapy for locally recurrent rectal cancer: Japan Carbon-ion Radiation Oncology Study Group (J-CROS) Study 1404 Rectum. *Radiother. Oncol.* 2019, *132*, 236–240. [CrossRef] [PubMed]
76. Yamada, S.; Kamada, T.; Ebner, D.K.; Shinoto, M.; Terashima, K.; Isozaki, Y.; Yasuda, S.; Makishima, H.; Tsuji, H.; Tsujii, H.; et al. Carbon-Ion Radiation Therapy for Pelvic Recurrence of Rectal Cancer. *Int. J. Radiat. Oncol. Biol. Phys.* 2016, *96*, 93–101. [CrossRef] [PubMed]
77. Regnier, A.; Ulbrich, J.; Münch, S.; Oechsner, M.; Wilhelm, D.; Combs, S.E.; Habermehl, D. Comparative Analysis of Efficacy, Toxicity, and Patient-Reported Outcomes in Rectal Cancer Patients Undergoing Preoperative 3D Conformal Radiotherapy or VMAT. *Front. Oncol.* 2017, *7*, 225. [CrossRef]
78. Van der Valk, M.J.; Marijnen, C.A.; van Etten, B.; Dijkstra, E.A.; Hilling, D.E.; Kranenbarg, E.M.; Putter, H.; Roodvoets, A.G.; Bahadoer, R.R.; Fokstuen, T.; et al. Compliance and tolerability of short-course radiotherapy followed by preoperative chemotherapy and surgery for high-risk rectal cancer—Results of the international randomized RAPIDO-trial. *Radiother. Oncol.* 2020, *147*, 75–83. [CrossRef]
79. Schulze, T.; Wust, P.; Gellermann, J.; Hildebrandt, B.; Riess, H.; Felix, R.; Rau, B. Influence of neoadjuvant radiochemotherapy combined with hyperthermia on the quality of life in rectum cancer patients. *Int. J. Hyperth.* 2006, *22*, 301–318. [CrossRef]

Article

Intensity-Modulated Radiotherapy with Regional Hyperthermia for High-Risk Localized Prostate Carcinoma

Sota Nakahara [1], Takayuki Ohguri [1,*], Sho Kakinouchi [1], Hirohide Itamura [1], Takahiro Morisaki [1], Subaru Tani [1], Katuya Yahara [2] and Naohiro Fujimoto [3]

1. Department of Therapeutic Radiology, University Hospital of Occupational and Environmental Health, Kitakyushu 807-8555, Japan; sotanakahara@med.uoeh-uoeh.ac.jp (S.N.); kakino365@gmail.com (S.K.); itamura@med.uoeh-u.ac.jp (H.I.); takam1989@med.uoeh-u.ac.jp (T.M.); s-tani@med.uoeh-u.ac.jp (S.T.)
2. Department of Radiotherapy, Kurashiki Medical Center, Kurashiki 710-8522, Japan; k-yahara@med.uoeh-u.ac.jp
3. Department of Urology, University of Occupational and Environmental Health, Kitakyushu 807-8555, Japan; n-fuji@med.uoeh-u.ac.jp
* Correspondence: ogurieye@med.uoeh-u.ac.jp; Tel.: +81-93-691-7264; Fax: +81-93-692-0249

Simple Summary: Several randomized controlled trials have shown that concurrent use of deep regional hyperthermia and radiotherapy results in a significant increase in local control of cervical and rectal cancer. Intensity-modulated radiotherapy (IMRT) plus androgen deprivation therapy (ADT) has recently become standard treatment for high-risk localized prostate carcinoma; however, as there is room for improvement in outcomes, we have been using hyperthermia to improve the effect of IMRT. This retrospective analysis shows that addition of regional hyperthermia to IMRT plus ADT is a promising approach as it improves clinical outcomes with acceptable toxicity. Importantly, a higher thermal dose was significantly correlated with better biochemical disease-free survival. Further investigations, including prospective trials with detailed treatment protocols, are needed.

Abstract: Background: The purpose of this study was to evaluate the efficacy and toxicity of adding regional hyperthermia to intensity-modulated radiotherapy (IMRT) plus neoadjuvant androgen deprivation therapy (ADT) for high-risk localized prostate carcinoma. Methods: Data from 121 consecutive patients with high-risk prostate carcinoma who were treated with IMRT were retrospectively analyzed. The total planned dose of IMRT was 76 Gy in 38 fractions for all patients; hyperthermia was used in 70 of 121 patients. Intra-rectal temperatures at the prostate level were measured to evaluate thermal dose. Results: Median number of heating sessions was five and the median total thermal dose of CEM43T90 was 7.5 min. Median follow-up duration was 64 months. Addition of hyperthermia to IMRT predicted better clinical relapse-free survival. Higher thermal dose with CEM43T90 (>7 min) predicted improved biochemical disease-free survival. The occurrence of acute and delayed toxicity ≥Grade 2 was not significantly different between patients with or without hyperthermia. Conclusions: IMRT plus regional hyperthermia represents a promising approach with acceptable toxicity for high-risk localized prostate carcinoma. Further studies are needed to verify the efficacy of this combined treatment.

Keywords: hyperthermia; intensity-modulated radiotherapy; prostate cancer; thermal dose

1. Introduction

Radiation therapy with androgen deprivation therapy (ADT) is the main treatment modality for patients with high-risk localized prostate cancer [1]. External radiation, such as intensity-modulated radiotherapy (IMRT), stereotactic body radiation therapy, and proton therapy, has been increasingly used in recent years to optimize dose concentration in tumors and reduce exposure to at-risk organs. The 5-year biochemical disease-free survival for external beam radiotherapy was reported to be 80–90% in the low-risk group, 70–80%

in the intermediate-risk group, and 50–70% in the high-risk group [2]. Clinical outcomes in the high-risk group can be improved, unlike in the low- to intermediate-risk groups.

Hyperthermia is known to be cytotoxic to cancer cells and acts as a radiosensitizer [3,4]. Radiation therapy-resistant tumor cells that are hypoxic, of low pH, nutritionally deprived, and in the S-phase are more sensitive to hyperthermia [3,5,6]. The clinical efficacy of radiotherapy plus hyperthermia have been demonstrated in randomized clinical trials in patients with advanced head and neck cancer, locally recurrent breast cancer, malignant melanoma, bladder cancer, rectal cancer, and cervical cancer [1]. In patients with prostate cancer, previous phase I/II clinical trials and retrospective studies have described the use of three-dimensional conformal radiation therapy in combination with regional hyperthermia to be both promising and feasible. Additionally, it does not cause severe toxicity [7–13].

In Japan, the safety and efficacy of hyperthermia in combination with radiotherapy using the 8-MHz capacitive device has been demonstrated since the 1980s, including in prospective phase I/II studies of patients with deep-seated malignant pelvic tumors [14–18]. Based on these results, and since the 1990s, electromagnetic hyperthermia for malignant tumors has been covered by public health insurance, irrespective of the type and stage of the malignant tumor. In Japan, all the people are covered by public health insurance. The patient is free to choose the medical institution and can receive advanced medical treatment at a low cost. In clinical practice, electromagnetic hyperthermia is mainly used in locally advanced cancers wherein further improvement of the antitumor effects of radiotherapy and/or chemotherapy is required, although only a limited number of hospitals are able to carry out the procedure. Hence, in our institution, combination therapy using IMRT and regional hyperthermia was initiated in 2011 to improve the clinical outcomes in patients with high-risk localized prostate cancer. To the best of our knowledge, there are no reports on clinical outcomes after such combination therapy; thus, the purpose of this study was to evaluate the efficacy and toxicity of IMRT plus regional hyperthermia for high-risk localized prostate carcinoma.

2. Materials and Methods
2.1. Patients

In the current study, we explained to the patients that the standard treatment for National Comprehensive Carcinoma Network (NCCN) high-risk prostate cancer combining IMRT and hormonal therapy results in biochemical recurrence in approximately 20–40% of patients, thereby requiring additional treatment. Furthermore, the possibility of improving the radiotherapeutic effect by performing hyperthermia and the possible side effects (mainly heat sensation, fatigue, and subcutaneous fat burns) were fully clarified. Finally, hyperthermia treatment can only be carried out after the patient had understood the advantages and disadvantages of and consented to the treatment by signing informed consent documents.

This retrospective study was conducted with the permission of the Institutional Review Board of the authors' university. All personal data, such as names and addresses, were anonymized so that the subjects could not be identified and stored in a locked vault together with their correspondence, under the strict control of the Principal Investigator, when investigating data from electronic medical records and treatment devices.

High-risk prostate carcinoma patients (n = 123), defined according to the NCCN, were treated with definitive IMRT between March 2011 and December 2018, at an institutional hospital. During the same period, according to our institution's treatment protocol aimed at improving clinical outcomes, a subset of the patients (70/123; 57%) were provided regional hyperthermia along with definitive IMRT (Figure 1); the remaining 53 patients were treated with definitive IMRT alone. Primary indications against the use of regional hyperthermia were as follows: patient refusal (n = 21), cerebral disease (n = 12), cardiovascular disease (n = 8), orthopedic disease (n = 5), presence of other disease (n = 4), and advanced age (n = 3). Two of the 123 patients were not able to complete the planned IMRT dose (76 Gy in 38 fractions) and were excluded from the study. Therefore, data from 70 patients treated with definitive IMRT plus regional hyperthermia, and 51 patients treated with definitive IMRT alone, were retrospectively analyzed (Figure 1). Patients with postoperative prostate carcinoma were not included in this study.

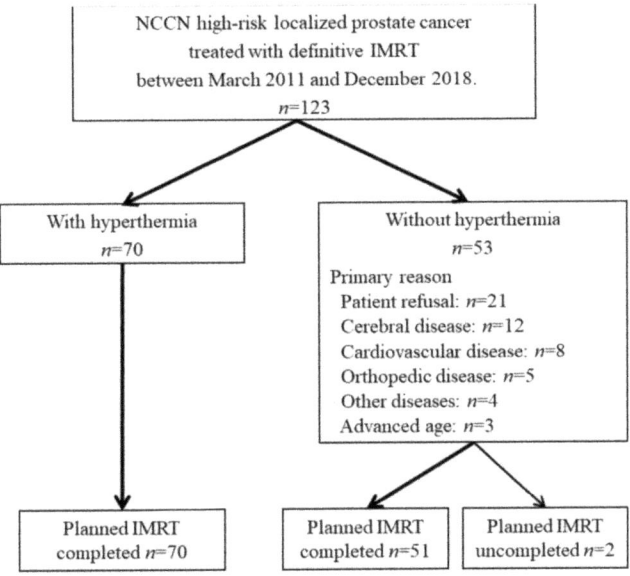

Figure 1. Patient flow diagram.

Patient baseline characteristics and treatments are listed in Table 1. All patients had pathologically confirmed prostate adenocarcinoma and initially underwent neoadjuvant ADT for a median duration of 9 months (interquartile range, 7–11 months). Adjuvant ADT was continued in 22 patients after completion of IMRT for a median duration of 24 months (interquartile range, 22–33 months). Median total duration of neoadjuvant plus adjuvant ADT was 10 months (interquartile range, 8–18 months).

Table 1. Patient characteristics.

Characteristics	With Hyperthermia	Without Hyperthermia	p
	$n = 70$ (%)	$n = 51$ (%)	
Age (median, range)	72 (54–80)	71 (54–83)	0.3381
Performance status			0.1948
0	41 (59)	25 (49)	
1	29 (41)	23 (45)	
2	0	2 (4)	
3	0	1 (2)	
T stage			0.8000
T1	25 (36)	18 (35)	
T2	31 (44)	25 (49)	
T3a	14 (20)	8 (16)	
N stage			
N0	72 (100)	51 (100)	
Gleason score			0.4774
≤7	17 (24)	14 (28)	
8	25 (36)	22 (43)	
9–10	28 (40)	15 (29)	

Table 1. Cont.

Characteristics	With Hyperthermia	Without Hyperthermia	p
Pretreatment PSA (ng/mL)			0.6095
<10	20 (29)	17 (33)	
10–20	19 (27)	16 (31)	
>20	31 (44)	18 (35)	
IMRT			
76 Gy, 38 fractions	72 (100)	51 (100)	
Total ADT duration			0.2296
<6 months	2 (3)	0 (0)	
6–11 months	46 (66)	29 (57)	
≥12 months	22 (31)	22 (43)	
Hyperthermia			
Number of sessions			
1	1 (1)	-	
2	1 (1)	-	
3	3 (4)	-	
4	2 (3)	-	
5	49 (70)	-	
6	12 (17)	-	
7	2 (3)	-	

PSA, prostate-specific antigen; IMRT, intensity-modulated radiotherapy; ADT, androgen deprivation therapy.

2.2. IMRT

Radiation treatment was provided to all patients with definitive intent using a 10-MV linear accelerator (ONCOR Impression Plus, Siemens Medical Systems, Concord, CA). The clinical target volume (CTV) included the entire prostate, gross extracapsular disease, and proximal seminal vesicles. The planning target volume (PTV) was delineated by contouring the CTV with a margin of 7 mm in all directions except posteriorly, where it was only 4 mm. Our dose prescription policy was based on D95 of the PTV, i.e., percentage of the prescribed dose covering 95% of the volume. The total planned dose for all patients was 76 Gy, with a fractional dose of 2.0 Gy once a day, five times/week. Patients were immobilized using Vac-Lok cushions in the supine position and were treated with step-and-shoot IMRT. A megavoltage cone beam CT system was used to match the patient's position. Dose-volume constraints for at-risk organs were as follows: rectum V50 Gy < 25%, V65 Gy < 17%; bladder V40 Gy < 50%, V65 Gy < 25%; femoral head D_{max} < 50 Gy, and small intestine D_{max} < 60 Gy.

2.3. Hyperthermia

Regional hyperthermia was provided using a 8 MHz radiofrequency capacitive device (Thermotron RF-8, Yamamoto Vinita Co., Osaka, Japan). The physical features of this instrument and its thermal distribution in a phantom model and the human body have been described previously [14,19]. Briefly, both the upper and lower electrodes were 30 cm in diameter and were placed on opposite sides of the pelvis with the patient in the prone position. The treatment goal was at least 30 min of continuous heating after the radiofrequency output was increased to the patient's tolerance threshold. Patients were carefully instructed to report any unpleasant sensations that were suggestive of a hot spot. Radiofrequency output was increased to the maximum level tolerated by the patient after appropriately adjusting treatment settings. The liquid in the regular boluses adhering to the metal electrode was 5% NaCl or 5% potassium sulfate, both having similar conductivity. To reduce any preferential heating of subcutaneous fat tissue, overlay boluses were applied in addition to regular boluses. Circulating liquid (0.5% NaCl or 0.5% potassium sulfate; both show similar conductivity) inside the overlay boluses was cooled by the RF-8 circulatory system during heating. Superficial cooling was performed using circulating liquid set at 5 °C in the overlay boluses. A gauze soaked in 10% NaCl was inserted in the intergluteal cleft to improve temperature distribution in the prostate. Exceptions occurred in 4 patients provided hyperthermia in 2012; they were included in a previous prospective clinical trial on optimization of deep heating area using this heating device and mobile insulator sheets [20].

Hyperthermia was provided once or twice a week, after radiotherapy. We directly measured intra-rectal temperature in all patients and during all hyperthermia sessions using a 4-point microthermocouple sensor that was inserted into the rectum at the level of the prostate. The thermal dose corresponding to the cumulative equivalent minutes at 43 °C for the T90 (CEM43T90) was obtained based on these intra-rectal temperatures during all hyperthermia sessions. The T90 is an index temperature that indicates either achieving or surpassing 90% of intra-rectal measurement points; similarly, T25 indicates either achievement of target temperature or that it has exceeded 25% of intra-rectal measurement points. The CEM43T90 has been extensively and successfully used in clinical trials to assess efficacy of heating [21–23] and provides data on the thermal isoeffect dose expressed in cumulative equivalent minutes at a reference temperature of 43 °C based on the lower end of temperature distribution (T90). The CEM43T90 is calculated from the time-temperature data as follows:

$$\text{CEM43T90} = \sum_{i=0}^{n} t_i R^{(43-T90i)}$$

When the temperature is higher than 43 °C, R = 0.5. When the temperature is lower than 43 °C, R = 0.25. In this protocol, t_i is the time interval of the *ith* sample (t_i = 1.0 min). Temperatures exceeding T90 of the intra-rectal measurement points during the *ith* minute was designated as T90i. We then used the CEM43T90 to convert each T90i into an equivalent time at 43 °C, and these were added over the entire treatment duration of "n" min.

2.4. Follow-Up

The length of follow-up was calculated from the IMRT start date. Patients were followed up at intervals of 1–3 months during the first year and at 3–6 months thereafter. At each follow-up visit, PSA was measured, and potential gastrointestinal (GI) and genitourinary (GU) morbidity were accessed. Biochemical relapse was defined as per the Phoenix definition [24]. The presence of bone metastasis was confirmed by bone scintigraphy, CT, or MRI, while soft tissue metastasis was confirmed by CT or MRI. Toxicity of the therapy was evaluated according to the Common Terminology Criteria for Adverse Events, version 4.0. The highest toxicity level for each patient during and after IMRT was used for toxicity analysis. Toxicity was classified as either acute (occurring during therapy or up to 3 months after therapy) or delayed (occurring more than 3 months after completion of therapy).

2.5. Statistical Analyses

The Chi-squared test or the Mann–Whitney U test was used to evaluate differences in clinical characteristics between patients with and without hyperthermia. Biochemical disease-free survival (bDFS) (Phoenix definition), clinical relapse-free survival (RFS), and overall survival (OS) rates were calculated from IMRT initiation using the Kaplan–Meier method. Any significant differences between the actuarial curves were assessed using the log-rank test. Hazard ratio and 95% confidence interval were calculated using the Wald test. Multivariate analyses using a Cox proportional hazards model were also performed to identify prognostic factors for the survivals. The Fisher's exact probability test was used to compare grade 2 or higher toxicity between patients with and without hyperthermia.

3. Results

3.1. Thermal Data

The number of heating sessions in each patient ranged from 1–7 (median, 5) and the median duration of heating per session was 50 min (range, 30–55 min). The thermal dose of CEM43T90 ranged from 0.1 to 32.1 min (median 7.5 min). Figure 2a shows CEM43T90 for each heating session with median values for the first, 2nd, 3rd, 4th, 5th, 6th, and 7th sessions being 0.9, 1.4, 1.3, 1.4, 1.9, 1.8, and 1.2 min, respectively. The CEM43T90 of the first session tended to be lower than of later sessions. Median T90 values for sessions 1–7 were 40.3, 40.5, 40.5, 40.3, 40.4, 40.4, and 40.2 °C, respectively, (Figure 2b) while those for T25 were 41.1, 41.2, 41.3, 41.3, 41.2, 41.2, and 40.9 °C, respectively (Figure 2c). Average heating time for each session is shown in Figure 2d.

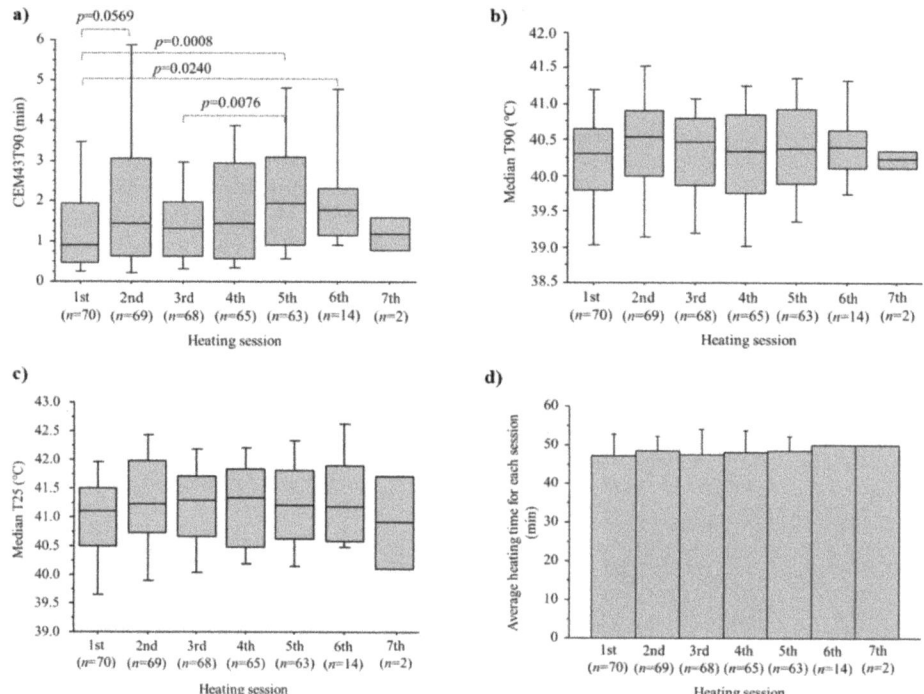

Figure 2. Thermal dose of CEM43T90 (**a**) median T90 (**b**) median T25 (**c**) and heating time (**d**) in each of the HT treatment sessions.

3.2. Efficacy and Prognostic Factors

Median follow-up time was 64 months (interquartile range, 49–83 months). Table 1 provides data on differences in patient characteristics between the two groups, and no significant differences were detected.

The 3-year and 5-year bDFS rates were 92.2% and 86.9%, respectively, for all 121 patients and biochemical relapse occurred in 6 patients in each group. Table 2 shows the results of univariate analyses of select factors affecting bDFS, and hyperthermia was not significant predictor of bDFS. Further, 5-year bDFS rate for patients with and without hyperthermia was similar at 89.8% and 82.9%, respectively (p = 0.2170, Figure 3a). However, the 5-year bDFS rate was 96.4% in the 39 patients with a CEM43T90 > 7 min, which was significantly better than 82.4% in the remaining 82 patients with a CEM43T90 $\leq$ 7 min or no hyperthermia treatment (Table 2). Table 3 lists the results of univariate analyses of factors affecting bDFS in 70 patients treated with IMRT plus regional hyperthermia, and a higher thermal dose of CEM43T90 > 7 min was a significant predictor of bDFS. Figure 3b shows that the 5-year bDFS rate of 96.4% in 39 patients with CEM43T90 > 7 min was significantly better than 81.5% in 31 patients with the CEM43T90 $\leq$ 7 min (p = 0.0316) and 82.9% in 51 patients not provided hyperthermia (p = 0.0370).

Table 2. Univariate analyses of certain factors for bDFS in 121 patients treated with IMRT with or without regional hyperthermia.

Variation	Patients (n)	5-y (%)	p (Log-Rank Test)	Hazard Ratio * (95% Confidence Interval)
T stage				
T1–T2	99	87.4	0.6978	0.777 (0.217–2.786)
T3a	22	84.0		
Gleason score				
≤8	78	86.8	0.8710	0.913 (0.306–2.726)
≥9	43	87.2		
Pretreatment PSA (ng/mL)				
≤20	72	88.4	0.4478	0.668 (0.234–1.905)
>20	49	84.8		
Total ADT (months)				
≤10	70	84.0	0.3344	0.569 (0.178–1.815)
>10	51	91.3		
Hyperthermia				
Yes	70	89.8	0.2170	0.519 (0.180–1.497)
None	51	82.9		
Hyperthermia				
CEM43T90 > 7	39	96.4	0.0296	0.144 (0.019–1.099)
None or CEM43T90 ≤ 7	82	82.4		

* Hazard ratio and 95% confidence interval were calculated using the Wald test.

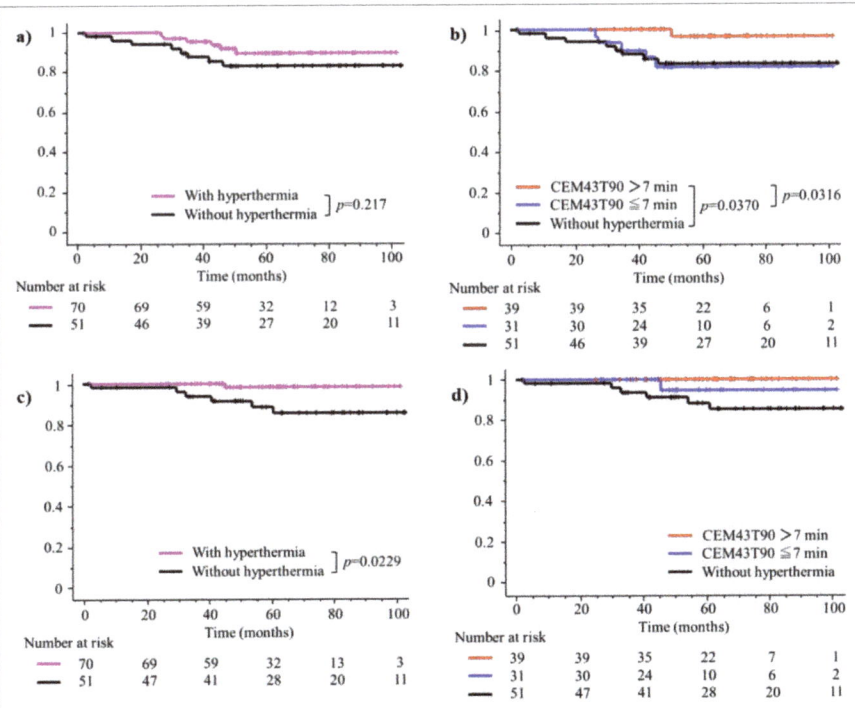

Figure 3. bDFS and clinical RFS rates. (**a**) bDFS with and without hyperthermia treatment. (**b**) bDFS among patients administered a thermal dose of CEM43T90 > 7 min, CEM43T90 ≤ 7 min, or no hyperthermia treatment. (**c**) Comparison of clinical RFS between the groups with and without hyperthermia treatment. (**d**) Comparison of clinical RFS among the patients with thermal dose CEM43T90 > 7 min, CEM43T90 ≤ 7 min, and no hyperthermia treatment.

Table 3. Univariate analyses of certain factors for bDFS in 70 patients treated with IMRT plus regional hyperthermia.

Variation	Patients (n)	5-y (%)	p (Log-Rank Test)	Hazard Ratio * (95% Confidence Interval)
T stage				
T1–T2	56	89.0	0.8403	0.802 (0.094–6.869)
T3a	14	92.9		
Gleason score				
≤8	42	91.2	0.5298	0.602 (0.121–2.984)
≥9	28	87.7		
Pretreatment PSA (ng/mL)				
≤20	39	89.7	0.784	0.800 (0.161–3.964)
>20	31	89.7		
Total ADT (months)				
≤10	42	86.3	0.2986	0.338 (0.039–2.894)
>10	28	96.3		
Hyperthermia CEM43T90 (min)				
≤7	31	81.5	0.0316	0.134 (0.016–1.152)
>7	39	96.4		

* Hazard ratio and 95% confidence interval were calculated using the Wald test.

Clinical relapse occurred in one patient treated with hyperthermia and in 4 patients without hyperthermia, and the sites of first clinical relapse were lymph node (n = 2), lymph node and lung (n = 2), and bone and lymph node (n = 1). The 3-year and 5-year clinical RFS rates were 97.4% and 93.9%, respectively, for all 121 patients. Table 4 shows the results of univariate and multivariate analyses of factors related to clinical RFS and additional hyperthermia was significant predictor of clinical RFS in both univariate and multivariate analyses. The 5-year clinical RFS rate was 98.0% for patients provided hyperthermia but 88.6% among patients without hyperthermia (p = 0.0229, Figure 3c). Further, 5-year clinical RFS rate was 100% in the 39 patients with CEM43T90 > 7 min and 95.0% in 31 patients with CEM43T90 ≤ 7 min (Figure 3d). The 5-year OS rate was 100% for patients who underwent hyperthermia and 95.9% among patients who did not undergo hyperthermia.

Table 4. Univariate and multivariate analyses of certain factors for clinical relapse-free survival in 121 patients treated with IMRT with or without regional hyperthermia.

Variation	Patients (n)	Univariate			Multivariate	
		5-y (%)	p *	Hazard Ratio ** (95% CI)	p	Hazard Ratio (95% CI)
T stage						
T1–T2	99	94.2	0.5391	0.601 (0.116–3.107)	0.564	0.600 (0.106–3.403)
T3a	22	93.3				
Gleason score						
≤8	78	95.7	0.5723	0.651 (0.145–2.920)	0.317	0.455 (0.097–2.125)
≥9	43	90.3				
Pretreatment PSA (ng/mL)						
≤20	72	92.8	0.5504	0.610 (0.118–3.144)	0.597	0.612 (0.100–3.766)
>20	49	95.5				
Total ADT (months)						
≤10	70	91.5	0.1592	0.246 (0.030–2.043)	0.121	0.170 (0.018–1.599)
>10	51	97.4				
Hyperthermia						
Yes	70	98.0	0.0229	0.126 (0.015–1.049)	0.035	0.099 (0.000–0.852)
None	51	88.6				

* Log-rank test. ** Hazard ratio and 95% confidence interval were calculated using the Wald test. CI, confidence interval; PSA, prostate-specific antigen; ADT, androgen deprivation therapy.

3.3. Toxicity

Acute toxicity (≥Grade 2) occurred in 70 patients treated with IMRT and hyperthermia and included grade 2 ($n = 11$, 15.7%) and grade 3 ($n = 2$; 2.8%) GU toxicity. In 51 patients treated with IMRT alone, acute toxicities were grade 3 GU toxicity in 3 (5.9%) patients and grade 2 GU toxicity in 6 (11.8%). The occurrence of acute toxicities ≥ grade 2 was not significantly different between patients with or without hyperthermia treatment. Skin burn, as a subcutaneous induration, was seen in two (2.9%) patients and it spontaneously disappeared after completion of combined therapy. Delayed toxicity ≥ grade 2 among 70 patients treated with IMRT with hyperthermia included grade 3 GI toxicity in one (1.4%) patient and grade 3 GU in one (1.4%) patient. Among 51 patients treated with IMRT alone, delayed toxicity ≥ grade 2 did not occur. Between patients with or without hyperthermia, the occurrence of delayed toxicity ≥ grade 2 was not significantly different.

4. Discussion

The results of the present study demonstrate the feasibility of combining IMRT (total 76 Gy in 38 fractions) and regional hyperthermia. This strategy appears to have promising efficacy in patients with high-risk localized prostate carcinoma as the addition of hyperthermia resulted in a significant improvement in clinical RFS. The strengths of this study are that total dose and fractionation of IMRT were identical in all patients, and that neoadjuvant hormone therapy was administered to all patients. Thus, this cohort of patients was suitable for evaluating the radio-sensitizing effect of hyperthermia and for reducing bias due to differences in treatment protocols for NCCN-defined high-risk localized prostate carcinoma. Additionally, temperature in the rectum of the dorsal prostate during heating was monitored in all patients, which permitted adequate analyses of the thermal dose provided.

IMRT is the standard radiation modality used in the treatment of high-risk localized prostate cancer. A recent study with IMRT at a dose of 76–80 Gy plus ADT, which was administrated in 78.5% of the patients with NCCN high-risk localized prostate carcinoma, reported 5-year bDFS and metastasis-free survival rates of 80.6% and 92.5%, respectively [25]. Simizu et al. (2017) have described clinical outcomes after IMRT (72.6–74.8 Gy in 2.2 Gy per fraction) plus ADT administrated to 61% of the patients with high-risk prostate carcinoma and report 5-year bDFS and clinical RFS rates of 77% and 87%, respectively [26]. Marvaso et al. (2018) conducted ultra-hypofractionated radiotherapy using image-guided IMRT (32.5 or 35 Gy in 5 fractions) plus ADT in 21 (75%) of the 28 patients with NCCN high-risk localized prostate carcinoma and report 3-year bDFS and clinical RFS rates of 66% and 87%, respectively [27]. We report higher and more promising 5-year bDFS and clinical RFS rates of 89.8% and 98.0%, respectively, after IMRT with 76Gy in 38 fractions plus regional hyperthermia and ADT (Figure 3a,c).

Previous reports of high-dose IMRT describe the occurrence of acute ≥ grade 2 toxicities to be 28% and that of delayed ≥ grade 2 GI and GU toxicities to be 4% and 15%, respectively, in 772 patients with prostate carcinoma [28]. We have previously reported that addition of regional hyperthermia to 3D-CRT (70 Gy in 35 fractions) did not increase the occurrence of acute or delayed toxicity in patients with prostate carcinoma [13]. Similarly, we now show that acute and delayed toxicities were comparable when regional hyperthermia was added to IMRT.

Maluta et al. (2007) have reported on the clinical outcomes of a prospective phase II study for locally advanced prostate carcinoma in a cohort of 144 patients treated with three-dimensional radiotherapy (74 Gy in 37 fractions) plus regional hyperthermia; additional ADT was administered to more than 60% of the patients [11]. In that study, 5-year OS was 87%, and 5-year bDFS was 49% and no severe toxicities were recorded. Hurwitz et al. (2011) also describe the results of a prospective phase II study for locally advanced prostate carcinoma in 37 patients treated with three-dimensional radiotherapy (66 Gy, daily dose of 1.8–2.0 Gy) plus two transrectal ultrasound hyperthermia treatments and ADT [12,29]; specifically, 5-year OS and bDFS were 93.5% and 60.6%, respectively. Although we only included patients with NCCN high-risk and not very high-risk, IMRT with 76 Gy in 38 fractions plus regional hyperthermia and ADT demonstrated a favorable clinical outcome, indicating that our treatment strategy is promising.

Several clinical randomized trials conducted in the 1990s have demonstrated that adding hyperthermia to radiotherapy improves local control and complete response rates in patients with superficial tumors, such as those involving recurrent breast carcinoma and malignant melanoma [30,31]. Importantly, detailed analyses of thermal data from those randomized trials of breast carcinoma as well as malignant melanoma treated with radiotherapy, with or without hyperthermia, showed significant improvements in local control rates in patients who achieved higher intra-tumor temperatures [32,33]. Previous clinical studies on deep-seated tumors, including cervical carcinoma of the uterus and rectal carcinoma that were treated with hyperthermia plus deep regional hyperthermia, also state that thermal parameters correlate with clinical outcomes [34–36]. For prostate carcinoma, we have previously demonstrated that the addition of regional hyperthermia with a higher thermal dose (CEM43T90 $\geq$ 1 min/heating session) for 3D-conformal radiotherapy improves bDFS [13]. Here, bDFS was significantly higher in patients treated with a higher combined thermal dose of CEM43T90 $\geq$ 7 min (Figure 3b).

Recent investigations on hyperthermia treatment planning have aimed to simulate temperature patterns as well as specific absorption rate (SAR) distributions, while helping operators visualize the effects of different steering strategies in modern locoregional radiofrequency hyperthermia treatments [37–39]. We have previously investigated the use of electromagnetic field numerical simulations for reducing subcutaneous fat overheating, which is a major drawback of deep heating using a capacitively coupled heating system [40]. Hence, optimization of temperature distribution in the deep regional hyperthermia in the pelvis is needed [40] and we used recommended optimal settings in the numerical simulation study, such as use of overlay boluses, electrical conductivity of the circulating coolant, prone position during hyperthermia, and intergluteal cleft gauze, which resulted in improved bDFS among patients who received a good thermal dose. Further improvements in heating methods and selection of patients suitable for hyperthermia represent future research directions.

The efficacy of brachytherapy combined with external beam radiotherapy and ADT as another method of improving the therapeutic effect of IMRT and ADT has been reported in prostate cancer. The ASCENDE-RT trial found that additional low-dose rate brachytherapy improved bDFS, but at the cost of higher, acute and late genitourinary toxicity [41]. Our proposed combination therapy with hyperthermia seems to be a promising method of improving the efficacy of external beam radiotherapy, given its noninvasiveness and the lack of a significant increase in side effects.

Despite these promising results, our study has a few limitations. As this was a retrospective study, the possibility of selection bias with respect to prognostic factors cannot be ruled out. However, as dose prescription for IMRT was constant and there were no differences in the major prognostic factors between patients with and without hyperthermia, the influence of selection bias can be presumed to be relatively small. The duration of ADT was a potential confounding factor. Although no significant difference was found in the duration of ADT between the patients with and without hyperthermia treatment, the duration of ADT was shorter in the hyperthermia group. Therefore, we speculate that the duration of ADT is unlikely to be a confounding factor in the results of this study. A formal prospective clinical trial is needed to determine the efficacy and prognostic factors associated with this approach of combined therapy in patients with high-risk localized prostate carcinoma.

5. Conclusions

To the best of our knowledge, this is the first report to assess efficacy, in terms of clinical outcomes, of a combination of IMRT and regional hyperthermia in patients with high-risk localized prostate carcinoma. We demonstrate that the use of definitive IMRT, combined with regional hyperthermia, is a promising treatment modality that is not associated with severe toxicity. Our results support further evaluation such as clinical trials evaluating IMRT with or without regional hyperthermia in patients with high-risk localized prostate carcinoma.

Author Contributions: Conceptualization, T.O. and S.N.; Data curation, T.O., S.N., S.K., H.I., T.M. and S.T.; Formal analysis, S.N. and T.O. Investigation, S.N., T.O., S.K., H.I., T.M. and S.T.; Methodology, T.O.; Project administration, T.O.; Validation, T.O.; Writing—original draft, S.N. and T.O.; Writing—review and editing, S.N., T.O., K.Y. and N.F. All authors have read and agreed to this tentative abstract. All authors have read and agreed to the published version of the manuscript.

Funding: This work was supported by JSPS KAKENHI Grant Number JP20K08146.

Institutional Review Board Statement: The study was conducted according to the guidelines of the Declaration of Helsinki, and approved by the Institutional Review Board of University of Occupational and Environmental Health (protocol code UOEHCRB19-073 and 13 February 2020).

Informed Consent Statement: Informed consent was obtained from all subjects involved in the study.

Data Availability Statement: The data presented in this study are available on request from the corresponding author.

Conflicts of Interest: Author T.O. received scholarship donation from Yamamoto Vinita Co., Ltd., Osaka, Japan.

References

1. Dal Pra, A.; Souhami, L. Prostate cancer radiation therapy: A physicians' perspective. *Phys. Med.* **2016**, *32*, 438–445. [CrossRef]
2. Grimm, P.; Billiet, I.; Bostwick, D.; Dicker, A.; Frank, S.; Immerzeel, J.; Keyes, M.; Kupelian, P.; Lee, W.R.; Machtens, S.; et al. Comparative analysis of prostate-specific antigen free survival outcomes for patients with low, intermediate and high risk prostate cancer treatment by radical therapy. Results from the Prostate Cancer Results Study Group. *BJU Int.* **2012**, *109* (Suppl. S1), 22–29. [CrossRef] [PubMed]
3. Datta, N.R.; Ordonez, S.G.; Gaipl, U.S.; Paulides, M.M.; Crezee, H.; Gellermann, J.; Marder, D.; Puric, E.; Bodis, S. Local hyperthermia combined with radiotherapy and-/or chemotherapy: Recent advances and promises for the future. *Cancer Treat. Rev.* **2015**, *41*, 742–753. [CrossRef] [PubMed]
4. Cihoric, N.; Tsikkinis, A.; van Rhoon, G.; Crezee, H.; Aebersold, D.M.; Bodis, S.; Beck, M.; Nadobny, J.; Budach, V.; Wust, P.; et al. Hyperthermia-related clinical trials on cancer treatment within the ClinicalTrials.gov registry. *Int. J. Hyperth.* **2015**, *31*, 609–614. [CrossRef] [PubMed]
5. Van der Zee, J. Heating the patient: A promising approach? *Ann. Oncol. Off. J. Eur. Soc. Med. Oncol.* **2002**, *13*, 1173–1184. [CrossRef] [PubMed]
6. Jones, E.L.; Samulski, T.V.; Vujaskovic, Z.; Leonard, R.P.; Dewhirst, M.W. Hyperthermia. *Principles and Practice of Radiation Oncology*, 4th ed.; Lippincott Williams & Wilkins: Philadelphia, PA, USA, 2003.
7. Anscher, M.S.; Samulski, T.V.; Leopold, K.A.; Oleson, J.R. Phase I/II study of external radio frequency phased array hyperthermia and external beam radiotherapy in the treatment of prostate cancer: Technique and results of intraprostatic temperature measurements. *Int. J. Radiat. Oncol. Biol. Phys.* **1992**, *24*, 489–495. [CrossRef]
8. Anscher, M.S.; Samulski, T.V.; Dodge, R.; Prosnitz, L.R.; Dewhirst, M.W. Combined external beam irradiation and external regional hyperthermia for locally advanced adenocarcinoma of the prostate. *Int. J. Radiat. Oncol. Biol. Phys.* **1997**, *37*, 1059–1065. [CrossRef]
9. Van Vulpen, M.; De Leeuw, A.A.; Raaymakers, B.W.; Van Moorselaar, R.J.; Hofman, P.; Lagendijk, J.J.; Battermann, J.J. Radiotherapy and hyperthermia in the treatment of patients with locally advanced prostate cancer: Preliminary results. *BJU Int.* **2004**, *93*, 36–41. [CrossRef]
10. Tilly, W.; Gellermann, J.; Graf, R.; Hildebrandt, B.; Weissbach, L.; Budach, V.; Felix, R.; Wust, P. Regional hyperthermia in conjunction with definitive radiotherapy against recurrent or locally advanced prostate cancer T3 pN0 M0. *Strahlenther Onkol.* **2005**, *181*, 35–41. [CrossRef]
11. Maluta, S.; Dall'Oglio, S.; Romano, M.; Marciai, N.; Pioli, F.; Giri, M.G.; Benecchi, P.L.; Comunale, L.; Porcaro, A.B. Conformal radiotherapy plus local hyperthermia in patients affected by locally advanced high risk prostate cancer: Preliminary results of a prospective phase II study. *Int. J. Hyperth.* **2007**, *23*, 451–456. [CrossRef]
12. Hurwitz, M.D.; Hansen, J.L.; Prokopios-Davos, S.; Manola, J.; Wang, Q.; Bornstein, B.A.; Hynynen, K.; Kaplan, I.D. Hyperthermia combined with radiation for the treatment of locally advanced prostate cancer: Long-term results from Dana-Farber Cancer Institute study 94-153. *Cancer* **2011**, *117*, 510–516. [CrossRef]
13. Yahara, K.; Ohguri, T.; Yamaguchi, S.; Imada, H.; Narisada, H.; Ota, S.; Tomura, K.; Sakagami, M.; Fujimoto, N.; Korogi, Y. Definitive radiotherapy plus regional hyperthermia for high-risk and very high-risk prostate carcinoma: Thermal parameters correlated with biochemical relapse-free survival. *Int. J. Hyperth.* **2015**, *3*, 600–608.

14. Abe, M.; Hiraoka, M.; Takahashi, M.; Egawa, S.; Matsuda, C.; Onoyama, Y.; Morita, K.; Kakehi, M.; Sugahara, T. Multi-institutional studies on hyperthermia using an 8-MHz radiofrequency capacitive heating device (Thermotron RF-8) in combination with radiation for cancer therapy. *Cancer* **1986**, *58*, 1589–1595. [CrossRef]
15. Hiraoka, M.; Jo, S.; Akuta, K.; Nishimura, Y.; Takahashi, M.; Abe, M. Radiofrequency capacitive hyperthermia for deep-seated tumors. I. Studies on thermometry. *Cancer* **1987**, *60*, 121–127. [CrossRef]
16. Kakehi, M.; Ueda, K.; Mukojima, T.; Hiraoka, M.; Seto, O.; Akanuma, A.; Nakatsugawa, S. Multi-institutional clinical studies on hyperthermia combined with radiotherapy or chemotherapy in advanced cancer of deep-seated organs. *Int. J. Hyperth.* **1990**, *6*, 719–740. [CrossRef] [PubMed]
17. Hiraoka, M.; Nishimura, Y.; Nagata, Y.; Mitsumori, M.; Okuno, Y.; Li, P.Y.; Abe, M.; Takahashi, M.; Masunaga, S.; Akuta, K.; et al. Site-specific phase I, II trials of hyperthermia at Kyoto University. *Int. J. Hyperth.* **1994**, *10*, 403–410. [CrossRef] [PubMed]
18. Masunaga, S.I.; Hiraoka, M.; Akuta, K.; Nishimura, Y.; Nagata, Y.; Jo, S.; Takahashi, M.; Abe, M.; Terachi, T.; Oishi, K.; et al. Phase I/II trial of preoperative thermoradiotherapy in the treatment of urinary bladder cancer. *Int. J. Hyperth.* **1994**, *10*, 31–40. [CrossRef]
19. Song, C.W.; Rhee, J.G.; Lee, C.K.; Levitt, S.H. Capacitive heating of phantom and human tumors with an 8 MHz radiofrequency applicator (Thermotron RF-8). *Int. J. Radiat. Oncol. Biol. Phys.* **1986**, *12*, 365–372. [CrossRef]
20. Tomura, K.; Ohguri, T.; Mulder, H.T.; Murakami, M.; Nakahara, S.; Yahara, K.; Korogi, Y. The usefulness of mobile insulator sheets for the optimisation of deep heating area for regional hyperthermia using a capacitively coupled heating method: Phantom, simulation and clinical prospective studies. *Int. J. Hyperth.* **2018**, *34*, 1092–1103. [CrossRef] [PubMed]
21. Oleson, J.R.; Samulski, T.V.; Leopold, K.A.; Clegg, S.T.; Dewhirst, M.W.; Dodge, R.K.; George, S.L. Sensitivity of hyperthermia trial outcomes to temperature and time: Implications for thermal goals of treatment. *Int. J. Radiat. Oncol. Biol. Phys.* **1993**, *25*, 289–297. [CrossRef]
22. Jones, E.L.; Oleson, J.R.; Prosnitz, L.R.; Samulski, T.V.; Vujaskovic, Z.; Yu, D.; Sanders, L.L.; Dewhirst, M.W. Randomized trial of hyperthermia and radiation for superficial tumors. *J. Clin. Oncol.* **2005**, *23*, 3079–3085. [CrossRef]
23. Dewhirst, M.W.; Viglianti, B.L.; Lora-Michiels, M.; Hanson, M.; Hoopes, P.J. Basic principles of thermal dosimetry and thermal thresholds for tissue damage from hyperthermia. *Int. J. Hyperth.* **2003**, *19*, 267–294. [CrossRef]
24. Roach, M., 3rd; Hanks, G.; Thames, H., Jr.; Schellhammer, P.; Shipley, W.U.; Sokol, G.H.; Sandler, H. Defining biochemical failure following radiotherapy with or without hormonal therapy in men with clinically localized prostate cancer: Recommendations of the RTOG-ASTRO Phoenix Consensus Conference. *Int. J. Radiat. Oncol. Biol. Phys.* **2006**, *65*, 965–974. [CrossRef] [PubMed]
25. Lopez-Torrecilla, J.; Pastor-Peidro, J.; Vicedo-Gonzalez, A.; Gonzalez-Sanchis, D.; Hernandez-Machancoses, A.; Almendros-Blanco, P.; García-Miragall, E.; Gordo-Partearroyo, J.C.; García-Hernández, T.; Brualla-González, L.; et al. Patterns of treatment failure in patients with prostate cancer treated with 76-80 Gy radiotherapy to the prostate and seminal vesicles +/− hormonotherapy. *Clin. Transl. Oncol.* **2021**, *23*, 481–490. [CrossRef] [PubMed]
26. Shimizu, D.; Yamazaki, H.; Nishimura, T.; Aibe, N.; Okabe, H. Long-term Tumor Control and Late Toxicity in Patients with Prostate Cancer Receiving Hypofractionated (2.2 Gy) Soft-tissue-matched Image-guided Intensity-modulated Radiotherapy. *Anticancer. Res.* **2017**, *37*, 5829–5835. [PubMed]
27. Marvaso, G.; Riva, G.; Ciardo, D.; Gandini, S.; Fodor, C.I.; Zerini, D.; Colangione, S.P.; Timon, G.; Comi, S.; Cambria, R.; et al. "Give me five" ultra-hypofractionated radiotherapy for localized prostate cancer: Non-invasive ablative approach. *Med. Oncol.* **2018**, *35*, 96. [CrossRef]
28. Zelefsky, M.J.; Fuks, Z.; Hunt, M.; Yamada, Y.; Marion, C.; Ling, C.; Amols, H.; Venkatraman, E.; A Leibel, S. High-dose intensity modulated radiation therapy for prostate cancer: Early toxicity and biochemical outcome in 772 patients. *Int. J. Radiat. Oncol. Biol. Phys.* **2002**, *53*, 1111–1116. [CrossRef]
29. Hurwitz, M.D.; Kaplan, I.D.; Hansen, J.L.; Prokopios-Davos, S.; Topulos, G.P.; Wishnow, K.; Manola, J.; Bornstein, B.A.; Hynynen, K. Hyperthermia combined with radiation in treatment of locally advanced prostate cancer is associated with a favourable toxicity profile. *Int. J. Hyperth.* **2005**, *21*, 649–656. [CrossRef]
30. Vernon, C.C.; Hand, J.W.; Field, S.B.; Machin, D.; Whaley, J.B.; van der Zee, J.; van Putten, W.L.; van Rhoon, G.C.; van Dijk, J.D.; Gonzales Gonzales, D.; et al. Radiotherapy with or without hyperthermia in the treatment of superficial localized breast cancer: Results from five randomized controlled trials. International Collaborative Hyperthermia Group. *Int. J. Radiat. Oncol. Biol. Phys.* **1996**, *35*, 731–744.
31. Overgaard, J.; Gonzalez Gonzalez, D.; Hulshof, M.C.; Arcangeli, G.; Dahl, O.; Mella, O.; Bentzen, S.M. Randomised trial of hyperthermia as adjuvant to radiotherapy for recurrent or metastatic malignant melanoma. *Eur. Soc. Hyperthermic Oncol. Lancet* **1995**, *345*, 540–543. [CrossRef]
32. Sherar, M.; Liu, F.F.; Pintilie, M.; Levin, W.; Hunt, J.; Hill, R.; Hand, J.; Vernon, C.; van Rhoon, G.; van der Zee, J.; et al. Relationship between thermal dose and outcome in thermoradiotherapy treatments for superficial recurrences of breast cancer: Data from a phase III trial. *Int. J. Radiat. Oncol. Biol. Phys.* **1997**, *39*, 371–380. [CrossRef]
33. Overgaard, J.; Gonzalez Gonzalez, D.; Hulshof, M.C.; Arcangeli, G.; Dahl, O.; Mella, O.; Bentzen, S.M. Hyperthermia as an adjuvant to radiation therapy of recurrent or metastatic malignant melanoma. *Eur. Soc. Hyperthermic Oncol. Int. J. Hyperth.* **1996**, *12*, 3–20. [CrossRef]

34. Franckena, M.; Fatehi, D.; De Bruijne, M.; Canters, R.A.M.; Van Norden, Y.; Mens, J.W.; Van Rhoon, G.C.; Van Der Zee, J. Hyperthermia dose-effect relationship in 420 patients with cervical cancer treated with combined radiotherapy and hyperthermia. *Eur. J. Cancer* **2009**, *45*, 1969–1978. [CrossRef] [PubMed]
35. Rau, B.; Wust, P.; Tilly, W.; Gellermann, J.; Harder, C.; Riess, H.; Budach, V.; Felix, R.; Schlag, P.M. Preoperative radiochemotherapy in locally advanced or recurrent rectal cancer: Regional radiofrequency hyperthermia correlates with clinical parameters. *Int. J. Radiat. Oncol. Biol. Phys.* **2000**, *48*, 381–391. [CrossRef]
36. Van Rhoon, G.C. Is CEM43 still a relevant thermal dose parameter for hyperthermia treatment monitoring? *Int. J. Hyperth.* **2016**, *32*, 50–62. [CrossRef] [PubMed]
37. Kok, H.; Wust, P.; Stauffer, P.; Bardati, F.; van Rhoon, G.; Crezee, J. Current state of the art of regional hyperthermia treatment planning: A review. *Radiat. Oncol.* **2015**, *10*, 196. [CrossRef]
38. Canters, R.A.M.; Paulides, M.; Franckena, M.F.; Van Der Zee, J.; Van Rhoon, G.C. Implementation of treatment planning in the routine clinical procedure of regional hyperthermia treatment of cervical cancer: An overview and the Rotterdam experience. *Int. J. Hyperth.* **2012**, *28*, 570–581. [CrossRef]
39. VilasBoas-Ribeiro, I.; Van Rhoon, G.C.; Drizdal, T.; Franckena, M.; Paulides, M.M. Impact of Number of Segmented Tissues on SAR Prediction Accuracy in Deep Pelvic Hyperthermia Treatment Planning. *Cancers (Basel)* **2020**, *12*, 2646. [CrossRef] [PubMed]
40. Ohguri, T.; Kuroda, K.; Yahara, K.; Nakahara, S.; Kakinouchi, S.; Itamura, H.; Morisaki, T.; Korogi, Y. Optimization of the clinical setting using numerical simulations of the electromagnetic field in an obese patient model for deep regional hyperthermia of an 8 MHz radiofrequency capacitively coupled device in the pelvis. *Cancers (Basel)* **2021**, *13*, 979. [CrossRef] [PubMed]
41. Rodda, S.; Tyldesley, S.; Morris, W.J.; Keyes, M.; Halperin, R.; Pai, H.; McKenzie, M.; Duncan, G.; Morton, G.; Hamm, J.; et al. ASCENDE-RT: An analysis of treatment-related morbidity for a randomized trial comparing a low-dose-rate brachytherapy boost with a dose-escalated external beam boost for high- and intermediate-risk prostate cancer. *Int. J. Radiat. Oncol. Biol. Phys.* **2017**, *98*, 286–295. [CrossRef]

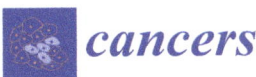

Article

Effects of Modulated Electro-Hyperthermia (mEHT) on Two and Three Year Survival of Locally Advanced Cervical Cancer Patients

Carrie Anne Minnaar [1,2], Innocent Maposa [3], Jeffrey Allan Kotzen [1,2] and Ans Baeyens [1,4,*]

1 Department of Radiation Sciences, University of the Witwatersrand, Johannesburg 2193, South Africa; carrie-anne.minnaar@wits.ac.za (C.A.M.); jeffrey.kotzen@wits.ac.za (J.A.K.)
2 Department of Radiation Oncology, Wits Donald Gordon Academic Hospital, Johannesburg 2193, South Africa
3 Department of Epidemiology & Biostatistics, University of the Witwatersrand, Johannesburg 2193, South Africa; innocent.maposa@wits.ac.za
4 Radiobiology, Department of Human Structure and Repair, Ghent University, 9000 Ghent, Belgium
* Correspondence: ans.baeyens@ugent.be

Citation: Minnaar, C.A.; Maposa, I.; Kotzen, J.A.; Baeyens, A. Effects of Modulated Electro-Hyperthermia (mEHT) on Two and Three Year Survival of Locally Advanced Cervical Cancer Patients. *Cancers* **2022**, *14*, 656. https://doi.org/10.3390/cancers14030656

Academic Editors: Stephan Bodis, Pirus Ghadjar and Gerard C. Van Rhoon

Received: 29 November 2021
Accepted: 26 January 2022
Published: 27 January 2022

Publisher's Note: MDPI stays neutral with regard to jurisdictional claims in published maps and institutional affiliations.

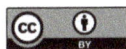

Copyright: © 2022 by the authors. Licensee MDPI, Basel, Switzerland. This article is an open access article distributed under the terms and conditions of the Creative Commons Attribution (CC BY) license (https://creativecommons.org/licenses/by/4.0/).

Simple Summary: More than 80% of global cervical cancer cases and deaths occur in Low-to-Middle-Income Countries. Improving the efficacy of treatments without increasing the costs in these regions is therefore imperative. The aim of our Phase III Randomised Controlled Trial was to investigate the effects of the addition of a mild heating technology, modulated electro-hyperthermia, to chemoradiotherapy protocols for the management of locally advanced cervical cancer patients in a resource-constrained setting. We previously reported on the positive outcomes on local disease control, quality of life, and early toxicity. Our recent results showed a significant improvement in two and three year disease free survival, without any significant changes to the toxicity profile, and with an improvement in quality of life, alongside a cost saving over three years. The effect was most significant in patients with Stage III disease, and a significant systemic effect was observed in patients with distant nodal metastases.

Abstract: (1) Background: Modulated electro-hyperthermia (mEHT) is a mild to moderate, capacitive-coupled heating technology that uses amplitude modulation to enhance the cell-killing effects of the treatment. We present three year survival results and a cost effectiveness analysis from an ongoing randomised controlled Phase III trial involving 210 participants evaluating chemoradiotherapy (CRT) with/without mEHT, for the management of locally advanced cervical cancer (LACC) in a resource constrained setting (Ethics Approval: M120477/M704133; ClinicalTrials.gov ID: NCT033320690). (2) Methods: We report hazard ratios (HR); odds ratio (OR), and 95% confidence intervals (CI) for overall survival and disease free survival (DFS) at two and three years in the ongoing study. Late toxicity, quality of life (QoL), and a cost effectiveness analysis (CEA) using a Markov model are also reported. (3) Results: Disease recurrence at two and three years was significantly reduced by mEHT (HR: 0.67, 95%CI: 0.48–0.93, $p = 0.017$; and HR: 0.70, 95%CI: 0.51–0.98, $p = 0.035$; respectively). There were no significant differences in late toxicity between the groups, and QoL was significantly improved in the mEHT group. In the CEA, mEHT + CRT dominated the model over CRT alone. (4) Conclusions: CRT combined with mEHT improves QoL and DFS rates, and lowers treatment costs, without increasing toxicity in LACC patients, even in resource-constrained settings.

Keywords: modulated electro-hyperthermia; abscopal effect; locally advanced cervical cancer; resource-constrained setting; radiosensitiser

1. Introduction

Around 602,127 new cases of cervical cancer and an estimated 341,831 deaths from cervical cancer were reported globally in 2020. More than 80% of these cases and deaths occurred in Low-to-Middle-Income-Countries (LMICs) [1], creating significant socio-economic stress in these resource-constrained settings [2]. The problem is compounded by poor screening programs [2], limited access to adequate treatments [3], and the high incidence of Human Immunodeficiency Virus (HIV) infections in these regions [4]. While developed countries are estimated to achieve the elimination goal of four cases per 100,000 women-years by 2060, LMICs are expected to only reach this goal towards the end of the century [2]. Improving treatment outcomes, without significantly increasing the costs, is therefore crucial to the management of the disease in these regions. Hyperthermia (HT) is a known radiosensitiser [5], and has proven to be a beneficial adjunct to radiotherapy (RT) and chemoradiotherapy (CRT) for the management for locally advanced cervical cancer (LACC) in developed settings [6]. Classical HT techniques include capacitive and radiative heating technologies, both of which have demonstrated efficacy at improving outcomes in cervical cancer [7–9]. Classical HT uses temperature-dependent dosing calculations such as CEM43 and TRISE [10,11] to optimise the treatment outcomes, although the optimal temperature and timing is still a topic of discussion [12,13].

There is emerging evidence that radiofrequency (RF) electromagnetic fields associated with some HT techniques have additional effects during the treatments [14]. Modulated electro-hyperthermia (mEHT) is a mild- to moderate-heating technology that applies 13.56 MHz RF waves generated by a capacitive coupling set-up between two electrodes. The amplitude of the waves is modulated with a signal equivalent to $1/f$ noise, where the power density ($S(f)$), (or power per frequency interval), of the $1/f$ amplitude-modulated signal is inversely proportional to the modulation signal: $S(f) \sim 1/f$. The amplitude modulation (AM), and the precise impedance matching (which allows for the cellular selection and the relatively low applied power), are the main differences between mEHT and classical capacitive HT technologies [15]. Pre-clinical studies have shown that the modulation induces a non-thermal field effect which enhances the cell–killing of the thermal effect by a factor of 3.2 [16]. This appears to make mEHT more effective when adjusted to the same temperature as other heating techniques in pre-clinical studies [17]. It has even been proposed that the AM could be the most important characteristic of mEHT [18]. Pre-clinical studies have shown several immune-related effects of mEHT, which, if applied clinically, could promote the recognition and the targeting of tumours by the immune system [19–22].

This technique proposes a dosing paradigm based on energy deposition and absorption, with thermal effects being an outcome of the treatment, and not the goal of the treatment. The biophysics of the technology are described in detail elsewhere in the literature [23,24]. The lower power output, lower temperatures achieved [25], and non-thermal dosing parameters negate the need for thermal monitoring as safety and dosing parameters during mEHT. This has led to opposing opinions regarding the grouping of mEHT with classical HT techniques.

While there are numerous Phase I/II trials on mEHT, and some small double arm studies [26], there have not been any completed Phase III Randomised Controlled Trials (RCT) on mEHT. We previously reported preliminary results from an ongoing Phase III RCT which is investigating the effects of CRT with or without mEHT for the management of LACC in a resource-constrained setting in South Africa. The primary outcome was two year overall survival (OS), and the secondary outcome was local disease control (LDC) at six months post-treatment. The LDC results, as summarised in Table 1 [27], and a detailed safety and toxicity analysis [28], have been reported previously. The Odds Ratios (OR) for achieving LDC and Local Disease Free Survival (LDFS) at six months post-treatment were 0.39 (95%CI: 0.20–0.77; $p = 0.006$) and 0.36 (95%CI: 0.19–0.69; $p = 0.002$), respectively, in favour of the administration of mEHT [27].

Table 1. Summary of the local disease control results at six months post-treatment [27].

210 Randomised Participants	Total		mEHT		Control		Chi Squared
	n	%	n	%	n	%	
Eligible for analysis	202	96.2%	101	50.0%	101	50.0%	
Alive at six months post-treatment	171	84.7%	88	87.1%	83	82.2%	$p = 0.329$
LDC achieved	60	29.7%	40	45.5%	20	24.1%	$p = 0.003$
LDFS achieved in those who survived six months post-treatment	59	29.2%	39	38.6%	20	19.8%	$p = 0.003$

Abbreviations: LDC: Local Disease Control; LDFS: Local Disease Free Survival; mEHT: Modulated electro-hyperthermia.

The addition of mEHT did not affect the early toxicity profile of the prescribed CRT. In the mEHT Group, 97% of the participants were able to receive ≥ 8 out of the 10 prescribed mEHT treatments, with 9.5% of participants in the mEHT group reporting grade 1–2 adipose burns, 2% reporting grade 1 surface burns, and 8.6% reporting pain during the mEHT treatments [28]. The average BMI of the participants was 27.8 [15–49]. A multivariate analysis showed that energy dose in kilojoules, HIV status, and Body Mass Index (BMI) were not significant predictors of adverse events. Body Mass Index was also not significantly predictive of LDC. This suggests that mEHT is able to penetrate thicker layers of adipose tissue than conventional capacitive heating technologies, without significant damage to the adipose tissue [28]. The addition of mEHT was also associated with a significantly greater improvement in cognitive function at six weeks post-treatment, a significant reduction in pain and fatigue, and a significant improvement in social and emotional functioning at three months post-treatment [28]. An unexpected observation was the potentiation of the abscopal effect. An analysis of the sub-group of participants with extra-pelvic nodal disease visualised on the pre-treatment ^{18}F-FDG PET/CT scans showed that 24.1% (13 out of 54) of those who were treated with mEHT had complete metabolic resolution of all disease on the follow-up ^{18}F-FDG PET/CT scans, compared to 5.6% (3 out of 54) of the participants who did not receive mEHT (Chi squared: $p = 0.013$). A multivariate analysis showed that the outcomes were not associated with the administration of cisplatin or with the participants' HIV-status. These results suggested the potentiation of an abscopal effect by mEHT, as the locally applied RT resulted in the resolution of distant disease, when combined with mEHT. These findings are elaborated in the paper by Minnaar et al. [29].

The preliminary results showed a significant short-term benefit with the addition of mEHT to CRT, without a significant increase in toxicity, in our resource-constrained setting. We present the two and three year OS results, and preliminary results from a cost effectiveness analysis (CEA) on the use of mEHT in public and private healthcare settings. Local disease control may be associated with a short-term improvement in quality of life and with OS; however, long-term DFS results hold more relevance as DFS may be associated with sustained improvements in quality of life and affect the socio-economic impact of the disease. The follow-up results presented in this paper are the first long-term results reported from a Phase III RCT on mEHT and they are an important contribution to the understanding of the long-term clinical impact of mEHT in the management of LACC. The CEA provides valuable insight into the feasibility of incorporating mEHT into clinical practice that can be applied to both developed and resource-constrained settings.

2. Materials and Methods

The trial (ClincialTrials.gov ID: NCT03332069), was approved by the Human Research and Ethics Committee (HREC) on 4 May 2012 (ID: M120477) and registered on the National Clinical Trial Database (ID: 3012) before recruitment began. Due to the significant improvement seen in the mEHT Group early on in the study, the follow-up period was extended from two to five years post treatment on 5 May 2017 (M704133). All patients (or their legal representatives) provided written informed consent before enrolment.

Participants: Inclusion criteria included females with treatment-naïve, histologically confirmed FIGO stage IIB (with invasion of the distal half of the parametrium) to IIIB squamous cell carcinoma of the uterine cervix (staged clinically using a chest X-ray, abdomino-pelvic ultrasound, and clinical examination); eligible for RT with radical intent; and a creatinine clearance > 60 mL/min (calculated according to the Cockcroft-Gault equation). Additional inclusion criteria included an Eastern Cooperative Oncology Group (ECOG) performance status < 2; estimated life expectancy of at least 12 months; adequate haematological function (absolute neutrophil count > 3000/mm^3, haemoglobin $\geq$ 10 g/dL; platelet count > 150/mm^3); and a negative pregnancy test and use of effective contraception in women of childbearing potential. Pre-treatment 18^F-FDG PET/CT scans were performed as part of the screening process. Patients with Vesicovaginal and vesicorectal fistulas; extra-pelvic visceral metastases, and bilateral hydronephrosis visualised on screening 18^F-FDG PET/CT scans, were excluded from the study, as were HIV-positive patients with a CD4 count < 200 cells/μL and/or not on antiretroviral therapy (ART) for at least six months and/or signs of ART resistance; contradictions or a known hypersensitivity to any of the prescribed treatments; life-threatening Acquired Immunodeficiency Syndrome (AIDS) defining illnesses (other than cervical carcinoma); prior invasive malignancy, other than LACC, diagnosed within the past 24 months; and pregnant or breast feeding women. For the analyses in this report, all participants who met the eligibility criteria, were randomised, were treated, and for whom data were available at two years and three years post-treatment, were included. Participants who were lost to follow-up are reported as "LTFU" and their last known disease status is included.

Treatment: As per institutional protocols, all participants received 50 Gy of external beam radiotherapy (EBRT) in 25 fractions, administered to the whole pelvis, using 2D planning with virtual simulation. High Dose Rate (HDR) brachytherapy (BT) (source used: Iridium-192), was administered in three fractions of 8 Gy for a total equivalent dose in 2 Gy fractions (for an alpha-beta ratio of 10) of 86 Gy. Further details of the RT method can be found in the paper by Minnaar et al. [27]. 2D planning for EBRT and HDR BT is standard in our facility and in resource-constrained settings due to the lack of access to sophisticated imaging techniques and due to limited resources and staff capacity available to manage the high volume of gynaecological oncology patients seen each year. All participants were prescribed two doses of 80 mg/m^2 cisplatin, administered 21 days apart (according to the institutional protocol), during EBRT (not administered on BT days or mEHT days). Participants in the study group received two mEHT treatments per week (Model: EHY2000+; Manufacturer: Oncotherm GmbH, Troisdorf, Germany), with a minimum of 48 h in between mEHT treatments, at a target power of 130 W for a minimum of 55 min. The EBRT was started within thirty minutes of completing mEHT treatments. Total Kilojoules administered per treatment were recorded.

Randomisation and Masking: After enrolment, participants were randomly assigned (stratum: HIV status; accounting for age and stage), to receive CRT alone, or in combination with mEHT, using the REDCap stratified secure online random-sampling tool. Although the trial was open-label, and participants were aware of which group they were in due to the challenges associated with setting up a sham hyperthermia treatment, physicians reporting on the pre- and six month post-treatment 18^F-FDG PET/CT scans were blinded to the group that the participants were in, as were the clinicians conducting the follow-up evaluations.

Data Collection and Management: The research co-ordinator was responsible for collecting the data and data were captured using the online REDCap electronic data capture tool hosted by the University of the Witwatersrand. The treatments were administered and the clinical evaluations were conducted by the clinical team, without the involvement of the research co-ordinator.

Outcomes: The primary outcome was Two Year OS. Two year DFS, defined as the time from the start of treatment until the time of first documented disease recurrence, is also reported. The first evaluation of LDC was done at six months post-treatment. If local disease was still visible on the six month 18^F-FDG PET/CT, then DFS was considered a failure from day one and the number of days spent disease free was considered to be zero. Three year OS and DFS are also reported. The DFS was censored for cancer specific deaths. Participants who demised with a disease free status, and who did not demise from a treatment related death, before the two or three year cut off, were allocated a positive disease free status at the exit date and the exit date was recorded as the date of death. Late toxicity was graded according the Common Toxicity Criteria for Adverse Events (CTCAE) version 4, and Quality of life (QoL) was measured using the validated European Organization for Research and Treatment of Cancer (EORTC) quality of life questionnaires (QLQ): C30 and Cx24 (cervical cancer specific). The QLQs were available in several local languages [30] and were administered at one and two years post-treatment. The results were compared to the baseline QLQ results and the scoring and reporting were done in accordance with the EORTC guidelines [31,32]. According to the EORTC guidelines, the scores were converted linearly to scores from 0–100, where a high score represents higher functioning or a higher symptom experience, and a lower score represents a lower symptom experience or a lower functioning [33]. Early toxicity and QoL at six months post treatment have been previously reported [27,28]. A CEA was performed, and the outcome was Cost per Quality Adjusted Life Year (QALY). After initial treatment costs, only disease progression and hospitalization costs are further incurred in the model. The private healthcare model included costs associated with Intensity-Modulated Radiation Therapy (IMRT), weekly cisplatin and a broader range of chemotherapy drugs for recurrent or residual disease, whereas the public healthcare model included only 3D-planning for radiotherapy, two doses of cisplatin during RT, and limited treatment options for recurrent or residual disease.

Statistical Analysis: The sample size was calculated based on the estimated required sample sizes for a two-sample comparison of survivors' functions at two years (statistical power of 90%). We estimated an expected reduction in mortality at two years of 50%, based on OS of 20% in the Control Group and 40% in the experimental group. The statistical significance is defined as a two-sided alpha < 0.05 for a log-rank test, with a constant Hazard Ratio (HR) of 0.5693. Cox proportional hazards models including each factor (treatment group, HIV status, age, stage of the disease) were performed to compare the time from the start of treatment to the first occurrence of any event (death or disease recurrence). We report the HR; Odds Ratio (OR), and 95% confidence interval. Log-rank statistics were used to compare both treatment arms with Kaplan–Meier survival curves plotted at two and three years (for OS; DFS), for stage IIB and stage III participants separately and combined. Overall type I error was considered at 5%, and the survival analysis was done by intention to treat. The initial survival analysis was planned for two years post-treatment. However, the positive results seen at two years post-treatment motivated an extension of the follow-up to five years post-treatment. In this paper, we therefore include the original planned two year analysis as well as the three year analysis, which was used for the evaluation of the cost effectiveness. Late toxicity was graded according to the CTCAE V.4 for bone, renal, bladder, skin, subcutaneous tissues, mucous membranes and gastrointestinal systems. The frequency of reported grade 1/2 late toxicity and grade 3/4 toxicity were compared by treatment group and by HIV status using frequency tables. Pearson's Chi squared test and Fisher's exact tests were used to determine the difference in frequencies between groups. Multivariable proportional hazards regression models were used to identify significant predictors (including arm, HIV status, and number of cisplatin doses), of grades 3/4 late toxicity. Two-sample independent t-tests with equal variances were used to evaluate QoL score change from baseline to 12 and 24 months post-treatment between the two treatment groups. The differences in score changes between the groups are assessed using paired t-tests. STATA 15.0 Statistics software program (Stata Corporation, College Station, TX, USA) was used to analyse the data.

The CEA was performed with a time horizon of three years, using a Markov model with a six month cycle length, from the perspective of a private healthcare funder (medical aid scheme), and a public healthcare funder (the state). The two-tiered healthcare system in South Africa is comprised of a state-funded public healthcare system and a private healthcare system that is mostly funded by private contributions to medical aid schemes. An estimated 70–80% of the population makes use of the public healthcare system [34], and this setting is underfunded and poorly equipped to manage the large volume of patients. The input costs of the treatments for the public healthcare CEA are based on the direct costs to the state for the treatments, as outlined in by the Department of Health [35], and therefore represents the cost versus benefit of the treatment of patients in a public healthcare facility, funded by the state. The input costs of the treatments in the private healthcare CEA include the regulated profit added to the cost of the treatments, charged by the privately owned hospitals and by the healthcare professionals in private practice, to the private medical aid schemes. The results of the private healthcare CEA therefore represent the costs to the private healthcare funders, versus the clinical benefit of the members or patients.

3. Results

3.1. Participants

A total of 271 patients were screened between January 2014 and November 2017, and 210 eligible participants were enrolled and randomised (mEHT Group: $n = 106$, Control Group: $n = 104$). Five participants were lost to follow-up either before, during, or immediately after treatment (mEHT Group: $n = 3$, Control Group: $n = 2$) and were excluded from OS and DFS analyses. Four participants were lost to follow-up after treatment and could not be contacted (mEHT: one lost to follow-up at six-, nine-, and 18 months post-treatment; Control group: one lost to follow-up at 24 months post-treatment). These participants were excluded from the survival analysis, and their last recorded disease status and follow-up date were used for the DFS analyses (Figure 1). There were no significant differences in participant characteristics and treatment characteristics between the mEHT and Control groups (Tables 2 and 3). Two thirds of the participants had FIGO Stage III disease and half of all the participants were HIV-positive with more than two thirds of the HIV-participants in the under 50 years old age group. The median age was 50.1 (27.3–74.8), and 79% of participants were unemployed. The median RT dose received was 74 Gy (range: 2–74) and the average dose of cisplatin received was 131 mg/m^2 per participant, with 12% of participants not receiving any cisplatin. In the mEHT Group, 97% of participants received 80% (8/10), or more of the prescribed mEHT treatments, with only 2% receiving 20% (2/10) or less of the prescribed mEHT treatments. All participants with a haemoglobin value < 10 g/dL at enrolment were transfused before treatment.

3.2. Two Year Survival

Survival data were available for 202 participants at two years post-treatment, (mEHT Group: $n = 100$; Control Group: $n = 102$), of which 53 [53%] and 43 [42%] participants in the mEHT Group and Control Group, respectively, were alive at the last follow-up. The frequency of participants achieving two year OS in the group with LDC at six months post-treatment (42/59 [71.2%]) was significantly higher than those who did not achieve LDC (17/59 [28.8%]; Pearson Chi2: $p < 0.001$). Local Disease Control is a significant predictor of two year OS (OR: 3.8; $p < 0.001$; 95%CI: 2.00–7.34). The risk of death was 30% lower in the mEHT group (HR: 0.70; $p = 0.074$; 95%CI: 0.48–1.03, adjusted for HIV status, age and FIGO stage) (Table 4, Figure 2a).

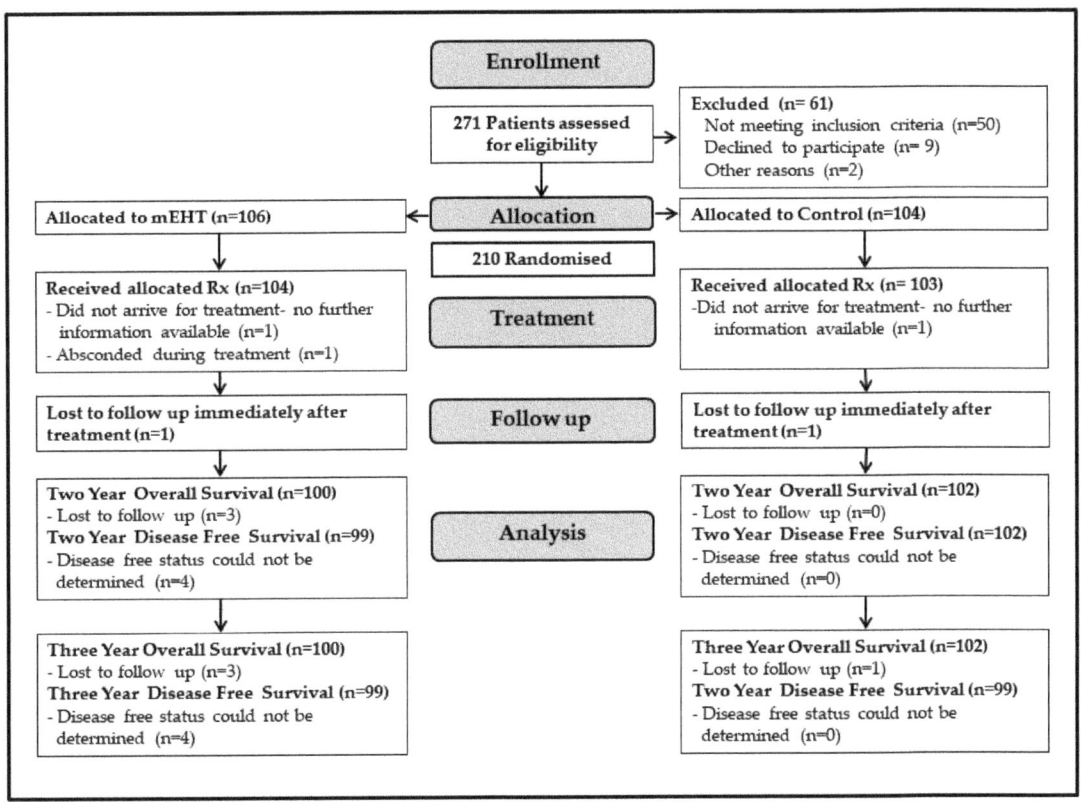

Figure 1. Trial profile. Abbreviations: mEHT: modulated electro-hyperthermia.

Table 2. Participant characteristics.

Participant Characteristic		mEHT		Control		p-Value
		106	(50.5%)	104	(49.5%)	
HIV Status	Positive	52	(49.1%)	55	(52.9%)	$p = 0.579$
	Negative	54	(50.9%)	49	(47.1%)	
Age Group	<50 years	52	(49.1%)	46	(44.2%)	$p = 0.483$
	≥50 years	54	(50.9%)	58	(55.8%)	
ECOG	0	3	(2.8%)	7	(6.7%)	$p = 0.184$
	1	103	(97.2%)	97	(93.3%)	
Race	African	98	(92.5%)	97	(93.3%)	
	Caucasian	4	(3.8%)	1	(1.0%)	
	Indian	0	(0.0%)	0	(0.0%)	$p = 0.335$
	Asian	0	(0.0%)	0	(0.0%)	
	Mixed Race	4	(3.8%)	6	(5.8%)	
Education	Primary	45	(43.3%)	50	(49.0%)	
	Secondary	55	(52.9%)	51	(50.0%)	$p = 0.334$
	Tertiary	4	(3.8%)	1	(1.0%)	
Employment	Unemployed	83	(78.3%)	82	(78.8%)	$p = 0.923$
	Employed	23	(21.7%)	22	(21.2%)	

Table 2. Cont.

Participant Characteristic		mEHT		Control		p-Value
		106	(50.5%)	104	(49.5%)	
FIGO Staging	IIB	40	(37.7%)	36	(34.6%)	
	IIIA	1	(0.9%)	1	(1.0%)	$p = 0.895$
	IIIB	65	(61.3%)	67	(64.4%)	
Histological Grade	1	7	(6.9%)	4	(4.1%)	
	2	70	(69.3%)	67	(69.1%)	$p = 0.759$
	3	24	(23.8%)	26	(26.8%)	
Tumour Dimensions (cm)	Median	7		7.1		
	Min	2.7		1.8		$p = 0.1429$
	Max	11.7		14.87		
Tumour SUV	Median	18.07		19.26		
	Min	7.01		6.07		$p = 0.7769$
	Max	63.25		97		
HB (g/dL)	Median	10.9		11		
	Min	5.7		5.2		$p = 0.9424$
	Max	16.2		16.2		
Age	Median	49.2		50.6		
	Min	27.3		29.2		$p = 0.3665$
	Max	70.8		74.8		
BMI	Median	27		26.5		
	Min	15		15		$p = 0.3883$
	Max	49		41.7		

Abbreviations: BMI: Body Mass Index; ECOG: Eastern Cooperative Oncology Group; FIGO: Fédération Internationale de Gynécologie et d'Obstétrique; HB: Haemoglobin; HIV: Human Immunodeficiency Virus; mEHT: Modulated Electro-Hyperthermia; SUV: Standard Uptake Value.

Table 3. Treatment characteristics.

Treatment Characteristics		mEHT		Control		p-Value
		106	(50.5%)	104	(49.5%)	
No of HDR BT doses	0	0	(0.0%)	0	(0.0%)	
	1	0	(0.0%)	2	(2.0%)	$p = 0.223$
	2	3	(2.9%)	1	(1.0%)	
	3	101	(97.1%)	99	(97.1%)	
No of Cisplatin Doses	0	14	(13.6%)	11	(10.7%)	
	1	42	(40.8%)	47	(45.6%)	$p = 0.727$
	2	47	(45.6%)	45	(43.7%)	
Total RT Dose	Median	74		74		
	Min	20		2		$p = 0.6133$
	Max	74		74		
Days between enrolment and Treatment	Median	37		37		
	Min	18		21		$p = 0.2241$
	Max	79		104		
No of mEHT doses	Median	10				
	Min	1				
	Max	10				

Abbreviations: HDR BT: High Dose Rate Brachytherapy; mEHT: Modulated Electro-Hyperthermia; RT: Radiotherapy.

Table 4. Multivariable Cox proportional hazards model for two year overall survival.

Overall	HR	p-Value	[95%CI]
mEHT	0.70	0.074	0.48–1.03
HIV-negative	0.82	0.328	0.54–1.23
Age at Enrolment	0.97	*0.007*	0.95–0.99
FIGO Stage III	1.01	0.785	0.71–1.57
FIGO Stage II	**HR**	***p*-Value**	**[95%CI]**
mEHT	0.88	0.677	0.47–1.64
HIV-negative	0.73	0.342	0.37–1.41
Age at Enrolment	0.99	0.401	0.96–1.02
FIGO Stage III	**HR**	***p*-Value**	**[95%CI]**
mEHT	0.61	0.047	0.37–0.99
HIV-negative	0.90	0.699	0.54–1.52
Age at Enrolment	0.96	0.006	0.94–0.99

Abbreviations: FIGO: Fédération Internationale de Gynécologie et d'Obstétrique; HIV: Human Immunodeficiency Virus; HR: Hazard Ratio; mEHT: Modulated Electro-Hyperthermia.

When considering participants with Stage II and Stage III disease separately, the risk of death within two years post-treatment, adjusted for age, disease stage, and HIV status, was significantly lower in the mEHT participants with Stage III disease compared to the Control participants with Stage III disease (mEHT Group: 34/61 [56%]; Control Group: 27/67 [40%]; HR: 0.61; p = 0.047; 95%CI: 0.37–0.99). Age was also a significant predictor of two year OS in the group of participants with Stage III disease (HR: 0.96, p = 0.006, 95%CI: 0.94–0.99) (Table 4).

When analysing the sample by treatment arm, age was a significant predictor of two year OS in the mEHT Group (HR: 0.95, p = *0.001*, 95%CI: 0.93–0.98), but not in the Control Group (HR: 0.98, p = 0.181, 95%CI: 0.96–1.01). We subsequently analysed participants according to their age group at the time of randomization (30 years; 30–50 years; >50 years). As there were only three participants younger than 30 years, we combined them with the group of participants between 30 and 50 years. Considering the participants younger than 50 years, and 50 years and older separately, the addition of mEHT had the most significant effect on two year OS in the age group 50 years and above (HR: 0.44, p = 0.011, 95%CI: 0.24–0.83).

Two year DFS was seen significantly more frequently in the mEHT Group (36/99 [36.4%]) than in the Control Group (14/102 [13.7%]; p < 0.0001), with participants treated with mEHT having 33% less risk of developing a recurrence during the first two years than the Control Group participants (HR: 0.67, 95%CI: 0.48–0.93. p = 0.017, adjusted for age, stage, and HIV status) (Table 5, Figure 2b). Participants treated with mEHT had an odds ratio of 3.59 of achieving disease free status at two years (p < 0.001; 95%CI: 1.79–7.21) compared to Control Group participants. When evaluated by disease stage, mEHT was not significantly predictive of two year DFS in participants with Stage II disease but remained significant for participants with Stage III disease (Table 5).

3.3. Three Year Survival

Three year OS was achieved by 33.7% (34/101) and 44% (44/100) of participants from the Control and mEHT Groups, respectively. The risk of death in the first three years was 28% lower for the participants who received mEHT, although this was not significant (HR: 0.72; 95%CI: 0.51–1.03, p = 0.74; adjusted for age, disease stage and HIV status) (Figure 3a), and when considering only the participants with Stage III disease, the risk was significantly lower (38%) in the mEHT group (HR: 0.62; p = 0.040; 95%CI: 0.40–0.98, adjusted for age, and HIV status) (Table 6).

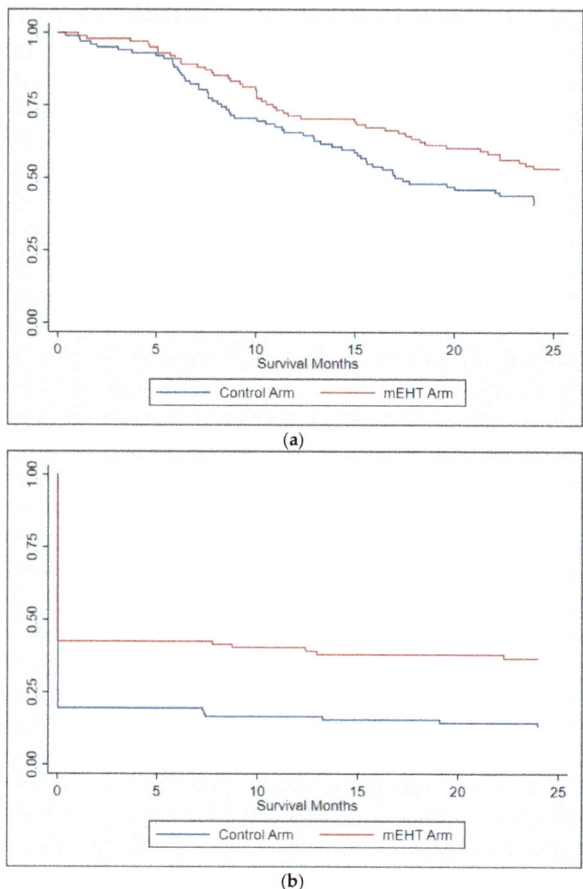

Figure 2. Kaplan–Meier survival curves at two years (**a**) two year overall survival; (**b**) two year disease free survival. The sharp drop of the DFS rates seen early on in 2b is a result of the higher rate of residual disease at six months post-treatment in the Control Group compared to mEHT Group. Participants with residual disease post-treatment were considered to have zero disease free survival days.

Table 5. Multivariable Cox proportional hazards model for two year disease free survival.

Overall	HR	p-Value	[95%CI]
mEHT	0.67	0.017	0.48–0.93
HIV-negative	0.99	0.257	0.72–1.48
Age at Enrolment	0.99	0.257	0.97–1.01
FIGO Stage III	0.99	0.944	0.79–1.38
FIGO Stage II	**HR**	**p-Value**	**[95%CI]**
mEHT	0.77	0.342	0.45–1.32
HIV-negative	1.18	0.569	0.66–2.01
Age at Enrolment	0.99	0.601	0.97–1.02
FIGO Stage III	**HR**	**p-Value**	**[95%CI]**
mEHT	0.62	0.025	0.41–0.94
HIV-negative	0.98	0.915	0.97–1.01
Age at Enrolment	0.99	0.301	0.97–1.01

Abbreviations: FIGO: Fédération Internationale de Gynécologie et d'Obstétrique; HIV: Human Immunodeficiency Virus; HR: Hazard Ratio; mEHT: Modulated Electro-Hyperthermia.

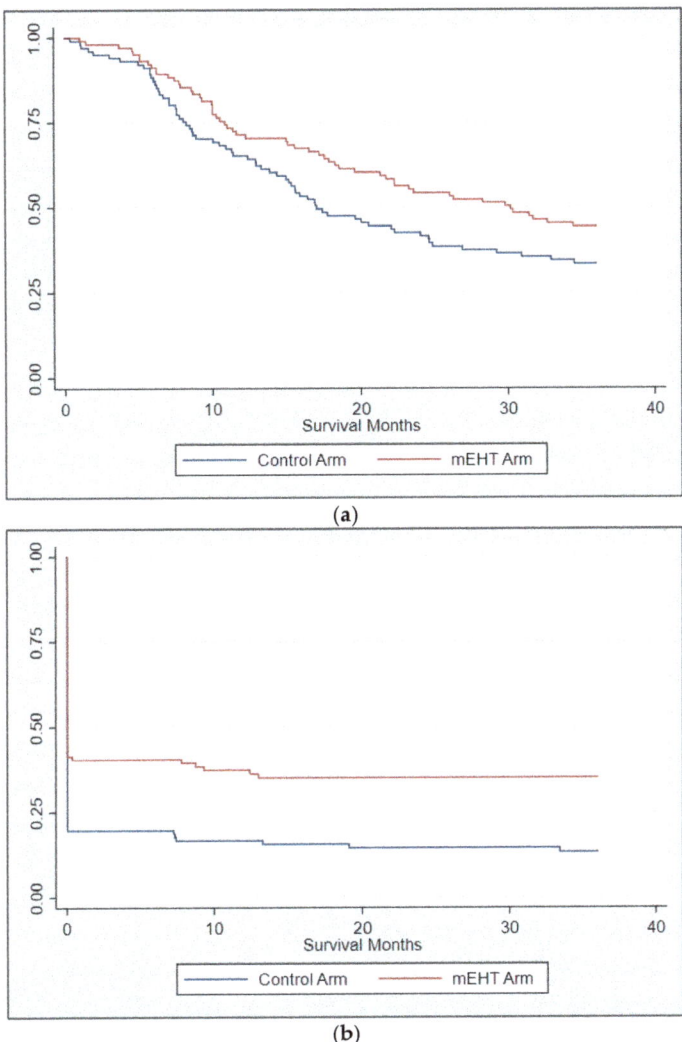

Figure 3. Kaplan–Meier survival curves at three years (**a**) three year overall survival; (**b**) three year disease free survival. The sharp drop off in DFS rates seen early on in 3b is again a result of the high rate of residual disease at six months post treatment.

The frequency of DFS remained significantly higher in the mEHT Group compared to the Control Group at three years post-treatment (mEHT: 35/99 [35.4%]; Control: 14/102 [13,7%]; Chi-squared: $p < 0.0001$) with an odds ratio of 3.4 of achieving DFS in favour of the mEHT Group ($p = 0.001$; 95%CI: 1.71–6.91) and a hazard ratio of 0.70 (95%CI: 0.51–0.97; $p = 0.035$, adjusted for age, stage and HIV status) (Figure 3b). When evaluated by stage of disease, the significance remained in participants with Stage III disease (Table 7).

Table 6. Multivariable Cox proportional hazards model for three year overall survival.

Overall	HR	p-Value	[95%CI]
mEHT	0.72	0.074	0.51–1.03
HIV-negative	0.84	0.366	0.58–1.23
Age at Enrolment	0.98	*0.019*	0.96–1.00
FIGO Stage	1.10	0.619	0.76–1.59
FIGO Stage II	**HR**	**p-Value**	**[95%CI]**
mEHT	0.91	0.748	0.51–1.64
HIV-negative	0.75	0.365	0.40–1.40
Age at Enrolment	0.99	0.468	0.96–1.02
FIGO Stage III	**HR**	**p-Value**	**[95%CI]**
mEHT	0.62	*0.040*	0.40–0.98
HIV-negative	0.93	0.777	0.58–1.50
Age at Enrolment	0.97	*0.018*	0.95–0.99

Abbreviations: FIGO: Fédération Internationale de Gynécologie et d'Obstétrique; HIV: Human Immunodeficiency Virus; HR: Hazard Ratio; mEHT: Modulated Electro-Hyperthermia.

Table 7. Multivariable Cox proportional hazards model for three year disease free survival.

Overall	HR	p-Value	[95%CI]
mEHT	0.70	0.035	0.51–0.98
HIV-negative	1.05	0.786	0.74–1.50
Age at Enrolment	0.99	0.240	0.97–1.01
FIGO Stage	0.98	0.913	0.70–1.37
FIGO Stage II	**HR**	**p-Value**	**[95%CI]**
mEHT	0.78	0.357	0.46–1.33
HIV-negative	1.20	0.538	0.68–2.11
Age at Enrolment	0.99	0.582	0.97–1.02
FIGO Stage III	**HR**	**p-Value**	**[95%CI]**
mEHT	0.66	0.040	0.43–0.98
HIV-negative	0.98	0.932	0.62–1.55
Age at Enrolment	0.99	*0.278*	0.97–1.01

Abbreviations: FIGO: Fédération Internationale de Gynécologie et d'Obstétrique; HIV: Human Immunodeficiency Virus; HR: Hazard Ratio; mEHT: Modulated Electro-Hyperthermia.

3.4. Late Toxicity

There was no significant difference in frequencies of reported late toxicity (grouped according to grades I/II and grades III/IV), between the two treatment groups or between the HIV-positive and HIV–negative participants at 9 months, 12 months, 18 months, and 24 months post-treatment. Multivariate Cox proportionate hazards models, including arm, HIV status and cisplatin doses, did not show any significant predictors of grades I/II or grades III/IV late toxicity.

3.5. Quality of Life

There were no statistically significant differences in QLQ scores between the two groups at baseline assessment [28]. When comparing the changes in scores from baseline to 24 months between groups, the reduction in pain was significantly higher in the mEHT Group ($p = 0.0368$), cognitive function was significantly improved in the mEHT group ($p = 0.0044$), and participants in the Control Group reported a reduction in role functioning while the mEHT Group participants reported an improvement in role functioning with a significant difference between the two groups ($p = 0.0172$). When assessing the change from baseline to 12 months within each group, there was an improvement in all scales except for role functioning in the mEHT Group, with significant improvements in Global Health Scale, Pain, Fatigue, and Emotional functioning. In the Control Group, there were significant improvements in the Visual Analogue Scale, Global Health Scale, Nausea and Vomiting, and Emotional Functioning, while Physical Functioning, Role Functioning and Cognitive Functioning decreased in the Control Group (Table 8). When assessing the change from baseline to 24 months within each group, the mEHT group reported a significant improved of all scales except for role function (which improved by a score of 9.4), while the Control Group only reported a significant change in five out of 11 scales, with a negative change in cognitive function (Table 9).

Table 8. Mean change in scores from baseline to 12 months in the mEHT and Control Group.

12 Months	mEHT				Control			
	Mean	SD	95%CI	p-Value	Mean	SD	95%CI	p-Value
Visual Analogue	5.4	31.6	−2.9 to 13.8	p = 0.1961	9.7	29.8	2.1 to 17.3	p = 0.0133
Global Health	10.2	34.3	1.2 to 19.2	p = 0.0275	13.8	36.3	4.4 to 23.1	p = 0.0047
Financial Burden	−7.1	50.7	−207 to 6.4	p = 0.2967	−6.1	48.0	−19.1 to 7.0	p = 0.3537
Symptom Scales								
Pain Reduction	−18.4	37.3	−28.2 to −8.6	p = 0.0004	−6.3	40.2	−16.6 to 4.0	p = 0.2264
Nausea/Vomiting	−5.5	23.4	−11.6 to 0.7	p = 0.0815	−6.5	19.1	−11.4 to −1.7	p = 0.0094
Fatigue reduction	−9.4	31.0	−17.5 to −1.2	p = 0.0247	−1.3	40.5	−11.6 to 9.1	p = 0.8065
Functional Scales								
Social	5.5	46.9	−6.9 to 17.8	p = 0.3787	2.6	55.2	−12.0 to 17.3	p = 0.7201
Cognitive	7.5	31.9	−0.9 to 15.9	p = 0.0795	−1.1	34.0	−10.1 to 7.3	p = 0.7542
Emotional	9.8	31.9	1.4 to 18.2	p = 0.0233	13.4	39.9	3.2 to 23.6	p = 0.0111
Role	−3.2	40.9	−13.9 to 7.6	p = 0.5583	−4.9	40.0	−15.2 to 5.3	p = 0.3401
Physical	2.3	29.9	−5.6 to 10.2	p = 0.5599	−4.0	27.7	−11.2 to 3.1	p = 0.2594

Abbreviations: CI: Confidence Interval; mEHT: Modulated Electro-Hyperthermia; SD: Standard Deviation.

Table 9. Mean change in scores from baseline to 24 months in the mEHT and Control Group.

	mEHT				Control			
	Mean	SD	95%CI	p-Value	Mean	SD	95%CI	p-Value
Visual Analogue	25.1	21.5	16.6 to 33.6	p < 0.0001	15.6	31.9	2.9 to 28.2	p = 0.0176
Global Health	23.2	31.7	11.7 to 35.6	p = 0.0002	17.3	29.1	6.0 to 28.6	p = 0.0041
Financial Burden	−26.1	60.9	−48.0 to 4.1	p = 0.0216	−16.7	46.7	−34.8 to 1.4	p = 0.0698
Symptom Scales								
Pain Reduction	−34.4	32.8	−46.2 to −22.6	p = 0.0001	−15.5	35.7	−29.3 to −16	p = 0.0298
Nausea/Vomiting	−13.0	27.7	−23.0 to −3.0	p = 0.0122	−1.2	18.7	−8.4 to 6.1	p = 0.7383
Fatigue reduction	−18.4	27.9	−28.5 to −8.4	p = 0.0008	−10.7	34.0	−23.9 to 2.4	p = 0.1071
Functional Scales								
Social	12.0	31.2	0.7 to 23.2	p = 0.0375	17.3	41.7	1.1 to 33.4	p = 0.0373
Cognitive	19.8	33.2	7.8 to 31.6	p = 0.0020	−4.2	28.9	−15.4 to 7.0	p = 0.4523
Emotional	27.3	30.3	16.4 to 38.3	p < 0.0001	17.9	34.2	4.6 to 31.1	p = 0.0101
Role Function	9.4	35.1	−3.3 to 22.1	p = 0.1415	7.1	35.0	6.4 to 20.7	p = 0.2893
Physical	11.7	21.2	4.0 to '9.3	p = 0.0040	2.6	27.2	−7.9 to 13.2	p = 0.6150

Abbreviations: CI: Confidence Interval; mEHT: Modulated Electro-Hyperthermia; SD: Standard Deviation.

3.6. The Abscopal Effect

We previously reported on an increased frequency of an abscopal effect seen in the mEHT participants at six months post-treatment [29]. The three year follow-up of these participants shows that 10 of the 14 mEHT participants with an abscopal effect were disease free at three years post-treatment, and three participants were deceased, two of whom were disease free at death (cause of death renal failure, DFS days 335 and 596), and one whom was disease free at the last follow-up with an unknown cause of death after 860 days. Of the three participants in the Control Group who had an abscopal response, two achieved three year DFS and one demised after 483 days, due to renal failure. The disease pattern and description of these participants are detailed in our previous paper on the abscopal effect seen at six months post-treatment [29].

3.7. Cost Effectiveness Analysis

The addition of mEHT to CRT increases the efficacy of the oncology treatments; however, it also increases the initial input costs. The base case CEA showed that the addition of mEHT to CRT dominated the model, compared to CRT alone, making the combined treatment (mEHT + CRT) less costly and more effective, from the perspective of both government and private healthcare funders. This result is driven by the difference in DFS and is due to the high costs of recurrent and progressive disease. This model did not use a societal costing perspective, which incorporates productivity-loss costs as well as dying costs, especially before retirement age. The incremental cost-effectiveness ratio (ICER) plane shows that CRT + mEHT produces more health effects at a lower cost over three years, in the government and private healthcare model, per disease free cycle (a half year lived in perfect health) (Figure 4). The probability that mEHT + CRT is cost-effective compared with CRT alone is about 82.2% in the government healthcare model and 77.7% in the private healthcare model, at no additional cost. The QALYs are summarised in Table 10.

Table 10. Quality adjusted life year data for private and government healthcare CEA models.

Perspective	Treatment	Cost in ZAR	QALYs Gained *	Incremental Cost	Incremental QALYs *	ICER
Government	mEHT	412,433.37	4.84			
	CRT	449,290.02	4.60	36,836.65	−0.24	Dominated
Private payer	mEHT	579,998.97	4.84			
	CRT	617,421.79	4.60	37,422.82	−0.24	Dominated

* QALYs gained in the two perspectives are the same since assumptions for health effects were the same. The only differences in the model inputs were the costs.

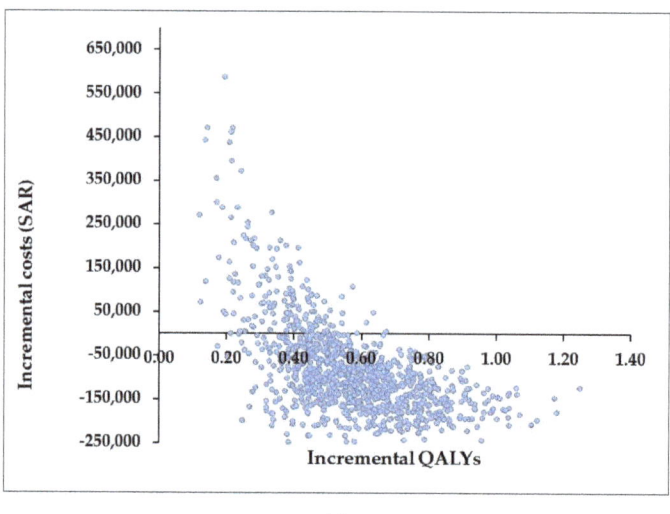

(a)

Figure 4. *Cont.*

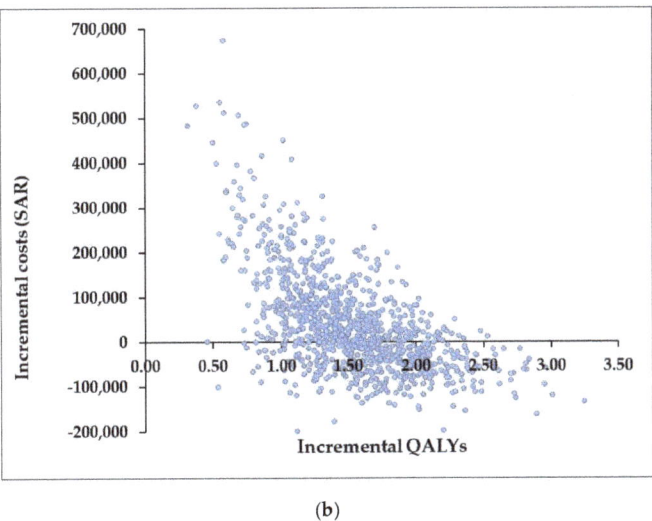

(b)

Figure 4. Incremental cost-effectiveness ratio (ICER) plane (**a**) government healthcare model; (**b**) private healthcare model. The Cost Effectiveness Analysis was done for both a Government-funded and a privately-funded healthcare model, for the same duration (three years), assuming the same health effects, with the only difference being the input costs. In the Government-funded healthcare model, the QALYs range from 0–1.4, with incremental costs mainly seen in the 4th Quadrant, showing improved clinical benefits and lower costs per QALY with the addition of mEHT. In the Privately funded healthcare model, the QALYs range from 0–3.5 with incremental costs falling in the lower portion of the 1st quadrant and the upper portion of the 4th quadrant, implying a clinical benefit with a high probability of cost saving with the addition of mEHT to chemoradiotherapy.

4. Discussion

The results from this study show a significant improvement in two and three year DFS with the addition of mEHT to CRT protocols for LACC, without any significant changes in late toxicity. This follows our previous paper describing the improvement in LDC with the addition of mEHT to CRT. The strict criteria for LDC evaluation is one of the strengths of the study. Evaluation of LDC was based on pre- and post-treatment ^{18}F-FDG PET/CT scans, examinations, and fine needle aspiration if indicated. Local disease control was considered a failure if any disease was confirmed in the pelvis [27]. We previously described the safety of mEHT in our paper on early toxicity, and reported high compliance rates to mEHT treatments in our high risk population. Other strengths of the study include the low variability in patient and treatment characteristics between the groups, the strict control between the groups, and the low number of participants lost to follow-up, even in the resource-constrained setting.

Our sample included HIV-positive participants, who are expected to have worse outcomes [36–38], and overweight participants [28]. Radiobiological data have previously suggested that HIV-positive patients may be more radiosensitive, and may therefore be at risk of increased toxicity from RT [39,40]. The evaluation of the early and late toxicity associated with RT combined with mEHT as a radiosensitiser in HIV-positive patients is therefore important in our setting where around 50% of LACC patients are HIV-positive. Heating pelvic tumours using capacitive HT techniques carries a high risk of adipose burns, especially when the treatment area includes a layer of adipose tissue thicker than 1.5 cm [41,42]. The safety demonstrated by mEHT for the management of cervical cancer, even in participants with above average BMIs, alongside the efficacy, indicates that mEHT is able to effectively and safely target deep tumours that would otherwise be difficult to treat using conventional capacitive HT. Factors which may contribute to the improved safety and efficacy of mEHT include the lower power output of mEHT (maximum of 130 W in our study), compared to other capacitive HT devices, the non-thermal effects [14] or field effects [16,43], and the AM of the RF waves in mEHT, which appears to contribute to the improved selectivity and enhanced effects in the tumour [18,25].

We initially estimated a reduction in two year mortality of 50% in order to achieve a power of 90% based on our sample size. While two year OS rates were not significantly improved, the reduction in disease recurrence at two years in the mEHT group was significant and was more than 50% (36.4% DFS in the mEHT Group and only 13.7% DFS in the Control Group), giving a statistical power of >90% for the DFS assessment. The effect of mEHT on outcomes was seen more significantly in the two year and three year DFS analyses than in the OS analyses, and the significance remained in both the HIV-positive and -negative participants and when considering participants based on age category. However, the significance was lost when considering only the participants with Stage II disease. In the OS analyses, the significance of the effects of mEHT on outcomes was less consistent. This may be a result of the inclusion of non-cancer related deaths in the OS analysis, which likely masked the effects of mEHT in the OS analyses. In our sample, the majority of the HIV-positive participants were younger than 50 years, and this may contribute to the improved OS outcomes seen in participants over the age of 50 years, compared to those younger than 50 years. This suggests that, while mEHT still improves the OS of HIV-positive participants, the effect is higher in HIV-negative participants as seen in the older group containing mostly HIV-negative women. In the group of participants who were 50 years and older, mEHT was a consistently significant predictor of DFS, regardless of HIV-status.

A limitation of the study is the substandard RT and BT administered as a result of a lack of sophisticated imaging and planning techniques in our setting, compared to developed settings. Due to resource constraints, the standard of care weekly cisplatin schedule was also not prescribed. Other limiting factors related to resource constraints include time to start EBRT, time to complete RT, and time between treatment completion and ^{18}F-FDG PET/CT scans. Delays were most frequently attributed to technical problems, machine down-time, and source supply problems (in the case of the ^{18}F-FDG PET/CT scans), as previously reported [27]. Another limitation of the study is the apparent high rate of under-staging of the patients using clinical staging techniques. The participants were all staged according to the recommended FIGO staging guidelines from 2014, and the institutional protocols at the time, using a chest X-ray, abdomino-pelvic ultrasound, and examination. The FIGO staging system was revised in 2018 to include more sophisticated imaging techniques which are able to include lymph node involvement and to improve the accuracy of the staging. The earlier FIGO staging criteria resulted in up to 40% of stage IB-IIIB cases being under diagnosed and as many as 64% of stage IIIB cases being over-diagnosed [44]. Funding was obtained for the addition of ^{18}F-FDG PET/CT scans pre-treatment and six months post-treatment to assess clinical response to treatment. The ^{18}F-FDG PET/CT scans were therefore not used for staging purposes in our study; however, participants with visceral and bone metastases and bilateral hydronephrosis on the ^{18}F-FDG PET/CT scans were still excluded as they required a change in the treatment protocol. The pre-treatment ^{18}F-FDG PET/CT scans indicated that more than half of the patients were in stage IVB disease, as seen by the high number of patients with extra-pelvic nodal involvement and local invasion of the bladder and rectum that was not detected during the routine clinical staging procedures. In a sub-group analysis of these participants, it was noted that there was complete metabolic resolution of all diseases, local and distant, in around a quarter of those who received mEHT. This suggests that mEHT may potentiate the abscopal effect induced by ionising radiation. This also provided an opportunity to assess the systemic effects of mEHT. The previously reported abscopal results [29], combined with the long term follow-up of the abscopal response reported in this paper, suggest that the preclinical immunological effects, observed in response to the administration of mEHT [45–47], could have clinical benefits in the management of systemic disease as well as local disease. If we consider that Stage IVB disease is generally considered incurable, then a disease free status in the participants with extra-pelvic disease at three years of 24.5% in the mEHT group compared to the 5.6% in the control group, even with sub-optimal RT delivery, is a significant and important outcome.

Only one Phase III study has investigated CRT with/without classical HT (using capacitive HT), for the management LACC, and they reported an improvement in five year DFS from 60.6% (95%CI, 45.3–72.9%) to 70.8% (95%CI, 55.5–81.7%), although the difference was not significant (HR: 0.517, 95%CI, 0.251–1.065, p = 0.073) [48]. While results from Phase III studies on RT with/without classical HT are positive, they are not comparable to our study, due to the differences in HT techniques and treatment protocols. Classical HT requires a substantial increase in local temperature in order to slow down DNA repair and induce tumour cell killing [12], and thermo-monitoring is a critical safety and efficiency measure [10], while mEHT aims to improve perfusion and support an immune response to the tumours [49], with a mild temperature increase, and without the need for thermo-monitoring as a measure of safety and efficiency.

The substantial improvements in quality of life are an important result to consider as prolonged life is not always associated with quality of life in cancer patients. The adverse effects from oncology treatments can negatively impact the quality of life even in patients who are disease free, while persistent and recurrent disease are often considered to be poor predators of quality of life. An increase in life expectancy, together with a decreased quality of life and increased costs of treatment for adverse effects and persistent/recurrent disease, can place additional burden on the healthcare system. The CEA performed confirms that the improvement in quality of life, and improvement in DFS, not only benefits the patients and the community, but also has the potential to reduce the economic burden of the disease in both private and public healthcare settings.

While it is unclear how much of an effect mEHT as a radiosensitiser would have when added to optimal RT and BT delivery for cervical cancer, it is encouraging to see such a large improvement in two and three year DFS with the addition of mEHT, even in sub-optimal conditions and in our high-risk population. There is still room for improvement in five year OS rates in cervical cancer patients with stage III and IV disease globally, even with sophisticated RT techniques, and a safe and effective radiosensitiser, such as mEHT, may still be a beneficial adjunct to RT in optimal settings. The continued monitoring of participants in the reported study will provide more insight into the effects of mEHT on five year survival. Modulated electro-hyperthermia is a feasible addition to LACC treatment protocols to improve outcomes, especially in settings in which sophisticated imaging and RT technologies are not accessible.

5. Conclusions

Modulated electro-hyperthermia enhances outcomes of LACC patients when added to CRT, without increasing the toxicity profile of treatments. The associated improvement in quality of life along with the reduction in healthcare costs makes this intervention a feasible and effective adjunct to CRT for the management of LACC. The addition of mEHT improved LDC and DFS in our sample, without additional toxicity, and with improved role functioning of the patients, benefiting both the patients, the community, and the already-strained healthcare system. Modulated electro-hyperthermia could therefore be considered as an adjunct to CRT, especially in resource-constrained settings and for cervical cancer patients with advanced disease. The five year follow-up results and detailed CEA will provide further insight into the long term benefits of mEHT as an adjunct to CRT. Further investigations into the immunological effects of mEHT could assist in the long-term goal of shifting RT from a local treatment, to a systemic treatment when combined with mEHT, offering additional options for patients with metastatic disease. Studies on the systemic effects of mEHT, as well as studies with the aim of better understanding the thermal and non-thermal effects of mEHT, are likely to shed more light on the mechanisms of action and further improve the application and recommendations for the use of mEHT in a clinical setting.

Author Contributions: Conceptualization, J.A.K. and C.A.M., methodology, J.A.K. and C.A.M.; software, C.A.M.; validation, A.B. and C.A.M.; formal analysis, I.M. and C.A.M.; investigation, C.A.M. and J.A.K.; resources, A.B. and J.A.K.; data curation, C.A.M.; writing—original draft preparation, C.A.M. and I.M.; writing—review and editing, C.A.M., I.M., J.A.K. and A.B.; visualization, J.A.K., A.B. and C.A.M.; supervision, A.B. and J.A.K.; project administration, A.B.; funding acquisition, J.A.K. All authors have read and agreed to the published version of the manuscript.

Funding: This research was funded by the National Research Foundation, Grant No. TP12082710852, awarded to J.A. Kotzen. The funder did not have any involvement in the protocol development, data collection, data analysis, or reporting.

Institutional Review Board Statement: The study was conducted according to the guidelines of the Declaration of Helsinki, and approved by the Institutional Review Board of the Charlotte Maxeke Johannesburg Academic Hospital and the Human Research and Ethics Committee of the University of the Witwatersrand on 4 May 2012 (M120477), and renewed on 5 May 2017 (M704133).

Informed Consent Statement: Informed consent was obtained from all subjects involved in the study.

Data Availability Statement: The data presented in this study will be made openly available in (repository name e.g., FigShare) upon acceptance of the paper for review.

Acknowledgments: The modulated electro-hyperthermia device was sponsored by Oncotherm GMBh, for the duration of the trial. ^{18}F-FDG was supplied at a reduced rate by NTP Radioisotopes SOC. The Radiation Oncology and Nuclear Medicine Department and all supportive staff involved in the patient care and management at the hospital at which the study took place, Charlotte Maxeke Johannesburg Academic Hospital, are acknowledged. We acknowledge and thank all of the participants, without whom this study would not be possible, who showed courage, grace, and determination throughout their journey, despite the difficulties that were faced with this under-resourced and poor socio-economic setting.

Conflicts of Interest: The authors declare no conflict of interest. The funders had no role in the design of the study; in the collection, analyses, or interpretation of data; in the writing of the manuscript, or in the decision to publish the results.

References

1. International Agency for Research on Cancer. *Cancer Today*; GLOBOCON: Lyon, France, 2020. Available online: https://gco.iarc.fr/today/home (accessed on 21 January 2022).
2. Arbyn, M.; Weiderpass, E.; Bruni, L.; De Sanjosé, S.; Saraiya, M.; Ferlay, J.; Bray, F. Estimates of incidence and mortality of cervical cancer in 2018: A worldwide analysis. *Lancet Glob. Health* **2020**, *8*, 191–203. [CrossRef]
3. Denny, L.; Anorlu, R. Cervical Cancer in Africa. *Cancer Epidemiol. Biomark.* **2012**, *21*, 1434–1439. [CrossRef] [PubMed]
4. Ghebre, R.G.; Grover, S.; Xu, M.J.; Chuang, L.T.; Simonds, H. Cervical cancer control in HIV-infected women: Past, present and future. *Gynecol. Oncol. Rep.* **2017**, *21*, 101–108. [CrossRef] [PubMed]
5. Horsman, M.R.; Overgaard, J. Hyperthermia: A Potent Enhancer of Radiotherapy. *Clin. Oncol.* **2007**, *19*, 418–426. [CrossRef]
6. Datta, N.R.; Rogers, S.; Klingbiel, D.; Gomez, S.; Puric, E.; Bodis, S. Hyperthermia and radiotherapy with or without chemotherapy in locally advanced cervical cancer: A systematic review with conventional and network meta-analyses. *Int. J. Hyperth.* **2016**, *6736*, 809–821. [CrossRef]
7. Van Der Zee, J.; González González, D. The Dutch Deep Hyperthermia trial: Results in cervical cancer. *Int. J. Hyperth.* **2002**, *18*, 1–12. [CrossRef]
8. Franckena, M.; Stalpers, L.J.A.; Koper, P.C.M.; Wiggenraad, R.G.J.; Hoogenraad, W.J.; van Dijk, J.D.P.; Wárlám-Rodenhuis, C.C.; Jobsen, J.J.; van Rhoon, G.C.; van der Zee, J. Long-Term Improvement in Treatment Outcome After Radiotherapy and Hyperthermia in Locoregionally Advanced Cervix Cancer: An Update of the Dutch Deep Hyperthermia Trial. *Int. J. Radiat. Oncol. Biol. Phys.* **2008**, *70*, 1176–1182. [CrossRef]
9. Harima, Y.; Nagata, K.; Harima, K.; Ostapenko, V.V.; Tanaka, Y.; Sawada, S. A randomized clinical trial of radiation therapy versus thermoradiotherapy in stage IIIB cervical carcinoma. *Int. J. Hyperth.* **2001**, *17*, 97–105. [CrossRef]
10. Franckena, M.; Fatehi, D.; de Bruijne, M.; Canters, R.A.; van Norden, Y.; Mens, J.W.; van Rhoon, G.C.; van der Zee, J. Hyperthermia dose-effect relationship in 420 patients with cervical cancer treated with combined radiotherapy and hyperthermia. *Eur. J. Cancer* **2009**, *45*, 1969–1978. [CrossRef]

11. Kroesen, M.; Mulder, H.T.; van Holthe, J.M.; Aangeenbrug, A.A.; Mens, J.W.M.; van Doorn, H.C.; Paulides, M.M.; Oomen-de Hoop, E.; Vernhout, R.M.; Lutgens, L.C.; et al. Confirmation of thermal dose as a predictor of local control in cervical carcinoma patients treated with state-of-the-art radiation therapy and hyperthermia. *Radiother. Oncol.* **2019**, *140*, 150–158. [CrossRef]
12. Crezee, H.; Kok, H.P.; Oei, A.L.; Franken, N.A.P.; Stalpers, L.J.A. The impact of the time interval between radiation and hyperthermia on clinical outcome in patients with locally advanced cervical cancer. *Front. Oncol.* **2019**, *9*, 412. [CrossRef] [PubMed]
13. Kroesen, M.; Mulder, H.T.; van Rhoon, G.C.; Franckena, M. Commentary: The Impact of the Time Interval Between Radiation and Hyperthermia on Clinical Outcome in Patients With Locally Advanced Cervical Cancer. *Front. Oncol.* **2019**, *9*, 1387. [CrossRef] [PubMed]
14. Wust, P.; Kortüm, B.; Strauss, U.; Nadobny, J.; Zschaeck, S.; Beck, M.; Stein, U.; Ghadjar, P. Non-thermal effects of radiofrequency electromagnetic fields. *Sci. Rep.* **2020**, *10*, 13488. [CrossRef] [PubMed]
15. Fiorentini, G.; Szasz, A. Hyperthermia today: Electric energy, a new opportunity in cancer treatment. *J. Cancer Res. Ther.* **2006**, *2*, 41. [CrossRef] [PubMed]
16. Andocs, G.; Renner, H.; Balogh, L.; Fonyad, L.; Jakab, C.; Szasz, A. Strong synergy of heat and modulated electromagnetic field in tumor cell killing. *Strahlenther. Onkol.* **2009**, *185*, 120–126. [CrossRef]
17. Yang, K.L.; Huang, C.C.; Chi, M.S.; Chiang, H.C.; Wang, Y.S.; Hsia, C.C.; Andocs, G.; Wang, H.E.; Chi, K.H. In vitro comparison of conventional hyperthermia and modulated electro-hyperthermia. *Oncotarget* **2016**, *7*, 84082–84092. [CrossRef]
18. Wust, P.; Ghadjar, P.; Nadobny, J.; Beck, M.; Kaul, D.; Winter, L.; Zschaeck, S. Physical analysis of temperature-dependent effects of amplitude-modulated electromagnetic hyperthermia. *Int. J. Hyperth.* **2019**, *36*, 1246–1254. [CrossRef]
19. Tsang, Y.W.; Huang, C.C.; Yang, K.L.; Chi, M.S.; Chiang, H.C.; Wang, Y.S.; Andocs, G.; Szasz, A.; Li, W.T.; Chi, K.H. Improving immunological tumor microenvironment using electro-hyperthermia followed by dendritic cell immunotherapy. *BMC Cancer* **2015**, *15*, 708. [CrossRef]
20. Andocs, G.; Meggyeshazi, N.; Okamoto, Y.; Balogh, L.; Szasz, O. Bystander Effect of Oncothermia. *Conf. Pap. Med.* **2013**, *2013*, 953482. [CrossRef]
21. Meggyeshazi, N.; Andocs, G.; Balogh, L.; Balla, P.; Kiszner, G.; Teleki, I.; Jeney, A.; Krenacs, T. DNA fragmentation and caspase-independent programmed cell death by modulated electrohyperthermia. *Strahlenther. Onkol.* **2014**, *190*, 815–822. [CrossRef]
22. Andocs, G.; Meggyeshazi, N.; Balogh, L.; Spisak, S.; Maros, M.E.; Balla, P.; Kiszner, G.; Teleki, I.; Kovago, C.; Krenacs, T. Upregulation of heat shock proteins and the promotion of damage-associated molecular pattern signals in a colorectal cancer model by modulated electrohyperthermia. *Cell Stress Chaperones* **2015**, *20*, 37–46. [CrossRef] [PubMed]
23. Szasz, O.; Szigeti, P.G.; Vancsik, T.; Szasz, A. Hyperthermia Dosing and Depth of Effect. *Open J. Biophys.* **2018**, *8*, 31–48. [CrossRef]
24. Papp, E.; Vancsik, T.; Kiss, E.; Szasz, O. Energy Absorption by the Membrane Rafts in the Modulated Electro-Hyperthermia (mEHT). *Open J. Biophys.* **2017**, *7*, 216–229. [CrossRef]
25. Lee, S.-Y.; Kim, J.-H.; Han, Y.-H.; Cho, D.-H. The effect of modulated electro-hyperthermia on temperature and blood flow in human cervical carcinoma. *Int. J. Hyperth.* **2018**, *34*, 953–960. [CrossRef] [PubMed]
26. Szasz, A.M.; Minnaar, C.A.; Szentmártoni, G.; Szigeti, G.P.; Dank, M. Review of the Clinical Evidences of Modulated Electro-Hyperthermia (mEHT) Method: An Update for the Practicing Oncologist. *Front. Oncol.* **2019**, *9*, 1012. [CrossRef] [PubMed]
27. Minnaar, C.A.; Kotzen, J.A.; Ayeni, O.A.; Naidoo, T.; Tunmer, M.; Sharma, V.; Vangu, M.D.T.; Baeyens, A. The effect of modulated electro-hyperthermia on local disease control in HIV-positive and -negative cervical cancer women in South Africa: Early results from a phase III randomised controlled trial. *PLoS ONE* **2019**, *14*, e0217894. [CrossRef] [PubMed]
28. Minnaar, C.A.; Kotzen, J.A.; Naidoo, T.; Sharma, V.; Vangu, M.; Baeyens, A.; Anne, C.; Kotzen, J.A.; Naidoo, T. Analysis of the effects of mEHT on the treatment- related toxicity and quality of life of HIV-positive cervical cancer patients. *Int. J. Hyperth.* **2020**, *37*, 263–272. [CrossRef]
29. Minnaar, C.A.; Kotzen, J.A.; Ayeni, O.A.; Vangu, M.; Baeyens, A. Potentiation of the Abscopal Effect by Modulated Electro-Hyperthermia in Locally Advanced Cervical Cancer Patients. *Front. Oncol.* **2020**, *10*, 376. [CrossRef]
30. Koller, M.; Aaronson, N.K.; Blazeby, J.; Bottomley, A.; Dewolf, L.; Fayers, P.; Johnson, C.; Ramage, J.; Scott, N.; West, K. Translation procedures for standardised quality of life questionnaires: The European Organisation for Research and Treatment of Cancer (EORTC) approach. *Eur. J. Cancer* **2007**, *43*, 1810–1820. [CrossRef]
31. Fayers, P.; Bottomley, A. Quality of life research within the EORTC—The EORTC QLQ-C30. *Eur. J. Cancer* **2002**, *38*, S125–S133. [CrossRef]
32. Aaronson, N.; Ahmedzai, S.; Bergman, B.; Bullinger, M.; Cull, A.; Duez, N.; Filiberti, A.; Flechtner, H.; Fleishman, S.; de Haes, J.; et al. The European Organisation for Research and Treatment of Cancer QLQ-C30: A quality-of-life instrument for use in international clinical trials in oncology. *J. Natl. Cancer Inst.* **1993**, *85*, 365–376. [CrossRef] [PubMed]
33. Fayers, P.; Aaronson, N.; Bjordal, K.; Groenvold, M.; Curran, D.; Bottomley, A. *The EORTC QLQ-C30 Scoring Manual*, 3rd ed.; European Organisation for Research and Treatment of Cancer: Brussels, Belgian, 2001.
34. Department of Statistics South Africa. *General Household Survey*; Pretoria, South Africa, 2021; Volume P0318. Available online: http://www.statssa.gov.za/publications/P0318/P03182020.pdf (accessed on 21 January 2022).
35. National Department of Health South Africa. *Uniform Patient Fee Schedule 2020*; Pretoria, South Africa, 2020. Available online: https://www.health.gov.za/uniform-patient-fee-schedule/ (accessed on 21 January 2022).

36. Coghill, A.E.; Newcomb, P.A.; Madeleine, M.M.; Richardson, B.A.; Mutyaba, I.; Okuku, F.; Phipps, W.; Wabinga, H.; Orem, J.; Casper, C. Contribution of HIV infection to mortality among cancer patients in Uganda. *AIDS* **2013**, *27*, 2933–2942. [CrossRef]
37. Coghill, A.E.; Shiels, M.S.; Suneja, G.; Engels, E.A. Elevated cancer-specific mortality among HIV-infected patients in the United States. *J. Clin. Oncol.* **2015**, *33*, 2376–2383. [CrossRef] [PubMed]
38. Dryden-Peterson, S.; Bvochora-Nsingo, M.; Suneja, G.; Efstathiou, J.A.; Grover, S.; Chiyapo, S.; Ramogola-Masire, D.; Kebabonye-Pusoentsi, M.; Clayman, R.; Mapes, A.C.; et al. HIV Infection and Survival Among Women With Cervical Cancer. *J. Clin. Oncol.* **2016**, *34*, 3749–3761. [CrossRef]
39. Herd, O.; Francies, F.; Kotzen, J.; Smith, T.; Nxumalo, Z.; Muller, X.; Slabbert, J.; Vral, A.; Baeyens, A. Chromosomal radiosensitivity of human immunodeficiency virus positive / negative cervical cancer patients in South Africa. *J. Mol. Med. Rep.* **2016**, *13*, 130–136. [CrossRef] [PubMed]
40. Baeyens, A.; Slabbert, J.P.; Willem, P.; Jozela, S.; Van Der Merwe, D.; Vral, A. Chromosomal radiosensitivity of HIV positive individuals. *Int. J. Radiat. Biol.* **2010**, *86*, 584–592. [CrossRef] [PubMed]
41. Kok, H.P.; Crezee, J. A comparison of the heating characteristics of capacitive and radiative superficial hyperthermia. *Int. J. Hyperth.* **2017**, *33*, 378–386. [CrossRef]
42. D'Ambrosio, V.; Dughiero, F. Numerical model for RF capacitive regional deep hyperthermia in pelvic tumors. *Med. Biol. Eng. Comput.* **2007**, *45*, 459–466. [CrossRef]
43. Andocs, G.; Rehman, M.U.; Zhao, Q.-L.; Tabuchi, Y.; Kanamori, M.; Kondo, T. Comparison of biological effects of modulated electro-hyperthermia and conventional heat treatment in human lymphoma U937 cells. *Cell Death Discov.* **2016**, *2*, 16039. [CrossRef]
44. Lee, S.I.; Atri, M. 2018 FIGO staging system for uterine cervical cancer: Enter cross-sectional imaging. *Radiology* **2019**, *292*, 15–24. [CrossRef]
45. Vancsik, T.; Forika, G.; Balogh, A.; Kiss, E.; Krenacs, T. Modulated electro-hyperthermia induced p53 driven apoptosis and cell cycle arrest additively support doxorubicin chemotherapy of colorectal cancer in vitro. *Cancer Med.* **2019**, *8*, 4292–4303. [CrossRef] [PubMed]
46. Vancsik, T.; Kovago, C.; Kiss, E.; Papp, E.; Forika, G.; Benyo, Z.; Meggyeshazi, N.; Krenacs, T. Modulated electro-hyperthermia induced loco-regional and systemic tumor destruction in colorectal cancer allografts. *J. Cancer* **2018**, *9*, 41–53. [CrossRef] [PubMed]
47. Jeon, T.W.; Yang, H.; Lee, C.G.; Oh, S.T.; Seo, D.; Baik, I.H.; Lee, E.H.; Yun, I.; Park, K.R.; Lee, Y.H. Electro-hyperthermia up-regulates tumour suppressor Septin 4 to induce apoptotic cell death in hepatocellular carcinoma. *Int. J. Hyperth.* **2016**, *32*, 648–656. [CrossRef] [PubMed]
48. Harima, Y.; Ohguri, T.; Imada, H.; Sakurai, H.; Ohno, T.; Hiraki, Y.; Tuji, K.; Tanaka, M.; Terashima, H. A multicentre randomised clinical trial of chemoradiotherapy plus hyperthermia versus chemoradiotherapy alone in patients with locally advanced cervical cancer. *Int. J. Hyperth.* **2016**, *32*, 801–808. [CrossRef] [PubMed]
49. Szasz, O.; Szasz, A. Heating, Efficacy and Dose of Local Hyperthermia. *Open J. Biophys.* **2016**, *6*, 10–18. [CrossRef]

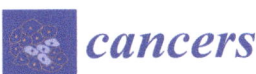

Article

Long-Term Feasibility of 13.56 MHz Modulated Electro-Hyperthermia-Based Preoperative Thermoradiochemotherapy in Locally Advanced Rectal Cancer

Yohan Lee [1,†], Sunghyun Kim [1,†], Hyejung Cha [1], Jae Hun Han [2], Hyun Joon Choi [1], Eun Go [3] and Sei Hwan You [1,4,*]

1. Department of Radiation Oncology, Wonju Severance Christian Hospital, Yonsei University Wonju College of Medicine, Wonju 26426, Korea; 2030john3636@gmail.com (Y.L.); tjdgus9410@naver.com (S.K.); hyejungcha@yonsei.ac.kr (H.C.); hjchoi1@yonsei.ac.kr (H.J.C.)
2. Department of Biostatistics, Yonsei University Wonju College of Medicine, Wonju 26426, Korea; cpflhan@yonsei.ac.kr
3. Department of Software, College of Software and Digital Healthcare Convergence, Yonsei University, Wonju 26493, Korea; 4him1@naver.com
4. Center of Evidence-Based Medicine, Institute of Convergence Science, Yonsei University, Seoul 03722, Korea
* Correspondence: ys3259@yonsei.ac.kr; Tel.: +82-33-741-1518
† These authors contributed equally to this work.

Simple Summary: We demonstrated that a 13.56 MHz modulated electro-hyperthermia (mEHT) boost is feasible in neoadjuvant treatment for rectal cancer. Herein, we attempted to present the long-term results for this phase 2 trial. Although there are many reports on the usefulness of thermoradiochemotherapy for loco-regional control, so far, only a few cases of survival benefit exist. Thus, this study assessed whether this limitation of hyperthermia could be overcome through the mEHT method featuring an applied energy variable. Following a median follow-up of 58 months for 60 patients, mEHT boost showed comparable results with conventional hyperthermia; potential therapeutic effects were also observed. Moreover, mEHT could be considered a useful tool in combination treatment with radiotherapy owing to its low thermotoxicity and improved treatment compliance.

Abstract: We evaluated the effect of 13.56 MHz modulated electro-hyperthermia (mEHT) boost in neoadjuvant treatment for cT3-4- or cN-positive rectal cancer. Sixty patients who completed the mEHT feasibility trial (ClinicalTrials.gov Identifier: NCT02546596) were analyzed. Whole pelvis radiotherapy of 40 Gy, mEHT boost twice a week during radiotherapy, and surgical resection 6–8 weeks following radiotherapy were performed. The median age was 59. The median follow-up period was 58 (6–85) months. Total/near total tumor regression was observed in 20 patients (33.3%), including nine cases of complete response. T- and N-downstaging was identified in 40 (66.6%) and 53 (88.3%) patients, respectively. The 5-year overall and disease-free survival were 94.0% and 77.1%, respectively. mEHT energy of $\geq$3800 kJ potentially increased the overall survival ($p = 0.039$). The ypN-stage and perineural invasion were possible significant factors in disease-free ($p = 0.003$ and $p = 0.005$, respectively) and distant metastasis-free ($p = 0.011$ and $p = 0.034$, respectively) survival. Tumor regression, resection margin status, and other molecular genetic factors showed no correlation with survival. Although a limited analysis of a small number of patients, mEHT was feasible considering long-term survival. A relatively low dose irradiation (40 Gy) plus mEHT setting could ensure comparable clinical outcomes with possible mEHT-related prognostic features.

Keywords: regional hyperthermia; rectal cancer; neoadjuvant chemoradiation; survival

Citation: Lee, Y.; Kim, S.; Cha, H.; Han, J.H.; Choi, H.J.; Go, E.; You, S.H. Long-Term Feasibility of 13.56 MHz Modulated Electro-Hyperthermia-Based Preoperative Thermoradiochemotherapy in Locally Advanced Rectal Cancer. *Cancers* 2022, 14, 1271. https://doi.org/10.3390/cancers14051271

Academic Editors: Stephan Bodis, Pirus Ghadjar and Gerard C. Van Rhoon

Received: 31 January 2022
Accepted: 24 February 2022
Published: 1 March 2022

Publisher's Note: MDPI stays neutral with regard to jurisdictional claims in published maps and institutional affiliations.

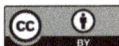

Copyright: © 2022 by the authors. Licensee MDPI, Basel, Switzerland. This article is an open access article distributed under the terms and conditions of the Creative Commons Attribution (CC BY) license (https://creativecommons.org/licenses/by/4.0/).

1. Introduction

Considering neoadjuvant treatment for rectal cancer, hyperthermia boost to radiochemotherapy reportedly produces excellent local control results; however, the long-term survival effects have not been sufficiently proven [1]. Attention is focused on whether this limitation of hyperthermia could be overcome by 13.56 MHz-based modulated electro-hyperthermia (mEHT), which possesses a potential cell killing effect by means of specific immunogenic pathways in addition to the traditional thermal effect [2–4].

mEHT has been demonstrated to possess effects at an average temperature of <39 °C [5,6]. In our previous early feasibility report for rectal cancer treatment, we demonstrated an excellent lymph node response by mEHT boost and a complementary nature of mEHT to radiation, thereby exploring the possibility of radiation dose reduction in combination with mEHT [7]. This study aimed to determine the follow-up results, focusing on the long-term survival of patients who faithfully received mEHT while undergoing neoadjuvant treatment for rectal cancer.

2. Materials and Methods

2.1. Patients

This single non-inferior prospective trial received approval of the Institutional Review Board of Wonju Severance Christian Hospital (Approval number: CR313035) and was registered with ClinicalTrials.gov (study number NCT02546596), a total of 60 patients with cT3-4 or cN positive rectal cancer faithfully underwent preoperative radiochemotherapy with concomitant mEHT boost between March 2014 and March 2017 (Figure 1). For pre-treatment staging, magnetic resonance imaging and computed tomography were performed. All patients had a general condition of ECOG performance status ≤2. Considering the thermal toxicity, cases in whom we anticipated thermal hypersensitivity, such as severe cardiac conditions or excessive subcutaneous fat, were fundamentally excluded. The above have been described in detail in the previous early clinical feasibility report [7]. Patient- and disease-related characteristics are shown in Table 1.

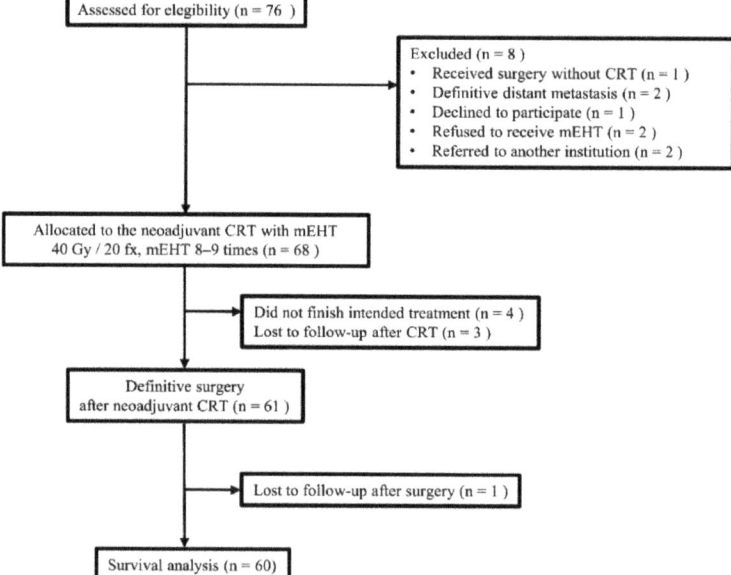

Figure 1. CONSORT diagram (CRT: chemoradiation, mEHT: modulated electro-hyperthermia).

Table 1. Patient- and disease-related characteristics at diagnosis ($n = 60$).

Characteristic		Value
Age (year)	<60	32 (53.3%)
	≥60	28 (46.7%)
Sex	Male	45 (75.0%)
	Female	15 (25.0%)
Pathologic diagnosis	Adenocarcinoma	57 (95.0%)
	Mucinous adenocarcinoma	2 (3.3%)
	Tubular adenocarcinoma	1 (1.7%)
Histological differentiation	Well-differentiated	8 (13.3%)
	Moderately differentiated	49 (81.7%)
	Poorly differentiated	3 (5.0%)
Primary tumor location from the anal verge (cm)	≤5	23 (38.3%)
	>5	37 (61.7%)
Primary tumor volume (cm^3)	<65	41 (68.3%)
	≥65	19 (31.7%)
Positive lymph node volume (cm^3)	≤5	34 (55.0%)
	>5	27 (45.0%)
cT stage	T3	46 (76.7%)
	T4	14 (23.3%)
cN stage	N1	28 (46.7%)
	N2	32 (53.3%)
Carcinoembryonic antigen (ng/mL)	≤5	39 (65.0%)
	>5	21 (35.0%)
Carbohydrate antigen 19–9 (U/mL)	≤37	50 (83.3%)
	>37	9 (15.0%)
	Not available	1 (1.7%)
KRAS mutation	Negative	27 (45.0%)
	Positive	14 (23.3%)
	Not available	19 (31.7%)
BRAF mutation	Negative	38 (63.3%)
	Positive	2 (3.3%)
	Not available	20 (33.3)
Microsatellite instability	Microsatellite-stable	38 (63.3%)
	Microsatellite instability-low	1 (1.7%)
	Microsatellite instability-high	1 (1.7%)
	Not available	20 (33.3%)

2.2. Overall Treatment Schedule

Three- or four-field linear accelerator-based 6–15 MV X-rays from three-dimensional planning were delivered to the whole pelvis area including the rectal tumor, mesorectum, and internal iliac/presacral lymph node chain up to the sacral promontory level in 2 Gy daily fractions up to a total dose of 40 Gy. Intravenous 5-fluorouracil (400 mg/m^2/day at the 1st and 5th weeks from the start of radiotherapy) or oral capecitabine (825 mg/m^2 based on the virtual period of the conventional 28-fraction radiation schedule) was administered concomitantly. According to the protocol, curative resection with lymph node dissection was planned at 6–8 weeks following completion of radiotherapy. Ultimately, the specific resection range was based on the surgeon's discretion considering the tumor location, sphincter function, or clinical response to preoperative treatment.

2.3. Modulated Electro-Hyperthermia

In addition to chemoradiation, eight sessions of mEHT were combined twice weekly during the radiotherapy period using 13.56 MHz capacitive coupled device (EHY2000, Oncotherm GmbH, Troisdorf, Germany). Treatment was performed such that a 30 cm-diameter electrode included the entire treatment area based on the center of the irradiation site while the patient was in a supine position. Treatment duration per session was 60 min, and the interval between mEHT and radiotherapy on the same day was <1 h. The power to be applied was 140 W; only for the first session, a gradual power increase method (starting at 100 W to increase in 20 W per 20 min) was used in consideration of the patient's adaptation status. In all subsequent sessions, the applied energy was partially adjusted when heat-related discomforts were recognized.

2.4. Treatment Response and Toxicities

Neoadjuvant treatment response and toxicity evaluation was performed as described in the previous early feasibility study [7,8]. The evaluation period of acute toxicity was from the start of neoadjuvant treatment to 90 days after ending radiotherapy, and toxic events that occurred thereafter were classified as late toxicity. Each toxicity grade during the period was based on the maximum value. Acute toxicity was assessed by NCI-CTCAE version 3.0 (NCI, Bethesda, MD, USA), while late toxicity was based on RTOG and EORTC criteria [9]. For the mEHT-related toxicity that mostly disappeared immediately after treatment, separate evaluation was conducted based on the Berlin scoring system, during the radiotherapy period only [10].

2.5. Statistical Analysis

In this study that assessed the follow-up results of the impact of mEHT boost on survival in a single-arm, non-inferiority trial, the primary endpoint (preoperative therapeutic response) assessment was by pathologic downstaging and tumor regression grade [7]. Survival rates were analyzed based on the baseline factors, in a median 58 (range, 6–85) months of follow-up. By definition, overall survival (OS) was the time interval from the day of radiotherapy to the day of death or last follow-up. Disease-free survival (DFS), loco-regional recurrence-free survival (LRRFS), and distant metastasis-free survival (DMFS) were determined to be from the day of surgery to the day of recurrence, death, or last follow-up, respectively. To examine the impact of each clinical parameter within a single group treated with radiotherapy plus mEHT, the difference in survival according to each parameter category was analyzed. Chi-square and Fisher's exact tests were used for categorical variable analysis, as appropriate. Cox proportional hazard regression analysis was used to calculate univariate/multivariate adjusted hazard ratios (HRs) and 95% confidence intervals (CIs) for each survival. Statistical significance was based on $p < 0.05$. Analyses were conducted using SAS software 9.4 (SAS, Cary, NC, USA) and R 4.0.5 (Institute for Statistics and Mathematics, Vienna, Austria).

3. Results

3.1. Clinicopathology- and Treatment-Related Indices

Factors that could affect the treatment outcomes, such as details of each treatment modality, response to preoperative treatment, and pathology after surgical resection, are shown in Table 2. The participants' median age was 59 (range, 33–83) years, and they were predominantly male (n = 45, 75%). The clinical tumor volume had a median of 52.7 (range, 22.4–233.1) cm^3. All patients completed their scheduled treatment course, including eight sessions of mEHT, whose median total energy was 3902 (range, 2704–4429) kJ (the energy value up to 8 sessions is shown in Figure 2a). At surgery, R0 resection was performed in 53 patients (88.3%); R2 resection was not performed. The proportion of lower ypT-stage (ypT0–2) and N-stage (ypN0) was 55.0% (33 patients) and 76.7% (46 patients), respectively. The number of relatively good treatment responses among patients (total and near total regression grade for primary tumors) was 20 (33.3%). All acute toxicity occurred within grade 2. As for late toxicity, there were no >grade 2 events other than grade 3 gastrointestinal toxicity in four cases. Among the analyzed patients, mEHT-related toxicity was mild in all but one grade 2 case (Table 3).

Table 2. Factors associated with neoadjuvant treatment and surgical outcomes ($n = 60$).

Characteristic		Value
Total dose of radiotherapy		40 Gy
Total number of mEHT session		Median 8 (range, 8–9)
Total energy of mEHT (kJ)	<3800	12 (20.0%)
	≥3800	48 (80.0%)
Chemotherapy regimen	5-fluorouracil/leucovorin	4 (6.7%)
	Capecitabine	55 (91.7%)
	Others	1 (1.7%)
Radiotherapy to surgery interval (day)		Median 52 (range, 41–70)
Types of Surgery	Low anterior resection	50 (83.3%)
	Abdominoperineal resection	4 (6.7%)
	Hartmann's procedure	3 (5.0%)
	Others	3 (5.0%)
Resection margin status	Negative	53 (88.3%)
	Positive	7 (11.7%)
ypT	CR, Tis, T1, T2	33 (55.0%)
	T3, T4	27 (45.0%)
ypN	N0	46 (76.7%)
	N1, N2	14 (23.3%)
Stage group	CR, 0(TisN0), I, II, III	26 (43.3%)
		34 (56.7%)
Tumor regression grade	Total, near total	20 (33.3%)
	Moderate, minimal	40 (66.7%)
Lymphatic invasion	Negative	41 (68.3%)
	Positive	5 (8.3%)
	Complete response	9 (15.0%)
	Not available	5 (8.3%)
Venous invasion	Negative	43 (71.7%)
	Positive	3 (5.0%)
	Complete response	9 (15.0%)
	Not available	5 (8.3%)
Perineural invasion	Negative	36 (60.0%)
	Positive	10 (16.7%)
	Complete response	9 (15.0%)
	Not available	5 (8.3%)
Tumor budding	Negative	16 (26.7%)
	Positive	26 (43.3%)
	Complete response	9 (15.0%)
	Not available	9 (15.0%)

mEHT: modulated electro-hyperthermia, SD: standard deviation, CR: complete response.

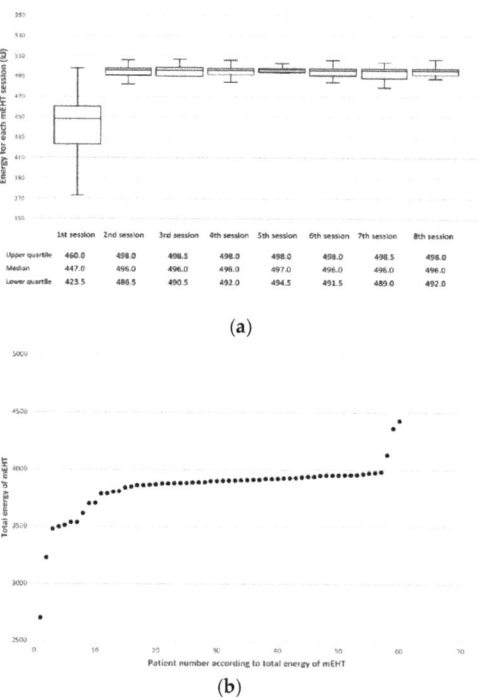

Figure 2. Energy profile of modulated electro-hyperthermia (mEHT) at each mEHT session (**a**) and from the perspective of total value line-up (**b**).

Table 3. Distribution of treatment-related toxicities (*n* = 60).

Toxicity Grade	0	1	2	3	4	5	NA
Acute GI	20	21	19	0	0	0	0
Acute GU	47	12	1	0	0	0	0
mEHT-related *	44	15	1	0	0	0	0
Late GI	16	16	15	4	0	0	9
Late GU	41	11	3	0	0	0	5

GI: gastrointestinal. GU: genitourinary. mEHT: modulated electro-hyperthermia. NA: not available. * Scoring system proposed by the Berlin group [10].

3.2. Survival

We included 60 patients for the log rank test and 52 patients for univariate/multivariate analysis, considering postoperative follow-up loss or missing values for various clinical factors. The 5-year OS, DFS, LRRFS, and DMFS rates were 94.0%, 77.1%, 96.4%, and 78.7%, respectively (Figure 3). A total of two loco-regional recurrences and 10 distant metastases occurred during the follow-up. Each recurrence site was the primary lesion (two patients) and peripheral lymph nodes (one patient), and one case of multiple recurrence or metastasis was observed. Two patients with loco-regional recurrence belonged to the low tumor regression group, one of whom had postoperative positive resection margin status. The distribution of the total mEHT energy showed a relatively rapid change around 3800 kJ, which was used as a cut-off value for the comparison of applied energy judged to be meaningful in terms of the relative balance between energy value categories except for the few extreme values (Figure 2b). When comparing 3800 kJ as a boundary, mEHT energy possibly affected the OS (Figure 4a). Differences according to molecular pathological factors, such as KRAS, BRAF, and microsatellite status, did not appear to affect survival in the mEHT-based group (Table 4). ypN-stage and perineural invasion (PNI) seemed to be related to DFS ($p = 0.003$ and $p = 0.005$, respectively for univariate analysis) and DMFS ($p = 0.011$ and $p = 0.034$, repectively for univariate analysis), which was more remarkable with the complete response group added (Figure 5b). Tumor regression and resection margin status, which are considered to be prognostic factors in preoperative chemoradiation, did not show significant correlation in our mEHT-based patient group (Table 4).

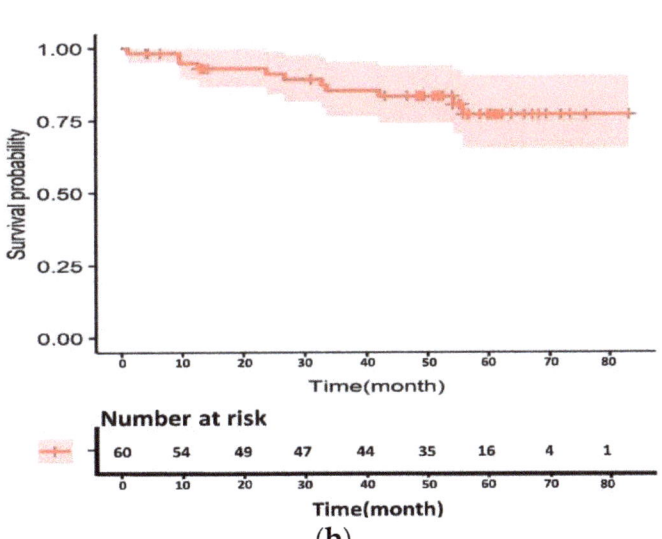

Figure 3. Cont.

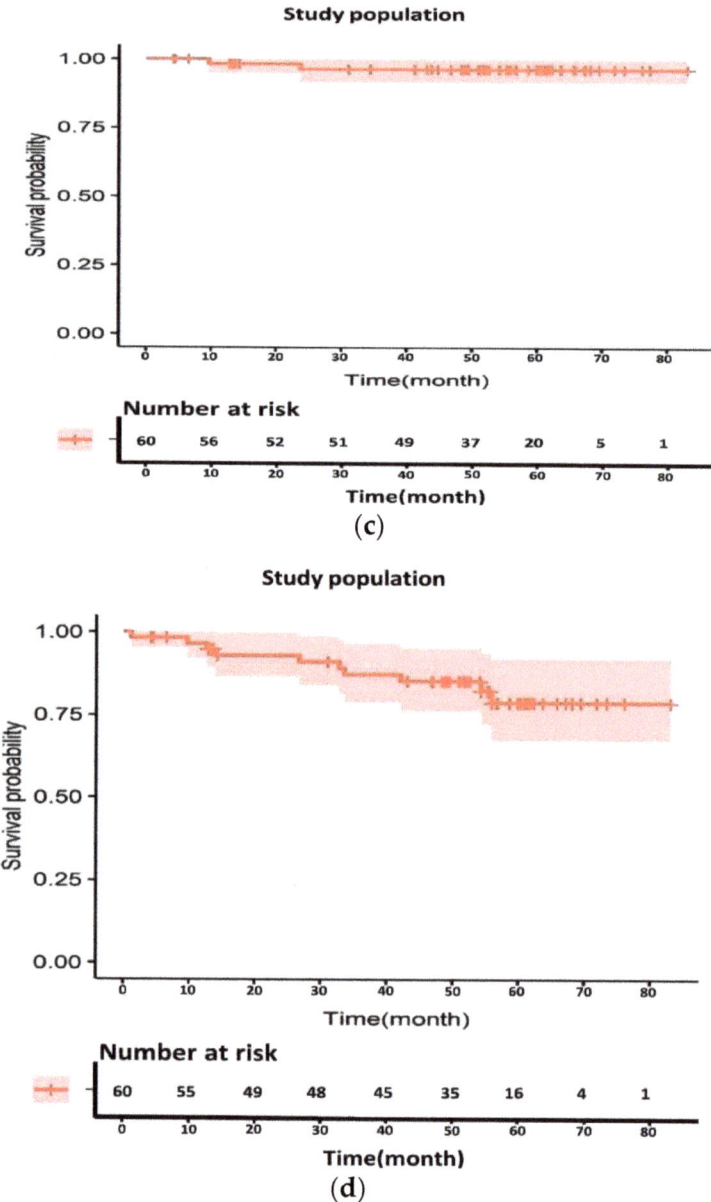

Figure 3. Survival analysis of the study population. (a) Overall survival, (b) disease-free survival, (c) loco-regional recurrence-free survival, and (d) distant metastasis-free survival.

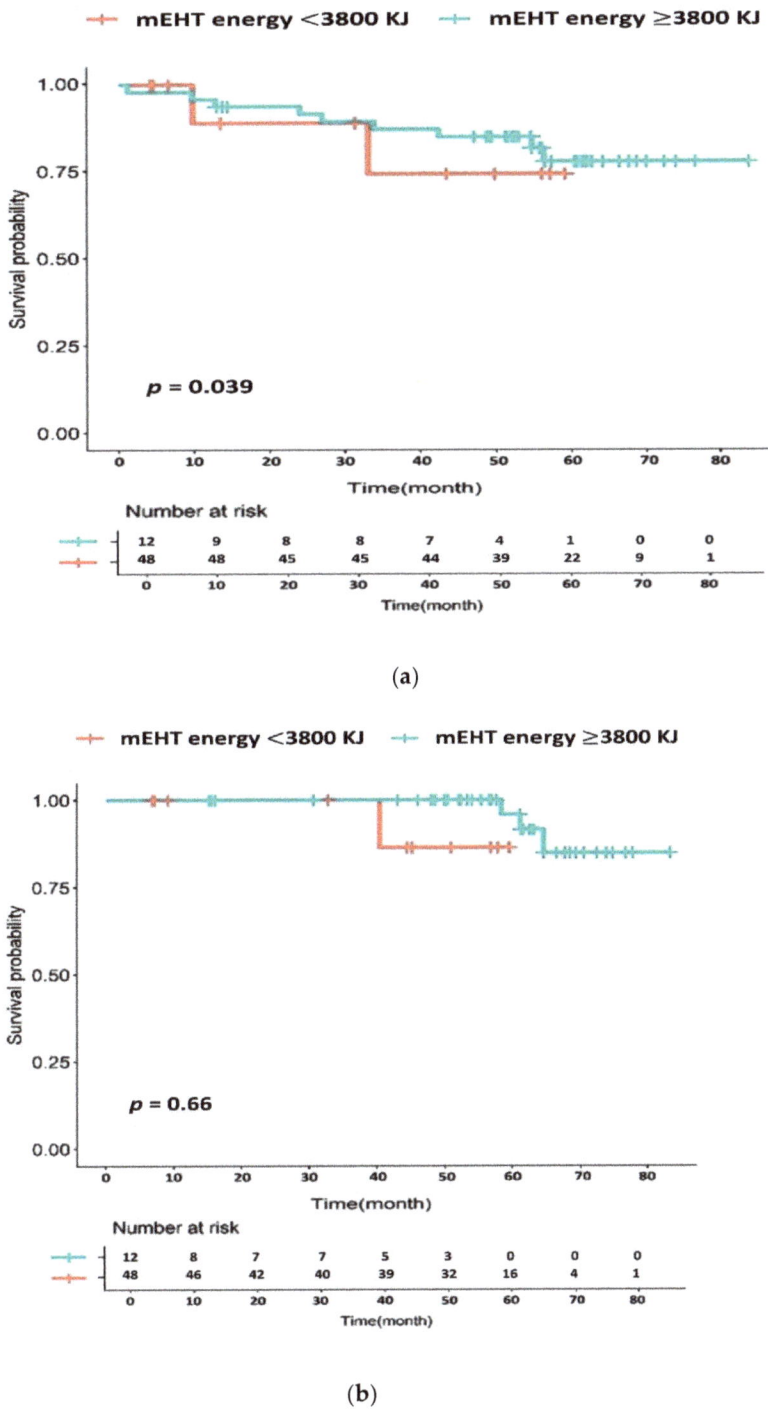

Figure 4. Survival comparison according to modulated electro-hyperthermia (mEHT) total energy by log rank test. (a) Overall survival, (b) disease-free survival.

Table 4. Univariate and multivariate analyses of the baseline variables.

Variable	Category	Univariate			Multivariate		
		HR	95% CI	p	HR	95% CI	p
Overall Survival							
Age (years)	<60 vs. ≥60	1.318	0.184–9.433	0.783	2.990	0.201–44.527	0.429
Sex	Male vs. Female	1.399	0.143–13.695	0.773	2.468	0.164–37.189	0.514
Resection margin status	Negative vs. Positive	9.200	0.575–147.73	0.117	59.458	0.150–23546.9	0.181
ypN-stage	0 vs. 1, 2	1.042	0.104–10.480	0.972	2.111	0.084–53.349	0.650
Tumor regression grade	Total, near total vs. Moderate, minimal	0.574	0.079–4.188	0.584	0.111	0.003–4.608	0.248
Total mEHT energy (kJ)	<3800 vs. ≥3800	0.103	0.006–1.869	0.124	0.402	0.008–19.397	0.645
Disease-free Survival							
Age (years)	<60 vs. ≥60	1.005	0.306–3.297	0.993	1.503	0.386–5.849	0.557
Sex	Male vs. Female	1.061	0.281–4.007	0.930	2.093	0.505–8.669	0.308
Resection margin status	Negative vs. Positive	2.057	0.442–9.568	0.358	5.623	0.375–84.259	0.211
ypN-stage	0 vs. 1, 2	6.630	1.916–22.934	0.003	5.831	0.955–35.594	0.056
Tumor regression grade	Total, near total vs. Moderate, minimal	1.538	0.407–5.811	0.526	0.223	0.036–1.396	0.109
Perineural invasion	Negative vs. Positive	5.744	1.687–19.559	0.005	4.487	0.818–24.630	0.084
Total mEHT energy (kJ)	<3800 vs. ≥3800	0.866	0.186–4.037	0.855	0.311	0.311–49.627	0.290
Loco-regional Recurrence-free Survival							
Age (years)	<60 vs. ≥60	1.239	0.077–19.802	0.880	5.232	0.078–349.23	0.440
Sex	Male vs. Female	2.622	0.164–41.953	0.496	7.443	0.185–298.65	0.287
Resection margin status	Negative vs. Positive	8.571	0.530–138.55	0.130	60.406	0.397–9196.8	0.110
ypN-stage	0 vs. 1, 2	3.087	0.193–49.355	0.425	5.937	0.305–115.46	0.240
Distant Metastasis-free Survival							
Age (years)	<60 vs. ≥60	0.793	0.224–2.811	0.719	0.928	0.229–3.758	0.917
Sex	Male vs. Female	1.208	0.311–4.687	0.784	2.093	0.498–8.793	0.313
Resection margin status	Negative vs. Positive	2.270	0.479–10.768	0.302	4.262	0.311–58.359	0.278
ypN-stage	0 vs. 1, 2	5.341	1.461–19.525	0.011	5.916	0.899–38.941	0.065
Tumor regression grade	Total, near total vs. Moderate, minimal	1.325	0.342–5.137	0.684	0.204	0.033–1.274	0.089
Perineural invasion	Negative vs. Positive	4.082	1.111–14.998	0.034	2.467	0.430–14.146	0.311
Total mEHT energy (kJ)	<3800 vs. ≥3800	0.737	0.155–3.498	0.701	2.221	0.219–22.515	0.500

HR: hazard ratio, CI: confidence interval, mEHT: modulated electro-hyperthermia.

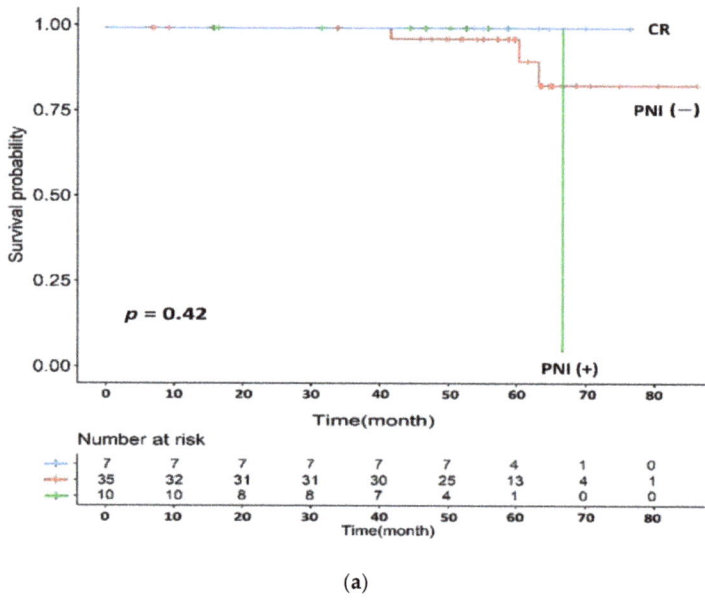

(a)

Figure 5. Cont.

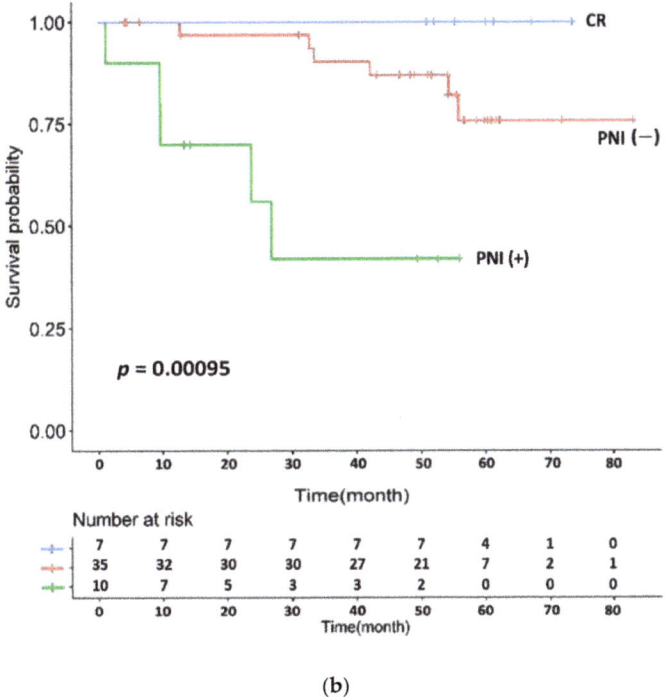

(b)

Figure 5. Survival comparison according to perineural invasion by log rank test. (a) Overall survival, (b) disease-free survival (CR: complete response, PNI: perineural invasion).

4. Discussion

In a recent retrospective analysis based on whether or not mEHT was supplemented, mEHT was effective in downstaging and tumor regression, which was more pronounced in large-sized tumors [11]. We attempted to assess how each clinical parameter affects the survival rates when mEHT is concurrently combined with radiation. This study was limited to ascertaining the significance of mEHT as it focused on descriptive data without a control group. Nevertheless, compared to previous studies on similar platforms, generally non-inferior survival outcomes were obtained. Although the patient characteristics were not completely consistent, 5-year OS and DFS of 94.0% and 77.1%, respectively, were similar to the results of survival improvement by conventional hyperthermia boost (Table 5). Generally, the addition of hyperthermia had excellent results for loco-regional control; however, it rarely resulted in an improvement in the survival rate [1,12].

Although mEHT-mediated survival gain was not clearly identified with a single-arm study, our non-inferior results at least demonstrated the usefulness of mEHT to some extent in the low radiation dose setting of 40 Gy. Despite attempts to improve the oncologic outcome through treatment intensification during chemoradiation, toxicity risk-related uncertainty still remains [13,14]. mEHT, which is relatively free from toxicity, is thought to be effective in more stable thermoradiotherapy. In addition, though very limited, the manageability of mEHT was revealed based on the concept of applied energy rather than intratumoral temperature without invasive parameter measurement. Recent mEHT studies have also reported good clinical cases regardless of temperature measurement [15,16]. Therefore, it is appropriate to investigate whether mEHT boost is a trigger for improving the clinical outcome through non-thermal effects, such as changes in the tumor microenvironment or immunogenicity, while being less affected by temperature.

Although limited, mEHT demonstrated the potential for survival improvement by increasing the total applied energy (Figure 4a). Unlike other previous clinical reports of hyperthermia, our study showed almost no variation in the mEHT-related parameters between patients as most patients possessed high treatment compliance and relatively uniform energy input above a certain level. Hence, the tendency in OS difference by energy level came from a structure wherein determining the prognosis was challenging owing to the tight energy distribution. Therefore, this result is thought to have its own clinical impact compared to the value obtained statistically, representing the importance of the input energy itself.

The low thermotoxicity of mEHT and its high therapeutic compliance are advantageous in terms of treatment management, including applied energy assessment. As originally planned, mEHT was performed in all patients twice a week. The energy for each session showed a slight increase generally up to the 8th session, which is directly contrary to common hyperthermia protocols (Figure 2a). Although the treatment compliance has been improving in conventional hyperthermia via technological advances [14], in most rectal cancer hyperthermia studies, the session number was insufficiently set to less than once a week or did not meet the schedule owing to thermotoxicity [10,12,17–20]. Therefore, mEHT application to the pelvic area is reportedly less associated with thermal toxicity, indicating that thermosensitive patients can adapt to the high-frequency energy as the session is repeated. The unexpectedly high heat sensitivity that appeared in some patients should be compensated by a more individualized approach. Another limitation of our study was that cases of severe obesity were excluded without clear criteria for heat sensitivity. If these cases are supplemented, discovery of biomarkers for mEHT indications and easier treatment application could be achieved.

Among molecular pathological factors, it was found that only PNI specifically affected the survival rates. PNI has been studied in several malignancies, including uterine cervical and head and neck cancers [21,22]; however, it has not been widely assessed in colorectal cancer. There have been limited reports in some colorectal cancer studies that PNI positivity could serve as a factor that lowers the survival rates [23–25]. Thus, a more in-depth study of PNI is needed in terms of the specific situation of mEHT-based neoadjuvant thermoradiotherapy.

In a previous retrospective analysis that included a control group (non-mEHT group), the resection margin status was one of the significant prognostic factors for survival [11]; however, this trend disappeared in this mEHT-dominant group. This could be the result of the difference in the follow-up period or the relatively small number of patients. However, the mEHT-mediated impact also needs to be confirmed, i.e., whether it is large enough to offset the influence of the resection margin, etc. Meanwhile, besides the role of mEHT, it is worth noting that 40 Gy radiation may be sufficient for the neoadjuvant treatment for rectal cancer, which is consistent with the latest report that 40–41.4 Gy was sufficient for esophageal cancer treatment [26,27]. Nevertheless, an index comparable to intratumoral temperature has not been established, which is a contemporary problem that needs to be continuously addressed in terms of the quality management of mEHT. These limitations in this study will have to be overcome through a large-scale prospective well-designed clinical trial in the future.

Table 5. Comparison of overall and disease-free survival in previous neoadjuvant thermoradiotherapy studies for rectal cancer.

References	Patient Enrollment	No. of Patients	Radiation Dose	Hyperthermia Machine	No. of Hyperthermia Session	Overall Survival	Disease-Free Survival
Maluta et al., 2010 [18]	Phase II	76	60 Gy (50 Gy + 10 Gy boost)/ 30 times	BSD-2000	Once a week (5 times)	86.5% (5 years)	74.5% (5 years)
Kang et al., 2011 [12]	Retrospective	98	Group A: 39.6 Gy /22 times, Group B: 45.0 Gy/25 times	Cancermia GHT-RF8	Twice a week (1–11 times)	73.9% (5 years)	75.1% (5 years)
Gani et al., 2016 [28]	Retrospective	60	50.4 Gy/28 times	BSD-2000	once or twice a week (1–9 times)	88.0% (5 years)	77.0% (5 years)
Gani et al., 2021 [29]	Phase II	78	50.4 Gy/28 times	BSD-2000	Twice a week (1–10 times)	94.0% (3 years)	81.0% (3 years)
Ott et al., 2021 [14]	Prospective	89	50.4 Gy/28 times	BSD-2000	Twice a week (1–11 times)	82.0% (5 years)	57.0% (5 years)
Current study	Phase II	60	40 Gy/20 times	Oncothermia EHY-2000	Twice a week (8–9 times)	94.0% (5 years)	77.1% (5 years)

5. Conclusions

A non-inferior effect of 40 Gy radiation plus mEHT combination was substantiated in the long-term survival of patients. In a slightly low-dose radiation platform, less thermotoxic mEHT can be considered to aid in rectal cancer treatment. In the long term, a segregated approach from conventional hyperthermia is warranted in the overall management with a reasonable consensus on the applied energy index.

Author Contributions: Conceptualization, S.H.Y.; methodology, J.H.H. and S.H.Y.; validation, Y.L., S.K. and S.H.Y.; formal analysis, Y.L., S.K., H.C. and S.H.Y.; data curation, J.H.H., S.K. and S.H.Y.; writing—original draft preparation, Y.L., S.K. and S.H.Y.; writing—review and editing, S.K., H.C., H.J.C., E.G. and S.H.Y.; visualization, J.H.H. All authors have read and agreed to the published version of the manuscript.

Funding: This research received no external funding.

Institutional Review Board Statement: The study was conducted according to the guidelines of the Declaration of Helsinki, and approved by the Institutional Review Board of Wonju Severance Christian Hospital (IRB No.: CR313035; date of approval: 18 February 2014).

Informed Consent Statement: Informed consent was obtained from all subjects involved in the study.

Data Availability Statement: Data used in this study can be provided by the corresponding authors upon request. Data cannot be shared publicly due to privacy concerns.

Conflicts of Interest: The authors declare no conflict of interest.

References

1. De Haas-Kock, D.F.; Buijsen, J.; Pijls-Johannesma, M.; Lutgens, L.; Lammering, G.; van Mastrigt, G.A.; De Ruysscher, D.K.; Lambin, P.; van der Zee, J. Concomitant hyperthermia and radiation therapy for treating locally advanced rectal cancer. *Cochrane Database Syst. Rev.* **2009**, *3*, CD006269. [CrossRef] [PubMed]
2. Vancsik, T.; Kovago, C.; Kiss, E.; Papp, E.; Forika, G.; Benyo, Z.; Meggyeshazi, N.; Krenacs, T. Modulated electro-hyperthermia induced loco-regional and systemic tumor destruction in colorectal cancer allografts. *J. Cancer* **2018**, *9*, 41–53. [CrossRef] [PubMed]
3. Kuo, I.M.; Lee, J.J.; Wang, Y.S.; Chiang, H.C.; Huang, C.C.; Hsieh, P.J.; Han, W.; Ke, C.H.; Liao, A.T.C.; Lin, C.S. Potential enhancement of host immunity and anti-tumor efficacy of nanoscale curcumin and resveratrol in colorectal cancers by modulated electro- hyperthermia. *BMC Cancer* **2020**, *20*, 603. [CrossRef] [PubMed]
4. Krenacs, T.; Meggyeshazi, N.; Forika, G.; Kiss, E.; Hamar, P.; Szekely, T.; Vancsik, T. Modulated electro-hyperthermia-induced tumor damage mechanisms revealed in cancer models. *Int. J. Mol. Sci.* **2020**, *21*, 6270. [CrossRef]

5. Andocs, G.; Renner, H.; Balogh, L.; Fonyad, L.; Jakab, C.; Szasz, A. Strong synergy of heat and modulated electromagnetic field in tumor cell killing. *Strahlenther. Onkol.* **2009**, *185*, 120–126. [CrossRef]
6. Lee, S.Y.; Kim, J.H.; Han, Y.H.; Cho, D.H. The effect of modulated electro-hyperthermia on temperature and blood flow in human cervical carcinoma. *Int. J. Hyperth.* **2018**, *34*, 953–960. [CrossRef]
7. You, S.H.; Kim, S. Feasibility of modulated electro-hyperthermia in preoperative treatment for locally advanced rectal cancer: Early phase 2 clinical results. *Neoplasma* **2020**, *67*, 677–683. [CrossRef]
8. Dworak, O.; Keilholz, L.; Hoffmann, A. Pathological features of rectal cancer after preoperative radiochemotherapy. *Int. J. Colorectal. Dis.* **1997**, *12*, 19–23. [CrossRef]
9. Cox, J.D.; Stetz, J.; Pajak, T.F. Toxicity criteria of the radiation therapy oncology group (rtog) and the european organization for research and treatment of cancer (eortc). *Int. J. Radiat. Oncol. Biol. Phys.* **1995**, *31*, 1341–1346. [CrossRef]
10. Rau, B.; Wust, P.; Hohenberger, P.; Loffel, J.; Hunerbein, M.; Below, C.; Gellermann, J.; Speidel, A.; Vogl, T.; Riess, H.; et al. Preoperative hyperthermia combined with radiochemotherapy in locally advanced rectal cancer: A phase ii clinical trial. *Ann. Surg.* **1998**, *227*, 380–389. [CrossRef]
11. Kim, S.; Lee, J.H.; Cha, J.; You, S.H. Beneficial effects of modulated electro-hyperthermia during neoadjuvant treatment for locally advanced rectal cancer. *Int. J. Hyperth.* **2021**, *38*, 144–151. [CrossRef]
12. Kang, M.K.; Kim, M.S.; Kim, J.H. Clinical outcomes of mild hyperthermia for locally advanced rectal cancer treated with preoperative radiochemotherapy. *Int. J. Hyperth.* **2011**, *27*, 482–490. [CrossRef]
13. Haddad, P.; Ghalehtaki, R.; Saeedian, A.; Farhan, F.; Babaei, M.; Aghili, M. Current approaches in intensification of long-course chemoradiotherapy in locally advanced rectal cancer: A review. *Radiat. Oncol. J.* **2021**, *39*, 83–90. [CrossRef]
14. Ott, O.J.; Gani, C.; Lindner, L.H.; Schmidt, M.; Lamprecht, U.; Abdel-Rahman, S.; Hinke, A.; Weissmann, T.; Hartmann, A.; Issels, R.D.; et al. Neoadjuvant chemoradiation combined with regional hyperthermia in locally advanced or recurrent rectal cancer. *Cancers* **2021**, *13*, 1279. [CrossRef]
15. Fiorentini, G.; Sarti, D.; Casadei, V.; Milandri, C.; Dentico, P.; Mambrini, A.; Nani, R.; Fiorentini, C.; Guadagni, S. Modulated electro-hyperthermia as palliative treatment for pancreatic cancer: A retrospective observational study on 106 patients. *Integr. Cancer Ther.* **2019**, *18*, 1534735419878505. [CrossRef]
16. Minnaar, C.A.; Kotzen, J.A.; Ayeni, O.A.; Naidoo, T.; Tunmer, M.; Sharma, V.; Vangu, M.D.; Baeyens, A. The effect of modulated electro-hyperthermia on local disease control in hiv-positive and -negative cervical cancer women in south africa: Early results from a phase iii randomised controlled trial. *PLoS ONE* **2019**, *14*, e0217894. [CrossRef]
17. Schroeder, C.; Gani, C.; Lamprecht, U.; von Weyhern, C.H.; Weinmann, M.; Bamberg, M.; Berger, B. Pathological complete response and sphincter-sparing surgery after neoadjuvant radiochemotherapy with regional hyperthermia for locally advanced rectal cancer compared with radiochemotherapy alone. *Int. J. Hyperth.* **2012**, *28*, 707–714. [CrossRef]
18. Maluta, S.; Romano, M.; Dall'oglio, S.; Genna, M.; Oliani, C.; Pioli, F.; Gabbani, M.; Marciai, N.; Palazzi, M. Regional hyperthermia added to intensified preoperative chemo-radiation in locally advanced adenocarcinoma of middle and lower rectum. *Int. J. Hyperth.* **2010**, *26*, 108–117. [CrossRef]
19. Tsutsumi, S.; Tabe, Y.; Fujii, T.; Yamaguchi, S.; Suto, T.; Yajima, R.; Morita, H.; Kato, T.; Shioya, M.; Saito, J.; et al. Tumor response and negative distal resection margins of rectal cancer after hyperthermochemoradiation therapy. *Anticancer Res.* **2011**, *31*, 3963–3967.
20. Kato, T.; Fujii, T.; Ide, M.; Takada, T.; Sutoh, T.; Morita, H.; Yajima, R.; Yamaguchi, S.; Tsutsumi, S.; Asao, T.; et al. Effect of long interval between hyperthermochemoradiation therapy and surgery for rectal cancer on apoptosis, proliferation and tumor response. *Anticancer Res.* **2014**, *34*, 3141–3146.
21. Cui, L.; Shi, Y.; Zhang, G.N. Perineural invasion as a prognostic factor for cervical cancer: A systematic review and meta-analysis. *Arch. Gynecol. Obstet.* **2015**, *292*, 13–19. [CrossRef] [PubMed]
22. Fagan, J.J.; Collins, B.; Barnes, L.; D'Amico, F.; Myers, E.N.; Johnson, J.T. Perineural invasion in squamous cell carcinoma of the head and neck. *Arch. Otolaryngol.-Head Neck Surg.* **1998**, *124*, 637–640. [CrossRef] [PubMed]
23. Huh, J.W.; Kim, H.R.; Kim, Y.J. Prognostic value of perineural invasion in patients with stage ii colorectal cancer. *Ann. Surg. Oncol.* **2010**, *17*, 2066–2072. [CrossRef] [PubMed]
24. Peng, J.; Sheng, W.; Huang, D.; Venook, A.P.; Xu, Y.; Guan, Z.; Cai, S. Perineural invasion in pt3n0 rectal cancer: The incidence and its prognostic effect. *Cancer* **2011**, *117*, 1415–1421. [CrossRef]
25. Liebig, C.; Ayala, G.; Wilks, J.; Verstovsek, G.; Liu, H.; Agarwal, N.; Berger, D.H.; Albo, D. Perineural invasion is an independent predictor of outcome in colorectal cancer. *J. Clin. Oncol.* **2009**, *27*, 5131–5137. [CrossRef]
26. Shapiro, J.; van Lanschot, J.J.B.; Hulshof, M.; van Hagen, P.; van Berge Henegouwen, M.I.; Wijnhoven, B.P.L.; van Laarhoven, H.W.M.; Nieuwenhuijzen, G.A.P.; Hospers, G.A.P.; Bonenkamp, J.J.; et al. Neoadjuvant chemoradiotherapy plus surgery versus surgery alone for oesophageal or junctional cancer (cross): Long-term results of a randomised controlled trial. *Lancet Oncol.* **2015**, *16*, 1090–1098. [CrossRef]
27. Yang, H.; Liu, H.; Chen, Y.; Zhu, C.; Fang, W.; Yu, Z.; Mao, W.; Xiang, J.; Han, Y.; Chen, Z.; et al. Neoadjuvant chemoradiotherapy followed by surgery versus surgery alone for locally advanced squamous cell carcinoma of the esophagus (neocrtec5010): A phase iii multicenter, randomized, open-label clinical trial. *J. Clin. Oncol.* **2018**, *36*, 2796–2803. [CrossRef]

28. Gani, C.; Schroeder, C.; Heinrich, V.; Spillner, P.; Lamprecht, U.; Berger, B.; Zips, D. Long-term local control and survival after preoperative radiochemotherapy in combination with deep regional hyperthermia in locally advanced rectal cancer. *Int. J. Hyperth.* **2016**, *32*, 187–192. [CrossRef]
29. Gani, C.; Lamprecht, U.; Ziegler, A.; Moll, M.; Gellermann, J.; Heinrich, V.; Wenz, S.; Fend, F.; Konigsrainer, A.; Bitzer, M.; et al. Deep regional hyperthermia with preoperative radiochemotherapy in locally advanced rectal cancer, a prospective phase ii trial. *Radiother. Oncol.* **2021**, *159*, 155–160. [CrossRef]

Review
Heterogeneous Heat Absorption Is Complementary to Radiotherapy

Andras Szasz

Biotechnics Department, Szent Istvan University, H-2040 Budaors, Hungary; Szasz.Andras@gek.szie.hu

Simple Summary: This review shows the advantages of heterogeneous heating of selected malignant cells in harmonic synergy with radiotherapy. The main clinical achievement of this complementary therapy is its extreme safety and minimal adverse effects. Combining the two methods opens a bright perspective, transforming the local radiotherapy to the antitumoral impact on the whole body, destroying the distant metastases by "teaching" the immune system about the overall danger of malignancy.

Abstract: (1) Background: Hyperthermia in oncology conventionally seeks the homogeneous heating of the tumor mass. The expected isothermal condition is the basis of the dose calculation in clinical practice. My objective is to study and apply a heterogenic temperature pattern during the heating process and show how it supports radiotherapy. (2) Methods: The targeted tissue's natural electric and thermal heterogeneity is used for the selective heating of the cancer cells. The amplitude-modulated radiofrequency current focuses the energy absorption on the membrane rafts of the malignant cells. The energy partly "nonthermally" excites and partly heats the absorbing protein complexes. (3) Results: The excitation of the transmembrane proteins induces an extrinsic caspase-dependent apoptotic pathway, while the heat stress promotes the intrinsic caspase-dependent and independent apoptotic signals generated by mitochondria. The molecular changes synergize the method with radiotherapy and promote the abscopal effect. The mild average temperature (39–41 °C) intensifies the blood flow for promoting oxygenation in combination with radiotherapy. The preclinical experiences verify, and the clinical studies validate the method. (4) Conclusions: The heterogenic, molecular targeting has similarities with DNA strand-breaking in radiotherapy. The controlled energy absorption allows using a similar energy dose to radiotherapy (J/kg). The two therapies are synergistically combined.

Keywords: loco-regional hyperthermia; oncology; modulated electro-hyperthermia; cellular selection; bioelectromagnetics; complexity; immune-effects

1. Introduction

Nowadays, oncology is one of the most complex interdisciplinary experimental and clinical research fields. Clinical success often relies on the sensitive balance between cure and toxicity, providing the most effective but at the same time the safest treatment. Hyperthermia (HT) has promised a simple way to solve the frequent dilemma of complementary treatment choice. Despite its promise and a long history with ancient roots, oncological hyperthermia has had a long and bumpy road to modern medicine, and even today, it has no complete acceptance among oncology professionals. The original ancient idea of hyperthermia is relatively simple: heat the tumor, which forces it to use more resources from the host tissue due to accelerated metabolism, but no extra supply is available. The "starving" tumor destroys itself by acidosis. A deep belief in the curative effect of the fever-like processes, which force self-control of the body, drives the medical concept of "Give me the power to produce fever and I will cure all diseases" [1]. Hippocrates successfully applied radiative heat to treat breast cancer [1]. In vitro measurements have proved this idea [2], measuring a significant impoverishment of Adenosine triphosphate (ATP) and lactate enrichment in treated tumors.

The large group of HT methods contains various therapies using various electromagnetic and mechanical (ultrasound) energy sources. The attention of hyperthermic oncology presently focuses on local-regional heating (LRHT) methods by electromagnetic effects. There are two basic categories of LRHT heating; Figure 1.

1. External radiation focused on the target, trying to heat the tumor mass as homogeneously as possible without considerably heating surroundings tissues. The heating intention is isothermal, but due to the heterogeneity of the target and the heat distribution dynamics controlled by blood flow, the temperature is not homogeneous (see later). The intensive heating of a larger volume (regional heating) achieves an approximately controllable condition in the tumor at the central position. The treatment evaluation involves the ratio of the isothermal areas. The specific power density (SAR) ranges from 4.6 to 89 W/kg [3], depending on the location and size of the tumor, determining the heated volume and its blood flow.

2. Heating good energy absorbers in a localized area by electromagnetic effects, which heats these materials extensively, and in the next step, the absorbers heat up their host tissues. The heating intention is heterogeneous, targets only the dedicated particles (like nanoparticles, seeds, rods, etc.). The dose homogeneity characterizes this method because of the dispersed absorbers. The particles heat up their environment by heat-conduction, realizing more localized heating in the volume. The SAR in nanoparticle methods is surprisingly large because the absorbers have only a tiny mass compared to the surrounding tissue. The small mass (ranging density of 1 mg/cm^3 specifically absorbs extra-large SAR >> 1 W/g = 1 kW/kg or higher [4], because of the absorption on the tiny target. When it heats the neighboring tissues, the average SAR corresponds to the isothermal heating conditions in the range of about a few W/kg. Targeting various chemical bonds uses even higher SAR because the absorbing mass is lighter than the metallic nanoparticle. These methods focus on molecular changes. The temperature is a possible cofactor.

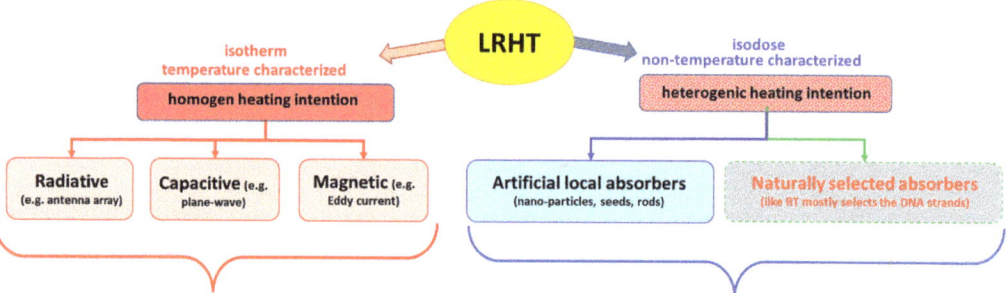

Figure 1. The two essential branches of electromagnetic LRHT methods. The majority of applications use the conventional focusing with isothermal intention. The method requests to measure the temperature as dose characterization. Heterogeneous (non-isothermal) heating is an emerging category of LRHT applications with nanoparticle insertion (mainly magnetic suspension). The heterogenic heating methods do not need direct temperature measurement. The dose measures the absorbed energy (J/kg = Ws/kg), so the tumor's temperature develops by the heat-conduction from the targeted particles. The figure does not show the popular non-electromagnetic LRHT methods (e.g., HIPEC and HiFu).

The success of LRHT is unquestionably conclusive. Results regarding many tumors, including breast [5], head and neck [6], cervix [7], pancreas [8], soft-tissue sarcoma [9], and others [10], provide convincing proof of its place in the field of oncotherapies. In particular, LRHT has had remarkable success, such as in a complementary application with radiation therapy (RT) [11–14], showing a solid synergy [15,16] and being applied successfully in various curative therapies [17–19]. The success of complementary RT + LRHT has a broad spectrum of clinical evidence [20–24], and has been well-reviewed in its details [25–28]. The introduced thermal enhancement ratio (TER) characterizes LRHT's additional gain over RT [29].

Together with the high rate of successes, challenges, of course, also appear. To fulfill our strong motivation to popularize LRHT among oncology professionals, we analyze some of the apparent controversies in LRHT applications, studying these challenges in the search for a solution. The challenges are not limiting but oppositely motivate us to solve the actual difficulties and thereby seize the extreme medical value of hyperthermia in oncology. The challenge guides us to new developments and improvements in the otherwise broad spectrum of hyperthermia facilities in oncology.

1.1. Heating Challenge

The skeptical opinion concerning hyperthermia in oncology was developed in parallel with expectations. A half-century ago, in 1964, a leading German oncosurgeon expressed his doubts [30]: "All of these methods impress the patient very much; they do not impress their cancer at all". His skepticism towards oncological hyperthermia became widespread among medical experts, who declared hyperthermia to be of no benefit to cancer patients and so did not propose it enter actual therapy protocols. Unfortunately, the method has to fight hard for its well-deserved place among stable routine therapies in oncology. Our task is to show the place of HT as the regular fourth column in the oncology arsenal, together with surgery, chemo, and radiotherapies.

The challenges always concern the complex behavior of living organisms, which balances multiple oppositional regulatory feedbacks. The balance gives a character a "double-edged sword", which determines a window of positive actions. When applied outside this window, the helpful actions act oppositely, the difference between support or degradation being only the dose.

The primary challenge connects hyperthermia to the standard systemic homeostatic thermal control according to the complexity. The body temperature provides fundamental conditions of the proper physiologic and molecular processes, so its stability is essential and ranges in a narrow 7/273 (~2.6%) interval in humans. The homeostatic control regulates the system, keeping it stable and adaptable. Heating locally or systemically attacks the regulatory stability, igniting non-linear physiological reactions to correct the system [31]. The body's homeostatic control monitors thermal conditions and regulates its temperature and parts compared to a set-point in the hypothalamus [32], trying to re-establish the unheated temperature. The feedback regulation non-linearly increases the blood-flow (BF) [33,34], as an effective heat exchanger, as well as the regulation intensifying other physiological mechanisms to control conditions [35]. The reactive BF change causes most of the challenges in LRHT applications.

On the other hand, the reaction to the growing temperature also has a supporting behavior. It induces relatively significant protective heat shock proteins (HSPs) in the targeted cells. The extra stress by heating increases the HSPs only slightly in the otherwise heavily stressed malignant cells but causes a drastic gain (8–10 times) in the healthy ones [36]. The difference makes the malignant cells more vulnerable to the temperature increase than the well adapting healthy cells.

1.2. Complementary Challenge

The correct dose application of LRHT is a critical issue in the future of hyperthermia in oncology [37]. Furthermore, the complementary therapy of LRHT and RT requires the precise dosing of both components to ensure safe and reproducible effectivity. RT has a traditional, well-applicable, accepted dose, which determines the isodose by the equal energy absorption in Gy ($= \frac{J}{kg}$) in the chosen target. The isodose energy absorption is not directly dependent on the size of the tumor. The dose is homogeneously distributed across the entire tumor volume, independently of its size; the same dose is maintained in all volume units. The treatment defines the isodose (e.g., fractional dose for daily application) equally, and the complete sum of fractions composes the final dose, which depends on the tumor conditions (localization, size, stage, conditions, cellular specialties, etc.). It is fixed through the planning process and the focusing adjustments realized.

LRHT uses the temperature as an active part of the treatment, applying it for dose characterization. Contrarily, RT regards it as an adverse effect, causing burns and fibrotic conditions [38,39]. A fundamental difference between RT and LRHT appears in their treatment length, and consequently, the applied energies. RT applies a short shot with only a negligible effect on the physiological regulation, while the LRHT treatment time is long (usually 60 min), so homeostatic control is activated. The radiation focus also shows significant differences: the heating produced with LRHT spreads into non-targeted volumes in conductive and convective ways, while RT remains local, being well focused on the planned volume. The frequency of the standard treatments differs too: while fractional RT treats daily, LRHT, due to the HSP protection that develops, cannot be applied so frequently, requiring at least a 48 h break between applications. Unfortunately, the LRHT-produced HSP could be associated with radioresistance too, but on the other hand, LRHT influences numerous other molecular parameters which could sensitize to the RT [40].

RT and LRHT achieve therapeutic synergy in their complementary application despite the differences. The LRHT supports the RT by the thermosensitizing [41] and oxygenation of the target [42]. The active arrest of the cell cycle can realize an essential synergy in different phases by the RT and LRHT. RT is most active in the mitosis phase, while moderate heat shock arrests G1/S and G2/M cell-cycle checkpoints [43]. The LRHT predominantly acts in the S phase of the cell cycle [44] in moderately acidic, hypoxic regions, complementing the cell cycle arrest. Various molecular parameters support the RT efficacy [45], e.g., a heat-induced decrease in DNA-dependent protein kinase [46].

The physiological regulation compensates for the heating effect of LRHT, increasing the BF by vasodilatation to maintain thermal homeostasis. The BF counterbalances the increased temperature by intensive heat-interchange, which in exchange delivers an extended oxygen supply for radio-effects, fixing the DNA breaks [47,48].

The possible synergy of RT and LRHT has a contradictory process. The high BF naturally opposes the Hippocratic "thermal starvation" concept. Nevertheless, the higher metabolic rate of the proliferating mass compensates for the missing supply by non-linearly increasing BF [49–51]. The effects of higher radiosensitivity compete with the increased volume of delivered nutrients due to vasodilation and the heat-promoted perfusion through the vessel walls. On the other hand, the neo-angiogenic arteries do not vasodilate in massive tumors, as they lack musculature in their vessel-wall [52].

Consequently, the reaction to heat differs in the healthy and malignant tissues, exhibiting approximately 38 °C when the BF in the tumor lags the BF in the healthy host [53]. Additionally, the temperature increase can produce vasoconstriction in certain tumors, which decreases the BF and the decrease in heat exchange offers a relatively higher temperature in these regions [54]. This effective heat trap [55] lowers the available oxygen, affecting the efficacy of RT. Parallel at the same time, vasodilatation in healthy tissues increases the relative BF, presenting more cooling media in the volume [56,57], and increases the RT effect in the healthy host tissue counterproductively to clinical safety.

The BF has a central role in maintaining the overall homeostasis. Besides the temperature, it regulates essential parameters like the acid-alkaline equilibrium, glucose delivery, immune actions, and numerous blood-delivered molecular feedback loops in the body. In the precise interaction of RT with LRHT, these parameters may also have remarkable modifying factors. The vascular response of tissues has a tumor-specific temperature threshold, indicated by the kink in the Arrhenius empirical plot [58,59], in consequence of a structural phase transition in the plasma membrane [60].

The above contradictory processes are natural in complex systems, where the suppressor–promoter pairs have an essential role in the dynamic regulation of the homeostatic balance. As always, the regulative processes balance the progressor and suppressor action, so not surprisingly, the radiotherapy-induced damage could cause the activation of damage-repair mechanisms, and survival signaling adds to other factors of tumor-resistive effects [61]. This complex dynamic behavior otherwise guarantees the robust stability of homeostasis as the regulator of healthy processes.

The complementary LRHT and RT synergy also require consideration of the system's complexity. The sum of its distinct parts does not describe the natural cooperating procedures. The interactions are essentially nonlinear, representing that the whole is more than the sum of the parts. The living structures, in their complexity, have a universal behavior: they are self-organized [62]. The basic synergistic possibilities of LRHT and RT are collected in Table 1.

Table 1. The synergistic possibility shows a broad range of advantages for combined therapy of LRHT and RT.

Tumor Characteristics	Oncological Hyperthermia Including All Technical Solutions	Synergy with Radiotherapy
Cell cycle	Arrests the cycle of cells at the S stage, activates the malignant cell from its dormant (G0) phase making attack possible for chemo- and radio-therapies	Radiotherapy arrests the M/G2 stages of the cell cycle well completes the arrest
pH dependence	Kills cancer cells in an acidic environment (Hippocrates' original idea)	It kills cancer cells in an alkaline environment, completes the cell desertion in all environmental conditions
Oxygenation	Acts in the hypoxic state	Acts in an oxygenated state
Increased temperature	Heated tumor mass increases the oxygen delivery	Makes strand breaks on DNA, the fixing of which means oxygen blocks the reparation

1.3. Dosing Challenge

The present dose of HT measured with cumulative equivalent minutes compared to the 43 °C basepoint, (CEM 43 °C) [63,64] fit to the complete necrotic cell killing in vitro [65]. This reference is far from the reality of human medicine. The principal challenge of this dose is that homogenous heating is only an illusion. The approximately isothermal x percent of the heated area at T temperature completes the correct dose. The $CEM\ 43\ °C\ T_x$ [65], where T_x refers to the $x\%$ of the heated mass is approximated with the isothermal condition at temperature T. The dose is, of course, lowered by the growing x value; Figure 2. The isothermal approach tries macroscopically equalizing the temperature with high SAR. The T_x estimation makes macro characterization and does not consider the tissue-defining microheterogeneity of the target.

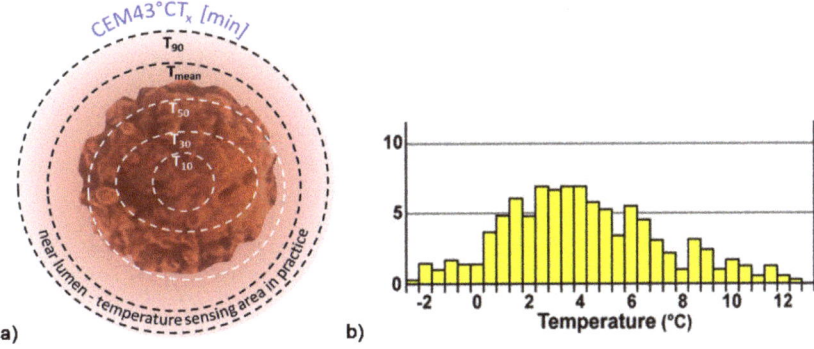

Figure 2. The heated focus rapidly spreads, so the temperature increases in a broader region. (**a**) The CEM43 dose depends on the isothermal areas, which differ by distance and develop by time. (**b**) The temperature distribution across the tumor after 64 min of treatment was measured by MRI (Pat.10. relapsed rectum carcinoma) [66].

The dosing of LRHT has serious challenges. It is much less reproducible and controllable than the dosing in RT. LRHT has huge anatomical, physiological, bio-electromagnetic, mechanical, and thermal heterogeneities, limiting the isodose-type approach of LRHT. The associated isothermal heating uses the temperature as a defining factor of the dose. However, the homogeneity and the lengthy treatment time do not maintain the otherwise precise focus. When the temperature stabilizes in a tiny region, the heat spreads from the targeted volume, and in this way, the intended isothermal region represents only a decreasing fraction of the target. The temporarily defined homogeneous volume may dynamically change by elapsed time; the situation is far from equilibrium [67], and the temperature and space distribution vary. The nonlinear BF and other homeostatic regulatory effects, together with the regular heat flow, destroy the homogeneity.

For example, when the measured temperature is actually T_{90} in 90% of the monitored sites (referred to as the thermal isoeffect dose in 90% of the area), considering the average (assumed homogenous) volume, the $T_{90} > T_{80} > \ldots > T_{10}$, and the T_{100} could be achieved only in a WBH situation. This construction certainly contradicts the homogenous idea.

Due to technical and safety issues in clinical conditions, achieving the 43 °C temperature requires enormous efforts. The challenge is heating the surrounding healthy host by the spread of heat that cannot be avoided with any precise focusing of the radiation beam. Clinical safety requests that the heating not exceed 42 °C in the healthy tissue. The blood flow increases more in the healthy host tissues than in the tumor, causing a particular gradient of the flow intensity to heat the tumor's boundary. The tumor periphery contains the most vivid, mostly proliferative malignant cells. The temperature differences at the tumor border develop a certain BF gradient, which could wash out the aggressive malignant cells, increasing the risk of dissemination.

The $CEM\ 43T_x$ dose has numerous principal challenges [68]. It failed to show the local control characterization of clinical results in soft tissue sarcomas [69] and does not correlate with clinical results for superficial tumors [70]. Complete homogeneity in the heating of living objects could be achieved only in the whole-body hyperthermia (WBH) process. It represents an entirely isothermal CEM 43 °C T_{100} situation. Contrary to isothermal heating, the non-isothermal LRHT shows better clinical results [71], and the results of complementary application to chemotherapy also remain behind the chemotherapy alone [72,73]. However, administering a dose of $CEM\ 43T_{90}$ LRHT also did not show a correlation between dose and clinical outcomes (such as local remissions, local disease-free survival, and overall survival) [74].

Measuring the isothermal situation, determining the $CEM\ 43T_x$ dose has practical challenges. Reliable temperature measurement is an unachievable goal; Figure 3.

1. The invasive temperature sensors available are point detectors. When the point is near the arteries of a highly vascularized area, the temperature is less than in the low vascularization part, so many independent sensors are necessary to attain objective results. However, this induces safety and treatment problems.
2. Usually, a near lumen (such as the esophagus, bronchus, colon, or vagina) offers the possibility to approximate the temperature in the distant tumor, but this is again far from the reality in the target.
3. The most effective temperature mapping can be done with MRI measurement, using a phantom for reference, usually unionized water. The MRI measurement depends on the temperature, but also strongly depends on the structure of the measured volume. In the temperature measurement, both factors are included in calculating the result, but the calibration does not consider a final element: the changes in the structure, which is the goal of the LRHT treatment.

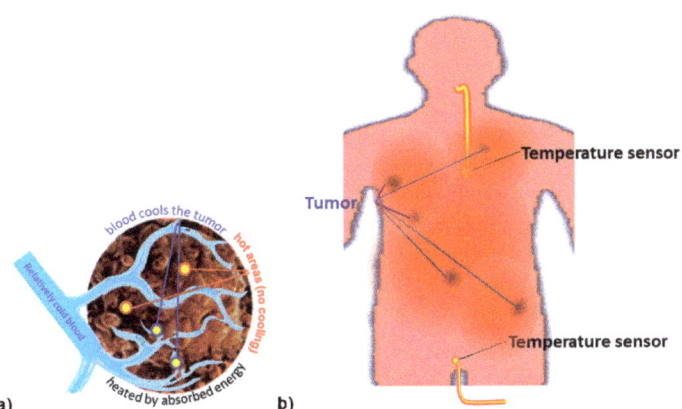

Figure 3. Challenges of temperature measurements: (**a**) the invasively inserted point sensors detect the very local temperature and not the average isothermal; (**b**) the semi-invasive temperature sensing catheters in lumens measure the temperature in near lumens, which could be far from the actual tumor temperature.

1.4. Challenge of the Heated Body

It looks evident that WBH offers the best heating possibility because of its easy control (measurements in body lumens) and the realized complete isothermal load on all the malignant cells and tissues. Notably, the WBH method does not show such good results in the high-temperature regime (≥ 41 °C). The prospective double-arm study shows that the overall survival was less in a combined hyperthermia application than in cases when only chemotherapy (ChT) was administered [72]. The same result was obtained in malignant pleural mesothelioma [73] when the toxicity was also higher in the combined treatments. Contrary to the 10+ times higher CEM 43 °C dose of WBH producing isothermal temperature (CEM 43 °C T_{100}), a fourfold development of metastases was measured in canine sarcomas with radiation therapy with or without WBH compared to the local heating [71]. The mild temperature WBH ($mWBH < 40$ °C and $dose_{mWBH} < \frac{2\ CEM43°CT_{100}}{treatment}$) was effective [75]. (The additional parameter T_{100} to CEM 43 °C denotes that 100% of the tumor received the dose). The mWBH activates the immune reactions, and so it could be a good complementary treatment for other therapies [76–78]. However, the demand for higher temperatures for direct cellular degradation challenges such applications and favors the LRHT application. Contrary to WBH, LRHT does not load the patient's heart, and negligible electrolyte loss happens, and consequently, the inclusion criteria allow more patients.

1.5. Challenge of Homogeneity

The challenge of LRHT differs from that of WBH. While WBH ensured a homogeneous loading of the tumor, achieving homogeneity in LRHT is complicated. The well-focused heated volume spreads by heat-conduction over time, heating larger and larger body regions. The spread of heat triggers BF and so supports the delivery of necessary nutrients (glucose and others) to the tumor. A further challenge is an increasing difference between the BF of the tumor and its healthy host, BF to the host increasing much more quickly than in the tumor. This flow gradient promotes the invasion and dissemination of the cancer cells from the most vivid near-surface region of the proliferating tumor. An early phase III clinical study faced this problem, the straightforward local advances of HT + RT compared to RT alone not appearing in the survival time in breast tumors [79]. Another study obtained the same controversy: local remission success and the opposite in the overall survival [80]. The development of distant metastases was also observed [81]. The same reason led to a debate about LRHT results for the cervix, showing both advantages [17] and disadvantages [82] in survival.

A further study of cervix carcinomas supports the survival benefit [83], but again a critic has questioned this result [84,85]. Another phase III trial of cervical carcinomas with HT plus brachytherapy involving 224 patients noticed the same controversies between survival time and local control [86]. The controversy was observed in a study of locally advanced non-small-cell lung cancer (NSCLC) having a significant response rate improvement, although there was no change in overall survival [87]. A multicenter phase III trial for NSCLC also showed no improvements in overall survival in the hyperthermia cohort [88]. The cause was directly shown: the appearance of distant metastases was five times higher (10/2; $p = 0.07$) in the HT + RT group than in the RT cohort [88]. The study of the surface tumors had the same contradiction between the local control and survival rate [89].

Most likely, the improved dissemination of malignant cells forming micro- and macro-metastases causes contradictory results. We must learn from the contradictions and follow the admonishment of Dr. Storm, a recognized specialist of hyperthermia: "The mistakes made by the hyperthermia community may serve as lessons, not to be repeated by investigators in other novel fields of cancer treatment" [90].

Our task is to improve the controllability of LRHT, ensure the stable, successful applicability of heat therapy combined with RT in oncology, and fulfill the authentic promise that LRHT is an excellent complementary tool for RT [91]. Serious analysis is necessary as has recently been started [92]. I would like to continue this approach and add biophysical aspects. The data showing a highly significant improvement of local control obtained with LRHT and RT represent facts that we must consider as the basis for the further development of oncological hyperthermia and the correction of the problems with overall survival. We must concentrate on blocking invasion and reducing dissemination to overcome the issues. The task is to prevent the formation of metastases caused by heating. Furthermore, we may eliminate the metastases formed earlier, prior to thermal treatment, with the primary tumor's local hyperthermia.

2. Materials and Methods

The radiation similarity of LRHT and RT induces the proposal to characterize the target volume with the isodose load. The isodose concept ensures reproducibility, safety, and efficacy too. The isodose in RT is simply the energy-dose of ionizing radiation measured in Gy ($= \frac{J}{kg}$) and applied to the tumor volume in daily fractions. The energy dosage may be reached in a session during a short time. The heating conditions limit the provision of the necessary energy. The LRHT needs a significantly longer time for a session than RT needs. Consider power, the applied energy per unit time (power, $P\ [\frac{J}{s} = W]$). The energy dose is the sum of the power P_i during the time τ_i when it is applied ($E = \sum_{i=0}^{t} P_i \tau_i$). The power in the unit of mass is the specific absorption rate ($SAR = P/m$, where m is the mass of the target) measured in $\frac{W}{kg}$ units. The energy (E/m) is the dose considering the duration of the SAR load in the target, measured in $\frac{J}{kg}$ units, like the dose Gy in RT. In this way, the SAR offers the possibility to unite the doses of LRHT and RT. The energy increases the temperature, so in an ideal case, the SAR could be applied as the isothermal dose of LRHT.

The heating process starts with an approximately linear rate of temperature growth. It is quasi adiabatic. The relatively slow homeostatic feedback does not disturb the heating [93], and the SAR is proportional with this development in time (t): $SAR \cong c\frac{dT}{dt}$ [31].

Physiological regulation and safety issues challenge this concept. The homeostatic regulation increases the BF in the targeted volume, and like a heat exchanger, cools it down. In this way, higher power is necessary than it otherwise would be desired without this physiological control. The systemic control increases rapidly and non-linearly [31] with different speeds as the BF changes. The treatment's safety requires an intensive cooling of the body surface where the heating power penetrates. The cooling takes away a large amount of the applied energy, not contributing to the heating. The cooling and other energy losses (like radiation, heat diffusion, convection, etc.) limit the application of E as the dose because the actual energy absorbed in the body is uncontrolled. Consequently, temperature measurement is mandatory to estimate the amount of the absorbed power (SAR) in the target.

A new paradigm solves the challenge when the heating does not target the whole mass of the tumor, but the individual malignant cells are in focus [94]. This case avoids overly intensive feedback of the homeostatic regulation, and the various other losses also become more easily manageable. The individual cellular heating breaks the homogeneous isothermal requirement. The absorption is heterogeneous and microscopically individual, using the tumor's natural thermal, electromagnetic, mechanical, and physiological heterogeneity [95].

The heterogeneous molecular actions in the selected volume do not contradict the isodose concept. The apparent contradiction originates from the false expectations of the isodose effect. The isodose does not mean that the action in the target involves all molecules and structures. It means that the isodose grants the desired molecular and structural changes in all isodose volumes. Nevertheless, the required molecular actions are individual and heterogenic. This homogenous-heterogenic vision is well observable in medication. When the body takes a dose intravenously, orally, or in other ways homogeneously in the body, the dose is calculated from the body's volumetric parameter (BMI). However, the expected action of the drug is heterogenic, selectively targeting molecular structures. The ionizing radiation-activated DNA damage is the heterogenic goal of RT. LRHT targets other molecular effects, but the expected effect is incidental due to the averaging of the energy by the isothermal conditions.

The crucial point of the new paradigm is to select the malignant cells and concentrate the energy absorption upon them. The new paradigm is electromagnetic heating, as most applied hyperthermia methods use radiofrequency (RF) current. The current delivers energy to depth, its parameters (amplitude, frequency, and phase) being chosen optimally to find the heterogeneities produced by the malignant cells; Figure 4. All three parameters have dynamic changes by time variation, improving the selection mechanisms. The carrier frequency is amplitude modulated, and the modulation frequency is not constant, but follows the demands of the homeostatic control, representing a spectrum suitable for the spatiotemporal distribution of the cancer cells.

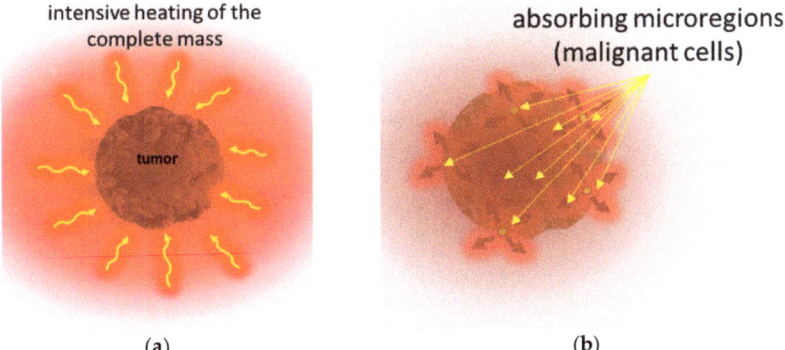

Figure 4. Draft presentation of the heating paradigms: (**a**) Homogeneous mass heating trying to achieve isothermal conditions. It intensively heats the surrounding healthy tissues as well. (**b**) Selective, heterogeneous (heterothermal) heating. It creates a high temperature in the absorbing points, but mild average temperature (<40 °C) in the surrounding healthy tissue.

The heterogeneous heating has a crucial behavior: it provides a high temperature for the selected malignant cells, but the average temperature of the tumor remains under 40 °C. A temperature of over 40 °C downregulates the cytotoxicity of innate immune attacks [96,97], including those of the natural killer cells (NKs) [98]. On the other hand, substantial cellular thermal damage has been observed at temperatures above 41–42 °C [99]. Modulated electro-hyperthermia's (mEHT's) heterogenic heating could harmonize these two otherwise contradictory demands.

Time-fractal modulated electro-hyperthermia (mEHT) supports the selection and induces programmed cell-killing processes, genuinely breaking the isothermal approach. Instead of homogenous heating of the target, mEHT uses excellent selection to force energy absorption on the malignant cells, heating them locally to the hyperthermia temperature to induce cellular changes in the targeted cells by thermal and nonthermal mechanisms [100]; Figure 5. The thermal component of the absorption heats the selected membrane rafts, which is the source of the temperature of the tumor, as is standard in heterogenic seeds or nanoparticle heating processes. In contrast, the nonthermal component causes molecular excitation for programmed cell death [101]. The excitation by electric field E has similar increase like the temperature increases the molecular reaction rate [102]. The cell-membrane represents decreasing impedance with increasing frequency, so the field penetrates the cell with improved intensity. The membrane practically shortcuts and does not significantly influence the RF current flow over ~25 MHz [103].

Nevertheless, the difference between the energy absorption between the membrane and intra- and extracellular electrolytes remains on high frequencies [104]. The primary energy absorption happens in the transmembrane proteins and their clusters on the rafts [105]. The density of membrane rafts is significantly higher than in the nonmalignant cells [106]. The absorbed energy makes the molecular excitation nonthermal and the temperature an essential joint conditional factor, promoting the reaction rate [107].

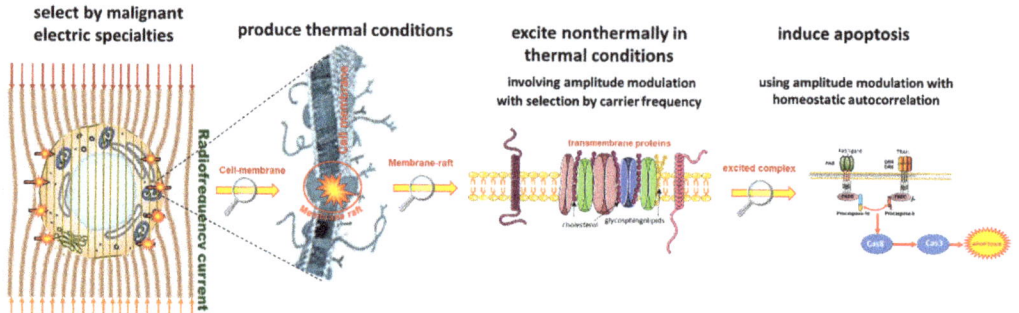

Figure 5. The transmembrane proteins of malignant cells absorb the energy in thermal and nonthermal forms. The amplitude-modulated carrier frequency's nonthermal effect gives the apoptotic signal pathway (see below in results). The carrier frequency delivers the modulated signal and selects the malignant cells, while the modulation with homeostatic autocorrelation (time-fractal) constrains the apoptotic pathway.

The applied selective energy-absorption works like RT and realizes isodose conditions, too, concentrating on very local (nanoscopic) molecular effects, mostly to break the DNA strands in the isodose-defined volume. In this meaning, mEHT and RT have a similar nano targeting philosophy; Figure 6. The target is the natural heterogeneity of the tissues, as RT targets the DNA. The method recognizes the particularities of tumor cells' microenvironment (TME) [108].

Two essential effects are considered for selection: thermal absorption and nonthermal excitation. The thermal component provides the appropriate temperature of the TME by heating the membrane rafts [105]. Another general thermal action affects the extracellular matrix (ECM) and a part thereof, the TME. This acts mechanically and molecularly [109], accompanying the thermal absorption of transmembrane protein clusters.

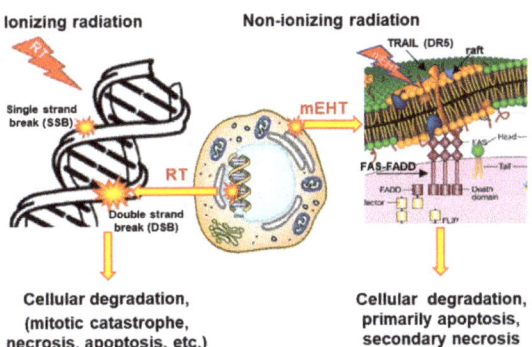

Figure 6. The conceptual similarity of RT and mEHT. Both therapies target molecular bonds, so the primary energy absorption is heterogenic. The result is cellular degradation in various ways.

The nonthermal effect happens when "under the influence of a field, the system changes its properties in a way that cannot be achieved by heating" [110]. The nonthermal component excites the membrane receptors of the cells. The well-chosen electric current can deliver energy for molecular excitations involving various ionic and molecular interactions [31]. The process only has a subtle thermal effect and excites the molecules or structures that fit the applied resonant conditions [111].

The apoptotic signal by the mEHT excited membrane receptors and the apoptosis by the single or double-strand breaking of DNA for cellular degradation are strong similarities of RT and mEHT. Nevertheless, despite conceptional similarities, RT and mEHT have an essential difference: the additional thermal component in HT, which is absent in RT. Thermal absorption is mostly an unwanted side effect in ionizing radiation. The goal is only the molecular effects.

The excitations of transmembrane proteins need low frequency [111], but their neuronal excitation, which may rise to 10 kHz [112], is not safe with the applied power. On the other hand, the frequency for selective heating is in the high RF frequency range. The mEHT solves the challenge of the contradictory simultaneous requirement of high and low frequencies. It uses the appropriate low frequency to modulate the high-frequency carrier; Figure 7 [113]. The membrane rectifies. The carrier frequency in the rectified signal remains active, but mainly at the cellular membrane (β-dispersion, see later). In this way, the original modulation signal makes the excitation process.

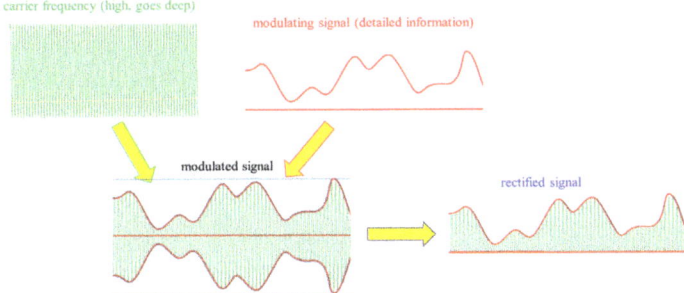

Figure 7. The modulation process compromises between the contradictory high- and low-frequency demands. The unification of the low-frequency modulating signal and the high-frequency carrier forms the modulated signal, a frequency spectrum on the carrier 13.56 MHz. The cell membrane rectifies and works for the excitation of apoptotic pathways. The high-frequency carrier gives the optimal thermal condition for the excitation by the low-frequency info signal in the selected cells.

mEHT is a complex method, which complicates its technical realization. The technical details (Figure 8) need further explanation. I will discuss it in the discussion section of this article.

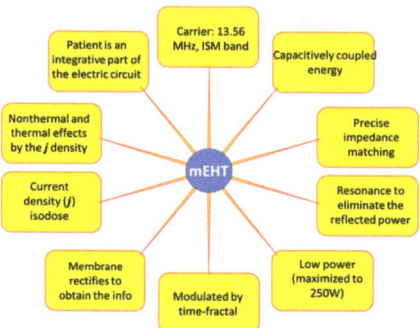

Figure 8. The technical conditions of mEHT. The realization of the method rigorously accommodates and utilizes the complexity of the heterogenic impact of mEHT to arrest the proliferation of cancer and degrade the developed tumor cells.

1. The chosen optimal carrier frequency is 13.56 MHz, which belongs to the freely applicable ISM band [114] and does not need shielding.
2. The energy is capacitively coupled, but it does not use the plane-wave approach. Plane-wave radiation is devoted to isothermal heating.
3. There is precise impedance matching [108] in the mEHT method. Proper impedance matching produces negligible reflected power (order of 1 W), mimicking the galvanic contact with the skin as much as possible.
4. It has resonant matching with micro-selection ability, which fits the impedance [109]. It eliminates the imaginary part of the impedance. It differs from the usually applied plane-wave matching.
5. The maximum adequate output power of mEHT is limited. The power limit depends on the size of the electrode. In device EHY2000+, the maximal power is 150 W, while in the model of EHY2030, which has optionally larger electrodes too, the limit is 250 W. The applied power in therapy depends on the localization and size of the tumor. The power limitation keeps the SAR less than for isothermal heating, but high enough to select and excite the membrane rafts of the malignant cells [100] and sensitizes to the RT [115,116].
6. The modulation spectrum is a low-frequency time-fractal [113], described by fractal physiology [117–120], which agrees with the homeostatic molecular temporal balance [113]. mEHT extensively uses the modulation technique to identify fractal structures in space and time (dynamics) in spatiotemporal identification [113]. The electric parameters (resistance and capacity) depend on the malignant status [121]. The selection between malignant and healthy cells was measured as a characteristic time-fractal [122]. The modulation delivers temporal information executing enzymatic processes at the cell membranes [123], promoting the consequence of the excitation.
7. The membrane rectifies [124,125], and considerably gains the strength of signal intracellularly [103,104]. The rectified signal acts in the low- and high-frequency ranges.
8. The correct impedance matching provides an appropriate electric field that ensures the current density (j). The j is the parameter of the isodose conditions, ensuring the constant current density in the target. A complex value describes the current depending on the phase shift from the applied signal voltage. The dominant dielectric actions (heating and excitation energies) produce thermal and nonthermal effects.
9. The modulated j-current density actively produces both the thermal and nonthermal effects.
10. The patient is interactively connected to the electric circuit, like a discrete element of the RF-net. This solution allows the real-time control of the patient due to the treated tumor being actively sensed and targeted as part of the tuned electric circuit.

Further technical details can be found elsewhere [108].

3. Results

The mEHT method is the focus of intensive research regarding all attributes. Phantom experiments show the proof of the thermal concept, measuring the temperature development in well-chosen chopped-meat phantoms [126,127], and computed results show the validity of heat selection using tissue heterogeneities, also proven in experimental setups [128].

These macro approaches are well completed with the micro-approach, calculating the nano-range thermal and nonthermal components [105].

In vitro experiments fixed the thermal effects to the reference calibration using the U937 human lymphoma cell line [95], and the HT29 and A431 [94] cell lines. The quantitative dose equivalence of mEHT with RT defines the harmonizing basis of cellular degradation in two different lung cancer cell lines, A549 and NCI-H1299 [129].

mEHT is a mild LRHT in the conventional meaning. The temperature dynamically grows in the mass of the liver when there is no tumor inside because selective targeting does not modify the distribution, as temperature measurement in the liver of an anesthetized pig shows [130]. The thermal component of mEHT heats the target, which may be used for temperature mapping in a preclinical murine model [131] at a mild level. A mild hyperthermia temperature level in humans could be measured in cervical cancer, which increases the peritumoral temperature to 38.5 °C, with proper blood flow for the complementary treatments [132].

The comparison of mEHT to wHT and to plane-wave fitted, non-modulated capacitive hyperthermia (cHT) at the same temperature shows a significant improvement of apoptosis with mEHT in the HepG2 cell line [133]. It showed that the wHT and cHT (the homogeneous heating) cause approximately the same low apoptotic rate, which reveals the advantage of the mEHT heterogeneous concept. The breaking of DNA measured with subG1 also significantly improves with mEHT as compared to the conventional homogeneous methods [133]. Radioresistant pancreatic cell lines show extensive DNA fragmentation measured with subG1 after mEHT [134].

The effect has given a possibility to make a reference calibration of mEHT compared to wHT on HepG2 cells shown at ~5 °C [133], while in the U937 cell-line [95], it shows a >3 °C shift to the advantage of mEHT over wHT (Figure 9), it is supposed that the difference indicates a 3+°C higher temperature of rafts than of the TME. The gain of tumor destruction at 42 °C is ≈4.9 fold, which corresponds well with the in vivo experiments (≈4.3) in HT29 colorectal carcinoma [135].

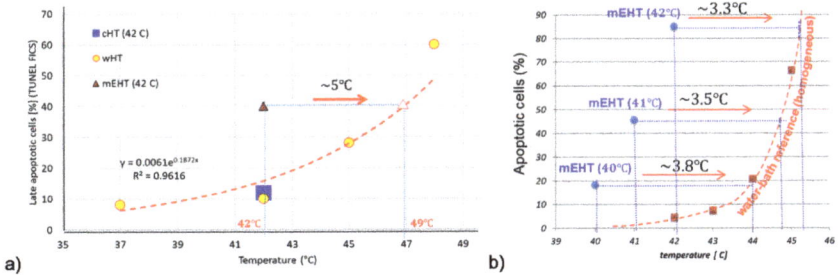

Figure 9. The calibration of the thermal factor of mEHT. (**a**) The homogeneous HT (water-bath hyperthermia, wHT) is used to calibrate apoptosis. The mEHT causes effective apoptosis at 42 °C, corresponding to the calibration at 5 °C higher (HepG2 cell-line) [133]. The mEHT affects the rafts on the cell-membrane with a 5 °C higher temperature than the average medium indicates. (**b**) Another calibration measurement with the U937 cell line [95,136]. The mEHT shows a >3 °C temperature difference in apoptotic efficacy at all measured points.

A critical thermal factor is that the possible touching point of two cells has a drastically increased heat-production due to the extensive SAR at that point [105]. The telophase of the cell cycle naturally forms a tight touching of the two just-created daughter-cells, where the increased SAR could block the finalizing of the cycle and cause the daughter to degrade [137]. Like all complex phenomena, the cytoskeleton's effect could also act oppositely. The reorganization of actin filaments and microtubules by an outside modulated electric field can support the proper polymerization of the cytoskeleton when the cell is only pre-malignant [138]. The close independent malignant cells attract each other by the induced dielectrophoretic forces and the vast electric field gradient between the cells [105]. This makes it possible to reconstruct the intercellular E-cadherin connection, allowing the regular networking of the cells [133]. The deformation of the cells by external field depends on the frequency [139]. The carrier of mEHT is high enough that the deformation is negligible due to the higher conductivity in the ECM than in the cytoplasm [104].

The molecular models concentrate on the membrane effects, showing the thermal and nonthermal results. The same heat conditions force the same processes in the cytosol ER and other cellular organelles, and the heat-sensitive transient receptor potential vanilloid receptor (TRPV) also senses the same temperature for action. The excess ionic concentration is caused by mEHT [140], which increases the influx of Ca^{2+} ions from the ECM to the cytosol. The high iCa^{2+} promotes apoptosis in the mitochondria-dependent intrinsic signal pathway [141]. The decreased membrane potential of mitochondria [136] well supports the mitochondria-associated apoptotic process. The mEHT induces the Ca^{2+} influx with the assistance of E2F1 [142], which regulates the HSPs without heat-shock [143], supporting the possible factors of the nonthermal effect of applied electric current.

Research of the nonthermal effects on HT29 and SW480 human colorectal cancer cell lines shows a significant nonthermal impact on the ionic fluxes, and mEHT has doubled the antiproliferative and anticlonogenic effects of conventional water-bath heating (wHT) at 42 °C [144].

There are tumor-specific thermal and nonthermal stresses with mEHT related to the metabolic profiles of the targeted malignant cells having elevated glycolysis [145]. The efficacy of mEHT may correlate with the tumor metabolic profile by the targeted selection [146].

The nonthermal activity causes structural changes affecting the intracellular polymerization of filaments [138]. The fluctuations also have an essential role in the electromagnetic interaction, showing thermal and electric noise limitation in the TME connected membrane [147].

mEHT applications focus on induced apoptosis [148,149]. The method may cause caspase-dependent paths through Cas8 (extrinsic way) and Cas9 (mitochondrial, intrinsic way) [133,150] and independent [151,152] apoptosis. A notable factor is the arrest of the XIAP effect to block the main path of caspase-dependent apoptosis by the secretion of SMAC/Diabolo [153] and Septin4 [154].

Experiments show that the aggressively radioresistant cell (L9) could be resensitized by mEHT [155], and also, radio-resistant pancreatic cells (Panc1, Capan1) show extended apoptosis when treated with mEHT [134,156,157]. mEHT also destroys these adenomacarcinoma cell lines [148]. The radiosensitization of mEHT significantly intensifies the autophagy and apoptosis in SCC VII and SAS cell lines compared to RT and wHT [158]. The massive apoptotic activity could be used for thermal dose calibration and energy-absorption-based temperature mapping [159].

Curiously, a notable reduction of apoptosis was measured with the addition of artificial gold suspension nanoparticles (NPS) to the targeted volume [160].

DNA fragmentation drives tumor-cell degradation [152]. The induced stress by mEHT upregulates the tumor suppressor p53 protein, a cell-cycle regulator, one of the key cell-cycle regulation and DNA repair players. mEHT activates DSB production. The phosphorylated form of histone family member X ($\gamma H2AX$) as a DSB marker can activate p53.

mEHT significantly upregulates the $\gamma H2AX$ producing DSB in treating a B16F10 melanoma murine tumor model [161], in C26 colorectal allografts [101]. The subG1 cell fraction grows significantly in a radioresistant ductal adenocarcinoma cell-line (Panc1) combined with mEHT + RT 24 h posttreatment [134]. In the same study, the cellular viability drastically decreased in these resistant tumors in mono and complementary therapies with mEHT. As independently expected [162], the thermal component of mEHT acts in synergy with the electric excitation, affecting the repair of DNA. The induced upregulation of cyclin-dependent kinase inhibitor protein ($p21_{waf1}$) and the reduced Ki67 proliferation marker correlates with $\gamma H2AX$, showing that the DSB is related to mEHT treatment [101,163]. The suppression of Ki67 and the significant growth inhibition has been shown in breast cancer murine isograft [164].

The heatmap of the gene expression chip shows the gene regulations of the mEHT-treated samples in an HT29 xenograft [165], in various gliomas [142], and also in vitro in the U937 cell line [136]. The gene map shows a distinct difference in the gene regulations between the homogeneous wHT and inhomogeneous mEHT treatments [136] at the same 42 °C temperature.

Extended research deals with the possible tumor-specific immune processes of the heterogenic thermal and nonthermal effects and supports the emerging science of immuno-oncology. This examination's direction is focused on the abscopal effect, an emerging approach in RT research [166], also recognized by the ASCO [167]. The expectation is a tumor-specific immune situation, considering that cancer precludes regular immune attacks. The mEHT being concentrated on the tumor cells provides immunogenic information for the adaptive immune system about the malignant state and simultaneously sensitizes the tumor to the innate immune attack. This situation could extend the RT + mEHT local synergy to be active in the entire system.

The research concentrates on the optimal liberation of the genetic information from the cancer cells during their degradation. We found that the best process to achieve our goals is "soft" killing, not degrading the secreted molecules with too large an energy load. So, we suppressed the necrosis and the observed apoptosis based on the immunogenic efforts. One particular type of apoptosis, immunogenic cell death (ICD), was the aim, which is associated with a damage-associated molecular pattern (DAMP) as expected in the abscopal activity of RT too [168]. The promotion of damage-associated molecular pattern signals in an HT29 xenograft clearly showed a DAMP when treated with mEHT [165]. In parallel research, the innate NK*-cell activation to attack the selected malignant cells was also proven in A2058 melanoma in a murine xenograft model [169].

DAMP productive mEHT has been supported with various immune supports, which otherwise had no impact on cancer alone. The support by dendritic cells (DCs) has shown to be an excellent addition to mEHT, despite its inactivity alone. The combined treatment showed a perfect abscopal effect on the preclinical murine model, using SCC VII malignant cell inoculation to the animal [170], detecting $CD3^+$, $CD4^+$, and $CD8^+$ T-cells resulting from DC maturation create antigen-presenting cells (APCs), increasing the S100 DC marker [171]. The presence of killer-T-cells ($CD8^+$) increased significantly. The mice had two distant tumor lesions (in the femoral and chest region) modeling metastases. The femoral region was treated, and the chest remained untreated. After multiple treatments, an apparent abscopal effect was observed, and the tumor growth was completely blocked in the untreated chest tumor and the treated femoral [170]. Importantly the T_{reg} protumoral activity was blocked as well, measured with Foxp3 suppression.

The abscopal effect of multiple mEHT treatments alone has been shown in B16F10 melanoma pulmonary metastases, where a significant anti-tumor effect, reducing the number of pulmonary metastatic nodules, and high immune cell infiltration was also present [163].

Similar results were obtained in another study, significantly improving the immunological tumor microenvironment with mEHT followed by dendritic cell immunotherapy [172]. This study also showed that no immune-effect happens with wHT at the same 42 °C temperature. A remarkable result of this study was that the rechallenge of the cured animals with the same malignant cell-line was rejected, observing the adaptation of the immune system, behaving like "tumor-vaccination".

A natural herbal immune-support, Marsdenia tenacissima (MTE), caused a similar arrest of the tumor development systemically after mEHT, despite it being ineffective alone [173,174].

mEHT's combination with the simple conventional tumor-suppressive drug Doxorubicin (Dox) shows a robust immune activation observed with ICD, DAMP, and APC production and having a solid synergy with mEHT in intensively producing DSB, measured by $\gamma H2AX$ [175].

The starting point of human applications is safety. One of the most sensitive organs, the brain, was tested by dose escalation to measure the safety in human glioma cases, proving the safety of mEHT [176]. Many RT-related clinical therapies combine the heat effects with radio-chemotherapy (ChRT). The reason is to be effective systemically by using the drug when LRHT and RT are only local. The ChRT could be a complete game-changer because the reaction rate of chemo-agents exponentially rises by reciprocal temperature (Arrhenius law) and makes cell death independent from RT or HT effects.

A Phase III trial comparing randomized cohorts of ChRT $\pm$ mEHT in clinical practice showed an excellent response to the combination with mEHT compared to the ChRT alone [177], and the toxicity was also low [178]. The abscopal effect was directly measured in addition to the Phase III study [179,180], showing a significant increase compared to the otherwise expected systemic effect of the ChRT. RT in combination with mEHT with checkpoint inhibitors also shows the abscopal effect in various tumors [116], supposing the immune-modulator function of mEHT [181]. Tumor-directed immunotherapy in the combination of RT and mEHT is also a possible option [182]. Table 2 lists 25 studies using mEHT complementarily to RT or ChRT, but the complete study list also contains monotherapy and chemotherapy.

Some recent reviews are available for references regarding conceptual [31,111], technical [94,108], preclinical [101,108], and clinical [183–185] aspects of the mEHT method, showing its efficacy in oncology.

Table 2. The table refers only to the clinical results obtained with mEHT complementary to RT or ChRT.

No.	Tumor Site	Number of Patients	Treatment Used	Results	Reference
1	Advanced gliomas	12	mEHT + RT + ChT	CR = 1, PR = 2, RR = 25%. Median duration of response = 10 m. Median survival = 9 m, 25% survival rate at 1 year.	Fiorentini, et al., 2006 [186]
2	Various brain-gliomas	140	mEHT + RT + ChT	OS = 20.4 m. mEHT was safe and well tolerated.	Sahinbas, et al., 2007 [187]
3	High-grade gliomas	179	mEHT + RT + ChT	Longstanding complete and partial remissions after recurrence in both groups.	Hager, et al., 2008 [188]
4	Glioblastoma & Astrocytoma	149	mEHT + RT + ChT (BSC, palliative range)	5y-OS = 83% (AST) in mEHT vs. 5y-OS = 25% by BSC. 5y-OS = 3.5% in mEHT vs. 5y-OS = 1.2% by BSC for GBM. Median OS = 14 m of mEHT for GBM and OS = 16.5 m for AST.	Fiorentini, et al., 2019b [189]
5	Advanced cervical cancer	236	Random. Phase III (RT + ChT ± mEHT) [preliminary data]	Preliminary data for the first 100 participants. A positive trend in survival and local disease control by mEHT. There were no significant differences in acute adverse events or quality of life between the groups.	Minnaar, et al., 2016 [190]
6	Advanced cervical cancer	72	mEHT + RT + ChT	CR + PR = 73.5%; SD = 14.7%. The addition of mEHT increased the QoL and OS.	Pesti, et al., 2013 [191]
7	Advanced cervical carcinoma	20	mEHT + RT + ChT	mEHT increases the peri-tumor temperature and blood flow in human cervical tumors, promoting the radiotherapy + chemotherapy	Lee, et al., 2018 [132]
8	Advanced cervical carcinoma	206	Random. Phase III (RT + ChT ± mEHT) [abscopal effect]	The abscopal effect grows significantly with mEHT complementary to ChRT.	Minnaar, et al., 2020 [178]

Table 2. Cont.

No.	Tumor Site	Number of Patients	Treatment Used	Results	Reference
9	Advanced cervical carcinoma	206	Random. Phase III (RT + ChT ± mEHT) [toxicity & Quality of life]	mEHT does not increase the toxicity of ChRT but increases the quality of life	Minnaar, et al., 2020 [178]
10	Advanced cervical carinoma	202	mEHT + RT + ChT	Six-month local disease-free survival (LDFS) = 38.6% for mEHT and LDFS = 19.8% without mEHT (p = 0.003). Local disease control (LDC) = 45.5% with mEHT LDC = 24.1% without mEHT; (p = 0.003).	Minnaar, et al., 2019 [177]
11	Advanced NSCLC	97	mEHT + RT + ChT	Median OS = 9.4 m with mEHT OS = 5.6 m without mEHT; (p < 0.0001). Median PFS = 3 m for mEHT and PFS = 1.85 m without mEHT; p < 0.0001.	Ou, et al., 2020 [192]
12	Advanced NSCLC	311 (61 +197 +53)	mEHT + RT + ChT	Two centers PFY (n = 61), HTT (n = 197) control (n = 53). 80% (PFY), 80% (HTT) had distant metastaises, conventional therapies failed. Median OS = 16.4 m (PFY), 15.6 m (HTT), 14 m (control); 1st y survival 67.2% (PFY), 64% (HTT), 26.5% (control).	Dani, et al., 2011 + Szasz, 2014 [193]
13	Advanced rectal cancer	76	mEHT + RT + ChT	Downstaging + tumor regression, ypT0, and ypN0 were better with mEHT than without. No statistical significance.	You et al., 2020 [194]
14	Various types of sarcoma	13	mEHT + RT + ChT	Primary, recurrent, and metastatic sarcomas responded to mEHT, the masses regressed.	Jeung, et al., 2015 [195]
15	Advanced pancreas carcinoma	106	mEHT + RT + ChT	After 3 m, PR = 22 (64.7%), SD = 10 (29.4%), PD = 2 (8.3%) with mEHT after 3 m of the therapy. In group without mEHT in the same time: PR = 3 (8.3%), SD = 10 (27.8%), PD = 23 (34.3%). The median OS = 18 m with mEHT and OS = 10.9 m without mEHT.	Fiorentini, et al., 2019 [196]
16	Advanced pancreas carcinoma	133 (26 +73 +34)	mEHT + RT + ChT	Two centers PFY (n = 26), HTT (n = 73) control (n = 34). 59% (PFY), 88% (HTT) had distant metastases, conventional therapies failed. Median OS = 12.0 m (PFY), 12.7 m (HTT), 6.5 m (control); 1st y survival 46.2% (PFY), 52.1% (HTT), 26.5% (control) QoL was improved.	Dani, et al., 2008 [197]
17	Metastatic cancers (colorectal, ovarian, breast)	23	mEHT + RT + ChT	OS and time to progression (TTP) were influenced by the number of chemotherapy cycles (p < 0.001) and mEHT sessions (p < 0.001). Bevacizumab-based chemotherapy with mEHT has a favorable tumor response, is feasible, and well-tolerated for metastatic cancer patients.	Ranieri, et al., 2017 [198]
18	Rectal cancer	120	mEHT + RT + surgery	In mEHT group, 80.7% showed down-staging compared with 67.2% in non-mEHT group.	Kim et al., 2021 [199]
19	Gliomas	164	mEHT + RT + ChT	CR + PR is 41.4% for mEHT and 33.4% for conventional therapies.	Fiorentini et al., 2020 [200]
20	Ovarian, cervical cancer		mEHT + RT + ChT	The feasibility and success of oncothermia is proven.	Wookyeom, et al., 2018 [201],
21	Various sites	784	mEHT + RT + ChT + surgery	Preliminary results show promising survival trajectories. mEHT is a safe treatment with very few adverse events or side effects, allowing patients to maintain a higher quality of life.	Parmar et al., 2020 [184]
22	Various sites		mEHT + RT + ChT	Planned trial.	Arrojo et al., 2020 [202]
23	Various sites		mEHT + RT + ChT	The feasibility and success of oncothermia are proven.	Szasz AM et al., 2019 [183]
24	Advanced glioblastoma	60	mEHT + RT + ChT	No added toxicity by immunotherapy. Median progression-free survival (PFS) = 13 m. Median follow-up 17 m, median OS was not reached. The estimated OS at 30 m was 58%.	Van Gool, et al., 2018 [203]
25	Different types of metastatic/recurrent cancers	33	mEHT + RT	CR = 2 (6.1%), Very good PR = 5 (15.2%), PR = 13 (39.4%), SD = 9 (27.3%), PD = 4 (12.1%). Three patients (9.1%) developed autoimmune toxicities. All these three patients had long-lasting abscopal responses outside the irradiated area.	Chi, et al., 2020 [116]

4. Discussion

All complex therapies overcome a contradictory process by considering one of the robust behaviors of this complexity: self-organization and the consequent self-similarity [204]. Recent decades have seen the development of various approaches describing the complexity of systems with self-organization [205,206]. The homogenous approach does not consider the natural heterogeneity of complex living systems. mEHT applies the selection of microtargets to distinguish the various parts and functions of the living organism.

4.1. The Electromagnetic Selection

The selection at the macro scale uses the intensive metabolic activity of the malignant cells to produce increased ionic density in the TME of the cells. In this way, the entire tumor has a higher complex conductivity (σ^*) for the electric current than its healthy environment [105,207–210]. The conductivity is proportional with the imaginary part of the complex dielectric function (ε^*), depending on the ionic density (strength) of the target. A part of the high conductivity could be followed using positron emission tomography (PET). The PET measures the intensified glucose metabolism, producing enhanced ionic concentration (primarily lactic acid). The PET results could be considered in the planning of RT [211], as it is a good addition for mEHT seeing the tumor activity, which is connected to the selectivity of the method. The electric current will choose the most accessible route (the most conductive one), flowing through the tumor.

Another electromagnetic selection mechanism concentrates on microregions (TMEs) using distinct structural heterogeneity. The individual autonomic development of cancer cells weakens the intercellular connections, breaking the E-cadherin protein connections. The malignant processes' breaking of the networking order also differentiates them in this parameter. In this way, the TME starts becoming gradually disordered by the development of the malignant network-breaking character shown in early observations by NMR measurements [212–214]. The disorder increases the dielectric permittivity (ε) of the microregion [215–218]. The high ε drives the mainly chosen radiofrequency (RF) current like the high σ does. The plasma membrane and the TME absorbs the central part of the energy in the MHz region of the RF current [104]. The microregion of the tumor cells has considerable gradients of the electrolyte constituents of the electrolyte. The TME is in direct contact with tumor cells, containing molecular bonds to the membrane surface, while ECM is wide. Its primary function is connected to the transport processes. The water content of the TME interacts with the membrane [219], having variant bonds [220], and critically alters the membrane effect, showing a low SAR but high voltage drop [221], which can help the signal's excitation of the raft proteins [222]. The electrostatic charge of the membrane attracts the ions from the ECM, whose very different effect is sufficient to establish a transmembrane potential [223].

The rafts operate as a trigger of the cellular processes [224]. The rafts collect dynamic proteins [225], including proteins with high lateral mobility in the membrane [226]. The cataphoretic forces generated by modulated electric fields induce lateral movements and are sensed by the rafts in the membrane [140]. The size of these clusters is in the nano range. It depends on the ratio of protein to lipid content, different ranges of their horizontal diameters have been measured: 10–100 nm [227]; 25–700 nm [228]; 100–200 nm [229]. The width of the membrane is 5 nm [230], but the thickness of rafts, due to their transmembrane proteins, has a larger size. Note that the temperature increase of the nanoparticle (NP) is proportional to the square of its radius [231], which gives an easy comparison of the temperature using the sizes of the particles. The standard applied SAR in nanoparticles, considering their weight heating is 100–1500 MW/kg [4]. The mEHT heats not only the rafts but heats the TME and also the tissues to a lesser extent. Rough approximation of the absorbed power of rafts by mEHT is SAR > 1 MW/kg [105]. However, the role of absorption differs in nanoparticle and raft heating. The absorbed energy in nanoparticles produces only heat, while in the rafts with excitable structures, the energy divides into thermal and nonthermal effects.

The relatively large rafts contain approximately half of the membrane mass because of their relatively large mass compared to the lipids, representing only 2% of the membrane components [104]. The targeting of the rafts induces accurate energy absorption. The incorporation of energy happens at clusters of transmembrane proteins [95,140]. The temperature of the selected rafts is over the thermal averaging of the tissue. On average, the relatively small SAR is high in the rafts, similarly to the nanoparticle selective heating.

The selection of mEHT is demonstrated in an experiment with artificial NPs added from suspension to the targeted volume [160]. The injecting gold NPs or other artificial good energy absorbers produce a higher quantity of energy absorption in the target. The temperature grows by the diffuse heating from these too. Despite the more intensive energy absorption, the observed apoptosis in these cases decreases [160]. Probably, the sharing of the energy between the membrane rafts and the NPs causes this contradictory effect. The phenomenon supports the proofs of the selection by mEHT.

The selection appears in the ECM too. The current which flows in the extracellular electrolyte heats it more in the areas of selected TMEs than in the membrane-isolated cytosol. The energy analysis of the heating differences explains how this effect contributes to cell-killing mechanisms [109].

Well-defined conditions limit the SAR in the target, which limits the average power provided.

1. The thermal effect happens in nanoscopic local "points", the rafts. These NPs are molecular clusters and sensitive to overheating. When the absorbed energy is too large, it destroys the rafts by overheating. The mEHT loses its most significant advantage, the excitation of signal-transports for apoptosis and immunogenic cell death (ICD).
2. The selection mechanisms of mEHT also limit the SAR, which forces temperature development. At high temperatures, the heat spreads extensively, and the microscopic differences vanish on average. A macroscopic average will characterize the target, as in WBH. The limited energy absorption is mandatory for the selection of rafts.
3. The appropriate frequency is selected around 10 MHz [94]. When the frequency is larger (>15 MHz), the membrane impedance becomes too small to select the disordered TME accurately. The current will flow through the entire target tissue almost homogeneously, neglecting the selection heterogenic selection factors of malignant cells. When the carrier frequency does not ensure selection, the modulation also activates the healthy cells. The significantly larger amount of membrane rafts between healthy and malignant cells [106] remain selective factors only.

4.2. Nonthermal Processes

Healthy dynamism realizes a certain and strictly ordered set of molecular signals in space and time to maintain homeostatic control. The functional signals repeatedly correlate with the given functions (for example, the metabolic cycles), causing an autocorrelation of the resultant signal [232,233]. Note that spatial autocorrelation is a valuable tool in studying the microarchitecture of TME [234]. A significant periodic component in a data set has data points in a time series that correlate with the preceding data points in time, consequently measuring the self-similarity of different delay times in the signal. The autocorrelation could be simply visualized in the particular self-overlapping value of the signal (how the signal correlates with its earlier values). Hence, when the signal is shifted with a time lag, it correlates with earlier values.

The autocorrelation makes preferences of bioeffect variants [235], changing chemical reactions, selecting them by their timing, and ordering them by the time required for the desired signal-pathway or enzymatic actions. The biological effects happen on a broad time-scale. An adequately chosen time-fractal modulation promotes the desired autocorrelation of the signal. This modulation noise regulates the biosystems to their normal homeostasis [236], and the spatial autocorrelation also ensures the harmlessness of white-noise excitation [237]. On the other hand, the otherwise healthy support has an opposite impact on malignant processes. It does not harmonize with the malignant processes, is absorbed in an anharmonic way (heating), and does not excite the molecular signals. The modulation signal selectively supports or blocks the cellular membrane's preferred (healthy) or avoidable (malignant) processes. This dynamic effect expands the electrodynamic selection mechanisms, taking effect not only in structural but also in dynamical malignant irregularities in the health system. Both the structure and dynamics of living organisms have a fractal pattern. The spatiotemporal structure and its consequence, the signal character measured by the fluctuations, differentiate malignant tissue from healthy [121] and are measurable by the RF current [122]. The fluctuation difference between malignant and healthy tissues grounds the applied modulation on the RF carrier. The mEHT therapy uses a pattern recognizing and harmonizing fractal modulation [113] to keep the natural homeostatic control as effective as possible. The well-chosen fractal modulation favors the healthy homeostatic control and combats malignancies outside this regulation [113]. The applied modulation in mEHT considers the natural heterogeneity in space and dynamics, including the autocorrelation of living processes.

Depending on the RF frequency, various processes happen in biomaterials, described by frequency dispersions [238]. The α-dispersion covers the low-frequency interactions (~10 Hz–~10 kHz). This dispersion affects the molecules near the cell membrane interacting with the TME, the various membrane components, and the transmembrane proteins. Ionic electrodiffusion affects the dielectric loss of bound water in molecules. Intercellular charging appears as the main change in α-dispersion. This region signifies our excitation activity. However, its direct application is limited by its missing selectivity and the risk of dangerous nerve stimulation. The task was to find a frequency that selects, does not make nerve stimuli safe, and penetrates deeply into the body. The higher frequencies are satisfactory, and the combination of those with low frequency in modulation solves this complex problem by applying 13.56 MHz carrier frequency and modulating it with a spectrum of frequencies in α-dispersion range.

The 13.56 MHz belongs to the β-dispersion. The broad range of β frequency dispersion [111,239] (known as the interfacial polarization effect) allows selective treatment [240].

The chosen 13.56 MHz select the cellular formations [241] interacting with the interface of membrane-electrolyte structures, using Maxwell-Wagner relaxation [239] causing interfacial polarization of the cell membranes [242]. It changes the charge distribution at the cellular or interfacial boundaries [219]. A part of β-dispersion takes effect in the torque of biological macro-molecules (like proteins) and orients these contrary to the thermal background [243].

The range of the δ-dispersion [244,245] overlaps with β-dispersion interacts with the dipolar moments of proteins and other large molecules (like cellular organelles, biopolymers) [246], and affects the suspended particles in TME [247]. The δ-dispersion is primarily selective for water-bonded lipid-protein complexes in the membrane rafts [219].

Important practical point to choose the carrier frequency in the β/δ interval, and internationally approved for industrial, scientific, and medical use. A total of 13.56 MHz was ideal for these requests. The model calculation also shows the importance of the 13.56 MHz [248]. The electrolyte and membrane differences between the malignant and healthy tissue [249,250] are involved in the selection. The membrane lipid targeting has recently come into focus, and it is recognized as having potential for cancer therapy [251]. Note that the rearranging (disordering) of the water structure at the membrane is clearly visible in the absorption spectra and needs energy [252], which could be obtained from the RF current density.

The carrier frequency's RF energy ensures the selection and absorbs on the membrane rafts [105]. The modulation in α-dispersion makes the requested excitation affects their receptors [140], which destructs the malignant cells dominantly in an apoptotic way [253]. Theoretical considerations also prove the nonthermal effect of mEHT, showing that the observed effects could not have a solely thermal origin [254]. The physical origin is also explained [255] and centers on the effect of the modulation.

The bioelectromagnetism determines various features of homeostasis [256]. The modulation is not a single frequency. It is a spectrum of $1/f$ spectral density in the audio range (<20 kHz), improving the electric field's homeostatic connection by a similar time-fractal structure. The autocorrelation of the signal prefers the external apoptotic pathway. The membrane gains the rectified signal [106], so the 10% modulation depth satisfies the expected signal excitation. The adaptation of this spectrum is in its $1/f$ ("pink") noise structure [236,237] which depends on the target and automatically modifies the effect of modulation by the noise structure in the TME [147].

This dynamic selection and distortion of malignant cells detect and treat. In this way, the mEHT is a kind of theranostic method.

4.3. Effect of RF Current Density and the Dynamic Heating

Impedance-matched mEHT uses the current density j as an isodose parameter. The current density does not depend on the technical losses outside of the target. It considers only the power which goes into the body. The isodose of j is approximative. It is rigorously true only for homogeneous targets. A large average statistically offers a quasi-homogeneity. This homogeneity expectation is a typical challenge in doses of chemotherapies, which expect the homogeneously transported drug in the body, which selectively destroys the malignancy. In the mEHT method, the same challenge appears in the homogeneity concept.

The j depends on the conductivity (σ) and the electric field strength vector (E): $j = \sigma E \left(\frac{A}{m^2}\right)$. The j vector and the σ conductivity are complex numbers, and due to the biomaterial not being a perfect conductor, it is lossy. The electric field drives both the thermal heating and the nonthermal excitation processes, and it is linearly proportional with the complex j, ($E = \frac{1}{\sigma}j$) so the current density well describes the amount of excitation, so linearly generates a nonthermal effect. In a good approximation, j does not depend on the size of the applied capacitor plates. The size of the plate defines the area $A = r^2\pi$ of the circular electrode with radius r. The current (I) depends on the electrode voltage (V) and the resistivity (R) between the electrodes: $I = \frac{V}{R}$. The current density $j = \frac{I}{A}$ while $R = \frac{d}{\sigma A}$, where d is the distance between the electrodes. Consequently, $j = \frac{V\sigma}{d}$, depends on only the constant parameters and does not depend on the area or radius of the electrode. The j can be kept constant when the electric potential is constant. The volume between the plates has an equal dose, as with the homogeneity principle of systemic chemotherapy.

The power (P) as the absorbed thermal energy depends on the square of the field: $P = \sigma E^2 = \frac{1}{\sigma} j^2 \left(\frac{W}{kg}\right)$. In homeostatic conditions, when the general energy loss is negligible, the measurement of the incident power (correlation with j^2) offers a dose identification. The dose, in this case, is the time summary of the power ($dose = \frac{energy}{mass} = \int P dt = \int \frac{j^2}{\sigma} dt, [\frac{J}{kg}]$). The high efficacy of current matching [257], and the low value of the cooling energy-loss allows this simple dose monitoring [68,258] instead of by the local temperature. Consequently, mEHT has no compulsory demand to measure the temperature. It has enough accuracy to measure the absorbed energy by the incident, not forced RF current density [68].

When the temperature grows, the heating period demands a higher dose than when keeping the temperature constant [150,159]. The higher power increases the dose by $j \sim \sqrt{P}$. The heating excites the selected molecular clusters and actively promotes the ICD and the essential immuno-related processes [31]. Maintaining the temperature compensates for the energy losses, so it needs a smaller dose. The unchanged temperature with lower current density produces significantly less apoptosis as the active heating period raises the temperature [259]; Figure 10. The amount of apoptosis increases by the synergy of the temperature dynamics and the electric field, but practically does not change when the temperature stabilizes and remains approximately constant. Stochastic explanation describes this phenomenon [31]. This complexity involves the similarity of the temperature and the electric field to improve the chemical reaction rate [102]. This effect provides a possibility to improve the heterogenic selective cell destruction by mEHT in clinical practices. The therapy needs a protocol that keeps the temperature development's dynamism [31]. Step-up heating considering the blood flow washing time (approximately 6 min) works approximately well.

Contrary to the homeostatic balancing, intensive cooling supports the growth of the incident power. Forced intensive cooling increases the current density because the incident power must increase quadratically, replacing the power taken by the cooling. Due to the applied cooling (energy loose), significantly modifying the incident power does not provide accurate dose measurement. The dose needs other direct registering, like temperature or current density j. The j flows through the patient practically independent from the energy losses, characterizes the absorbed SAR only. Consequently, the direct measurement of the current density appears as the dose in an intensive cooling process instead of the power.

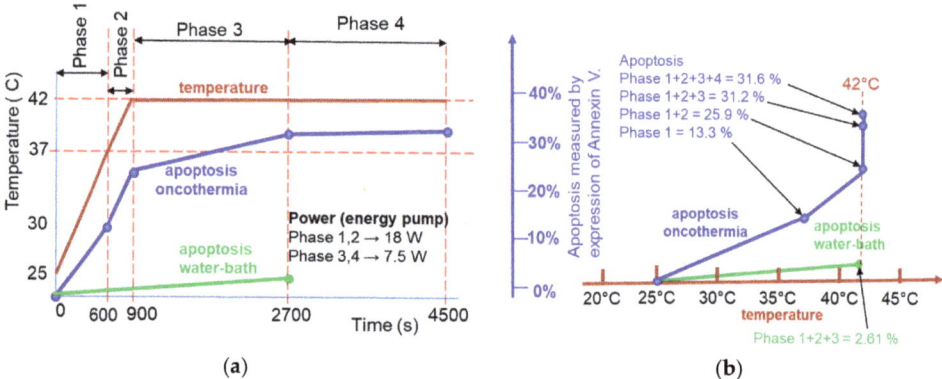

Figure 10. The effect of heating and maintaining the temperature on apoptosis. The mEHT had significantly higher apoptotic cells than the wHT at the same temperature. (**a**) The apoptosis saturated when the temperature became constant at the temperature maintenance period of treatment. (**b**) The temperature dependence of apoptosis shows a limit at the saturated temperature.

The apoptosis of malignant cells shows the efficacy of mEHT therapy. The apoptotic cellular degradation could be used for dosing in the active heating period [259]; Figure 11. Consequently, the connection of the apoptotic cell degradation and current density appears like an essential task of the new dose when the j is enhanced by cooling.

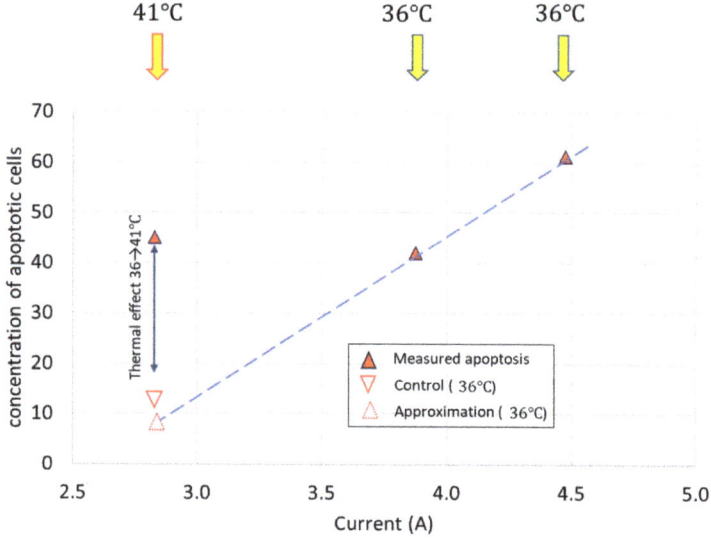

Figure 11. The apoptosis linearly increases by the increase of current density. The higher current density was reached by intensive cooling of the sample, keeping the medium at 36 °C, while the standard treatment was at 41 °C. The difference in the approximated apoptosis at low current at 36 and at 41 °C is produced by the thermal effect.

The current density is proportional to the percentage of apoptosis. Measurements on the U937 cell line well prove this concept [136]. The concentration of apoptotic cells grows linearly with the current density j of mEHT; Figure 11. The standard mEHT treatment was performed at 41 °C, with a standard current density. The control is a sham experiment, which fits a linear line. The heat effect of the standard treatment could be approximated from this experiment.

The current density j appears as an optimal dose of mEHT. On the other hand, the j does not offer a dose solution for conventional LRHT methods, where the patient impedance matching is far from the resonance. The measured current density in LRHT does not show the effective targeting of the tumor, having reflected imaginary parts and various other impedance losses. Temperature measurement remains mandatory in the conventional homogeneous mass heating of LRHT.

The percentage of the apoptotic processes induced by mEHT grows by increasing current density, which participates in both fundamental processes of this method: in the thermal and nonthermal action components. The thermal effects ensure the conditions for optimal nonterminal (excitation) processes and the rates of chemical reactions (mostly enzymatic assistances) afterward. We may regard the current density as a treatment dose, having the same role in mEHT as the ionizing isodose in RT.

The j represents an isodose distribution in the target with mEHT, like the beam isodose in the RT method. Note that this dose could happen only when the energy loss is low, and the overall energy intake is not as high as the heterogeneity differences that may appear with massive heating. Hence, the sensing heterogeneity limits the incident power. When the heating forces isothermal conditions, the $SAR \sim j^2$ dominates, and the heterogenic structure becomes thermally homogeneous. The isothermal temperature overshadows the electrical differences in the target. The electromagnetic differences become gradually visible when the incoming energy decreases. The electromagnetic effects distinguish the electrical differences when its average absorption intensity does not exceed the distinct energy levels of the difference between the absorption values of the desired differentiable units, so when the $j \geq j^2$. So, in conditions when $j \leq 1$, the selection of tumor cells is effective.

The proper modulated signal may trigger resonant excitations of the proteins [111], which initiates extrinsic signal pathways for apoptosis [101,253] in a dose-dependent way [259]. Consequently, the thermal factor generating hyperthermia temperatures creates an appropriate condition for the nonthermal electric field effect by optimizing the reaction rates and enzymatic reactions. The direct thermal and nonthermal effects complete each other, creating a complex synergy of mEHT actions; Figure 12.

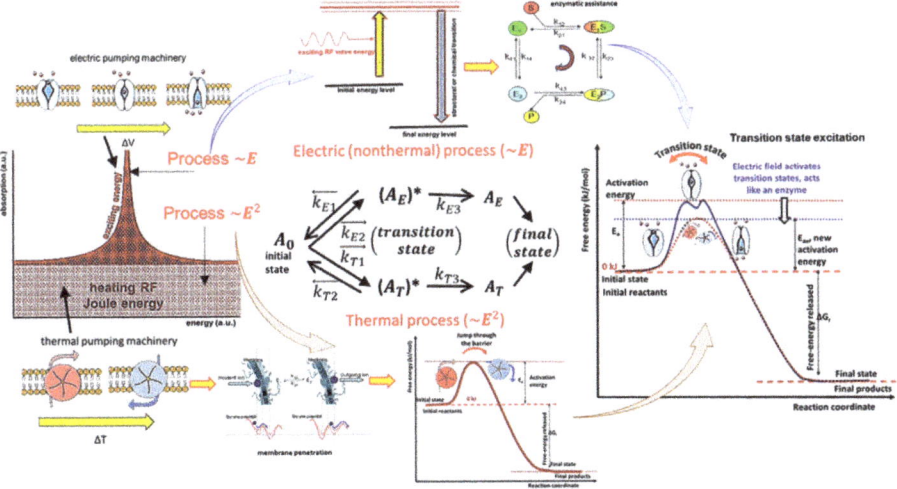

Figure 12. The measured thermal and nonthermal effects of mEHT. The thermal effect has an Arrhenius character, while the nonthermal effects are quantum-mechanical, promoting enzymatic processes, pushing through the transitional state. The nonthermal processes use the thermal conditions for optimal reaction rates. (For details, see in the text.). The * denotes metastable transitional state.

4.4. Complementary to Radiotherapy

The temperature distribution in the hyperthermic process also has complex balancing. The homogeneously high temperatures (>42 °C) in LRHT could block the enzyme activity [260] and so arrest the DNA-repairing enzymes and optimize the cellular degradation of malignant cells [261]. However, they produce massive necrosis, which makes the DAMP release unstable, as well as the high temperature (>40 °C) blocking the immune-cell activity [96], which would be necessary for APC production to form tumor-specific processes. The heterogenic heating of mEHT unites the advantages of the high cellular temperature with the mild average. The thermal component of mEHT (T_{mEHT}) produces a mild hyperthermic average (38 °C $\leq T_{mEHT} <$ 40 °C), which is enough for a blood-flow increase [132] to sensitize the RT, but less than the immune-cell inactivation limit [96]. The temperature of the selected cells (T_{cell}) is well over the average ($T_{cell} \gg T_{mEHT}$), at least by 3 °C as obtained from the apoptotic rate [95,133] and tumor degradation [135,150] (see Figure 9).

Complex balancing appears in various features of the hyperthermia processes. LRHT accelerates the distortions of malignant cells, reducing the α/β ratio in the linear-quadratic model (LQM) of cell-survival in RT [262]. The LQM neglects the third term of the Taylor expansion of the function of dose ($f(D)$) in an exponential dependence from the efficacy (RT_{eff}), which is reciprocal with the cellular survival ($S_{cell} = \frac{1}{RT_{eff}}$), supporting $S_{cell} = e^{-f(D)} \cong e^{-\alpha D - \beta D^2}$. High efficacy means a quick decrease of the S_{cell} by the applied RT dose, so the quadratic term is expected to be high. The hypo- or hyper-fractionating tries to fit the α/β ratio to the survival of cellular variants [263].

It is predicted that LRHT optimizes the α/β ratio [264], which can be used for quantitative reference for an equivalent radiation dose of mEHT [129]. Due to the LRHT effect varying by types of cancer cells, the quantitative dose reference was measured on two different lung cancer cell lines, A549 and NCI-H1299. The dose escalation by mEHT well fits LQM and made it possible to estimate the reference dose determined by equivalence.

The daily RT fractions destabilize the cellular membrane [265], which is a possible general target for cancer therapy [266]. The mEHT attacks the membrane by thermal and electric field load, supporting the membrane destabilization. The double stress of mEHT (heat and field) probably also destabilizes the plasma membrane. The observed intensive apoptosis in many mEHT measurements in various tumors and the synergy with fractional RT concludes that the membrane destabilization helps the apoptosis and does not lead to necrotic cell death. The tripling of the apoptotic bodies in radioresistant pancreas tumors in mono-mEHT and mEHT + RT combined therapies [134] supports the idea that the destabilized membrane helps form apoptotic bodies.

Both the RT and the mEHT induce reactive oxygen species (ROS) as well as damaging subcellular structures and organelles (such as the cytoplasmic membrane, endoplasmic reticulum (ER), ribosome, mitochondria, and lysosome), affecting various biological activities globally altering the living processes of cancer cells, and possibly promoting autophagy too [61]. Results show the intensive promotion of autophagy with mEHT and mEHT + RT to produce apoptosis [158].

The synergy has been proven clinically in the combination of mEHT compared to RT or ChRT alone [116,179]. The frequency of LRHT and the timing with RT are essential considerations in the clinical practice of complementary therapy. The combined application of these methods has synergy, considering the complex regulations connected with both parts. The central focus of the RT makes a single or double break of a DNA strand (SSB or DSB). Inhibiting the DNA repair is the expected primary support from LRHT. RT needs radiosensitive conditions to fulfill its task, while LRHT (as shown with mEHT too [132]) gives oxygenation for the inhibition of the repair and/or arrests the activity of repair enzymes. The $\gamma H2AX$ monitors the repair after RT is connected to the DSB of DNA.

4.5. Sequences and Timing of Treatments in Complementary Therapy

Both therapies, mEHT and RT, could cause cellular destruction in their stand-alone application, inducing necrosis. mEHT in monotherapy produces massive apoptosis [134,142,150], even in radioresistant cases [148]. These distortion mechanisms are mostly independent of the subsequent therapy, while in the application as the second in the sequence, a strong dependence could be formed.

The optimal timing between RT and mEHT has a spatiotemporal complexity, challenging the sequencing and frequency of the combination. The RT defines the application sequence:

- When the oxygenation (blood flow intensity) is high, we expect sensitivity for RT, so apply it first. The maximal frequency of mEHT is every second day.
- When the tumor has hypoxic conditions (low oxygen content), apply the first mEHT to increase it and sensitize the RT.

Further considerations can modify the above sequences depending on the tumor and its grade. The temperature effect also modifies the clinical issues, so we list some features in general for HT effects, where mEHT could also be involved.

- When HT is applied first, it sensitizes the RT by oxygenation of the tumor, but there could also be an inhibitory effect when HT induces hypoxic conditions, which may happen at higher temperatures than 43 °C, which usually does not happen with mEHT.
- Both HT and RT produce heat shock proteins (HSPs). The RT-induced stress also produces these chaperone proteins in different amounts and types. For example, HSP70 and HSP27 are involved in regulating the base excision repair (BER) enzymes in response to RT stress [267].
- Developing an antiapoptotic HSP70 chaperone defines the minimal time between the repeated HT treatments. Due to the HSP70 back to the baseline 48 h post-treatment. Consequently, every second day is recommended as the most frequent application. The maximal time between the HT treatments is one week when the possible buildup of the adaptive immune system finishes.
- HT has effects that are not dependent on enzyme activity, such as a variety of irreparable DNA mismatches, heat-activated methylation, hydrolysis, mono- or di-adduct damages, etc. The activity of repairing enzymes grows by temperatures, but at high temperatures (generally 43 °C) it blocks their activity. The enzyme block could be helpful. The high temperature causes intense hypoxia in the tumor and suppresses the RT efficacy, so mild heating of mEHT is optimal.
- HT at lower temperatures is sufficient to enhance perfusion [70] and the formation of numerous reactive oxygen species (ROS), such as hydrogen peroxide, superoxide anions, nitric oxide, hydroxyl radical, etc. Superoxide dismutase (SOD) forms an essential component in the defense against ROS. Heat stress could cause a decrease in SOD levels, which also leads to cell death [268].
- There is a risk that HT could support the activity of DNA repairing enzymes when it is applied after RT, even also when the end temperature is as high to block the enzymatic activity, because the first part of the heating is a "warming up", presenting a preheating, which could increase the activity of reparation enzymes [269].

The DSBs are typically repaired within two to six hours following RT. A higher rate of the $\gamma H2AX$ expression was observed at three hours as compared to one hour post-RT treatment, signaling that the DSBs are still left unrepaired [270] 3 h posttreatment. However, this could depend on the type of malignant cells [271]. By 6 h posttreatment, $\gamma H2AX$ decreases approximately to half the amount [272]. Combining LRHT with 2 Gy radiation, the concentration of $\gamma H2AX$ after 1 h at 42 °C is higher than at 39 °C [273], and it is observed that a shorter time between the treatment parts results in a higher number of $\gamma H2AX$.

A 90 min timing between LRHT and RT significantly decreases the treatment efficacy in clinical practice compared to a shorter (60 min) delay [274]. The subsequent in vitro modeling on SiHa and HeLa cell lines [275] did not significantly impact the time interval as in the clinical data, while earlier in vitro studies showed a significant difference preferring the treatments to follow each other quickly [276]. Another in vitro experiment supports quick sequences, observing that the DSB of DNA, measured with $\gamma H2AX$, vanishes after

2 h of RT [274]. Earlier, it was shown that simultaneous application has the highest efficacy [277].

A high number of patients was studied, and a large impact of timing between LRHT and RT of 4 h was not observed [278]. This contradictory result started an intensive debate between the research groups [279,280]. The discussed disagreement of the two clinical studies is confusing indeed. The reasons could have multiple components. The different devices, the sequence order of the treatments, and the frequency of the LRHT application could represent differences between the therapies and lead to a contradictory conclusion. The first thirty minutes of "warming up" could be considered preheating, which could increase the activity of reparation enzymes, including a risk that LRHT increases the DNA-repairing enzyme activity and supports the repair of DNA when LRHT is applied second in the sequence [269]. The warming-up period is mostly technically dependent, but depends on the nonlinear physiologic control of the complex regulation of the patient, which could rely on the bolus cooling and other device-dependent conditions. The warming-up period with the non-homogeneous thermal effect by mEHT behaves oppositely than conventional LRHT. mEHT generates the most significant apoptotic activity in the warming-up period [259]. When the LRHT-induced temperature is high enough (>42.5 °C), it could imply the blocking of the repairing enzymes. However, the necrotic cell-killing is also intensive in this high-temperature regime so that the DNA damage could have secondary importance in cellular degradation.

Note, the murine models in vivo (C3H mammary carcinoma) [281] show the thermal enhancement ratio (TER) extensively decreases and at the end vanishes after 4 h in both sequences when the LRHT precedes or follows RT, while the tumor control has a much narrower (30 min) and non-symmetric interval.

The cell-cycle arrest is connected to the electric field activity and is primarily non-thermal [282]. A part of the electric field penetrates the cell through the voltage-sensitive phosphatase (VSP) [283] and modifies the cytoskeletal polymerization [138]. The field-controlled phosphorous hydrolysis could have an essential role in cytoskeleton restructuring and resonant-type behavior phenomena. The amplitude-modulated carrier frequency can produce stochastic resonance, selectively inducing biological enzymatic reactions and polymerization [111].

With care about the physiologic complexity, mEHT takes this contradictory situation seriously and defines the clinical guideline for the complementary therapy, considering the BF as the primary factor [284]. When the BF is low, the RT efficacy is suboptimal; the guideline proposes applying mEHT first, increasing the oxygenation, and helping the set of RT reactions be more effective with the higher reaction rate of molecular changes promoting the fixing of the strand break in the DNA. The mild hyperthermic factor of mEHT optimizes the blood-perfusion to support the RT, and the most optimal frequency of mEHT is every two to three days [285], which well correlates with the timing relaxation of the induced protective HSP70 in the heated malignant cells [253]. This frequency of mEHT treatment fits well with the clinical evaluations, which are fixed in the internationally accepted guideline of mEHT therapy [284].

When LRHT or mEHT is the first in the chosen sequence, it provides oxygenation, which sensitizes the RT and produces protecting HSPs. The RT-induced stress also produces repairing chaperone proteins, like HSP70 and HSP27, which regulate the base excision repair (BER) enzymes in response to RT stress [267]. In addition, the heat effect has other enzyme-independent effects such as sensitizing to the RT: it could cause a variety of irreparable DNA mismatches, heat-activated methylation, hydrolysis, etc.

Mild heating also produces a sufficient enhancement of blood perfusion [70] and enhances the formation of numerous reactive oxygen species (ROS), such as hydrogen peroxide, superoxide anions, nitric oxide, hydroxyl radicals, etc. The heat stress could decrease the superoxide dismutase (SOD) level, weakening the defense against ROS, leading to cell death [268]. mEHT increases the ROS level more extensively than homogeneous (isothermal) heating [136], supporting the RT. Other physiological effects of heating (such as the increase in the electrolyte transport systems like the blood flow and lymph) could enhance the success of RT, together with the increased oxygenation. However, there could also be an inhibitory effect when LRHT induces hypoxic conditions, which may happen at higher temperatures, while mEHT reduces the hypoxic level [286], vastly promoting the better efficacy of RT.

4.6. Immunogenetic Effects

The heat and electrical stresses produce HSP chaperone proteins with mEHT to protect the cells from stress damage. The most characteristic protein family of chaperones, HSP70, acts like a "double edge sword" [287,288], exhibiting both inflammatory and anti-inflammatory, protumoral or antitumoral, immune stimulator or immune suppressor, etc. functions. The role of HSPs depends on the conditions of their activity forming "friends or foes" [289–291]. The primary function of intracellular HSPs (iHSPs) is to avoid the cell's apoptosis and protect the cell's living conditions irrespective of its malignant or healthy state. Nevertheless, certain conditions may promote the secretion of HSPs in the transmembrane position (mHSPs) or their escape extracellularly to the TME milieu (eHSPs). mHSPs may signal to make malignant cells recognizable to NK cells [169]. eHSPs could offer even more help in the elimination of malignancies. The mHSP70 carries an "info signal" [292], with the genetic properties for producing antigen-presenting cells (APCs) and creating killer T-cells [293], by the maturation of dendritic cells (DCs) [294]. This process requires that the destruction of the cell is "gentle enough" and does not degrade the DAMP proteins. When the appropriate molecules have a particular spatiotemporal order (immunogenic cell death, ICD), the set of molecules ensures that the mHSP70 becomes a forceful "friend" losing its "double-edge sword" behavior, and the genetic info well matures the DCs forming APCs. The process directly applies immune-oncology principles, and so ICD is of tremendous clinical interest [295].

The major achievement of mEHT is activating the innate and adaptive immune system to eliminate tumor cells both locally and systemically in the whole body. The induced mHSPs mark cancer such as to be recognized by the innate immune action with NK cells [169]. The secretion of eHSPs and the correct spatiotemporal set of DAMP may develop tumor-specific adaptive immune processes to attack the cancer cells all over the body.

In such a way, mEHT turns the local treatment systemic (abscopal), as proven preclinically [170,174] and clinically too [116,179,296].

The abscopal effect was discovered in RT more than 60 years ago [297], but its application was hindered because it was observable only in low radiation doses, limiting the expected direct local degradation. The recent rediscovering of the abscopal effect with RT shifts the idea from myth to reality [298] and sees it explained by molecular processes [299]. The synergy of RT with the emerging checkpoint inhibitor and antibody immune-therapies provides new curative possibilities [300–302]. This field could have a new combination: mEHT supported TSI develops immune adaptation by the tumor antigens providing an abscopal addition to local RT.

The synergy of mEHT and RT turns these local treatments systemic, creating tumor-specific immune processes (TSI) that extend the abscopal effect. The immunotherapy strategy optimizes the RT with mEHT for the best efficacy [303] and highest safety [178]. The abscopal effect could renew the complementary applications of RT with this theranostic synergy and well fits to the emerging trend of immuno-oncology too. This function connects mEHT to the emerging trend in the field, to immuno-oncology [304]. The in-situ feedback loop of the immune effects of mEHT is shown in Figure 13.

Finally, we may conclude that the thermal and nonthermal effects represent the nonlinear ($\sim j^2$) and linear ($\sim j$) dependence of the current density and in consequence of the electric field, but their functions differ. The thermal effect ensures the general energy background, while the nonthermal is resonant; Figure 14.

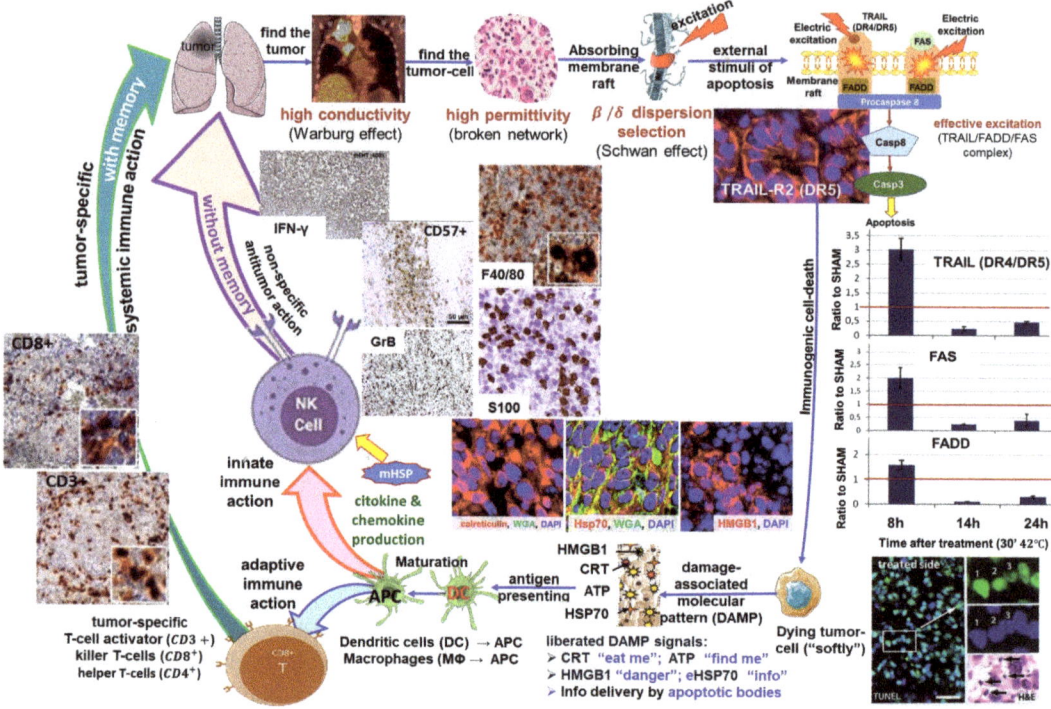

Figure 13. The negative feedback structure of the abscopal effect shows a complex loop from recognizing the antigens to their use in tumor-specific immune processes. The experiments are from various publications. The loop summary only demonstrates how the loop works. The measurements are from the following publications: the selection line reviewed [101], TRAIL-R2-FAS-FADD complex [153]; apoptosis [133,150], ICD [305]; DAMP [174], APC [163] immune [172], NK, Granzyme [169], IFN-γ [182], CD3+, CD8+ [163,170].

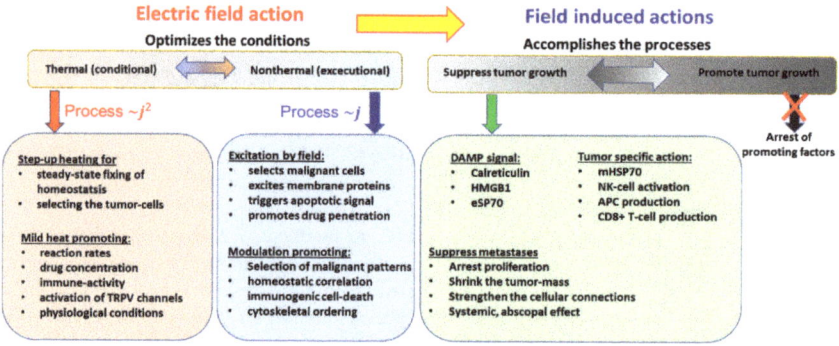

Figure 14. The processes of thermal and nonthermal effects of selective, heterogenic heating. The field-induced actions are complex, requiring both the thermal (conditional) and nonthermal (excitation) processes.

The synergy of mEHT with radiotherapy completes the advantages with essential factors additionally to the conventional heating processes; Table 3.

Table 3. The essential addition of mEHT to the synergistic RT-with-hyperthermia methods.

	Synergistic Addition of Modulated Electrohyperthermia
Nanoscopic action	Selects malignant cells and nonthermally excites, marginal heating of the healthy cells renders less vulnerable to ionizing radiation
Apoptotic effect	Mostly natural apoptosis, no inflammation, no large cytokine liberation, no extra injury current, no extra pH hypoxia
Immune effect	Immunogenic processes, abscopal effect. Both the innate and adaptive immune system are activated, vaccination facility (patented)
Homeostatic effect	Harmonized with homeostatic controls, the temperature increase in the nuclei is moderate, does not make an additional enzymatic activity for reparation
Side effects	Lower incident power puts less load on the skin, which is anyway irritated by radiotherapy, so the synergy has fewer adverse effects
Quality of life	Improves quality of life by reducing side effects
The broad range of application	Possible to combine with radiotherapy in localizations which were not possible with radiative hyperthermia (like the brain)
Applicable for palliative conditions	Resensitizes to radiotherapy in highly metastatic advanced refractory cases, when conventional therapies are ineffective
Long-time application	mEHT is applicable as a chronic treatment for as long as is necessary with radiotherapy complementation
Applicability	mEHT is applicable with most comorbidities as well as in combination with any other oncotherapies

5. Summary

To solve the challenges of conventional LRHT, mEHT has modified the isothermal concept of oncological hyperthermia, focusing on the cellular distortion of malignant cells. The new paradigm strongly considers the goal of LRHT, concentrates on the malignant cells, and destroys them in the targeted volume. The principal idea is to use the natural heterogeneity of the cancerous tissue, using the particular living conditions of malignant cells, making them different from healthy cells and healthy host tissue. mEHT has an isodose. The RF current density is defined similarly to the ionizing isodose in RT practice. The degradation of the malignant cells and controllable stable dosing guides the efforts in synergy with RT.

Modulated electro-hyperthermia complements radiotherapy with the precise heterogenic cellular selection of malignant cells. The transmembrane protein clusters (rafts) are excited by mEHT and heated in synergy with the double-strand breaking of the DNA by RT. The synergistic harmony of ionizing, thermal, and nonthermal effects allows the immunogenic cell death of the malignant cells and develops tumor-specific immune actions in both the innate and adaptive immune system in situ during the treatment. The recognition characteristic is amalgamated with the curative therapy, so the mEHT + RT synergy is theranostic.

The selection process of mEHT uses the malignant attributes that characterize all malignancies: the metabolic, dynamic, and structural differences. This universality of mEHT does not depend on the mutation variants of cancer. Consequently, mEHT—like RT—independently breaks the DNA strands of various malignant mutants, so the synergy of the two methods may form a forceful cancer therapy. The final result is a systemic (abscopal) effect that destroys the malignant cells in the entire body irrespective of the possibility of its visual imaging. The complex integrating effect of mEHT + RT triggers physiologic and cellular changes by thermal and ionizing components. Additionally, the complementary application to RT triggers molecular and immunological changes with resonant and ionizing excitation. All complex balances have progenitors of functioning promoters and suppressors for balancing.

mEHT changes the LRHT paradigm from homogeneous mass heating to a heterogeneous selective one. The difference between the two approaches has been proven in various experiments. Figure 15 shows a rough comparison of mass heating with selective heating.

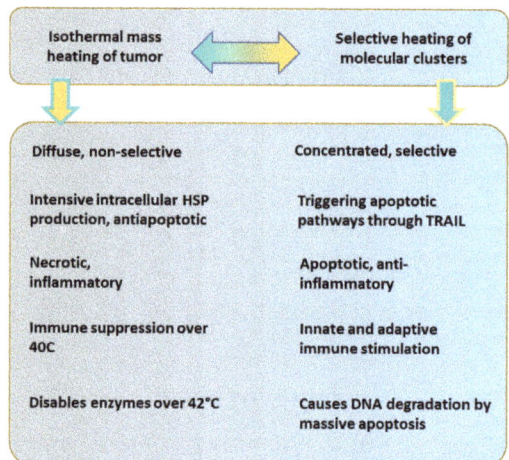

Figure 15. The major differences between isothermal and selective paradigm heating are listed in the columns.

6. Conclusions

mEHT results well prove the nanothermia efficacy and its conceptual success. The synergy with RT delivers effective cell degradation in tumors and develops an abscopal effect, using the homeostatic adaptation of the healthy immune regulation to degrade the malignant cells systemically in the entire body. The synergy is verified by preclinical and validated by clinical results.

Funding: This work was supported by the Hungarian National Research Development and Innovation Office PIACI KFI grant: 2019-1.1.1-PIACI-KFI-2019-00011.

Conflicts of Interest: Andras Szasz is the Chief Scientific Officer of Oncotherm Kft. Hungary/Oncotherm GmbH Germany.

References

1. Seegenschmiedt, M.H.; Vernon, C.C. A Historical Perspective on Hyperthermia in Oncology. In *Thermoradiotherapy and Thermochemotherapy*; Seegenschmiedt, M.H., Fessenden, P., Vernon, C.C., Eds.; Springer: Berlin/Heidelberg, Germany, 1995; Volume 1, pp. 3–44.
2. Vaupel, P.W.; Kelleher, D.K. Metabolic status and reaction to heat of normal and tumor tissue. In *Thermoradiotherapy and Thermochemiotherapy*; Seegenschmiedt, M.H., Fessenden, P., Vernon, C.C., Eds.; Springer: Berlin/Heidelberg, Germany, 1995; Volume 1, pp. 157–176.
3. Griffiths, H.; Ahmed, A.; Smith, C.W.; Moore, J.L.; Kerby, I.J.; Davies, R.M.E. Specific absorption rate and tissue temperature in local hyperthermia. *Int. J. Radiat. Oncol. Biol. Phys.* **1986**, *12*, 1997–2002. [CrossRef]
4. Dutz, S.; Hergt, R. Magnetic nanoparticle heating and heat transfer on a microscale: Basic principles, realities and physical limitations of hyperthermia for tumour therapy. *Int. J. Hyperth.* **2013**, *29*, 790–800. [CrossRef] [PubMed]
5. Datta, N.R.; Puric, E.; Klingbiel, D.; Gomez, S.; Bodis, S. Hyperthermia and Radiation Therapy in Locoregional Recurrent Breast Cancers: A Systematic Review and Meta-analysis. *Int. J. Radiat. Oncol.* **2016**, *94*, 1073–1087. [CrossRef] [PubMed]
6. Datta, N.R.; Rogers, S.; Ordonez, S.G.; Puric, E.; Bodis, S. Hyperthermia and radiotherapy in the management of head and neck cancers: A systematic review and meta-analysis. *Int. J. Hyperth.* **2016**, *32*, 31–40. [CrossRef] [PubMed]
7. Datta, N.R.; Rogers, S.; Klingbiel, D.; Gomez, S.; Puric, E.; Bodis, S. Hyperthermia and radiotherapy with or without chemotherapy in locally advanced cervical cancer: A systematic review with conventional and network meta-analyses. *Int. J. Hyperth.* **2016**, *32*, 809–821. [CrossRef]
8. Rogers, S.J.; Datta, N.R.; Puric, E.; Timm, O.; Marder, D.; Khan, S.; Mamot, C.; Knuchel, J.; Siebenhüner, A.; Pestalozzi, B.; et al. The addition of deep hyperthermia to gemcitabine-based chemoradiation may achieve enhanced survival in unresectable locally advanced adenocarcinoma of the pancreas. *Clin. Transl. Radiat. Oncol.* **2021**, *27*, 109–113. [CrossRef]

9. Issels, R.D.; Lindner, L.H.; Verweij, J.; Wessalowski, R.; Reichardt, P.; Wust, P.; Ghadjar, P.; Hohenberger, P.; Angele, M.; Salat, C.; et al. Effect of Neoadjuvant Chemotherapy Plus Regional Hyperthermia on Long-term Outcomes Among Patients with Localized High-Risk Soft Tissue Sarcoma. *JAMA Oncol.* **2018**, *4*, 483–492. [CrossRef]
10. Falk, M.H.; Issels, R.D. Hyperthermia in oncology: Invited Review. *Int. J. Hyperth.* **2001**, *17*, 1–18. [CrossRef]
11. Streffer, C.; van Beuningen, D.; Dietzel, F.; Röttinger, E.; Robinson, J.E.; Scherer, E.; Seeber, S.; Trott, K.R. *Cancer Therapy by Hyperthermia and Radiation*; Urban and Schwarzenberg: Baltimore, MD, USA; Munich, Germany, 1978.
12. Seegenschmiedt, M.H.; Fessenden, P.; Vernon, C.C. *Thermoradiotherapy and Thermochemotherapy, Volume 2: Clinical Applications*; Springer: Berlin/Heidelberg, Germany, 1996.
13. Kosaka, M.; Sugahara, T.; Schmidt, K.L.; Simon, E. *Thermotherapy for Neoplasia, Inflammation, and Pain*; Springer: Tokyo, Japan, 2001.
14. Matsuda, T. *Cancer Treatment by Hyperthermia, Radiation and Drugs*; Taylor & Francis: London, UK; Bristol, PA, USA, 1993.
15. Urano, M.; Douple, E. *Hyperthermia and Oncology: Volume 2, Biology of Thermal Potentiation of Radiotherapy*; VSP BV: Utrecht, The Netherlands, 1992.
16. Hehr, T.; Wust, P.; Bamberg, M.; Budach, W. Current and potential role of thermoradiotherapy for solid tumors. *Onkologie* **2003**, *26*, 295–302.
17. van der Zee, J.; Gonzalez, D.G.; van Rhoon, G.C.; van Dijk, J.D.; van Putten, W.L.; Hart, A.A.; The Dutch Deep Hyperthermia Group. Comparison of radiotherapy alone with radiotherapy plus hyperthermia in locally advanced pelvic tumors: A prospective, randomised, multicentre trial. *Lancet* **2000**, *355*, 1119–1125. [CrossRef]
18. Wust, P.; Hildebrandt, B.; Sreenivasa, G.; Rau, B.; Gellermann, J.; Riess, H.; Felix, R.; Schlag, P.M. Hyperthermia in combined treatment of cancer. *Lancet Oncol.* **2002**, *3*, 487–497. [CrossRef]
19. Overgaard, J.; Gonzalez, D.; Hulshof, M.C.; Arcangeli, G.; Dahl, O.; Mella, O.; Bentzen, S.M. Randomised trial of hyperthermia as adjuvant to radiotherapy for recurrent or metastatic malignant melanoma. *Lancet* **1995**, *345*, 540–543. [CrossRef]
20. van der Zee, J.; Truemiet-Donker, A.D.; The, S.K.; Helle, P.A.; Seldenrath, J.J.; Meerwaldt, J.H.; Wijnmaalen, A.J.; van den Berg, A.P.; van Rhoon, G.C.; Broekmeyer-Reurink, M.P.; et al. Low-dose reirradiation in combination with hyperthermia: A palliative treatment for patients with breast cancer recurring in previously irradiated areas. *Int. J. Radiat. Oncol. Biol. Phys.* **1988**, *15*, 1407–1413. [CrossRef]
21. Vernon, C.C.; Harrison, M. Hyperthermia with low-dose radiotherapy for recurrent breast carcinoma. *Lancet* **1991**, *337*, 59. [CrossRef]
22. Bicher, J.I.; Al-Bussam, N.; Wolfstein, R.S. Thermotherapy with curative intent–breast, head, and neck, and prostate tumours. *Dtsch. Z. Fur Oncol.* **2006**, *38*, 116–122.
23. Peeken, J.C.; Vaupel, P.; Combs, S.E. Integrating Hyperthermia into Modern Radiation Oncology: What Evidence Is Necessary? *Front. Oncol.* **2017**, *7*, 132. [CrossRef]
24. Horsman, M.R.; Overgaard, J. Hyperthermia: A Potent Enhancer of Radiotherapy. *Clin. Oncol.* **2007**, *19*, 418–426. [CrossRef]
25. Molls, M. Hyperthermia—The actual role in radiation oncology and future prospects. *Strahlenther. Oncol.* **1992**, *168*, 183–190.
26. Seegenschmiedt, M.H.; Feldmann, H.J.; Wust, P. Hyperthermia–Its actual role is radiation oncology. *Strahlenther. Oncol.* **1995**, *171*, 560–572.
27. Emami, B.; Scott, C.; Perez, C.A.; Asbell, S.; Swift, P.; Grigsby, P.; Montesano, A.; Rubin, P.; Curran, W.; Delrowe, J.; et al. Phase III study of interstitial thermoradiotherapy compared with interstitial radiotherapy alone in the treatment of recurrent or persistent human tumours: A prospectively controlled randomized study by radiation therapy oncology group. *Int. J. Radiat. Oncol. Biol. Phys.* **1996**, *34*, 1097–1104. [CrossRef]
28. Wust, P.; Rau, B.; Gremmler, M.; Schlag, P.; Jordan, A.; Löffel, J.; Riess, H.; Felix, R. Radio-Thermotherapy in Multimodal Surgical Treatment Concepts. *Oncologie* **1995**, *18*, 110–121. [CrossRef]
29. Overgaard, J. The current and potential role of hyperthermia in radiotherapy. *Int. J. Radiat. Oncol. Biol. Phys.* **1989**, *16*, 535–549. [CrossRef]
30. Bauer, K.H. *Das Krebsproblem*; Springer: Berlin/Heidelberg, Germany, 1964.
31. Szasz, O.; Szasz, A. Approaching Complexity: Hyperthermia Dose and Its Possible Measurement in Oncology. *Open J. Biophys.* **2021**, *11*, 68–132. [CrossRef]
32. Romanovsky, A.A. Thermoregulation: Some concepts have changed. Functional architecture of the thermoregulatory system. *Am. J. Physiol. Integr. Comp. Physiol.* **2007**, *292*, R37–R46. [CrossRef]
33. Vaupel, P.W.; Hammersen, F. *Mikrozirkulation in malignen Tumoren. 6. Jahrestagung der Gesellschaft für Mikrozirkulation e.V., München, November 1982*; Karger: Basel, Switzerland, 1983; ISBN 978-3-8055-3762-9.
34. Charkoudian, N. Skin Blood Flow in Adult Human Thermoregulation: How It Works, When It Does Not, and Why. *Mayo Clin. Proc.* **2003**, *78*, 603–612. [CrossRef]
35. Zhao, Z.; Yang, W.Z.; Gao, C.; Fu, X.; Zhang, W.; Zhou, Q.; Chen, W.; Ni, X.; Lin, J.-K.; Yang, J.; et al. A hypothalamic circuit that controls body temperature. *Proc. Natl. Acad. Sci. USA* **2017**, *114*, 2042–2047. [CrossRef]
36. Watanabe, M.; Suzuki, K.; Kodama, S.; Sugahara, T. Normal human cells at confluence get heat resistance by efficient accumulation of HSP72 in nucleus. *Carcinogenesis* **1995**, *16*, 2373–2380. [CrossRef]
37. Jones, E.; Thrall, D.; Dewhirst, M.W.; Vujaskovic, Z. Prospective thermal dosimetry: The key to hyperthermia's future. *Int. J. Hyperth.* **2006**, *22*, 247–253. [CrossRef]

38. di Lalla, V.; Chaput, G.; Williams, T.; Sultanem, K. Radiotherapy Side Effects: Integrating a Survivorship Clinical Lens to Better Serve Patients. *Curr. Oncol.* **2020**, *27*, 107–112. [CrossRef]
39. Majeed, H.; Gupta, V. *Adverse Effects of Radiation Therapy*; StatPearls Publishing: Treasure Island, FL, USA, 2021. Available online: https://pubmed.ncbi.nlm.nih.gov/33085406/ (accessed on 11 December 2021).
40. Kaur, P.; Hurwitz, M.D.; Krishnan, S.; Asea, A. Combined Hyperthermia and Radiotherapy for the Treatment of Cancer. *Cancers* **2011**, *3*, 3799–3823. [CrossRef]
41. Rao, W.; Deng, Z.-S.; Liu, J. A Review of Hyperthermia Combined with Radiotherapy/Chemotherapy on Malignant Tumors. *Crit. Rev. Biomed. Eng.* **2010**, *38*, 101–116. [CrossRef]
42. Elming, P.B.; Sorensen, B.S.; Oei, A.L.; Franken, N.A.P.; Crezee, J.; Overgaard, J.; Horsman, M.R. Hyperthermia: The optimal treatment to overcome radiation resistant hypoxia. *Cancers* **2019**, *11*, 60. [CrossRef] [PubMed]
43. Kühl, N.M.; Rensing, L. Heat shock effects on cell cycle progression. *Cell. Mol. Life Sci. CMLS* **2000**, *57*, 450–463. [CrossRef] [PubMed]
44. Roti, J.L.; Laszlo, A. The effects of hyperthermia on cellular macromolecules. In *Hyperthermia and Oncology Volume 1, Thermal Effects on Cells and Tissues*; Urano, M., Douple, E., Eds.; VSP: Utrecht, The Netherlands, 1988; pp. 13–56.
45. Pandita, T.K.; Pandita, S.; Bhaumik, S.R. Molecular parameters of hyperthermia for radiosensitization. *Crit. Rev. Eukaryot. Gene Expr.* **2009**, *19*, 235–251. [CrossRef] [PubMed]
46. Okumura, Y.; Ihara, M.; Shimasaki, T.; Takeshita, S.; Okiachi, K. Heat inactivation of DNA-dependent protein kinase: Possible mechanism of hyperthermic radiosensitization. In *Thermotherapy for Neoplasia, Inflammation, and Pain*; Kosaka, M., Sugahara, T., Schmidt, K.L., Kosaka, M., Sugahara, T., Simon, E., Eds.; Springer: Tokyo, Japan, 2001; pp. 420–423.
47. Vujaskovic, Z.; Song, C.W. Physiological mechanisms underlying heat-induced radiosensitization. *Int. J. Hyperth.* **2004**, *20*, 163–174. [CrossRef]
48. Song, C.W.; Shakil, A.; Osborn, J.L.; Iwata, K. Tumour oxygenation is increased by hyperthermia at mild temperatures. *Int. J. Hyperth.* **2009**, *25*, 91–95. [CrossRef] [PubMed]
49. Dudar, T.E.; Jain, R.K. Differential response of normal and tumor microcirculation to hyperthermia. *Cancer Res.* **1984**, *44*, 605–612. [PubMed]
50. Song, C.W.; Lokshina, A.; Rhee, J.G.; Patten, M.; Levitt, S.H. Implication of blood-flow in hyperthermic treatment of tumors. *IEEE Trans. Biomed. Eng.* **1984**, *31*, 9–16. [CrossRef] [PubMed]
51. Pence, D.M.; Song, C.W. Effect of heat on blood-flow. In *Hyperthermia in Cancer Treatment*; Anghileri, L.J., Robert, J., Eds.; CRC Press Inc.: Boca Raton, FL, USA, 1986; Volume 2, pp. 1–17.
52. Vaupel, P. Pathophysiological mechanism of hyperthermia in cancer therapy. In *Methods of Hyperthermia Control, Clinical Thermology*; Gautherie, M., Ed.; Springer: Berlin/Heidelberg, Germany, 1990; pp. 73–134.
53. Erdmann, B.; Lang, J.; Seebass, M. Optimization of temperature distributions for regional hyperthermia based on a nonlinear heat transfer model. *Ann. NYAS* **1998**, *858*, 36–46.
54. Vaupel, P.; Kallinowski, F.; Okunieff, P. Blood flow, oxygen and nutrient supply, and metabolic microenvironment of human tumours: A review. *Cancer Res.* **1989**, *49*, 6449–6465.
55. Takana, Y. Thermal responses of microcirculation and modification of tumour blood flow in treating the tumours. In *Theoretical and Experimental Basis of Hyperthermia. Thermotherapy for Neoplasia, Inflammation, and Pain*; Kosaka, M., Sugahara, T., Schmidt, K.L., Simon, E., Eds.; Springer: Tokyo, Japan, 2001; pp. 408–419.
56. Song, C.W.; Choi, I.B.; Nah, B.S.; Sahu, S.K.; Osborn, J.L. Microvasculature and perfusion in normal tissues and tumours. In *Thermoradiometry and Thermochemotherapy*; Seegenschmiedt, M.H., Fessenden, P., Vernon, C.C., Eds.; Springer: Berlin/Heidelberg, Germany, 1995; Volume 1, pp. 139–156.
57. Song, C.W.; Park, H.; Griffin, R.J. Theoretical and experimental basis of hyperthermia. In *Thermotherapy for Neoplasia, Inflammation, and Pain*; Kosaka, M., Sugahara, T., Schmidt, K.L., Simon, E., Eds.; Springer: Tokyo, Japan, 2001; pp. 394–407.
58. Lindholm, C.E. Hyperthermia and Radiotherapy. Ph.D. Thesis, Lund University, Malmo, Sweden, 1992.
59. Hafström, L.; Rudenstam, C.M.; Blomquist, E.; Ingvar, C.; Jönsson, P.E.; Lagerlöf, B.; Lindholm, C.; Ringborg, U.; Westman, G.; Ostrup, L. Regional hyperthermic perfusion with melphalan after surgery for recurrent malignant melanoma of the extremities. *J. Clin. Oncol.* **1991**, *9*, 2091–2094. [CrossRef] [PubMed]
60. Dewey, W.C.; Hopwood, L.E.; Sapareto, S.A.; Gerweck, L.E. Cellular Responses to Combinations of Hyperthermia and Radiation. *Radiology* **1977**, *123*, 463–474. [CrossRef] [PubMed]
61. Kim, W.; Lee, S.; Seo, D.; Kim, D.; Kim, K.; Kim, E.; Kang, J.; Seong, K.M.; Youn, H.; Youn, B. Cellular Stress Responses in Radiotherapy. *Cells* **2019**, *8*, 1105. [CrossRef] [PubMed]
62. Walleczek, J. *Self-Organized Biological Dynamics & Nonlinear Control*; Cambridge University Press: Cambridge, UK, 2000.
63. Dewhirst, M.W.; Viglianti, B.L.; Lora-Michiels, M.; Hanson, M.; Hoopes, P.J. Basic principles of thermal dosimetry and thermal thresholds for tissue damage from hyperthermia. *Int. J. Hyperth.* **2003**, *19*, 267–294. [CrossRef] [PubMed]
64. Perez, C.A.; Sapareto, S.A. Thermal dose expression in clinical hyperthermia and correlation with tumor response/control. *Cancer Res.* **1984**, *44*, 4818–4825.
65. Dewey, W.C. Arrhenius relationships from the molecule and cell to the clinic. *Int. J. Hyperth.* **1994**, *10*, 457–483. [CrossRef]
66. Gellerman, J. Nichtinvasive Thermometrie bei lokoregionaler Tiefenhyperthermie, Noninvasive thermometry in loco-regional deep hyperthermia. In Proceedings of the Oncothermia Symposia, 2016, Cologne, Germany, 22–23 September 2006.

67. Hegyi, G.; Vincze, G.; Szasz, A. On the Dynamic Equilibrium in Homeostasis. *Open J. Biophys.* **2012**, *2*, 60–67. [CrossRef]
68. Lee, S.-Y.; Szigeti, G.P.; Szasz, A.M. Oncological hyperthermia: The correct dosing in clinical applications. *Int. J. Oncol.* **2018**, *54*, 627–643. [CrossRef]
69. Maguire, P.D.; Samulski, T.V.; Prosnitz, L.R.; Jones, E.L.; Rosner, G.L.; Powers, B.; Layfield, L.W.; Brizel, D.M.; Scully, S.P.; Herrelson, M.; et al. A phase II trial testing the thermal dose parameter CEM43° T$_{90}$ as a predictor of response in soft tissue sarcomas treated with pre-operative thermorasiotherapy. *Int. J. Hyperth.* **2001**, *17*, 283–290. [CrossRef]
70. Dewhirst, M.W.; Vujaskovic, Z.; Jones, E.; Thrall, D. Re-setting the biologic rationale for thermal therapy. *Int. J. Hyperth.* **2005**, *21*, 779–790. [CrossRef]
71. Thrall, D.E.; Prescott, D.M.; Samulski, T.V.; Rosner, G.L.; Denman, D.L.; Legorreta, R.L.; Dodge, R.K.; Page, R.L.; Cline, J.; Lee, J.; et al. Radiation plus local hyperthermia versus radiation plus the combination of local and whole-body hyperthermia in canine sarcomas. *Int. J. Radiat. Oncol.* **1996**, *34*, 1087–1096. [CrossRef]
72. Hildebrandt, B.; Dräger, J.; Kerner, T.; Deja, M.; Löffel, J.; Stroszczynski, C.; Ahlers, O.; Felix, R.; Riess, H.; Wust, P. Whole-body hyperthermia in the scope of von Ardenne's systemic cancer multistep therapy (sCMT) combined with chemotherapy in patients with metastatic colorectal cancer: A phase I/II study. *Int. J. Hyperth.* **2004**, *20*, 317–333. [CrossRef] [PubMed]
73. Bakhshandeh, A.; Wiedemann, G.; Zabel, P.; Dalhoff, K.; Kohlmann, T.; Penzel, R.Z.; Wagner, T.; Peters, S. Randomized trial with ICE (ifosfamide, carboplatin, etoposide) plus whole body hyperthermia versus ICE chemotherapy for malignant pleural mesothelioma. *J. Clin. Oncol.* **2004**, *22*, 7288. [CrossRef]
74. de Bruijne, M.; van der Holt, B.; van Rhoon, G.C.; van der Zee, J. Evaluation of CEM43°CT90 thermal dose in superficial hyperthermia: A retrospective analysis. *Strahlenther. Onkol. Radiother. Oncol.* **2010**, *186*, 436–443. [CrossRef] [PubMed]
75. Kraybill, W.G.; Olenki, T.; Evans, S.S.; Ostberg, J.R.; O'Leary, K.A.; Gibbs, J.F.; Repasky, E.A. A phase I study of fever-range whole body hyperthermia (FR-WBH) in patients with advanced solid tumors: Correlation with mouse models. *Int. J. Hyperth.* **2002**, *18*, 253–266. [CrossRef] [PubMed]
76. Toyota, N.; Strebel, F.R.; Stephens, L.C.; Matsuda, H.; Bull, J.M.C. Long-duration, mild whole body hyperthermia with cisplatin: Tumour response and kinetics of apoptosis and necrosis in a metastatic rat mammary adenocarcinoma. *Int. J. Hyperth.* **1997**, *13*, 497–506. [CrossRef] [PubMed]
77. Sakaguchi, Y.; Makino, M.; Kaneko, T.; Stephens, L.C.; Strebel, F.R.; Danhauser, L.L.; Jenkins, G.N.; Bull, J.M. Therapeutic efficacy of long duration-low temperature whole body hyperthermia when combined with tumor necrosis factor and carboplatin in rats. *Cancer Res.* **1994**, *54*, 2223–2227.
78. Ostberg, R.; Repasky, E.A. Use of mild, whole body hyperthermia in cancer therapy. *Immunol. Investig.* **2000**, *29*, 139–142. [CrossRef]
79. International Collaborative Hyperthermia Group; Vernon, C.C.; Hand, J.W.; Field, S.B.; Machin, D.; Whaley, J.B.; van der Zee, J.; van Putten, W.L.; van Rhoon, G.C.; van Dijk, J.D.; et al. Radiotherapy with or without hyperthermia in the treatment of superficial localized breast cancer: Results from five randomized controlled trials. *Int. J. Radiat. Oncol. Biol. Phys.* **1996**, *35*, 731–744. [CrossRef]
80. Sherar, M.; Liu, F.-F.; Pintilie, M.; Levin, W.; Hunt, J.; Hill, R.; Hand, J.; Vernon, C.; van Rhoon, G.; van der Zee, J.; et al. Relationship between thermal dose and outcome in thermoradiotherapy treatments for superficial recurrences of breast cancer: Data from a phase III trial. *Int. J. Radiat. Oncol.* **1997**, *39*, 371–380. [CrossRef]
81. Sharma, S.; Patel, F.D.; Sandhu, A.P.S.; Gupta, B.D.; Yadav, N.S. A prospective randomized study of local hyperthermia as a supplement and radiosensitiser in the treatment of carcinoma of the cervix with radiotherapy. *Endocurietherapy/Hyperth. Oncol.* **1989**, *5*, 151–159.
82. Vasanthan, A.; Mitsumori, M.; Park, J.H.; Zhi-Fan, Z.; Yu-Bin, Z.; Oliynychenko, P.; Tatsuzaki, H.; Tanaka, Y.; Hiraoka, M. Regional hyperthermia combined with radiotherapy for uterine cervical cancers: A multi-institutional prospective randomized trial of the international atomic energy agency. *Int. J. Radiat. Oncol.* **2005**, *61*, 145–153. [CrossRef]
83. Harima, Y.; Nagata, K.; Harima, K.; Ostapenko, V.V.; Tanaka, Y.; Sawada, S. A randomized clinical trial of radiation therapy versus thermoradiotherapy in stage IIIB cervical carcinoma. *Int. J. Hyperth.* **2009**, *25*, 338–343. [CrossRef]
84. Roussakow, S.V. A randomized clinical trial of radiation therapy versus thermoradiotherapy in stage IIIB cervical carcinoma of Yoko Harima et al. (2001): Multiple biases and no advantage of hyperthermia. *Int. J. Hyperth.* **2018**, *34*, 1400. [CrossRef]
85. Harima, Y. A randomised clinical trial of radiation therapy versus thermoradiotherapy in stage IIIB cervical carcinoma of Yoko, Harima et al. (2001): A response letter to the editor of comments from Dr. Roussakow. *Int. J. Hyperth.* **2018**, *34*, 1401. [CrossRef]
86. Zolciak-Siwinska, A.; Piotrokowicz, N.; Jonska-Gmyrek, J.; Nicke-Psikuta, M.; Michalski, W.; Kawczyńska, M.; Bijok, M.; Bujko, K. HDR brachytherapy combined with interstitial hyperthermia in locally advanced cervical cancer patients initially treated with concomitant radiochemotherapy–A phase III study. *Radiother. Oncol.* **2013**, *109*, 194–199. [CrossRef]
87. Kay, C.S.; Choi, I.B.; Jang, J.Y.; Choi, B.O.; Kim, I.A.; Shinn, K.S. Thermoradiotherapy in the treatment of locally advanced nonsmall cell lung cancer. *Radiat. Oncol. J.* **1996**, *14*, 115–122.
88. Mitsumori, M.; Zhi-Fan, Z.; Oliynychenko, P.; Park, J.H.; Choi, I.B.; Tatsuzaki, H.; Tanaka, Y.; Hiraoka, M. Regional hyperthermia combined with radiotherapy for locally advanced non-small cell lung cancers: A multi-institutional prospective randomized trial of the International Atomic Energy Agency. *Int. J. Clin. Oncol.* **2007**, *12*, 192–198. [CrossRef]
89. Jones, E.L.; Oleson, J.R.; Prosnith, L.R.; Prosnitz, L.R.; Samulski, T.V.; Vujaskovic, Z.; Yu, D.; Sanders, L.L.; Dewhirst, M.W. Randomized trial of hyperthermia and radiation for superficial tumors. *J. Clin. Oncol.* **2005**, *23*, 3079–3085. [CrossRef]

90. Storm, F.K. What happened to hyperthermia and what is its current status in cancer treatment? *J. Surg. Oncol.* **1993**, *53*, 141–143. [CrossRef]
91. van der Zee, J. Heating the patient: A promising approach? *Ann. Oncol.* **2002**, *13*, 1173–1184. [CrossRef] [PubMed]
92. Datta, N.R.; Kok, H.P.; Crezee, H.; Gaipl, U.S.; Bodis, S. Integrating Loco-Regional Hyperthermia into the Current Oncology Practice: SWOT and TOWS Analyses. *Front. Oncol.* **2020**, *10*, 819. [CrossRef] [PubMed]
93. Wildeboer, R.R.; Southern, P.; Pankhurst, Q.A. On the reliable measurement of specific absorption rates and intrinsic loss parameters in magnetic hyperthermia materials. *J. Phys. D Appl. Phys.* **2014**, *47*, 495003. [CrossRef]
94. Szasz, A.; Szasz, N.; Szasz, O. *Oncothermia: Principles and Practices*; Springer Science: Heidelberg, Germany, 2010. [CrossRef]
95. Andocs, G.; Rehman, M.U.; Zhao, Q.L.; Papp, E.; Kondo, T.; Szasz, A. Nanoheating without Artificial Nanoparticles Part II. Experimental support of the nanoheating concept of the modulated electro-hyperthermia method, using U937 cell suspension model. *Biol. Med.* **2015**, *7*, 1–9. [CrossRef]
96. Beachy, S.H.; Repasky, E.A. Toward establishment of temperature thresholds for immunological impact of heat exposure in humans. *Int. J. Hyperth.* **2011**, *27*, 344–352. [CrossRef]
97. Shen, R.-N.; Lu, L.; Young, P.; Shidnia, H.; Hornback, N.B.; Broxmeyer, H.E. Influence of elevated temperature on natural killer cell activity, lymphokine-activated killer cell activity and lectin-dependent cytotoxicity of human umbilical cord blood and adult blood cells. *Int. J. Radiat. Oncol.* **1994**, *29*, 821–826. [CrossRef]
98. Hietanen, T.; Kapanaen, M.; Kellokumpu-Lehtinen, P.-L. Restoring natural killer cell cytotoxicity after hyperthermia alone or combined with radiotherapy. *Anticancer. Res.* **2016**, *36*, 555–563.
99. Repasky, E.; Issels, R. Physiological consequences of hyperthermia: Heat, heat shock proteins and the immune response. *Int. J. Hyperth.* **2002**, *18*, 486–489. [CrossRef]
100. Szasz, A. Thermal and nonthermal effects of radiofrequency on living state and applications as an adjuvant with radiation therapy. *J. Radiat. Cancer Res.* **2019**, *10*, 1–17. [CrossRef]
101. Krenacs, T.; Meggyeshazi, N.; Forika, G.; Kiss, E.; Hamar, P.; Szekely, T.; Vancsik, T. Modulated Electro-Hyperthermia-Induced Tumor Damage Mechanisms Revealed in Cancer Models. *Int. J. Mol. Sci.* **2020**, *21*, 6270. [CrossRef]
102. Vincze, G.; Szasz, A. Similarities of modulation by temperature and by electric field. *Open J. Biophys.* **2018**, *8*, 95–103. [CrossRef]
103. Gowrishankar, T.R.; Weaver, J.C. An approach to electrical modeling of single and multiple cells. *Proc. Natl. Acad. Sci. USA* **2003**, *100*, 3203–3208. [CrossRef] [PubMed]
104. Kotnik, T.; Miklavcic, D. Theoretical evaluation of the distributed power dissipation in biological cells exposed to electric fields. *Bioelectromagnetics* **2000**, *21*, 385–394. [CrossRef]
105. Papp, E.; Vancsik, T.; Kiss, E.; Szasz, O. Energy absorption by the membrane rafts in the modulated electro-hyperthermia (mEHT). *Open J. Biophys.* **2017**, *7*, 216–229. [CrossRef]
106. The Physical Sciences-Oncology Centers Network; Agus, D.B.; Alexander, J.F.; Arap, W.; Ashili, S.; Aslan, J.; Austin, R.H.; Backman, V.; Bethel, K.; Bonneau, R.; et al. A physical sciences network characterization of non-tumorigenic and metastatic cells. *Sci. Rep.* **2013**, *3*, 01449. [CrossRef]
107. Arrhenius, S. On the reaction rate of the inversion of non-refined sugar upon souring. *Z Phys. Chem.* **1889**, *4*, 226–248. [CrossRef]
108. Szasz, A. The Capacitive Coupling Modalities for Oncological Hyperthermia. *Open J. Biophys.* **2021**, *11*, 252–313. [CrossRef]
109. Szasz, A.; Vincze, G.; Szasz, O.; Szasz, N. An Energy Analysis of Extracellular Hyperthermia. *Electromagn. Biol. Med.* **2003**, *22*, 103–115. [CrossRef]
110. Fröhlich, H. What are non-thermal electric biological effects? *Bioelectromagnetics* **1982**, *3*, 45–46. [CrossRef]
111. Szasz, A. Therapeutic Basis of Electromagnetic Resonances and Signal-Modulation. *Open J. Biophys.* **2021**, *11*, 314–350. [CrossRef]
112. Neudorfer, C.; Chow, C.T.; Boutet, A.; Loh, A.; Germann, J.; Elias, G.J.; Hutchison, W.D.; Lozano, A.M. Kilohertz-frequency stimulation of the nervous system: A review of underlying mechanisms. *Brain Stimul.* **2021**, *14*, 513–530. [CrossRef] [PubMed]
113. Szasz, A.; Szasz, O. Time-fractal modulation of modulated electro-hyperthermia (mEHT). In *Book Challenges and Solutions of Oncological Hyperthermia*; Szasz, A., Ed.; Cambridge Scholars: Newcastle upon Tyne, UK, 2020; pp. 377–415.
114. Rec. ITU-R SM.1056-1. 1 RECOMMENDATION ITU-R SM.1056-1. Limitation of Radiation from Industrial, Scientific and Medical (ISM) Equipment (Question ITU-R 70/1). Available online: https://www.itu.int/dms_pubrec/itu-r/rec/sm/R-REC-SM.1056-1-200704-I!!PDF-E.pdf (accessed on 31 October 2021).
115. Yeo, S.-G. Definitive radiotherapy with concurrent oncothermia for stage IIIB non-small-cell lung cancer: A case report. *Exp. Ther. Med.* **2015**, *10*, 769–772. [CrossRef] [PubMed]
116. Chi, M.-S.; Mehta, M.P.; Yang, K.-L.; Lai, H.-C.; Lin, Y.-C.; Ko, H.-L.; Wang, Y.-S.; Liao, K.-W.; Chi, K.-H. Putative Abscopal Effect in Three Patients Treated by Combined Radiotherapy and Modulated Electrohyperthermia. *Front. Oncol.* **2020**, *10*, 254. [CrossRef] [PubMed]
117. Deering, W.; West, B.J. Fractal physiology. *IEEE Comput. Graph. Appl.* **1992**, *11*, 40–46. [CrossRef]
118. West, B.J. *Fractal Physiology and Chaos in Medicine*; World Scientific: Singapore; London, UK, 1990.
119. Bassingthwaighte, J.B.; Leibovitch, L.S.; West, B.J. *Fractal Physiology*; Oxford University Press: New York, NY, USA; Oxford, UK, 1994.
120. Musha, T.; Sawada, Y. *Physics of the Living State*; IOS Press: Amsterdam, The Netherlands, 1994.
121. Lovelady, D.C.; Friedman, J.; Patel, S.; Rabson, D.A.; Lo, C.-M. Detecting effects of low levels of cytochalasin B in 3T3 fibroblast cultures by analysis of electrical noise obtained from cellular micromotion. *Biosens. Bioelectron.* **2009**, *24*, 2250–2254. [CrossRef]

122. Lovelady, D.C.; Richmond, T.C.; Maggi, A.N.; Lo, C.-M.; Rabson, D.A. Distinguishing cancerous from noncancerous cells through analysis of electrical noise. *Phys. Rev. E* **2007**, *76*, 041908. [CrossRef]
123. Astumian, R.D.; Chock, P.B.; Tsong, T.Y.; Westerhoff, H.V. Effects of oscillations and energy-driven fluctuations on the dynamics of enzyme catalysis and free-energy transduction. *Phys. Rev. A* **1989**, *39*, 6416–6435. [CrossRef]
124. Astumian, R.D.; Weaver, J.C.; Adair, R.K. Rectification and signal averaging of weak electric fields by biological cells. *Proc. Natl. Acad. Sci. USA* **1995**, *92*, 3740–3743. [CrossRef]
125. Sabah, N.H. Rectification in Biological Membranes. *IEEE Eng. Med. Biol.* **2000**, *19*, 106–113. [CrossRef]
126. Nagy, G.; Meggyeshazi, N.; Szasz, O. Deep temperature measurements in oncothermia processes. In Proceedings of the Conference of the International Clinical Hyperthermia Society 2012, Budapest, Hungary, 12–14 October 2012.
127. Orczy-Timko, B. Phantom measurements with the EHY-2030 device. In *Challenges and Solutions of Oncological Hyperthermia*; Szasz, A., Ed.; Cambridge Scholars: Newcastle upon Tyne, UK, 2020; pp. 416–428.
128. Hossain, M.T.; Prasad, B.; Park, K.S.; Lee, H.J.; Ha, Y.H.; Lee, S.K.; Kim, J.K. Simulation and experimental evaluation of selective heating characteristics of 13.56 MHz radiofrequency hyperthermia in phantom models. *Int. J. Precis. Eng. Manuf.* **2016**, *17*, 253–256. [CrossRef]
129. Prasad, B.; Kim, S.; Cho, W.; Kim, J.K.; Kim, Y.A.; Kim, S.; Wu, H.G. Quantitative estimation of the equivalent radiation dose escalation using radiofrequency hyperthermia in mouse xenograft models of human lung cancer. *Sci. Rep.* **2019**, *9*, 3942. [CrossRef] [PubMed]
130. Balogh, L.; Polyák, A.; Pöstényi, Z.; Kovács-Haász, V.; Gyöngy, M.; Thuróczy, J. Temperature increase induced by modulated electrohyperthermia (onco-thermia®) in the anesthetized pig liver. *J. Cancer Res. Ther.* **2016**, *12*, 1153–1159. [PubMed]
131. Kim, J.K.; Prasad, B.; Kim, S. Temperature mapping and thermal dose calculation in combined radiation therapy and 13.56 MHz radiofrequency hyperthermia for tumor treatment. In *SPIE 10047, Optical Methods for Tumor Treatment and Detection: Mechanisms and Techniques in Photodynamic Therapy XXVI, Proceedings of the SPIE Conferences and Exhibitions, San Francisco, CA, USA, 28 January–2 February 2017*; SPIE: Bellingham, WA, USA, 2017.
132. Lee, S.-Y.; Kim, J.-H.; Han, Y.-H.; Cho, D.-H. The effect of modulated electro-hyperthermia on temperature and blood flow in human cervical carcinoma. *Int. J. Hyperth.* **2018**, *34*, 953–960. [CrossRef] [PubMed]
133. Yang, K.-L.; Huang, C.-C.; Chi, M.-S.; Chiang, H.-C.; Wang, Y.-S.; Hsia, C.-C.; Andocs, G.; Wang, H.-E.; Chi, K.-H. In vitro comparison of conventional hyperthermia and modulated electro-hyperthermia. *Oncotarget* **2016**, *7*, 84082–84092. [CrossRef]
134. Forika, G.; Balogh, A.; Vancsik, T.; Zalatnai, A.; Petovari, G.; Benyo, Z.; Krenacs, T. Modulated Electro-Hyperthermia Resolves Radioresistance of Panc1 Pancreas Adenocarcinoma and Promotes DNA Damage and Apoptosis In Vitro. *Int. J. Mol. Sci.* **2020**, *21*, 5100. [CrossRef]
135. Andocs, G.; Renner, H.; Balogh, L.; Fonyad, L.; Jakab, C.; Szasz, A. Strong synergy of heat and modulated electro-magnetic field in tumor cell killing, Study of HT29 xenograft tumors in a nude mice model. *Strahlenther. Onkol.* **2009**, *185*, 120–126. [CrossRef]
136. Andocs, G.; Rehman, M.U.; Zhao, Q.-L.; Tabuchi, Y.; Kanamori, M.; Kondo, T. Comparison of biological effects of modulated electro-hyperthermia and conventional heat treatment in human lymphoma U937 cells. *Cell Death Discov.* **2016**, *2*, 16039. [CrossRef]
137. Kirson, E.D.; Gurvich, Z.; Schneiderman, R.; Dekel, E.; Itzhaki, A.; Wasserman, Y.; Schatzberger, R.; Palti, Y. Disruption of Cancer Cell Replication by Alternating Electric Fields. *Cancer Res.* **2004**, *64*, 3288–3295. [CrossRef]
138. Vincze, G.; Szasz, A. Reorganization of actin filaments and microtubules by outside electric field. *J. Adv. Biol.* **2015**, *8*, 1514–1518.
139. Dimova, R.; Bezlyepkina, N.; Jordö, M.D.; Knorr, R.L.; Riske, K.A.; Staykova, M.; Vlahovska, P.M.; Yamamoto, T.; Yang, P.; Lipowsky, R. Vesicles in electric fields: Some novel aspects of membrane behavior. *Soft Matter* **2009**, *5*, 3201–3212. [CrossRef]
140. Vincze, G.; Szigeti, G.; Andocs, G.; Szasz, A. Nanoheating without Artificial Nanoparticles. *Biol. Med.* **2015**, *7*, 249.
141. Guo, J.; Lao, Y.; Chang, D.C. Calcium and Apoptosis. In *Handbook of Neurochemistry and Molecular Neurobiology*; Lajtha, A., Mikoshiba, K., Eds.; Springer: Boston, MA, USA, 2009. [CrossRef]
142. Cha, J.; Jeon, T.-W.; Lee, C.G.; Oh, S.T.; Yang, H.-B.; Choi, K.-J.; Seo, D.; Yun, I.; Baik, I.H.; Park, K.R.; et al. Electro-hyperthermia inhibits glioma tumorigenicity through the induction of E2F1-mediated apoptosis. *Int. J. Hyperth.* **2015**, *31*, 784–792. [CrossRef] [PubMed]
143. Li, J.; Chauve, L.; Phelps, G.; Brielmann, R.M.; Morimoto, R.I. E2F coregulates an essential HSF developmental program that is distinct from the heat-shock response. *Genes Dev.* **2016**, *30*, 2062–2075. [CrossRef] [PubMed]
144. Wust, P.; Kortüm, B.; Strauss, U.; Nadobny, J.; Zschaeck, S.; Beck, M.; Stein, U.; Ghadjar, P. Non-thermal effects of radiofrequency electromagnetic fields. *Sci. Rep.* **2020**, *10*, 13488. [CrossRef] [PubMed]
145. Krenacs, T.; Benyo, Z. Tumor specific stress and immune response induced by modulated electrohyperthermia in relation to tumor metabolic profiles. *Oncothermia J.* **2017**, *20*, 264–272.
146. Forika, G.; Vancsik, T.; Kiss, E.; Hujber, T.; Sebestyen, A.; Krencz, I.; Benyo, Z.; Hamar, P.; Krenacs, T. The efficiency of modulated electro-hyperthermia may correlate with the tumor metabolic profiles. *Oncothermia J.* **2017**, *20*, 228–235.
147. Vincze, G.; Szasz, N.; Szasz, A. On the thermal noise limit of cellular membranes. *Bioelectromagnetics* **2004**, *26*, 28–35. [CrossRef]
148. Forika, G.; Balogh, A.; Vancsik, T. Elevated apoptosis and tumor stem cell destruction in a radioresistant pancreatic adenocarcinoma cell line when radiotherapy is combined with modulated electrohyperthermia. *Oncothermia J.* **2019**, *26*, 90–98.
149. Meggyeshazi, N.; Andocs, G.; Krenacs, T. Modulated electro-hyperthermia induced programmed cell death in HT29 colorectal carcinoma xenograft. *Virchows Arch.* **2012**, *461* (Suppl. 1), S131–S132.

150. Danics, L.; Schvarcz, C.A.; Viana, P.; Vancsik, T.; Krenács, T.; Benyó, Z.; Kaucsár, T.; Hamar, P. Exhaustion of Protective Heat Shock Response Induces Significant Tumor Damage by Apoptosis after Modulated Electro-Hyperthermia Treatment of Triple Negative Breast Cancer Isografts in Mice. *Cancers* **2020**, *12*, 2581. [CrossRef]
151. Meggyeshazi, N.; Andocs, G.; Spisak, S.; Krenacs, T. Modulated electrohyperthermia causes caspase independent programmed cell death in HT29 colon cancer xenografts. *Virchows Arch.* **2013**, *463*, 329.
152. Meggyesházi, N.; Andocs, G.; Balogh, L.; Balla, P.; Kiszner, G.; Teleki, I.; Jeney, A.; Krenács, T. DNA fragmentation and caspase-independent programmed cell death by modulated electrohyperthermia. *Strahlenther. Onkol.* **2014**, *190*, 815–822. [CrossRef] [PubMed]
153. Meggyeshazi, N.; Andocs, G.; Spisak, S.; Krenacs, T. Early changes in mRNA and protein expression related to cancer treatment by modulated electro-hyperthermia. *Hindawi Publ. Corp. Conf. Pap. Med.* **2013**, *2013*, 249563.
154. Jeon, T.-W.; Yang, H.; Lee, C.G.; Oh, S.T.; Seo, D.; Baik, I.H.; Lee, E.H.; Yun, I.; Park, K.R.; Lee, Y.-H. Electro-hyperthermia up-regulates tumour suppressor Septin 4 to induce apoptotic cell death in hepatocellular carcinoma. *Int. J. Hyperth.* **2016**, *32*, 648–656. [CrossRef] [PubMed]
155. McDonald, M.; Corde, S.; Lerch, M.; Rosenfeld, A.; Jackson, M.; Tehei, M. First in vitro evidence of modulated electro-hyperthermia treatment performance in combination with megavoltage radiation by clonogenic assay. *Sci. Rep.* **2018**, *8*, 16608. [CrossRef] [PubMed]
156. Forika, G. Radiotherapy and modulated electro-hyperthermia effect on Panc1 and Capan1 pancreas adenocarcinoma cell lines. *Oncothermia J.* **2018**, *24*, 455–463.
157. Forika, G.; Balogh, A.; Vancsik, T.; Benyo, Z.; Krenács, T. Apoptotic response and DNA damage of the radioresistant Panc1 pancreas adenocarcinoma to combined modulated electro hyperthermia and radiotherapy. *Oncothermia J.* **2020**, *29*, 103–109.
158. Yoshikata, M.; Junki, H.; Yuta, S. Radiosensitization effect of novel cancer therapy, oncothermia toward overcoming treatment resistance. *Oncothermia J.* **2019**, *25*, 68–84.
159. Prasad, B.; Kim, S.; Cho, W.; Kim, S.; Kim, J.K. Effect of tumor properties on energy absorption, temperature mapping, and thermal dose in 13.56-MHz radiofrequency hyperthermia. *J. Therm. Biol.* **2018**, *74*, 281–289. [CrossRef]
160. Chen, C.-C.; Chen, C.-L.; Li, J.-J.; Chen, Y.-Y.; Wang, C.-Y.; Wang, Y.-S.; Chi, K.-H.; Wang, H.-E. Presence of Gold Nanoparticles in Cells Associated with the Cell-Killing Effect of Modulated Electro-Hyperthermia. *ACS Appl. Bio Mater.* **2019**, *2*, 3573–3581. [CrossRef]
161. Besztercei, B.; Vancsik, T.; Benedek, A.; Major, E.; Thomas, M.J.; Schvarcz, C.A.; Krenács, T.; Benyó, Z.; Balogh, A. Stress-Induced, p53-Mediated Tumor Growth Inhibition of Melanoma by Modulated Electrohyperthermia in Mouse Models without Major Immunogenic Effects. *Int. J. Mol. Sci.* **2019**, *20*, 4019. [CrossRef] [PubMed]
162. Oei, A.L.; Vriend, L.E.M.; Crezee, J.; Franken, N.A.P.; Krawczyk, P.M. Effects of hyperthermia on DNA repair pathways: One treatment to inhibit them all. *Radiat. Oncol.* **2015**, *10*, 165. [CrossRef] [PubMed]
163. Thomas, M.B.; Major, E.; Benedek, A.; Horváth, I.; Máthé, D.; Bergmann, R.; Szasz, A.M.; Krenacs, T.; Benyo, Z. Suppression of metastatic melanoma growth in lung by modulated electro-hyperthermia monitored by a minimally invasive heat stress testing approach in mice. *Cancers* **2020**, *12*, 3872. [CrossRef] [PubMed]
164. Schvarcz, C.; Danics, L.; Krenács, T.; Viana, P.; Béres, R.; Vancsik, T.; Nagy, Á.; Gyenesei, A.; Kun, J.; Fonović, M.; et al. Modulated Electro-Hyperthermia Induces a Prominent Local Stress Response and Growth Inhibition in Mouse Breast Cancer Isografts. *Cancers* **2021**, *13*, 1744. [CrossRef]
165. Andocs, G.; Meggyeshazi, N.; Balogh, L.; Spisak, S.; Maros, M.E.; Balla, P.; Kiszner, G.; Teleki, I.; Kovago, C.; Krenacs, T. Upregulation of heat shock proteins and the promotion of damage-associated molecular pattern signals in a colorectal cancer model by modulated electrohyperthermia. *Cell Stress Chaperones* **2014**, *20*, 37–46. [CrossRef]
166. Daguenet, E.; Louati, S.; Wozny, A.-S.; Vial, N.; Gras, M.; Guy, J.-B.; Vallard, A.; Rodriguez-Lafrasse, C.; Magné, N. Radiation-induced bystander and abscopal effects: Important lessons from preclinical models. *Br. J. Cancer* **2020**, *123*, 339–348. [CrossRef]
167. Piana, R. The Abscopal Effect: A Reemerging Field of Interest. The ASCO Post 2018. Available online: https://ascopost.com/issues/november-25-2018/the-abscopal-effect-a-reemerging-field-of-interest/ (accessed on 12 December 2021).
168. Hu, Z.I.; McArthur, H.L.; Ho, A.Y. The Abscopal Effect of Radiation Therapy: What Is It and How Can We Use It in Breast Cancer? *Curr. Breast Cancer Rep.* **2017**, *9*, 45–51. [CrossRef]
169. Vancsik, T.; Máthé, D.; Horváth, I.; Várallyaly, A.A.; Benedek, A.; Bergmann, R.; Krenács, T.; Benyó, Z.; Balogh, A. Modulated Electro-Hyperthermia Facilitates NK-Cell Infiltration and Growth Arrest of Human A2058 Melanoma in a Xenograft Model. *Front. Oncol.* **2021**, *11*, 590764. [CrossRef]
170. Qin, W.; Akutsu, Y.; Andocs, G.; Suganami, A.; Hu, X.; Yusup, G.; Komatsu-Akimoto, A.; Hoshino, I.; Hanari, N.; Mori, M.; et al. Modulated electro-hyperthermia enhances dendritic cell therapy through an abscopal effect in mice. *Oncol. Rep.* **2014**, *32*, 2373–2379. [CrossRef]
171. Lee, Y.J.; Kang, S.Y.; Jo, M.S.; Suh, D.S.; Kim, K.H.; Yoon, M.S. S100 expression in dendritic cells is inversely correlated with tumor grade in endometrial carcinoma. *Obstet. Gynecol. Sci.* **2014**, *57*, 201–207. [CrossRef]
172. Tsang, Y.W.; Huang, C.C.; Yang, K.L.; Chi, M.-S.; Chiang, H.-C.; Wang, Y.-S.; Andocs, G.; Szasz, A.; Li, W.-T. Improving immunological tumor microenvironment using electro-hyperthermia followed by dendritic cell immunotherapy. *BMC Cancer* **2015**, *15*, 708. [CrossRef] [PubMed]

173. Vancsik, T.; Kiss, E.; Kovago, C.; Meggyeshazi, N.; Forika, G.; Krenacs, T. Inhibition of proliferation, induction of apoptotic cell death and immune response by modulated electro-hyperthermia in C26 colorectal cancer allografts, thermometry. *Oncothermia J.* **2017**, *20*, 277–292.
174. Vancsik, T.; Kovago, C.; Kiss, E.; Papp, E.; Forika, G.; Benyo, Z.; Meggyeshazi, N.; Krenacs, T. Modulated electro-hyperthermia induced loco-regional and systemic tumor destruction in colorectal cancer allografts. *J. Cancer* **2018**, *9*, 41–53. [CrossRef] [PubMed]
175. Vancsik, T.; Forika, G.; Balogh, A.; Kiss, E.; Krenacs, T. Modulated electro-hyperthermia induced p53 driven apoptosis and cell cycle arrest additively support doxorubicin chemotherapy of colorectal cancer in vitro. *Cancer Med.* **2019**, *8*, 4292–4303. [CrossRef]
176. Wismeth, C.; Dudel, C.; Pascher, C.; Ramm, P.; Pietsch, T.; Hirschmann, B.; Reinert, C.; Proescholdt, M.A.; Rümmele, P.; Schuierer, G.; et al. Transcranial electro-hyperthermia combined with alkylating chemotherapy in patients with relapsed high-grade gliomas: Phase I clinical results. *J. Neuro-Oncol.* **2009**, *98*, 395–405. [CrossRef]
177. Minnaar, C.A.; Kotzen, J.A.; Ayeni, O.A.; Naidoo, T.; Tunmer, M.; Sharma, V.; Vangu, M.-D.-T.; Baeyens, A. The effect of modulated electro-hyperthermia on local disease control in HIV-positive and -negative cervical cancer women in South Africa: Early results from a phase III randomized controlled trial. *PLoS ONE* **2019**, *14*, e0217894. [CrossRef]
178. Minnaar, C.A.; Kotzen, J.A.; Naidoo, T.; Tunmer, M.; Sharma, V.; Vangu, M.-D.-T.; Baeyens, A. Analysis of the effects of mEHT on the treatment-related toxicity and quality of life of HIV-positive cervical cancer patients. *Int. J. Hyperth.* **2020**, *37*, 263–272. [CrossRef]
179. Minnaar, C.A.; Kotzen, J.A.; Ayeni, O.A.; Vangu, M.-D.-T.; Baeyens, A. Potentiation of the Abscopal Effect by Modulated Electro-Hyperthermia in Locally Advanced Cervical Cancer Patients. *Front. Oncol.* **2020**, *10*, 376. [CrossRef]
180. Minnaar, C.A.; Kotzen, J.A.; Baeyens, A. Possible potentiation of the abscopal effect of ionising radiation by modulated electro-hyperthermia in locally advanced cervical cancer patients. *Oncothermia J.* **2018**, *24*, 122–132.
181. Minnaar, C.; Kotzen, J. Modulated electro hyperthermia as an immune modulator with checkpoint inhibitors and radiotherapy. *Eur. J. Cancer* **2019**, *110*, S19–S20. [CrossRef]
182. Chi, K.H. Tumor-directed immunotherapy: Combined radiotherapy and oncothermia. *Oncothermia J.* **2018**, *24*, 196–235.
183. Szasz, A.M.; Minnaar, C.A.; Szentmartoni, G.; Szigeti, G.P.; Dank, M. Review of the clinical evidences of modulated electro-hyperthermia (mEHT) method: An update for the practicing oncologist. *Front. Oncol.* **2019**, *9*, 1012. [CrossRef] [PubMed]
184. Parmar, G.; Rurak, E.; Elderfield, M.; Li, K.; Soles, S.; Rinas, A. 8-year observational study on naturopathic treatment with modulated electro-hyperthermia (mEHT): A single-centre experience. In *Challenges and Solutions of Oncological Hyperthermia*; Szasz, A., Ed.; Cambridge Scholars: Newcastle upon Tyne, UK, 2020; pp. 227–266.
185. Fiorentini, G.; Sarti, D.; Gadaleta, C.D.; Ballerini, M.; Fiorentini, C.; Garfagno, T.; Ranieri, G.; Guadagni, S. A Narrative Review of Regional Hyperthermia: Updates from 2010 to 2019. *Integr. Cancer Ther.* **2020**, *19*, 1–13. [CrossRef] [PubMed]
186. Fiorentini, G.; Giovanis, P.; Rossi, S.; Dentico, P.; Paola, R.; Turrisi, G.; Bernardeschi, P. A phase II clinical study on relapsed malignant gliomas treated with electro-hyperthermia. *Vivo* **2006**, *20*, 721–724.
187. Sahinbas, H.; Groenemeyer, D.H.W.; Boecher, E.; Szasz, A. Retrospective clinical study of adjuvant electro-hyperthermia treatment for advanced brain-gliomas. *Dtsch. Z. Für Onkol.* **2007**, *39*, 154–160. [CrossRef]
188. Hager, E.D.; Sahinbas, H.; Groenemeyer, D.H.; Migeod, F. Prospective phase II trial for recurrent high-grade gliomas with capacitive coupled low radiofrequency (LRF) hyperthermia. *J. Clin. Oncol.* **2008**, *26*, 2047. [CrossRef]
189. Fiorentini, G.; Sarti, D.; Milandri, C.; Dentico, P.; Mambrini, A.; Fiorentini, C.; Mattioli, G.; Casadei, V.; Guadagni, S. Modulated Electrohyperthermia in Integrative Cancer Treatment for Relapsed Malignant Glioblastoma and Astrocytoma: Retrospective Multicenter Controlled Study. *Integr. Cancer Ther.* **2018**, *18*, 1–11. [CrossRef]
190. Minnaar, C.; Baeyens, A.; Kotzen, J. O34. Update on phase III randomized clinical trial investigating the effects of the addition of electro-hyperthermia to chemoradiotherapy for cervical cancer patients in South Africa. *Phys. Med.* **2016**, *32*, 151–152. [CrossRef]
191. Pesti, L.; Dankovics, Z.; Lorencz, P.; Csejtei, A. Treatment of advanced cervical cancer with complex chemoradio–hyperthermia. *Hindawi Publ. Corp. Conf. Pap. Med.* **2013**, *2013*, 192435. [CrossRef]
192. Ou, J.; Zhu, X.; Chen, P.; Du, Y.; Lu, Y.; Peng, X.; Bao, S.; Wang, J.; Zhang, X.; Zhang, T.; et al. A randomized phase II trial of best supportive care with or without hyperthermia and vitamin C for heavily pretreated, advanced, refractory non-small-cell lung cancer. *J. Adv. Res.* **2020**, *24*, 175–182. [CrossRef]
193. Szasz, A. Current Status of Oncothermia Therapy for Lung Cancer. *Korean J. Thorac. Cardiovasc. Surg.* **2014**, *47*, 77–93. [CrossRef] [PubMed]
194. You, S.H.; Kim, S. Feasibility of modulated electro-hyperthermia in preoperative treatment for locally-advanced rectal cancer: Early phase 2 clinical results. *Neoplasma* **2019**, *67*, 677–683. [CrossRef] [PubMed]
195. Jeung, T.S.; Ma, S.Y.; Choi, J.; Yu, J.; Lee, S.Y.; Lim, S. Results of Oncothermia Combined with Operation, Chemotherapy and Radiation Therapy for Primary, Recurrent and Metastatic Sarcoma. *Case Rep. Clin. Med.* **2015**, *04*, 157–168. [CrossRef]
196. Fiorentini, G.; Sarti, D.; Casadei, V.; Milandri, C.; Dentico, P.; Mambrini, A.; Nani, R.; Fiorentini, C.; Guadagni, S. Modulated electro-hyperthermia as palliative treatment for pancreas cancer: A retrospective observational study on 106 patients. *Integr. Cancer Ther.* **2019**, *18*, 1–8. [CrossRef]
197. Dani, A.; Varkonyi, A.; Magyar, T.; Szasz, A. Clinical study for advanced pancreas cancer treated by oncothermia. *Forum Hyperthermie* **2008**, *1*, 13–20.

198. Ranieri, G.; Ferrari, C.; di Palo, A.; Marech, I.; Porcelli, M.; Falagario, G.; Ritrovato, F.; Ramuni, L.; Fanelli, M.; Rubini, G.; et al. Bevacizumab-Based Chemotherapy Combined with, Regional Deep Capacitive Hyperthermia in Metastatic Cancer Patients: A Pilot Study. *Int. J. Mol. Sci.* **2017**, *18*, 1458. [CrossRef]
199. Kim, S.; Lee, J.H.; Cha, J.; You, S.H. Beneficial effects of modulated electro-hyperthermia during neoadjuvant treatment for locally advanced rectal cancer. *Int. J. Hyperth.* **2021**, *38*, 144–151. [CrossRef]
200. Fiorentini, G.; Sarti, D.; Casadei, V.; Milandri, C.; Dentico, P.; Mambrini, A.; Guadagni, S. Modulated electro-hyperthermia for the treatment of relapsed brain gliomas. In *Challenges and Solutions of Oncological Hyperthermia*; Szasz, A., Ed.; Cambridge Scholars: Newcastle upon Tyne, UK, 2020; pp. 110–125.
201. Wookyeom, Y.; Han, G.H.; Shin, H.Y.; Lee, E.-J.; Cho, H.; Chay, D.B.; Kim, J.-H. Combined treatment with modulated electro-hyperthermia and an autophagy inhibitor effectively inhibit ovarian and cervical cancer growth. *Int. J. Hyperth.* **2018**, *36*, 9–20.
202. Arrojo, E.E. The position of modulated electro-hyperthermia (oncothermia) in combination with standard chemo- and radio-therapy in clinical practice–Highlights of upcoming phase III clinical studies in hospital Universitario Marqués de Val-decilla (HUMV). In *Challenges and Solutions of Oncological Hyperthermia*; Szasz, A., Ed.; Cambridge Scholars: Newcastle upon Tyne, UK, 2020; pp. 91–104.
203. van Gool, S.W.; Makalowski, J.; Feyen, O.; Prix, L.; Schirrmacher, V.; Stuecker, W. The induction of immunogenic cell death (ICD) during maintenance chemotherapy and subsequent multimodal immunotherapy for glioblastoma (GBM). *Austin Oncol. Case Rep.* **2018**, *3*, 1–8.
204. Kurakin, A. The self-organizing fractal theory as a universal discovery method: The phenomenon of life. *Theor. Biol. Med Model.* **2011**, *8*, 1–66. [CrossRef] [PubMed]
205. Haken, H. Self-Organization and Information. *Phys. Scr.* **1987**, *35*, 247–254. [CrossRef]
206. Sornette, D. *Chaos, Fractals, Self-Organization and Disorder: Concepts and Tools*; Springer: Berlin/Heidelberg, Germany; Los Angeles, CA, USA, 2000.
207. Sha, L.; Ward, E.R.; Stroy, B. A Review of Dielectric Properties of Normal and Malignant Breast Tissue. In Proceedings of the IEEE Southeast Con. 2002, Columbia, SC, USA, 5–7 April 2002; pp. 457–462.
208. Scholz, B.; Anderson, R. On electrical impedance scanning-principles and simulations. *Electromedica* **2000**, *68*, 35–44.
209. Haemmerich, D.; Staelin, S.T.; Tsai, J.Z.; Tungjitkusolmun, S.; Mahvi, D.M.; Webster, J.G. In vivo electrical conductivity of hepatic tumors. *Physiol. Meas.* **2003**, *24*, 251–260. [CrossRef]
210. Smith, S.R.; Foster, K.R.; Wolf, G.L. Dielectric Properties of VX-2 Carcinoma Versus Normal Liver Tissue. *IEEE Trans. Biomed. Eng.* **1986**, *33*, 522–524. [CrossRef]
211. Gregorie, V.; Chiti, A. PET in radiotherapy planning: Particularly exquisite test or pending and experimental tool? *Radiother. Oncol.* **2010**, *96*, 275–276. [CrossRef]
212. Cope, F.W. A review of the applications of solid state physics concepts to biological systems. *J. Biol. Phys.* **1975**, *3*, 1–41. [CrossRef]
213. Damadian, R. Tumor Detection by Nuclear Magnetic Resonance. *Science* **1971**, *171*, 1151–1153. [CrossRef]
214. Hazlewood, C.F.; Nichols, B.L.; Chamberlain, N.F. Evidence for the Existence of a Minimum of Two Phases of Ordered Water in Skeletal Muscle. *Nature* **1969**, *222*, 747–750. [CrossRef]
215. Durney, C.H.; Johnson, C.C.; Barber, P.W.; Massoudi, H.; Iskander, M.F.; Allen, S.J.; Mitchell, J.C. Descriptive summary: Radiofrequency radiation dosimetry handbook-Second edition. *Radio Sci.* **1979**, *14*, 5–7. [CrossRef]
216. Szent-Györgyi, A. The living state and cancer. *Physiol. Chem. Phys.* **1980**, *12*, 99–110. [CrossRef]
217. Szent-Györgyi, A. *Electronic Biology and Cancer*; Marcel Dekker: New York, NY, USA, 1998.
218. Szent-Györgyi, A. *Bioelectronics, a Study on Cellular Regulations, Defense and Cancer*; Acadamic Press: New York, NY, USA; London, UK, 1968.
219. Pething, R. *Dielectric and Electronic Properties of Biological Materials*; John Wiley and Sons: New York, NY, USA, 1979.
220. Volkov, V.V.; Palmer, D.J.; Righini, R. Distinct Water Species Confined at the Interface of a Phospholipid Membrane. *Phys. Rev. Lett.* **2007**, *99*, 078302. [CrossRef] [PubMed]
221. Liu, L.M.; Cleary, S.F. Absorbed Energy Distribution from Radiofrequency Electromagnetic Radiation in a Mammalian Cell Model: Effect of Membrane-Bound Water. *Bioelectromagnetics* **1995**, *16*, 160–171. [CrossRef] [PubMed]
222. Hendry, B. *Membrane Physiology and Membrane Excitation*; Croom Helm: London, UK, 1981.
223. Ma, Y.; Poole, K.; Goyette, J.; Gaus, K. Introducing Membrane Charge and Membrane Potential to T Cell Signaling. *Front. Immunol.* **2017**, *8*, 1513. [CrossRef] [PubMed]
224. Horváth, I.; Multhoff, G.; Sonnleitner, A.; Vígh, L. Membrane-associated stress proteins: More than simply chaperones. *Biochim. Biophys. Acta* **2008**, *1778*, 1653–1664. [CrossRef] [PubMed]
225. Nicolau, D.V.; Burrage, K.; Parton, R.G.; Hancock, J.F. Identifying Optimal Lipid Raft Characteristics Required to Promote Nanoscale Protein-Protein Interactions on the Plasma Membrane. *Mol. Cell. Biol.* **2006**, *26*, 313–323. [CrossRef]
226. Nicolson, G.L. The Fluid—Mosaic Model of Membrane Structure: Still relevant to understanding the structure, function and dynamics of biological membranes after more than 40 years. *Biochim. Biophys. Acta* **2014**, *1838*, 1451–1466. [CrossRef]
227. Gramse, G.; Dols-Perez, A.; Edwards, M.A.; Fumagalli, L.; and Gomila, G. Nanoscale Measurement of the Dielectric Constant of Supported Lipid Bilayers in Aqueous Solutions with Electrostatic Force Microscopy. *J. Biophys.* **2013**, *104*, 1257–1262. [CrossRef]

228. Dharia, S. Spatially and Temporally Resolving Radio-Frequency Changes in Effective Cell Membrane Capacitance. Ph.D. Thesis, University of Utah, Salt Lake City, UT, USA, 2011.
229. Pike, L.J. Lipid rafts: Bringing order to chaos. *J. Lipid Res.* **2003**, *44*, 655–667. [CrossRef]
230. Andersen, O.S.; Koeppe, I.I.; and Roger, E. Bilayer Thickness and Membrane Protein Function: An Energetic Perspective. *Annu. Rev. Biophys. Biomol. Struct.* **2007**, *36*, 107–130. [CrossRef]
231. Govorov, A.O.; Richardson, H.H. Generating heat with metal nanoparticles. *Nano Today* **2007**, *2*, 30–38. [CrossRef]
232. Potoyan, D.A.; Wolynes, P.G. On the dephasing of genetic oscillators. *Proc. Natl. Acad. Sci. USA* **2014**, *111*, 2391–2396. [CrossRef] [PubMed]
233. Ptitsyn, A.A.; Zvonic, S.; Gimble, J.M. Digital Signal Processing Reveals Circadian Baseline Oscillation in Majority of Mammalian Genes. *PLOS Comput. Biol.* **2007**, *3*, e120. [CrossRef] [PubMed]
234. Carey, S.P.; Kraning-Rush, C.M.; Williams, R.M.; Reinhart-King, C.A. Biophysical control of invasive tumor cell behavior by extracellular matrix microarchitecture. *Biomaterials* **2012**, *33*, 4157–4165. [CrossRef]
235. Wang, Y.; Wang, X.; Wohland, T.; Sampath, K. Extracellular interactions and ligand degradation shape the nodal morphogen gradient. *Elife* **2016**, *5*, e13879. [CrossRef]
236. Szendro, P.; Vincze, G.; Szasz, A. Pink noise behaviour of the biosystems. *Eur. Biophys. J.* **2001**, *30*, 227–231. [CrossRef]
237. Szendro, P.; Vincze, G.; Szasz, A. Bio-response to white noise excitation. *Electro- Magn.* **2001**, *20*, 215–229. [CrossRef]
238. Nasir, N.; Al Ahmad, M. Cells Electrical Characterization: Dielectric Properties, Mixture, and Modeling Theories. *J. Eng. 2020*, *2020*, 1–17. [CrossRef]
239. Cole, K.S. *Membranes, Ions and Impulses*; University of California Press: Berkeley, CA, USA, 1968.
240. Schwan, H.P. Determination of biological impedances. In *Physical Techniques in Biological Research*; Academic Press: New York, NY, USA, 1963; pp. 323–406.
241. Schwan, H.P.; Takashima, S. Dielectric behavior of biological cells and membranes. *Bull. Inst. Chem. Res.* **1991**, *69*, 459–475.
242. Anderson, J.C. *Dielectrics*; Chapman & Hall: London, UK, 1964.
243. Grant, E.H.; Sheppard, R.J.; South, S.P. *Dielectric Behavior of Biological Molecules in Solution*; Clarendon Press: Oxford, UK, 1978. [CrossRef]
244. Pennock, B.E.; Schwan, H.P. Further observations on the electrical properties of hemoglobin-bound water. *J. Phys. Chem.* **1969**, *73*, 2600–2610. [CrossRef]
245. Pethig, R.R. *Dielectrophoresis: Theory, Methodology and Biological Applications*; John Wiley & Sons: Hoboken, NJ, USA, 2017.
246. Asami, K. Characterization of biological cells by dielectric spectroscopy. *J. Non-Cryst. Solids* **2002**, *305*, 268–277. [CrossRef]
247. Pauly, H.; Schwan, H.P. Über die Impedanz einer Suspension von kugelförmigen Teilchen mit einer Schale. *Z. Für Nat. B* **1959**, *14*, 125–131. [CrossRef]
248. Stubbe, M.; Gimsa, J. Maxwell's Mixing Equation Revisited: Characteristic Impedance Equations for Ellipsoidal Cells. *Biophys. J.* **2015**, *109*, 194–208. [CrossRef] [PubMed]
249. Pliquett, F.; Pliquett, U. Tissue impedance, measured by pulse deformation. In Proceedings of the 8th International Conference on Electrical Bio-impedance, University of Kuopio, Kuopio, Finland, 28–31 July 1992; pp. 179–181.
250. Loft, S.M.; Conway, J.; Brown, B.H. Bioimpedance and cancer therapy. In Proceedings of the 8th International Conference on Electrical Bio-impedance, University of Kuopio, Kuopio, Finland, 28–31 July 1992; pp. 119–121.
251. Tan, L.T.-H.; Chan, K.-G.; Pusparajah, P.; Lee, W.-L.; Chuah, L.-H.; Khan, T.M.; Lee, L.-H.; Goh, B.-H. Targeting membrane lipid a potential cancer cure? *Front. Pharmacol.* **2017**, *8*, 12. [CrossRef] [PubMed]
252. Chidambaram, R.; Ramanadham, M. Hydrogen bonding in biological molecules—An update. *Phys. B Condens. Matter* **1991**, *174*, 300–305. [CrossRef]
253. Meggyeshazi, N. Studies on Modulated Electrohyperthermia Induced Tumor Cell Death in a Colorectal Carcinoma Model. Ph.D. Thesis, Pathological Sciences Doctoral School, Semmelweis University, Budapest, Hungary, 2015.
254. Wust, P.; Ghadjar, P.; Nadobny, J.; Beck, M.; Kaul, D.; Winter, L.; Zschaeck, S. Physical analysis of temperature-dependent effects of amplitude-modulated electromagnetic hyperthermia. *Int. J. Hyperth.* **2019**, *36*, 1245–1253. [CrossRef] [PubMed]
255. Wust, P.; Nadobny, J.; Zschaeck, S.; Ghadjar, P. Physics of hyperthermia–Is physics really against us? In *Challenges and Solutions of Oncological Hyperthermia*; Szasz, A., Ed.; Cambridge Scholars: Newcastle upon Tyne, UK, 2020; pp. 346–376.
256. Romanenko, S.; Begley, R.; Harvey, A.R.; Hool, L.; Wallace, V. The interaction between electromagnetic fields at megahertz, gigahertz and terahertz frequencies with cells, tissues and organisms: Risks and potential. *J. R. Soc. Interface* **2017**, *14*, 20170585. [CrossRef]
257. Szasz, O.; Szasz, A. Heating, Efficacy and Dose of Local Hyperthermia. *Open J. Biophys.* **2016**, *6*, 10–18. [CrossRef]
258. Szasz, O. Bioelectromagnetic Paradigm of Cancer Treatment—Modulated Electro-Hyperthermia (mEHT). *Open J. Biophys.* **2019**, *9*, 98–109. [CrossRef]
259. Kao, P.H.J.; Chen, C.H.; Chang, Y.W.; Lin, C.-S.; Chiang, H.-C.; Huang, C.-C.; Chi, M.-S.; Yang, K.-L.; Li, W.-T.; Kao, S.-J.; et al. Relationship between energy dosage and apoptotic cell death by modulated electro-hyperthermia. *Sci. Rep.* **2020**, *10*, 8936. [CrossRef]
260. Almeida, V.M.; Marana, S.R. Optimum temperature may be a misleading parameter in enzyme characterization and application. *PLoS ONE* **2019**, *14*, e0212977. [CrossRef]

261. Eppink, B.; Krawczyk, P.M.; Stap, J.; Kanaar, R. Hyperthermia induced DNA repair deficiency suggests novel therapeutic anti-cancer strategies. *Int. J. Hyperth.* **2012**, *28*, 509–517. [CrossRef] [PubMed]
262. Datta, N.R.; Bodis, S. Hyperthermia with radiotherapy reduces tumor alpha/beta: Insights from trials of thermoradiotherapy vs radiotherapy alone. *Radiother. Oncol.* **2019**, *138*, 1–8. [CrossRef] [PubMed]
263. Fowler, J.F. The linear-quadratic formula and progress in fractionated radiotherapy. *Br. J. Radiol.* **1989**, *62*, 679–694. [CrossRef] [PubMed]
264. Kok, H.P.; Crezee, J.; Franken, N.; Stalpers, L.J.; Barendsen, G.W.; Bel, A. Quantifying the Combined Effect of Radiation Therapy and Hyperthermia in Terms of Equivalent Dose Distributions. *Int. J. Radiat. Oncol.* **2014**, *88*, 739–745. [CrossRef] [PubMed]
265. Wang, J.-S.; Wang, H.-J.; Qian, H.-L. Biological effects of radiation on cancer cells. *Mil. Med. Res.* **2018**, *5*, 1–10. [CrossRef]
266. Zalba, S.; Ten Hagen, T.L.M. Cell membrane modulation as adjuvant in cancer therapy. *Cancer Treat. Rev.* **2016**, *52*, 48–57. [CrossRef]
267. Mendez, F.; Sandigursky, M.; Franklin, W.A.; Kenny, M.K.; Kureekattil, R.; Bases, R. Heat-Shock Proteins Associated with Base Excision Repair Enzymes in HeLa Cells. *Radiat. Res.* **2000**, *153*, 186–195. [CrossRef]
268. Gaitanaki, C.; Mastri, M.; Aggeli, I.-K.S.; Beis, I. Differential roles of p38-MAPK and JNKs in mediating early protection or apoptosis in the hyperthermic perfused amphibian heart. *J. Exp. Biol.* **2008**, *211*, 2524–2532. [CrossRef]
269. Daniel, R.M.; Danson, M.J. Temperature and the catalytic activity of enzymes: A fresh understanding. *FEBS Lett.* **2013**, *587*, 2738–2743. [CrossRef]
270. Vashum, S.; Singh, I.R.R.; Das, S.; Azharuddin, M.; Vasudevan, P. Quantification of DNA double-strand break induced by radiation in cervix cancer cells: In vitro study. *J. Radiother. Pract.* **2019**, *18*, 55–62. [CrossRef]
271. Macphail, S.H.; Banáth, J.P.; Chu, E.H.M.; Lambur, H.; Olive, P.L. Expression of phosphorylated histone H2AX in cultured cell lines following exposure to X-rays. *Int. J. Radiat. Biol.* **2003**, *79*, 351–359. [CrossRef] [PubMed]
272. Banáth, J.P.; MacPhail, S.H.; Olive, P.L. Radiation sensitivity, H2AX phosphorylation, and kinetics of repair of DNA strand breaks in irradiated cervical cancer cell lines. *Cancer Res.* **2004**, *64*, 7144–7149. [CrossRef] [PubMed]
273. Mei, X.; Ten Cate, R.; van Leeuwen, C.M.; Rodermond, H.M.; de Leeuw, L.; Dimitrakopoulou, D.; Stalpers, L.J.A.; Crezee, J.; Kok, H.P.; Franken, N.A.P.; et al. Radiosensitization by hyperthermia: The effects of temperature, sequence, and time interval in cervical cell lines. *Cancers* **2020**, *12*, 582. [CrossRef] [PubMed]
274. van Leuwen, C.M.; Oei, A.L.; Chin, K.W.T.K.; Crezee, J.; Bel, A.; Westerman, A.M.; Buist, M.R.; Franken, N.A.P.; Stalpers, L.J.A.; Kok, H.P. A short time interval between radiotherapy and hyperthermia reduces in-filed recurrence and mortality in women with advanced cervical cancer. *Radiat. Oncol.* **2017**, *12*, 1–8. [CrossRef]
275. van Leuwen, C.M.; Oei, A.L.; Ten Cate, R.; Franken, N.A.P.; Bel, A.; Stalpers, L.J.A.; Crezee, J.; Kok, H.P. Measurement and analysis of the impact of time interval temperature and radiation dose on tumor cell survival and its application in thermoradiotherapy plan evaluation. *Int. J. Hyperth.* **2018**, *34*, 30–38. [CrossRef]
276. Raaphorst, G.P. Thermal radiosensitization in vitro. In *Hyperthermia and Oncology*; Urano, M., Douple, E., Eds.; VSP: Utrecht, The Netherlands, 1994; Volume 2, pp. 17–51.
277. Overgaard, J. Simultaneous and sequential hyperthermia and radiation treatment of an experimental tumor and its surrounding normal tissue in vivo. *Int. J. Radiat. Oncol.* **1980**, *6*, 1507–1517. [CrossRef]
278. Kroesen, M.; Mulder, H.T.; van Holthe, J.M.L.; Aangeenbrug, A.A.; Mens, J.W.M.; van Doorn, H.C.; Paulides, M.M.; Oomen-de Hoop, E.; Vernhout, R.M.; Lutgens, L.C.; et al. The Effect of the Time Interval Between Radiation and Hyperthermia on Clinical Outcome in 400 Locally Advanced Cervical Carcinoma Patients. *Front. Oncol.* **2019**, *9*, 134. [CrossRef]
279. Crezee, H.; Kok, H.P.; Oei, A.L.; Franken, N.A.P.; Stalpers, L.J.A. The Impact of the Time Interval Between Radiation and Hyperthermia on Clinical Outcome in Patients with Locally Advanced Cervical Cancer. *Front. Oncol.* **2019**, *9*, 412. [CrossRef]
280. Kroesen, M.; Mulder, H.T.; van Rhoon, G.C.; Franckena, M. Commentary: The Impact of the Time Interval Between Radiation and Hyperthermia on Clinical Outcome in Patients with Locally Advanced Cervical Cancer. *Front. Oncol.* **2019**, *9*, 1387. [CrossRef]
281. Horsman, M.R.; Overgaard, J. Thermal radiosensitization in animal tumors: The potential for therapeutic gain. In *Hyperthermia and Oncology*; Urano, M., Douple, E., Eds.; VSP: Utrecht, The Netherlands, 1989; Volume 2, pp. 113–145.
282. Aguilar, A.; Ho, M.; Chang, E.; Carlson, K.; Natarajan, A.; Marciano, T.; Bomzon, Z.; Patel, C. Permeabilizing Cell Membranes with Electric Fields. *Cancers* **2021**, *13*, 2283. [CrossRef]
283. Okamura, Y.; Kawanabe, A.; Kawai, T. Voltage-Sensing Phosphatases: Biophysics, Physiology, and Molecular Engineering. *Physiol. Rev.* **2018**, *98*, 2097–2131. [CrossRef] [PubMed]
284. Szasz, A.M.; Arkosy, P.; Arrojo, E.E.; Bakacs, T.; Balogh, A.; Barich, A.; Borbenyi, E.; Chi, K.H.; Csoszi, T.; Daniilidis, L.; et al. Guidelines for local hyperthermia treatment in oncology. In *Challenges and Solutions of Oncological Hyperthermia*; Szasz, A., Ed.; Cambridge Scholars: Newcastle upon Tyne, UK, 2020; pp. 32–71.
285. Griffin, R.J.; Dings, R.P.M.; Jamshidi-Parsian, A.; Song, C.W. Mild temperature hyperthermia and radiation therapy: Role of tumor vascular thermotolerance and relevant physiological factors. *Int. J. Hyperth.* **2010**, *26*, 256–263. [CrossRef] [PubMed]
286. Kim, W.; Kim, M.S.; Kim, H.J.; Lee, E.; Jeong, J.-H.; Park, I.; Jeong, Y.K.; Jang, W.I. Role of HIF-1α in response of tumors to a combination of hyperthermia and radiation in vivo. *Int. J. Hyperth.* **2017**, *34*, 276–283. [CrossRef]
287. Hance, M.W.; Nolan, K.D.; Isaacs, J.S. The Double-Edged Sword: Conserved Functions of Extracellular Hsp90 in Wound Healing and Cancer. *Cancers* **2014**, *6*, 1065–1097. [CrossRef]

288. Tittelmeier, J.; Nachman, E.; Nussbaum-Krammer, C. Molecular Chaperones: A Double-Edged Sword in Neurodegenerative Diseases. *Front. Aging Neurosci.* **2020**, *12*, 581374. [CrossRef]
289. Giri, B.; Sethi, V.; Modi, S.; Garg, B.; Banerjee, S.; Saluja, A.; Dudeja, V. Heat shock protein 70 in pancreatic diseases: Friend or foe. *J. Surg. Oncol.* **2017**, *116*, 114–122. [CrossRef]
290. Pockley, A.G.; Multhoff, G. Cell Stress Proteins in Extracellular Fluids: Friend or Foe? *Ciba Found. Symp. Nat. Sleep* **2008**, *291*, 86–100. [CrossRef]
291. Wu, T.; Tanguay, R. Antibodies against heat shock proteins in environmental stresses and diseases: Frend or foe? *Cell Stress Chaper.* **2006**, *11*, 1–12. [CrossRef]
292. Taha, E.A.; Ono, K.; Eguchi, T. Roles of Extracellular HSPs as Biomarkers in Immune Surveillance and Immune Evasion. *Int. J. Mol. Sci.* **2019**, *20*, 4588. [CrossRef]
293. Derer, A.; Deloch, L.; Rubner, Y.; Fietkau, R.; Frey, B.; Gaipl, U.S. Radio-Immunotherapy-Induced Immunogenic Cancer Cells as Basis for Induction of Systemic Anti-Tumor Immune Responses–Pre-Clinical Evidence and Ongoing Clinical Applications. *Front. Immunol.* **2015**, *6*, 505. [CrossRef]
294. Stagg, A.J.; Knight, S.C. Antigen-Presenting Cells, Nature. 2001. Available online: http://labs.icb.ufmg.br/lbcd/pages2/bernardo/Bernardo/Artigos/Antigen-presenting%20Cells.pdf (accessed on 7 October 2020).
295. Rapoport, B.L.; Anderson, R. Realizing the Clinical Potential of Immunogenic Cell Death in Cancer Chemotherapy and Radiotherapy. *Int. J. Mol. Sci.* **2019**, *20*, 959. [CrossRef] [PubMed]
296. Szasz, O. Local treatment with systemic effect: Abscopal outcome. In *Challenges and Solutions of Oncological Hyperthermia*; Szasz, A., Ed.; Cambridge Scholars: Newcastle upon Tyne, UK, 2020; pp. 192–205.
297. Mole, R.H. Whole body irradiation-radiology or medicine? *Br. J. Radiol.* **1953**, *26*, 234–241. [CrossRef] [PubMed]
298. Yilmaz, M.T.; Elmali, A.; Yazici, G. Abscopal Effect, From Myth to Reality: From Radiation Oncologists' Perspective. *Cureus* **2019**, *11*, e3860. [CrossRef] [PubMed]
299. Craig, D.J.; Nanavay, N.S.; Devanaboyina, M.; Stanbery, L.; Hamouda, D.; Edelman, G.; Dworkin, L.; Nemunaitis, J.J. The abscopal effect of radiation therapy. *Future Oncol.* **2021**, *17*, 1683–1694. [CrossRef] [PubMed]
300. Liu, Y.; Dong, Y.; Kong, L.; Shi, F.; Zhu, H.; Yu, J. Abscopal effect of radiotherapy combined with immune checkpoint inhibitors. *J. Hematol. Oncol.* **2018**, *11*, 1–15. [CrossRef]
301. Reynders, K.; Illidge, T.; Siva, S.; Chang, J.Y.; de Ruysscher, D. The abscopal effect of local radiotherapy: Using immunotherapy to make a rare event clinically relevant. *Cancer Treat. Rev.* **2015**, *41*, 503–510. [CrossRef]
302. Dewan, M.Z.; Galloway, A.E.; Kawashima, N.; Dewyngaert, J.K.; Babb, J.S.; Formenti, S.C.; Demaria, S. Fractionated but not single dose radiotherapy induces an immune-mediated abscopal effect when combined with anti-CTLA-4 antibody. *Clin. Cancer Res.* **2009**, *15*, 5379–5388. [CrossRef]
303. Chi, K.H. Tumour-directed immunotherapy: Clinical results of radiotherapy with modulated electro-hyperthermia. In *Challenges and Solutions of Oncological Hyperthermia*; Szasz, A., Ed.; Cambridge Scholars: Newcastle upon Tyne, UK, 2020; pp. 206–226.
304. Dank, M.; Meggyeshazi, N.; Szigeti, G.; Andocs, G. Immune effects by selective heating of membrane rafts of cancer-cells. *J. Clin. Oncol.* **2016**, *34*, e14571. [CrossRef]
305. Andocs, G.; Meggyeshazi, N.; Okamoto, Y.; Balogh, L.; Kovago, C.; Szasz, O. Oncothermia treatment induced immunogenic cancer cell death. *Oncothermia J.* **2013**, *9*, 28–37.

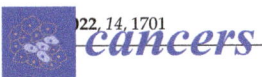

Review

Accurate Three-Dimensional Thermal Dosimetry and Assessment of Physiologic Response Are Essential for Optimizing Thermoradiotherapy

Mark W. Dewhirst [1,*], James R. Oleson [1,†], John Kirkpatrick [1] and Timothy W. Secomb [2]

1 Department of Radiation Oncology, Duke University School of Medicine, Durham, NC 27710, USA; jncoleson@bellsouth.net (J.R.O.); john.kirkpatrick@duke.edu (J.K.)
2 Department of Physiology, University of Arizona, Tucson, AZ 85724, USA; secomb@u.arizona.edu
* Correspondence: mark.dewhirst@duke.edu
† Retired.

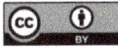

Simple Summary: Many clinical trials have shown benefit for adding hyperthermia (heat) treatment to radiotherapy. Despite overall success, some patients do not derive maximum benefit from this combination treatment. Tumor hypoxia (low oxygen concentration) is a major cause for radiotherapy treatment resistance. In this paper, we examine the question of whether hyperthermia reduces hypoxia and, if so, whether reduction in hypoxia is associated with treatment outcome. The review is focused mainly on several clinical trials conducted in humans and companion dogs with cancer treated with hyperthermia and radiotherapy. Detailed measurements of temperature, hypoxia and perfusion were made and compared with treatment outcome. These analyses show that reoxygenation after hyperthermia occurs in patients and is related to treatment outcome. Further, reoxygenation is most likely caused by variable intra-tumoral temperatures that improve perfusion and reduce oxygen consumption rate. Directions for future research on this important issue are indicated.

Abstract: Numerous randomized trials have revealed that hyperthermia (HT) + radiotherapy or chemotherapy improves local tumor control, progression free and overall survival vs. radiotherapy or chemotherapy alone. Despite these successes, however, some individuals fail combination therapy; not every patient will obtain maximal benefit from HT. There are many potential reasons for failure. In this paper, we focus on how HT influences tumor hypoxia, since hypoxia negatively influences radiotherapy and chemotherapy response as well as immune surveillance. Pre-clinically, it is well established that reoxygenation of tumors in response to HT is related to the time and temperature of exposure. In most pre-clinical studies, reoxygenation occurs only during or shortly after a HT treatment. If this were the case clinically, then it would be challenging to take advantage of HT induced reoxygenation. An important question, therefore, is whether HT induced reoxygenation occurs in the clinic that is of radiobiological significance. In this review, we will discuss the influence of thermal history on reoxygenation in both human and canine cancers treated with thermoradiotherapy. Results of several clinical series show that reoxygenation is observed and persists for 24–48 h after HT. Further, reoxygenation is associated with treatment outcome in thermoradiotherapy trials as assessed by: (1) a doubling of pathologic complete response (pCR) in human soft tissue sarcomas, (2) a 14 mmHg increase in pO2 of locally advanced breast cancers achieving a clinical response vs. a 9 mmHg decrease in pO2 of locally advanced breast cancers that did not respond and (3) a significant correlation between extent of reoxygenation (as assessed by pO2 probes and hypoxia marker drug immunohistochemistry) and duration of local tumor control in canine soft tissue sarcomas. The persistence of reoxygenation out to 24–48 h post HT is distinctly different from most reported rodent studies. In these clinical series, comparison of thermal data with physiologic response shows that within the same tumor, temperatures at the higher end of the temperature distribution likely kill cells, resulting in reduced oxygen consumption rate, while lower temperatures in the same tumor improve perfusion. However, reoxygenation does not occur in all subjects, leading to significant uncertainty about the thermal–physiologic relationship. This uncertainty stems from limited knowledge about the spatiotemporal characteristics of temperature and physiologic response. We conclude with recommendations for future research with emphasis on retrieving co-registered thermal and physiologic data before and after HT in order to begin to unravel complex thermophysiologic interactions that appear to occur with thermoradiotherapy.

Keywords: thermal dosimetry; hypoxia; hyperthermia; radiation therapy; reoxygenation; perfusion; oxygen consumption rate; local tumor control; biomarker

1. Introduction

Key meta-analyses have been published on locally advanced cervix cancer [1], head and neck cancer [2] and chest wall recurrences of breast cancer [3], showing therapeutic benefit in terms of improvement of either/or local tumor control, progression free and overall survival after combining local-regional HT with radiotherapy. An important randomized trial comparing multi-agent chemotherapy +/− HT showed improvements in progression free and overall survival in patients with locally advanced high-risk soft tissue sarcomas in the arm receiving HT [4,5].

Despite the overall success of many trials, a therapeutic benefit was not obtained in all patients and some randomized trials did not show a statistically significant therapeutic benefit of HT [6–8]. Even in those patients in which there was some benefit, it may not have been maximally optimized. Demonstration of enhanced anti-tumor effect with HT would increase its wider acceptance as a viable adjuvant therapy. Thus, there is strong rationale for investigating mitigating factors that may play a role in treatment outcome.

HT induces a number of biologic and physiologic effects on tumors. HT inhibits multiple DNA damage repair mechanisms, which play a major role in heat radiosensitization. The inhibition of DNA repair provides a rationale for combining HT with HSP90 (heat shock protein-90) and/or PARP (poly (ADP-ribose) polymerase) inhibitors [9]. Heat shock proteins, HSP70 and HSP27, bind to enzymes to facilitate base excision repair [10]. This heat shock protein association may enhance DNA damage repair after HT. Substantiating this hypothesis is the observation that enhancement of repair of heat induced double strand breaks is linked to HSP70 and HSP27 association with heat labile DNA polymerase beta in thermotolerant cells [11]. The thermotolerance-induced enhancement of DNA damage repair could reduce the effectiveness of radiotherapy treatments administered when cells are thermotolerant [12,13]. If so, such an effect could reduce the impact of reoxygenation observed 24–48 h post HT, which is the main subject of this review. It is unknown whether this mechanism of thermotolerance-induced radioresistance is clinically relevant. Further research would be needed to answer this question.

Maximal thermal enhancement of radiotherapy in pre-clinical and theoretical models occurs when the two modalities are given simultaneously or within a short time interval between the two [14]. The effect of time interval on radiosensitization is the result of the effects of HT on DNA damage repair [14]. Retrospective analysis of the impact of time interval between HT and radiotherapy has been controversial for cervix cancer [15–18]. A call for standardization of methods and results reporting has been recently published [19]. Standardization of reporting will contribute significantly toward understanding how to optimize thermoradiotherapy from the perspective of methods of delivery and documentation of results.

Hyperthermia also induces a number of immunostimulatory effects in both the innate and adaptive immune systems [20] that are likely important for its biological effectiveness when combined with radiotherapy. HT is cytotoxic itself, with the extent of cytotoxicity being dependent upon the time and temperature of heating [21]. Further, the cytotoxicity of HT is not dependent upon oxygen availability, so it is complementary to radiation in this respect, since hypoxia causes significant reduction in cytotoxicity of radiotherapy [22].

In this review, we will focus on the clinical observation that HT can reduce hypoxia up to at least 1–2 days after HT. Further, the reoxygenation is associated with treatment outcome in patients with locally advanced breast cancer and soft tissue sarcomas in humans and in companion dogs. These observations suggest that positive interactions between HT and radiotherapy can occur outside the short time window suggested for maximal interaction from pre-clinical studies.

Tumor hypoxia is well-established as a cause for radioresistance and treatment failure [23–26]. Hypoxia is also known to negatively influence treatment response to chemotherapy [27] and immunotherapy [20,28], as well as contributing to tumor aggressiveness [29–33]. A recent *Special Issue in Cancers* contained several original reports and contemporary review papers on the subject of tumor hypoxia [34–48]. In this review, we will consider how thermal dose affects tumor hypoxia and, in turn, whether changes in hypoxia in response to thermoradiotherapy can influence treatment outcome.

Extensive pre-clinical studies have been conducted in tumor-bearing rodents with cancer, and these studies revealed important trends in defining the relationship between conditions of thermal exposure and changes in perfusion and hypoxia [49–51]. It has been shown that heating rates in the range of 1 °C/min are: (1) more cytotoxic in vitro [52] and (2) more damaging to tumor microvasculature than slower heating rates [53]. Further, reduced perfusion and enhanced anti-tumor effect after HT alone has been shown to be associated with faster heating rates [54]. It is unknown whether faster heating rates impact reoxygenation 24–48 h post HT in either pre-clinical models or clinically. Heating rate effects have not been studied in conjunction with radiotherapy. If faster heating rates cause vascular damage and hypoxia, then they may result in radioresistance.

For the most part, pre-clinical studies were not designed to test whether changes in perfusion and hypoxia in individual subjects were associated with individual treatment outcome. Such information is required for perfusion or hypoxia measurements to be clinically translatable. Therefore, we will review studies conducted primarily in humans and companion dogs with cancer, where detailed thermometry and physiologic data were acquired for each individual. In most cases, treatment outcome was also documented.

For the purposes of this review, we define 30–60 min of "mild heating" as temperatures from 40 to 42 °C, because minimal direct cell killing occurs in this range. A number of other effects occur in this temperature range, however, including increases in perfusion [22,55] and vascular permeability [56], alterations in cell signaling [9,57–59], inhibition of DNA damage repair [9], inhibition of the HPV viral oncoprotein, E6 [60] and immunologic effects [20]. "Moderate heating" is defined as temperatures >42 and <44 °C. In this moderate temperature range, direct thermal cytotoxicity occurs [61], in addition to many of the effects described above in the mild heating range. "High heating" occurs at temperatures >44 °C and <50 °C. We truncate the high temperature heating at 50 °C to distinguish it from thermal ablation, which occurs at temperatures higher than 60 °C. We have adopted this classification because temperatures >44 °C can increase tumor hypoxia in canine soft tissue sarcomas, whereas below this threshold, hypoxia is either not affected or is reduced [62,63]. Others have used adjectival descriptors of mild (40–42 °C), moderate (42–45 °C) and T > 45 °C as causing irreversible damage [64]. This classification is similar to what we describe. We have chosen 30–60 min heating because that is the range over which HT is most often administered clinically.

2. Hypoxia Is Caused by Imbalance between Oxygen Delivery and Oxygen Consumption Rate

The pO2 of any location within a tissue is governed by the balance between oxygen delivery and oxygen consumption. Oxygen delivery is influenced by the flow rate of microvessels, oxygen content, vascular density and vessel orientation surrounding the location [65]. An important question to ask is which of these factors has the greatest influence on development of hypoxia. Computer generated sensitivity studies were used to address the question of whether increasing oxygen delivery or reducing oxygen consumption rate would be more effective in reducing tumor hypoxia [66,67]. These simulations were based on in vivo measurements of the parameters listed above. Reducing oxygen consumption rate was more efficient by factors of 10–30-fold, compared with increasing blood flow rate or oxygen content of blood, respectively [66]. It has been shown in vitro that elevation of glucose concentration reduces oxygen consumption rate as cells switch to anaerobic metabolism. Induction of hyperglycemia with hyperoxic gas breathing was synergistic in reducing tumor hypoxia in computer simulations [68] and in vivo [69]. Similarly, the combination of HT and carbogen breathing was shown to significantly increase tumor pO2 and enhance radiotherapeutic response [70,71]. HT can also affect oxygen consumption rates, so it is important to consider such effects when evaluating how HT affects tumor hypoxia.

In this review, we address questions about effects of HT on:

- hypoxia,
- perfusion,
- metabolism and oxygen consumption rate and
- necrosis.

Some pre-clinical data will be presented as background. However, the main focus will be on what clinical evidence exists for HT affecting factors that influence tumor hypoxia and whether such changes influence thermoradiotherapeutic treatment outcome.

3. Challenges to Relating Temperatures Achieved during HT with Physiologic Response

3.1. Difference in Temperature Distributions between Rodent and Human Tumors

In rodent tumors, water bath heating exposes the skin and normal tissue around the tumor to the highest temperatures because they are immediately adjacent to the water in the bath; intra-tumoral temperatures are somewhat lower and relatively uniform [72]. In human tumors, there can be large variations in temperature (several degrees above and below the median value) within tumors. The tumor margin and surrounding normal tissue may not be heated appreciably, while the interior of the tumor is hotter [73]. The spatial variation in temperature in human tumors is related to non-uniformities in power deposition from heating devices, with spatial variations in: (1) tissue properties and (2) peri- and intra-tumoral perfusion [74–78]. The differences in the temperature distribution between rodent and human tumors may contribute to differences in physiologic response to HT (Figure 1).

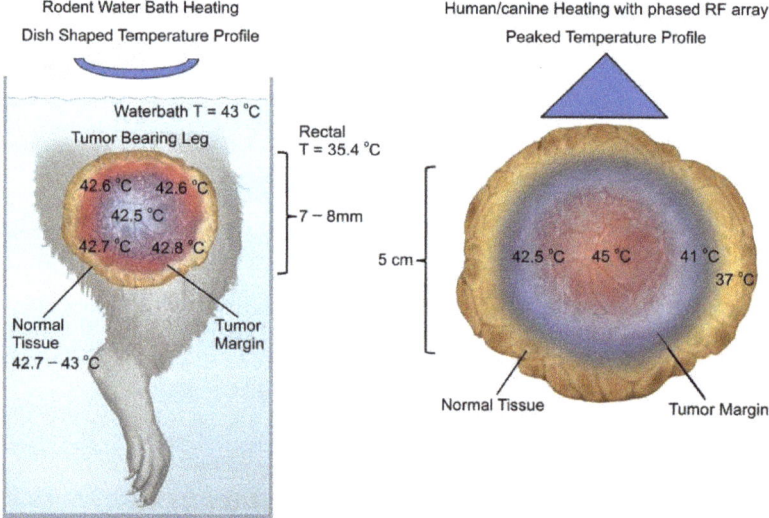

Figure 1. Schematic comparison of temperature distributions for rodent water bath heating vs. temperatures seen in canine and human tumors heated with radiofrequency or microwave devices.

(**Left Panel**) Temperature distributions in rodent tumors heated with water baths tend to be relatively uniform [profiles are dish-shaped], with highest temperatures at the margin of the tumor, while intra-tumoral temperatures are slightly cooler and relatively uniform. Depicted data are taken from a paper by O'Hara et al., where detailed intra-tumoral temperatures were documented using microthermocouples [72]. Although not shown in color for clarity, the whole leg is at elevated temperature. This is described numerically at the left side of the figure. (**Right Panel**) Temperature distributions in human and canine sarcomas heated with phased radiofrequency devices have a peaked temperature distribution in which the temperatures closer to the center are higher than those at the tumor edge. Typically, some surrounding normal tissue is heated to mild temperatures, as depicted. Note also that maximum intra-tumoral temperatures are higher than what is seen in rodent tumors. This is a schematic representation of non-invasive thermometry obtained in human sarcomas [79–81].

3.2. Thermometry in Human Tumors Is Mainly Acquired from Implanted Thermal Probes

Since temperatures in human tumors are heterogeneous, thermometry is essential to assess the therapeutic value of a treatment. The vast majority of clinical thermal data to date has been derived from direct intra-tumoral measurements. Typically, one to two catheters are placed into the tumor and temperatures are measured as thermometers are pushed back and forth within the catheter [82]. The resultant data are depicted by descriptors of the temperature distribution, such as T_{90} [10th percentile of distribution], T_{50} [distribution median] or T_{10} [90th percentile] [82]. Descriptors of the temperature distribution do not reveal anything about the spatial distribution of temperature, but rather provide an overall summary for the tumor as a whole. Non-invasive thermometry can provide spatially encoded thermal data, and this method has been implemented in some patients [78,81,82]. In the future, combinations of non-invasive thermometry with imaging of physiologic response may reveal whether intra-tumoral heterogeneity of physiologic response in tumors is dictated by local temperature variation.

4. Effects of Hyperthermia on Tumor Metabolism

It has been reported previously that enzyme activity increases with temperature and time of heating until the point where enzyme denaturation occurs [83]. These effects are observed during heating and could influence oxygenation during HT. However, effects occurring during HT may not be related to what happens 24–48 h later. There are two documented effects in tumors after HT that could influence oxygen consumption rate: (1) switch to anaerobic metabolism and (2) direct cytotoxicity by hyperthermia.

4.1. Switch to Anaerobic Metabolism after Hyperthermia Treatment

Kelleher utilized a near-IR heating device to heat DS-sarcomas in rats for 60 min [84]. This device yielded temperature distributions analogous to what is seen clinically, with T_{90}, T_{50} and T_{10} values of 42.6, 43.8 and 44.8 °C, respectively. Using a bioluminescence method in snap frozen tissues, lactate and glucose levels were significantly increased, whereas ATP concentrations were decreased after HT. The depletion in ATP concentration is consistent with a reduction in oxidative phosphorylation, whereas the increase in lactate concentration is consistent with a switch to anaerobic metabolism. This switch to anaerobic metabolism is associated with reduction in oxygen consumption rate.

Others have used 31-P Magnetic resonance spectroscopy to monitor ATP concentrations immediately after HT at various temperatures and times of heating [85,86]. They showed significant temperature and heating time-dependent reductions in ATP/Pi (Pi = inorganic phosphate) ratio at temperatures between 43 and 44 °C. In canine sarcomas, depletion in ATP/Pi ratio at 24 h post HT was dependent upon $CEM43T_{50}$ and $CEM43T_{90}$ during heating [87]. Further, reduction in ATP/PME [phosphomonoester] was significantly correlated with probability of pathologic complete response rate (pCR rate) in humans with soft tissue sarcomas [87]. Although the time intervals after HT when measurements were made in rodents and these spontaneous sarcomas are different, there is remarkable similarity in the temperature dependence of ATP depletion.

We conducted a phase II study in human soft tissue sarcomas, where we hypothesized that reaching a pre-determined thermal dose would lead to >75% incidence of pCR rate [88]. We failed to prove the hypothesis, but in parallel studies conducted in the same patient series, we found that pre-treatment metabolic factors, such as hypoxia, phosphodiester/inorganic phosphate (PDE/Pi) and phosphomonoester/Pi (PME/Pi) ratios, were associated with pCR rate [89]. We speculated that in this particular trial, pre-treatment physiology interfered with our ability to show the hypothesized thermal dose–response relationship.

Moon et al. examined potential underlying mechanisms for the apparent switch to anaerobic metabolism after 42 °C HT [57]. HT increased hypoxia inducible factor-1α (HIF-1α) for several hours after HT. HIF-1 is a heterodimer, consisting of HIF-1α and HIF-1β subunits. When bound together, HIF-1 enters the nucleus and initiates transcription of many genes, including PDK1 (3-phosphoinositide-dependent kinase 1), which controls the switch to anaerobic metabolism. Normally, HIF-1α is efficiently degraded by prolyl hydroxylases that initiate degradation of HIF-1α so that the heterodimer does not form [65]. HIF-1α is stabilized during hypoxia because the prolyl hydroxylases require oxygen for their action. However, in the case of HT, inactivation of HIF-1α degradation was associated with an increase in oxidative stress. The switch to anaerobic metabolism would reduce oxygen consumption rate, since anaerobic metabolism does not rely on oxygen to produce ATP.

Radiotherapy is also known to increase HIF-1 dependent transcription, but underlying mechanisms for HIF-1 upregulation are different from HT and are radiation dose dependent. For doses in the range of conventionally fractionated radiotherapy, HIF-1 dependent transcription is upregulated in response to increased oxidative stress associated with reoxygenation [90], followed by prolonged HIF-1 upregulation in response to massive nitric oxide production by infiltrating macrophages [91]. Higher single radiotherapy doses, in the range of 15Gy, decrease perfusion and increase hypoxia by causing microvascular damage; HIF-1 dependent transcription is subsequently upregulated by hypoxia [92]. Mild temperature heating immediately after high dose radiation reduces the radiation induced upregulation of HIF-1α caused by vascular damage by radiotherapy [92]. These differing effects of HT and radiotherapy dose on HIF-1 expression may be important in affecting tumor metabolism and treatment response.

Another method for assessing metabolic response to HT is 18-FDG-PET. Glucose uptake would be expected to increase if there is a switch to anaerobic metabolism, in the absence of extensive tumor cell killing by treatment. Some studies have been conducted in human patients prior to and after HT. However, these reports involved repeat scans taken weeks into the treatment course or even after treatment was completed. These studies showed that reductions in 18-FDG-PET uptake are associated with pathologic response in patients with esophageal cancer [93], rectal cancer [94] and soft tissue sarcomas [95]. The results are more likely dominated by extent of cell killing than by HT induced changes in cellular glucose uptake.

4.2. Direct Cytotoxicity of HT

The cytotoxic effects of HT are logarithmically related to temperature and linearly to the time of heating [96]. Sapareto and Dewey were the first to develop means to relate any time–temperature history into an equivalent number of minutes of heating at 43 °C [61]. This formulation has proven useful in describing tissue damage across a range of tissue types and temperature time histories as long as temperature is less than 50 °C [21,96]. The acronym for cumulative equivalent number of minutes at 43 °C is referred to as CEM43. An important question is whether there is enough direct cytotoxicity from HT to influence oxygen consumption rates.

Rosner et al. [97] conducted a theoretical study asking how much cell killing would be expected from a non-uniform temperature distribution typical of what is observed clinically.

The temperature distributions were derived from a finite element heat transfer model of a simulated subcutaneous tumor, where power was delivered from a microwave applicator. Cytotoxicity was predicted based on a stochastic model of cell killing probability, based on survival curve data from CHO cells. For 60 min HT, the simulations revealed that 30–50% of cells would be directly killed by HT with a T_{90} of 41 °C. This occurs because of cell killing temperatures higher than the T_{90}. Simulated temperatures above the T_{90} ranged up to 45.5 °C. Thermal killing of 30–50% of tumor cells would be sufficient to have an important impact on oxygen consumption rate and tumor hypoxia [66].

Below, we provide additional clinical results, addressing the question of whether increases in perfusion and/or direct cell killing by HT contributes to reoxygenation.

5. Effects of Hyperthermia on Tumor Perfusion and Hypoxia

Most of the published pre-clinical data have focused on effects of HT on perfusion and hypoxia during or immediately after treatment. However, there is a second body of work that has focused on effects that occur 24–48 h after treatment. Both will be discussed.

5.1. Physiologic Effects during or Immediately after Heating

The effects of HT on tumor perfusion and hypoxia have been studied extensively at the pre-clinical level. Pre-clinical data demonstrate an increase in perfusion and oxygenation during and shortly after heating at mild temperatures (39–42 °C) at heating times of 30–60 min [98,99]. At temperatures >43–46 °C for 30–60 min there is significant damage to vasculature, leading to hypoxia, anoxia and necrosis [100]. Thus, at the pre-clinical level, the physiologic response of tumors during or immediately after HT is bi-phasic. If reoxygenation occurs only during the application of HT, then taking advantage of it with radiotherapy would require simultaneous application of radiotherapy with HT.

5.2. Physiologic Effects Occurring after Heating

In his Robinson Award manuscript, Oleson hypothesized that the enhanced effectiveness of HT + radiotherapy compared with radiotherapy alone had to be a result of reoxygenation [101]. The effectiveness of radiotherapy fractions given 24 h after HT could be influenced by HT induced reoxygenation. Part of his rationale was based on the observation that the prognostically important temperatures from clinical trials are at the lower end of the temperature distribution, where little direct cell killing occurs. Subsequent to Oleson's paper, several papers were published, showing results that are consistent with his hypothesis.

Shakil et al. [98] were the first to report on reoxygenation occurring 24 h after mild temperature water bath HT of the R3230Ac rat mammary tumor to 40.5–43.5 °C for 30–60 min. Perfusion increased by 10–33% at the end of 30 min HT. At 24 h post HT, perfusion was further increased by two-fold over baseline. Immediately after HT, pO2 values increased two-fold, compared with baseline. At 24 h post HT, pO2 remained elevated, although lower than that seen immediately after HT. Similar effects were seen in other tumor models [99,102].

It has been speculated that reoxygenation rarely occurs hours to days after HT in human subjects; if it does occur, it has little to do with enhancing cell killing by radiotherapy [14]. Given the complexity of physiologic effects that occur in tumors in response to HT, this challenge requires rigorous and critical thought. This question will be addressed in the following discussion of clinical results.

5.3. Human Studies of Reoxygenation Post HT

Brizel et al. [103] reported that reoxygenation occurs at 24 h post heating in a portion of 38 patients with soft tissue sarcomas treated with pre-operative thermoradiotherapy (50 Gy in 2 Gy fractions, 5 fractions per week and 1–2 fractions of HT per week, given 1–2 h post radiotherapy). Oxygenation (Eppendorf pO2 histography) did not change after the first week of conventionally fractionated radiotherapy. However, median pO2 24–48 h after the first HT (given during second week of radiotherapy) increased from 6.2 mmHg to

12.4 mmHg, which was statistically significant. There was a significant correlation between reoxygenation and percent necrosis in the resected tumors. The median T_{90} in these tumors was 39.9 °C in tumors that had <90% necrosis, vs. 40.0 °C for tumors that achieved >90% necrosis [pathologic complete response; pCR—this small difference was not significant]. T_{90} values were lower than temperatures required for direct cell killing by HT [96]. This argues against the idea that pCR was a result of direct cell killing by HT, as hypothesized by others [14]. Although the results are provocative, a rigorous examination between thermal dose achieved and extent of reoxygenation and treatment outcome was not undertaken in this series.

Vujaskovic reported on a series of women with locally advanced breast cancer who received neoadjuvant chemotherapy consisting of liposomal doxorubicin [Myocet™ and paclitaxel] combined with HT [104]. The rationale for this treatment was to take advantage of effects of HT on vascular permeability and liposomal extravasation [105,106]. pO2 measurements were made, using Eppendorf pO2 histography, prior to and 24 h after the second HT, which coincided with the second chemotherapy treatment course. Eleven of eighteen tumors were hypoxic (median pO2 < 10 mmHg). In the hypoxic tumors, eight out of eleven exhibited reoxygenation [median pO2 = 19.2 mmHg]. The response rate for hypoxic tumors that reoxygenated was higher than a sub-group that did not reoxygenate. There was no correlation between extent of reoxygenation and thermal dose in this group of patients, but there was a trend indicating that chances of reoxygenation were greater if median T_{50} remained between 39.5 and 41 °C [104]. This trend, showing a better chance for response with relatively low T_{50} values, was consistent with a separate group of patients with locally advanced breast cancer who were treated with pre-operative HT, radiotherapy and taxol [107]. Tumors that achieved either a partial or complete response were well oxygenated at baseline or reoxygenated by a median of 18 mmHg. Those tumors that had no response to treatment showed a reduction of pO2, by a median of 9 mmHg. In this clinical series, temperatures were not high enough to cause appreciable direct cell killing by HT.

5.4. Canine Studies of Reoxygenation Post HT

Vujaskovic also reported on changes in tumor oxygenation in a series of 13 dogs with soft tissue sarcomas treated with thermoradiotherapy [62]. Oxygen measurements were made prior to and 24 h after the first HT. The Oxford Optronix™ fluorescence lifetime probe was used to measure pO2 in multiple locations by placing the probe deep in the tumor and then recording pO2 during using a pull-back. Reduction in hypoxic fraction (HF) was observed for T_{50} values ranging from 39.5 to 44 °C. HF increased when T_{50} values were >44 °C. Consistent with the human studies, mild temperature HT improved tumor oxygenation, whereas higher temperatures contributed to apparent vascular damage, with an increase in tumor hypoxia. In this study, correlations between the oxygenation measurements with treatment outcome were not made.

Thrall et al. [108] conducted a randomized thermal dose escalation clinical trial that compared long term local tumor control in 122 dogs with soft tissue sarcomas that were randomized into two different thermal dose groups in combination with fractionated radiotherapy (2.25 Gy/fx, 25Fx). There was a 17-fold higher CEM43T_{90} in the high vs. the low HT dose group (Figure 2A). The difference in thermal dose was achieved by generating higher temperatures and longer heating times in the high thermal dose group (Figure 2B,C). Duration of local tumor control was significantly longer in the high thermal dose group, with a hazard ratio of 2.3 in multivariate analysis.

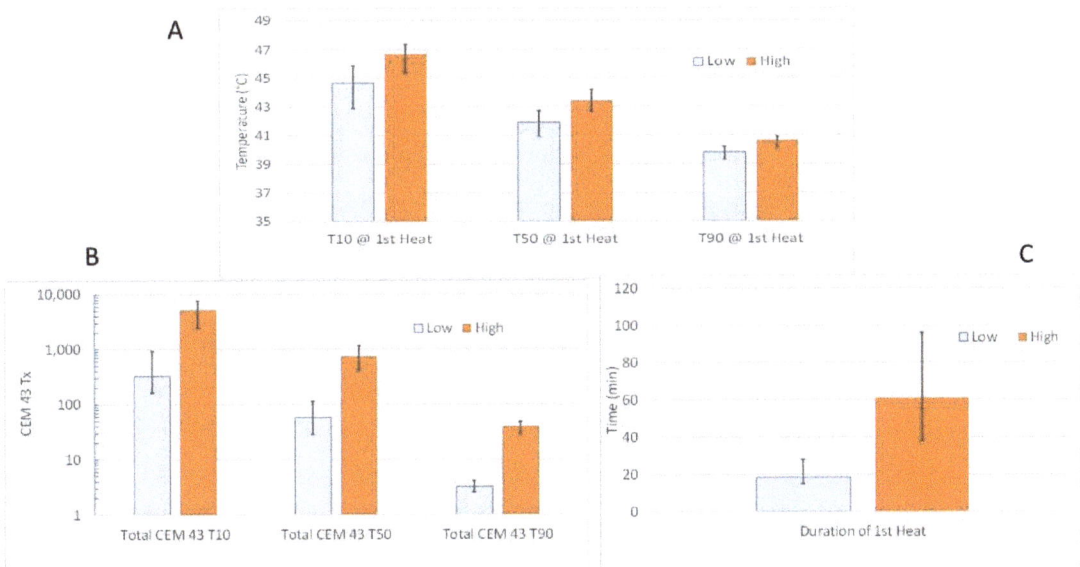

Figure 2. Thermal dose characteristics of thermal dose escalation trial of Thrall et al. [108] (**A**) Comparison of CEM43T$_{10}$, T$_{50}$ and T$_{90}$ values. The trial was designed to deliver approximately a 20-fold difference in CEM43T$_{90}$ between the low and high dose groups. (**B**) To achieve this difference in CEM43T$_{90}$, and CEM43T$_{10}$, T$_{50}$ throughout the tumors were higher. (**C**) Heating times were also longer. $N = 21$ Low dose group; $N = 18$ High dose group. Data from the subjects for which physiologic data were reported (Lora-Michaels et al. [109]).

Hypoxia was measured in subgroups of animals in this trial. These results have not been published previously. The Oxford Optronix™ fluorescence lifetime probe was used prior to and 24 h after the first HT to determine change in median pO2 and HF in 11 subjects (% measurements < 10 mmHg). There were significant correlations (Pearson correlation) between increased median pO2 ($p = 0.0230$) or reduced HF ($p = 0.007$) and duration of local control (Table 1). This observation was corroborated in another subgroup of 16 animals that were given pimonidazole prior to and 24 h after the first HT. Immunohistochemistry was used to determine the hypoxic fraction, as described by Cline et al. [110,111]. Reduction in the % pimonidazole positive area was inversely associated with increased time to local failure. Caution has to be used, given the small number of patients in these analyses. However, the similarity between the oxygen probe results and the pimonidazole data suggest that reoxygenation after the first HT is likely predictive of time to local failure. Additional studies would be required for validation.

Table 1. Physiological Predictors of Time to Local Failure: Thermal Dose Escalation Trial.

Variable	Parameter Estimate	Hazard Ratio	Score p-Value	Wald p-Value
HF Post-Pre	−0.0643	0.94	0.0070	0.0340
Median pO2 Post-Pre	0.0896	1.09	0.0230	0.0710
Pimo % area	−6.549	0.00	0.038	0.0510
PDE/ATP	0.2246	1.25	0.0490	0.0640

HF = Hypoxic Fraction—fraction of measurements <10 mmHg; $N = 11$ for HF and Median pO2; $N = 16$ Pimo area; $N = 13$ PDE/ATP; Pimo = pimonidazole; (PDE/ATP data previously published, Lora-Michaels et al. [109]).

Thrall et al. reported on another trial of 37 dogs with soft tissue sarcomas that were treated with two different HT dose fractionation schedules (5Fx ($n = 21$) vs. 20Fx ($n = 16$)), in conjunction with fractionated radiotherapy (2.25 Gy/Fx, 25Fx) [63]. The goal of this thermal dose fractionation trial was to achieve equivalent $CEM43T_{90}$ for both fractionation schedules. The working hypothesis was that the 20Fx group would achieve better anti-tumor effect compared with the 5Fx group. In the final analysis, $CEM43T_{90}$ was slightly and significantly higher in the 5Fx HT arm (29.9 vs. 24.9 $CEM43T_{90}$ for the 5 vs. 20 HT fractions, respectively). To accomplish near equivalence in total $CEM43T_{90}$ between the treatment groups, the duration of heating for the 5Fx HT group was six-fold longer per treatment. Although T_{50} and T_{10} values were higher for the 5Fx HT group than the 20Fx HT group, the total CEM 43 T_{10} and T_{50} values were higher in the 20Fx HT group. This was a product of the larger number of HT fractions in this group (Tables S1 and S2). Multiple physiologic endpoints were measured in these subjects, pre and 24 h after the first HT: pO2, contrast enhanced perfusion with MRI, apparent diffusion coefficient (ADC) with MRI, and genomic analysis [112]. Contrary to the hypothesis, the 5Fx HT group showed greater volume reduction than the 20Fx HT group ($p = 0.0022$). The physiologic endpoints associated with treatment group were change in ADC after the treatment course and change in perfusion at 24 h after the first HT. Additionally, there was a significant correlation between HF change 24 h after the first HT and tumor volume change at the end of therapy; as hypoxic fraction was reduced, tumor volume was reduced. The 5Fx HT group showed a trend toward a reduction in ADC. In contrast, the 20Fx HT group showed increased ADC values (Figure S1). Increases in ADC values at the end of therapy were associated with changes in gene expression at 24 h post first HT, consistent with induction of inflammation [112]. Thus, the increase in ADC with the 20Fx HT group may be associated with increased edema as a result of inflammation. There was also a significant difference in perfusion response after the first HT between the two arms. The 5Fx HT arm exhibited increases in perfusion, whereas the 20Fx HT arm exhibited decreases in perfusion.

Further analyses of data from this trial, which have not been published previously, suggest that the reoxygenation observed in these tumors is linked to the distribution of thermal dose. The results of this analysis are shown in Tables 2 and 3.

1. Higher $CEM43T_{10}$ was associated with an improvement in average pO2 ($p = 0.0214$) and reduction in HF (% points < 10 mmHg; $p = 0.0451$), 24 h after the first HT.
2. There was a significant positive correlation between $CEM43T_{90}$ and perfusion at 24 h post first hyperthermia fraction.
3. Increases in average pO2 and perfusion at 24 h after the first HT were correlated with tumor volume reduction at the end of treatment.
4. Higher Total $CEM43T_{10}$ and Total $CEM43T_{50}$ were associated with change in ADC at the end of treatment ($p = 0.007$ and $p = 0.0007$, respectively), but the trends were different for the 5Fx HT vs. 20Fx HT groups. Reduction in ADC is associated with lower diffusion coefficient of water, which can be interpreted as a relative decrease in water mobility. It has been reported that early onset of apoptosis or apoptosis mixed with necrosis is associated with increased ADC [113,114]. However, in situations where there is necrosis in the absence of apoptosis, chronic necrosis or fibrosis, ADC tends to decrease [115,116]. The increase in ADC associated with relatively high $CEM43T_{10}$ and $-T_{50}$ in the 20Fx HT group is consistent with the notion that higher cumulative thermal doses cause cell killing and increased edema. Extensive cell death could reduce oxygen consumption rate across a tumor, thereby contributing to improved oxygenation.
5. Higher $CEM43T_{10}$ and $-T_{50}$ were significantly negatively correlated with greater tumor volume reduction at the end of therapy.

Table 2. CEM43Tx vs. change in volume, ADC, pO2, HF, iAUC: Thermal Dose Fractionation Trial.

Variable	N	CEM43T$_{10}$		CEM43T$_{50}$		CEM43T$_{90}$	
		Coefficient	p-Value	Coefficient	p-Value	Coefficient	p-Value
Change ADC Pre-post *	29	−0.53	0.0030	−0.56	0.0015	0.11	0.5665
iAUC change 24 h ^	17	0.07	0.7798	0.23	0.3599	0.5109	0.0311
Median pO2 change at 24 h ^	38	0.38	0.0214	0.27	0.1087	−0.07	0.9829
Change HF 24 h ^	38	−0.34	0.0451	−0.27	0.1074	−0.07	0.674
Volume change Pre-Post *	38	−0.42	0.0084	−0.36	0.0258	0.2983	0.17

* Total CEM43Tx; ^ CEM43Tx first HT; HF = % measurements < 10mmHg; iAUC = DCE-MRI perfusion parameter; HF = hypoxic fraction.

Table 3. Physiological Predictors of Tumor Volume Change: Thermal Dose Fractionation Trial.

Variable	N	Coefficient	p-Value
iAUC median change 24 h	17	−0.47	0.0472
Median pO2 change 24 h	38	−0.040	0.0146

iAUC = DCE-MRI perfusion parameter.

These results provide a direct link between characteristics of the temperature distribution, potential mechanisms of reoxygenation and treatment response. We hypothesize that the reduction in hypoxia is associated with a reduction in oxygen consumption rate associated with the higher end of the thermal dose distribution (CEM43T$_{10}$, -T$_{50}$), combined with an increase in perfusion associated with the lower end of the temperature distribution (CEM43T$_{90}$) (Figure 3).

There are some conundrums in the results, however. Contrary to the correlation between T$_{10}$ and ADC change at the end of treatment, there was no correlation between T$_{10}$ and ADC change at 24 h post treatment [117]. These results could be interpreted as indicating that cell killing does not contribute to reoxygenation 24 h after the first HT. It is possible that this lack of correlation of T$_{10}$ with ADC change at 24 h post HT has to do with the relatively small volume of tumor represented by the T$_{10}$ (90% of measurements would be <T$_{10}$). If there was direct cytotoxicity after the first HT in the volume represented by the T$_{10}$, it may not have impacted the overall median ADC. Another option to consider is that temperatures >T$_{50}$ interfered with respiration, thereby reducing oxygen consumption rate. As discussed earlier in this review, respiration is relatively thermosensitive and is reduced in the temperature range of T$_{10}$ and T$_{50}$ (see Figure 2). A reduction in oxygen consumption rate, even in a small sub-volume of the tumor, would be sufficient to impact oxygen transport and reduce hypoxic fraction. Additional evidence for a reduction in oxygen consumption rate as a contributor to reoxygenation comes from observations that HIF-1 regulated genes and proteins were upregulated after HT [63,112] in these subjects. Increases in HIF-1 would cause a switch to anaerobic metabolism [57,118]. Finally, it was not possible to follow these individuals to ascertain long term local tumor control or progression free survival. Clearly, further research is required.

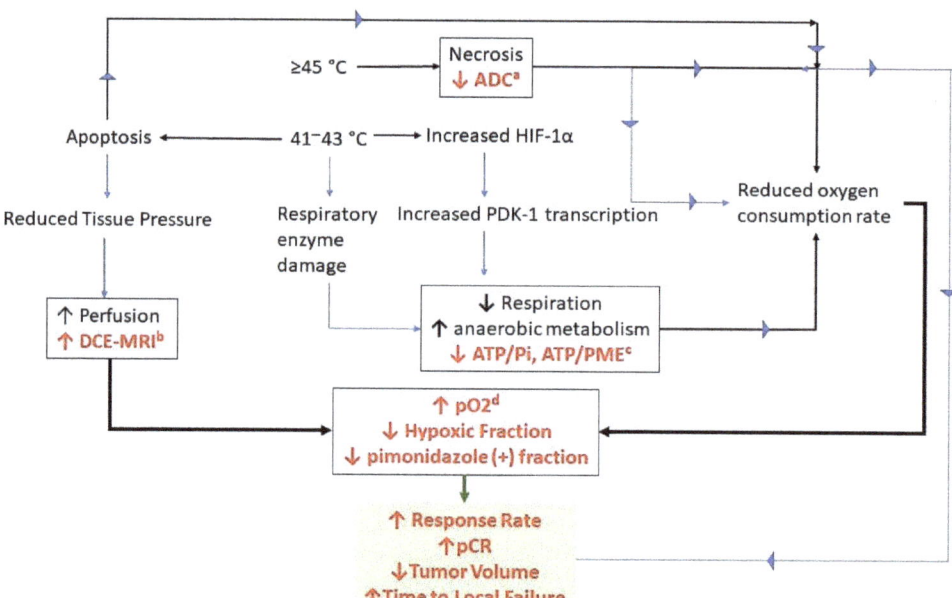

Figure 3. Potential mechanisms for reoxygenation following HT. The boxes in this figure contain putative mechanisms for reoxygenation, along with supportive data acquired from canine soft tissue sarcomas and/or human patients with soft tissue sarcomas or locally advanced breast cancer. The terms highlighted in red font are observations that support the proposed mechanisms. The box highlighted in green lists treatment responses that are linked back to the physiologic response observations. The superscripted letters next to the individual measurements refer back to the papers in which the observations were reported. a—[63]; b—[62,63]; c—[87]; d—[62,63,104,107,119]. The temperatures listed are linked to typical heating times of 60 min per HT fraction.

Viglianti et al. [120] examined tumor perfusion using DCE/MRI [dynamic contrast enhanced MRI] prior to and 24 h post first HT in the canine soft tissue sarcomas treated with thermoradiotherapy. Perfusion was measured prior to and 24 h after the first HT, [120]. Although perfusion increased in some subjects after HT, there was no association with local tumor control. Vaupel suggested that integrated temperature–time combination could be associated with biphasic vascular effects of HT [51]. Further work would be needed to verify that physiologic effects are associated with this measure of thermal dose. The integrated time–temperature approach has been reported to be associated with treatment outcome to thermoradiotherapy, however [121,122].

Recently, Thomsen et al. [123] reported on changes in oxygenation of the chest wall skin of normal subjects and patients with chest-wall recurrences of breast cancer. Water-filtered infrared-A-irradiation was used to heat this superficial tumor site. Hyperspectral imaging was used to ascertain hemoglobin saturation. Implanted fiber optic oxygen sensors (Oxford Optronix™, fluorescence life time probe) were used to measure pO2 directly. In normal volunteers, tissue oxygenation increased during HT to reach an elevated plateau and slowly declined after power was turned off. Measurements of Hb_{sat} followed a similar pattern, with elevations persisting up to 15 min post heating [123]. Preliminary patient data were also provided, suggesting a similar time course for change in oxygenation. These data are provocative. We await follow up reports as to whether improvements in oxygenation in these tumor bearing subjects are associated with treatment outcome.

Waterman et al. [124] measured perfusion in superficial human tumors during HT using a thermal diffusion method based on monitoring the rate of decline in temperature during brief periods of turning off microwave applicator power. He also observed increases in perfusion during heating [124]. These patients were treated with thermoradiotherapy, but the authors did not report whether the changes in perfusion were associated with tumor response.

Thrall et al. [119] reported on changes in tumor hypoxia in a series of seven dogs over a five-week course of thermoradiotherapy. Hypoxia was measured using the Oxford Optronix™ fluorescence lifetime probe 3–4× per week. In four out of five tumors that were hypoxic at baseline, reduction in hypoxia observed after the first HT continued to be observed throughout the treatment course. This included measurements that were made during several day intervals when HT was not administered. In a fifth marginally hypoxic tumor at baseline, pO2 values dropped to near zero at 24 h post first HT and remained that way for the duration of the treatment course. The remaining three tumors were not hypoxic to start with and the treatment course did not cause hypoxia. In this series of tumors, T_{90} values were far below those that would cause appreciable direct cell killing by HT.

6. A Look Backward and Future Directions

As indicated in the beginning of this review, there were concerns raised as to whether reoxygenation occurs in 1–2 days after HT and, if so, whether it has any influence on radiobiologically significant hypoxia [14]. We can say without reservation that reoxygenation can occur up to 24 h and perhaps even longer after HT. We showed this was the case in: (1) human soft tissue sarcomas [103], (2) four separate series involving canine soft tissue sarcomas [62,63,109,119] and (3) in two clinical trials of women with locally advanced breast cancer [104,107]. Concerns were raised as to whether clinical responses, such as pathologic CR rate, were simply caused by HT induced necrosis as opposed to reoxygenation having an effect on radiosensitivity [14]. Although we show clear evidence that $CEM43T_{10}$ and $CEM43T_{50}$ are associated with necrosis induction, temperatures at the lower end of the distribution are too low to cause direct cell killing by HT (Figure 2 and Table S1). Similar results were reported previously in human sarcomas [73]. Thus, it seems implausible to explain complete pathologic response or early tumor response by simple necrotic cell killing, as has been suggested by others [14].

We have speculated that reoxygenation occurs as a result of direct HT cytotoxicity of aerobic cells, which in turn reduces overall oxygen consumption rate across the tumor. One cannot rule out that the main effect is simply the result of preferential HT killing of hypoxic tumor cells and that oxygen consumption rate is not important here. However, we argue that oxygen consumption does occur in relatively hypoxic tumor subregions. Hypoxic regions are not totally hypoxic. They are composed of many microscopic foci of hypoxia that also contain well-oxygenated cells near blood vessels [125]. Less hypoxic subregions contain less of these hypoxic foci. Such patterns are readily discernable by looking at the distribution of hypoxia marker drug retention in tumor sections stained immunohistochemically for hypoxia marker drug–protein adducts [126,127]. Killing of aerobic cells lying within relatively hypoxic subregions would contribute to reduced oxygen consumption across a whole tumor. Killing of cells could be by direct coagulative necrosis in regions near the T_{10} values, which are at or above 45 °C. On the other hand, moderate temperature thermal killing (T_{50} values of 42–43 °C) could reduce oxidative phosphorylation [87,109] and/or induce apoptosis in aerobic tumor cells, thereby contributing to reduced oxygen consumption as well as reducing tissue pressure to enhance perfusion [128]. However, we acknowledge that further work would be needed to resolve whether direct hypoxic tumor cell killing alone or in combination with reduced oxygen consumption rate contributes to reoxygenation. One method that could be used to resolve this question is ^{15}O PET [129].

Importantly, reoxygenation does not occur in all subjects. In fact, hypoxia is exacerbated 24 h post HT in some subjects [104,107,119]. Mechanisms for this heterogeneous response are not currently delineated. It is possible that the microvasculature in some subjects is less mature and more thermally sensitive. Immature microvasculature is devoid of pericyte coverage and lacks strong endothelial cell junction connections. Such microvessels are sensitive to VEGF withdrawal [130] and are more thermally sensitive [131–133]. Selective destruction of such vessels by HT would lead to necrosis and hypoxia. Alternatively, induction of hypoxia could occur as a result of vascular steal. Vascular steal has been described as being responsible for reduced perfusion and increased tumor hypoxia in response to some vasoactive drugs, for example. Upon drug treatment, vasodilation of surrounding normal vasculature occurs [134,135]. Tumor vessels, on the other hand, are often devoid of smooth muscle and cannot vasodilate. Vascular steal occurs because of the shift in flow resistance between normal and tumor tissue, which thereby shunts perfusion to the surrounding normal tissue [135]. Arterioles and venules in normal tissue are more thermally resistant than tumor arterioles [53]. This relative difference in thermal resistance to permanent stasis could increase flow in normal tissue at temperatures that cause vascular stasis in tumors. Further work is needed to more fully explain why reoxygenation occurs in some subjects, while in others, hypoxia is exacerbated. In any case, the heterogeneous response of tumors to HT in different subjects points to the need to measure extent of hypoxia before and during HT treatment regimens in order to differentiate those subjects who benefit from HT-induced reoxygenation vs. for which HT is contraindicated. As described earlier, high rates of heating could also contribute to vascular damage and persistent hypoxia [53,54].

It is likely that the characteristics of the temperature distribution and/or tumor location have an important role in the physiologic response to HT in human subjects. Perfusion was measured prior to and immediately after HT in a subject with cervix and rectal cancer, using $H_2{}^{15}O$-PET [136]. Increases in perfusion were not observed. There was an increase in water partition coefficient, which the authors speculated could influence oxygen transport. The temperatures achieved were lower than those seen in sarcomas, averaging 40.7 ± 0.6 °C vs. median temperatures of 41–42 °C in sarcomas [121].

It is also important to consider whether HT induced reoxygenation plays a role in immune surveillance. Both HT and radiotherapy are known to enhance immune surveillance by a range of mechanisms [20,137]. However, both hypoxia and lactic acidosis exert a negative influence on the innate and adaptive immune systems [20,28]. Reoxygenation induced by HT, therefore, could be playing an important role in the enhanced anti-tumor effect of thermoradiotherapy. An increase in perfusion along with killing of hypoxic tumor cells could reduce lactate levels (and increase pHe) as well, thereby contributing to enhanced immunity. We have previously shown a direct positive correlation between HT induced increases in perfusion at 24 h post HT and increases in pHe [120]. We did not find a correlation of these changes with local tumor control after thermoradiotherapy to soft tissue sarcomas in dogs, but increases in pHe 24 h post HT were associated with prolonged metastasis free survival. Low baseline pHe was associated with shorter time to metastasis, as well [109]. Perhaps these differences in tumor acidity at baseline or after HT were associated with tumor immunity. Further work needs to be conducted to define underlying mechanisms.

Although the results shown here support underlying mechanisms for reoxygenation following HT, they are limited by lack of spatially registered data. Functional imaging holds potential to uncover how spatially varying thermal doses affect tumor physiologic response. Using MRI, it is possible to acquire temperature distributions, serial measurements of perfusion distribution and ADC distribution in the same tumor. Oxygen sensitive MR imaging methods and/or ^{18}F-misonidazole PET imaging [138] could reveal information about the spatial distribution of hypoxia. Using such data, it would then be possible to estimate the efficiency of cell killing across a tumor.

A preliminary effort was conducted to ascertain the efficiency of cytotoxicity following a thermoradiotherapy treatment in a human soft tissue sarcoma, where non-invasive thermometry was used to ascertain the temperature distribution, and radiation treatment planning revealed the spatial distribution of RT dose within the same tumor. Effects of the varied temperature distribution on cell survival were estimated using extensive cytotoxicity data of CHO cells by Loshek, who measured the time dependence of cell killing for 42 °C

HT alone, RT alone and the combination [139]. All of the temperature data within the heated volume of the example case were converted to equivalent minutes at 42 °C, using the Sapareto and Dewey CEM formalism [61]. For further details about the methods for determining cell survival, please see Text S1 for further information. The soft tissue sarcoma in the calf of a human patient is depicted in Figure 4. Figure 4A shows the location of the tumor, as imaged by ADC. Figure 4B shows the temperature distribution, measured by proton resonance frequency shift MRI [81]. Figure 4C depicts the radiation dose distribution from treatment planning. The predicted cell kill within each image pixel from a single dose of radiation is in the range of 50% and is uniform within the irradiated volume because the spatial distribution of radiation was set to be uniform by treatment planning (Figure 4E).

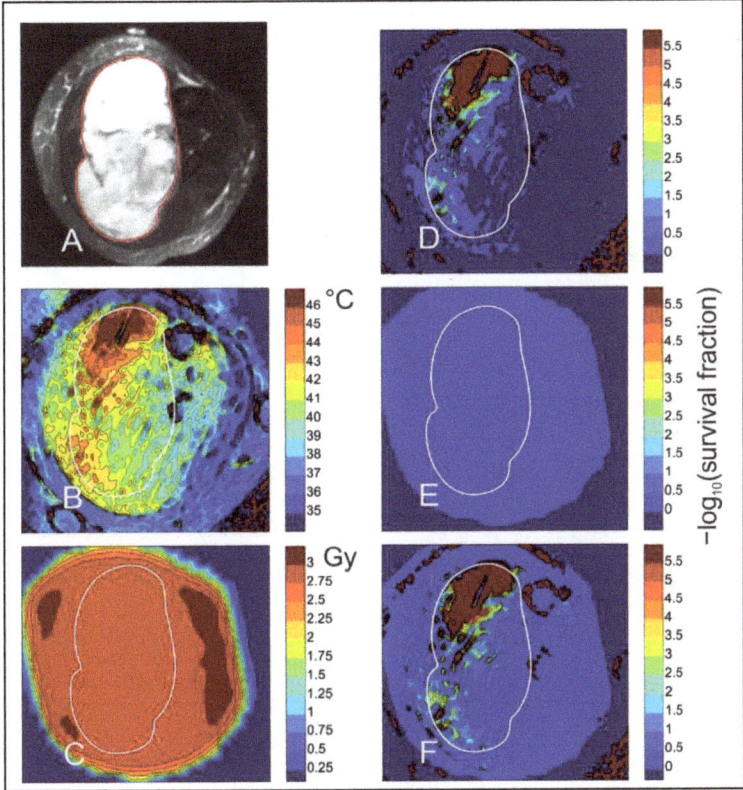

Figure 4. Imaging and simulation of combined HT and radiation treatment of a sarcoma. Images show a cross-section through a human patient's calf. Simulations are based on results of Loshek et al. [139] for dependence of survival fraction of Chinese hamster ovary cells on doses of combined radiation and heating, together with results of Sapareto and Dewey [61] for the dependence of thermal dose on temperature. The period of heating was 54 min. Details of the simulation are provided in Text S1. (**A**) Diffusion weighted MRI image of thigh cross-section. Tumor region is outlined in red and transferred to other images. (**B**) Temperature distribution in tissue during hyperthermia, obtained by non-invasive MRI thermometry. (**C**) Radiation dose derived from treatment plan. (**D**) Predicted cell kill from HT alone. All cell kill values are expressed in terms of −log10 (survival fraction). (**E**) Predicted cell kill from radiation alone. (**F**) Predicted cell kill from combined HT and radiation.

The impact of the varied temperature distribution on cell killing (as depicted by −log10 (survival)) shows highly efficient killing in the hottest tumor regions, along with virtually no killing in the cooler regions of the tumor (Figure 4D). The influence of thermoradiosensitization on cell killing is seen in Figure 4F. Careful examination shows enhanced killing efficiency around areas of cell killing by HT alone (Figure 4D). These data reveal interesting insights into the influence of temperature variation on the distribution of cell killing. First, the extent of cell killing is much greater for HT than for a 2 Gy dose of RT alone within the hotter tumor regions. The greatest cell killing, on the order of 5 logs/pixel, occurs in 10–15% of the tumor region. Killing in these hotter regions would be expected to reduce oxygen consumption rate, thereby contributing to reoxygenation in the rest of the tumor hours to days after HT. Second, although thermoradiosensitization is evident, it is not as extensive as one might project, particularly in the cooler regions of the tumor. Even this one example case suggests that more simulations of this type should be considered, especially if information about hypoxia is added.

We have also conducted a series of simulations of tumor control probability [TCP] based on the Loshek data referred to above [139]. We considered the impact of once weekly HT induced radiosensitization (Text S2 and Figures S2 and S3) on cell survival and TCP over a six- or seven-week course of conventionally fractionated radiotherapy. Secondly, we considered the impact of a portion of hypoxic tumor cells moving to the aerobic compartment 24 h post HT (Text S2 and Figure 5). These simulations are based on observations that we made in canine sarcomas [119]. Even a 30% shift after each weekly HT leads to a TCP nearing 100%. On the other hand, TCP drops quite significantly if a tumor becomes more hypoxic after HT, as we have observed in some subjects. Lack of reoxygenation is predicted to render the tumor described as incurable with the radiotherapy doses described.

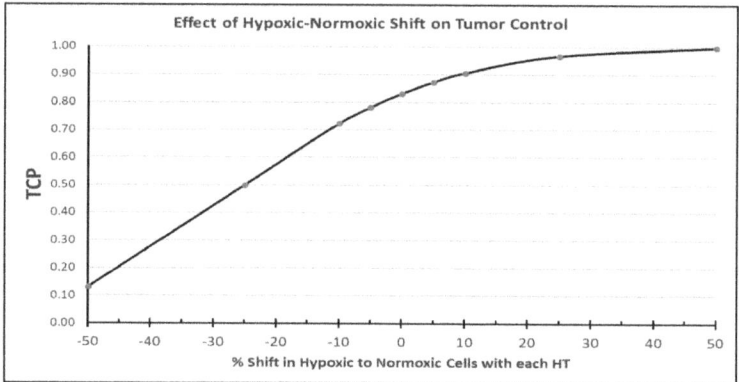

Figure 5. Predicted tumor control probability [TCP] for conventionally fractionated radiotherapy + HT, where HT is administered once weekly. The impact of HT induced reoxygenation at 24 h post HT is depicted, as the proportion of hypoxic cells that reoxygenate vs. proportion of aerobic cells that become more hypoxic after each HT. TCP reaches nearly 100% if even 30% of hypoxic tumor cells reoxygenate 24 h after each HT, thereby affecting cytotoxicity of the radiotherapy fraction given the day after HT. On the other hand, TCP drops quickly in a condition where aerobic tumor cells become more hypoxic 24 h after HT. Although reoxygenation occurs more frequently with HT, one must remain aware of the smaller population of tumors that become more hypoxic after HT, as such effects are predicted to substantially reduce TCP. Details of these simulations are shown in Text S2.

Despite clear evidence that reoxygenation can occur up to 24–48 h after HT in some canine and human tumors, it is not definitively known whether reoxygenation occurring in an individual's tumor is associated with long-term treatment outcome. We report on two small subset analyses in canine soft tissue sarcomas suggesting that reoxygenation after the first HT can influence duration of local tumor control after thermoradiotherapy. However, validation is required in larger patient series. Future studies should be directed toward answering whether changes in oxygenation after HT correlate with local tumor control and progression free and overall survival. We also caution that the human sarcoma and locally advanced breast cancer and canine sarcoma data reported in the review are based on several small studies. Further clinical trials, with greater numbers of subjects, would be needed for validation of the observation that reoxygenation after HT results in better anti-tumor effect.

It is also important to note that many other factors, independent of reoxygenation or thermal dose, per se, may influence treatment response to thermoradiotherapy. Examples include: (1) technical variations in application of HT [19,78], (2) variations in sequence and/or time interval between HT and radiotherapy [19], (3) rate of heating [54]; other physiologic factors such as pH, perfusion and/or metabolism and patient specific factors such as age [140,141], smoking history [142,143] and genomic variation [112,144]. Thus, as we have attempted to tease out how hypoxia and reoxygenation influence treatment outcome, it is important to keep in mind that many factors can play into the ultimate outcome for a specific patient. Trials conducted in the future could benefit from data acquisition of as many potential mitigators as possible.

7. Returning Back to Differences in Temperature Distributions between Rodent and Human Tumors

Finally, we need to come back to our original premise that differences in temperature distribution between rodent tumors vs. human and canine tumors are physiologically important. We show that thermal doses at the higher end of the distribution in human and canine sarcomas create ADC changes that are consistent with induction of necrosis and, ironically, reoxygenation. In contrast, temperatures in the lower end of the distribution are associated with increased perfusion. These physiologic changes are associated with treatment response. Such heterogeneity in physiologic response within human and canine tumors would not have been seen in rodent tumors, where water bath heating yields a fairly uniform temperature distribution. This raises the question, then, of why reoxygenation has been observed in some rodent tumors and not in others after uniform mild temperature water bath heating? There are two potential explanations for this: (1) It has been shown that mild temperature HT increases HIF-1α expression in some tumors [57]. HIF-1, in turn, upregulates PDK-1, which controls the switch from aerobic to anaerobic metabolism. This switch would reduce oxygen consumption rate, thereby contributing to reoxygenation. (2) Mild temperature heating has been reported to induce apoptosis and/or senescence in some tumor cell types in vitro and in vivo [145,146]. The induction of apoptosis and senescence would reduce oxygen consumption rate. Apoptosis could also contribute to improved perfusion as a result of reduced tissue pressure [128]. The preponderance of apoptosis appears to be temperature dependent, with increases occurring with temperature up to 43 °C for 30–40 min [147]; above this, necrosis becomes the primary cell death mechanism [147]. It is likely that the aforementioned putative mechanisms of reoxygenation occur in some tumor lines, but not all. Uncovering mechanisms for variation creates a clear framework for future pre-clinical research, as mechanisms may very well be associated with treatment responses in human tumors as well.

It is also important to consider potential reasons for variation in treatment response, within specific tumor lines. Examination of individual variability in tumor response has rarely been examined in pre-clinical models. One example is provided that involved HT. Palmer et al. examined individual responses of the ovarian tumor model, SKOV-3, to a thermosensitive liposome containing doxorubicin [148]. The tumors were heated to 42 °C for 60 min by water bath. Using optical spectroscopy, they measured hemoglobin saturation [Hb_{sat}], total hemoglobin and drug concentration in heated tumors. The primary outcome variable was growth time [time to reach 3 times treatment volume]. Hb_{sat} and drug concentration were significantly related to growth time. Further, cluster analysis revealed that tumors with both low Hb_{sat} and low total Hb had relatively short growth times. Total Hb is related to blood volume and perfusion rate. Although optical spectroscopy is not widely available, there are many other ways to non-invasively measure parameters related to tumor hypoxia, perfusion and ADC in mice, using MRI or PET [24,149]. It is recommended that pre-clinical study designs involving monitoring of individual treatment responses be considered for future research. Additionally, it is advised to use heating methods that yield peaked temperature distributions that mirror what is seen clinically. For example, Kelleher used a near infrared method that achieved a peaked temperature distribution in a rat tumor line [84]. Such studies could prove invaluable in setting the stage for future human clinical trial designs.

8. Conclusions

In this review, we provide convincing evidence that HT causes prolonged reoxygenation lasting at least 24–48 h in both human and canine cancers. Further, we show that reoxygenation is likely caused by increased perfusion as well as a putative reduction in oxygen consumption rate. Importantly, these effects are linked to characteristics of the peaked temperature distribution that usually accompany HT treatment of solid cancers in the clinic. The higher end of the temperature distribution is associated with evidence of cell killing and/or reduced oxygen consumption rate, whereas temperatures at the lower end of the distribution are associated with increases in perfusion. These effects appear to be occurring simultaneously in tumors after HT.

We hypothesize that the relative lack of validation of such results in pre-clinical models is due to the fact that rodent tumor heating is usually performed in water baths that do not yield peaked temperature distributions seen in the clinic.

Finally, we end with a suggestion for future clinical studies that carefully examine the impact of HT on cell killing and physiology by combining functional imaging with estimates of cell survival based on in vitro cell survival curve data. Such studies are likely to provide important insights into which features of HT+RT (direct cell killing by HT, direct cell killing by RT, reoxygenation influence on RT cell killing and heat radiosensitization) will have the greatest influence on local tumor control.

Supplementary Materials: The following supporting information can be downloaded at: https://www.mdpi.com/article/10.3390/cancers14071701/s1, Table S1: Temperatures obtained during 1st HT: Thermal dose fractionation trial^, Table S2: Key Thermal Characteristics: Thermal dose fractionation trial^, Figure S1: Total CEM43T$_{10}$ vs. Relative Change in ADC Mean Post/Pre; Text S1: Supplemental Methods pertaining to Figure 4, Text S2: Supplemental Materials related to Figure 5; Figure S2: Predicted clonogenic survival vs. day of treament, taking into account heat radiosensitization; Figure S3: Predicted tumor control probability vs. Day of Treatment. This figure depicts the theoretical tumor control probability vs. day of treatment for the two scenarios shown in Figure S2.

Author Contributions: Conceptualization, M.W.D.; formal analysis, J.K. and T.W.S.; investigation, M.W.D.; data curation, M.W.D.; writing—original draft preparation, M.W.D.; writing—review and editing, J.R.O.; visualization, M.W.D., funding acquisition, M.W.D. All authors have read and agreed to the published version of the manuscript.

Funding: The previously unpublished data in this paper were generated during canine clinical trials supported by a grant from NIH/NCI P01CA42745.

Data Availability Statement: Previously unpublished data presented in this paper can be provided upon request.

Acknowledgments: The authors recognize the invaluable contributions made by members of the Duke Hyperthermia program that generated the data shown in this paper. Special thanks go to Thaddeus Samulski, Paul Stauffer, Oana Craciunescu, Zeljko Vujaskovic, Leonard Prosnitz, Ellen Jones, David Brizel, Donald Thrall, Susan LaRue, Edward Gillette, Greg Palmer, and Gary Rosner. In addition, thanks to Greg Palmer for graphical and editorial assistance in the preparation of this paper.

Conflicts of Interest: The authors declare no conflict of interest.

References

1. Datta, N.R.; Bodis, S. Hyperthermia with radiotherapy reduces tumour alpha/beta: Insights from trials of thermoradiotherapy vs. radiotherapy alone. *Radiother. Oncol.* **2019**, *138*, 1–8. [CrossRef]
2. Datta, N.R.; Rogers, S.; Ordonez, S.G.; Puric, E.; Bodis, S. Hyperthermia and radiotherapy in the management of head and neck cancers: A systematic review and meta-analysis. *Int. J. Hyperth.* **2016**, *32*, 31–40. [CrossRef]
3. Datta, N.R.; Puric, E.; Klingbiel, D.; Gomez, S.; Bodis, S. Hyperthermia and Radiation Therapy in Locoregional Recurrent Breast Cancers: A Systematic Review and Meta-analysis. *Int. J. Radiat. Oncol.* **2015**, *94*, 1073–1087. [CrossRef]
4. Issels, R.D.; Lindner, L.H.; Verweij, J.; Wessalowski, R.; Reichardt, P.; Wust, P.; Ghadjar, P.; Hohenberger, P.; Angele, M.; Salat, C.; et al. Effect of Neoadjuvant Chemotherapy Plus Regional Hyperthermia on Long-term Outcomes Among Patients With Localized High-Risk Soft Tissue Sarcoma: The EORTC 62961-ESHO 95 Randomized Clinical Trial. *JAMA Oncol.* **2018**, *4*, 483–492. [CrossRef]
5. Issels, R.D.; Lindner, L.; Verweij, J.; Wust, P.; Reichardt, P.; Schem, B.-C.; Abdel-Rahman, S.; Daugaard, S.; Salat, C.; Wendtner, C.-M.; et al. Neo-adjuvant chemotherapy alone or with regional hyperthermia for localised high-risk soft-tissue sarcoma: A randomised phase 3 multicentre study. *Lancet Oncol.* **2010**, *11*, 561–570. [CrossRef]
6. Perez, C.A.; Pajak, T.; Emami, B.; Hornback, N.B.; Tupchong, L.; Rubin, P. Randomized Phase III Study Comparing Irradiation and Hyperthermia with Irradiation Alone in Superficial Measurable Tumors. *Am. J. Clin. Oncol.* **1991**, *14*, 133–141. [CrossRef]
7. Harima, Y.; Ohguri, T.; Imada, H.; Sakurai, H.; Ohno, T.; Hiraki, Y.; Tuji, K.; Tanaka, M.; Terashima, H. A multicentre randomised clinical trial of chemoradiotherapy plus hyperthermia versus chemoradiotherapy alone in patients with locally advanced cervical cancer. *Int. J. Hyperth.* **2016**, *32*, 801–808. [CrossRef]
8. Vasanthan, A.; Mitsumori, M.; Park, J.H.; Zhi-Fan, Z.; Yu-Bin, Z.; Oliynychenko, P.; Tatsuzaki, H.; Tanaka, Y.; Hiraoka, M. Regional hyperthermia combined with radiotherapy for uterine cervical cancers: A multi-institutional prospective randomized trial of the international atomic energy agency. *Int. J. Radiat. Oncol.* **2005**, *61*, 145–153. [CrossRef]
9. Oei, A.L.; Vriend, L.E.M.; Crezee, J.; Franken, N.A.P.; Krawczyk, P.M. Effects of hyperthermia on DNA repair pathways: One treatment to inhibit them all. *Radiat. Oncol.* **2015**, *10*, 165. [CrossRef]
10. Mendez, F.; Sandigursky, M.; Franklin, W.A.; Kenny, M.K.; Kureekattil, R.; Bases, R. Heat-Shock Proteins Associated with Base Excision Repair Enzymes in HeLa Cells. *Radiat. Res.* **2000**, *153*, 186–195. [CrossRef]
11. Takahashi, A.; Yamakawa, N.; Mori, E.; Ohnishi, K.; Yokota, S.-I.; Sugo, N.; Aratani, Y.; Koyama, H.; Ohnishi, T. Development of thermotolerance requires interaction between polymerase-β and heat shock proteins. *Cancer Sci.* **2008**, *99*, 973–978. [CrossRef] [PubMed]
12. Raaphorst, G.P.; Yang, D.P.; Bussey, A.; Ng, C.E. Cell killing, DNA polymerase inactivation and radiosensitization to low dose rate irradiation by mild hyperthermia in four human cell lines. *Int. J. Hyperth.* **1995**, *11*, 841–854. [CrossRef] [PubMed]
13. Stege, G.; Kampinga, H.; Konings, A. Heat-induced Intranuclear Protein Aggregation and Thermal Radiosensitization. *Int. J. Radiat. Biol.* **1995**, *67*, 203–209. [CrossRef] [PubMed]
14. Elming, P.B.; Sørensen, B.S.; Oei, A.L.; Franken, N.A.P.; Crezee, J.; Overgaard, J.; Horsman, M.R. Hyperthermia: The Optimal Treatment to Overcome Radiation Resistant Hypoxia. *Cancers* **2019**, *11*, 60. [CrossRef]
15. Van Leeuwen, C.M.; Oei, A.L.; Chin, K.W.T.K.; Crezee, J.; Bel, A.; Westermann, A.M.; Buist, M.R.; Franken, N.A.P.; Stalpers, L.J.A.; Kok, H.P. A short time interval between radiotherapy and hyperthermia reduces in-field recurrence and mortality in women with advanced cervical cancer. *Radiat. Oncol.* **2017**, *12*, 75. [CrossRef]
16. Kroesen, M.; Mulder, H.T.; Van Holthe, J.M.L.; Aangeenbrug, A.A.; Mens, J.W.M.; Van Doorn, H.C.; Paulides, M.M.; Oomen-de Hoop, E.; Vernhout, R.M.; Lutgens, L.C.; et al. The Effect of the Time Interval Between Radiation and Hyperthermia on Clinical Outcome in 400 Locally Advanced Cervical Carcinoma Patients. *Front. Oncol.* **2019**, *9*, 134. [CrossRef]
17. Kroesen, M.; Mulder, H.T.; Van Rhoon, G.C.; Franckena, M. Commentary: The Impact of the Time Interval Between Radiation and Hyperthermia on Clinical Outcome in Patients With Locally Advanced Cervical Cancer. *Front. Oncol.* **2019**, *9*, 1387. [CrossRef]
18. Crezee, J.; Oei, A.L.; Franken, N.A.P.; Stalpers, L.J.A.; Kok, H.P. Response: Commentary: The Impact of the Time Interval Between Radiation and Hyperthermia on Clinical Outcome in Patients With Locally Advanced Cervical Cancer. *Front. Oncol.* **2020**, *10*. [CrossRef]
19. Ademaj, A.; Veltsista, D.P.; Ghadjar, P.; Marder, D.; Oberacker, E.; Ott, O.J.; Wust, P.; Puric, E.; Hälg, R.A.; Rogers, S.; et al. Clinical Evidence for Thermometric Parameters to Guide Hyperthermia Treatment. *Cancers* **2022**, *14*, 625. [CrossRef]
20. Repasky, E.A.; Evans, S.S.; Dewhirst, M.W. Temperature Matters! And Why It Should Matter to Tumor Immunologists. *Cancer Immunol. Res.* **2013**, *1*, 210–216. [CrossRef]
21. Yarmolenko, P.S.; Moon, E.J.; Landon, C.; Manzoor, A.; Hochman, D.W.; Viglianti, B.L.; Dewhirst, M.W. Thresholds for thermal damage to normal tissues: An update. *Int. J. Hyperth.* **2011**, *27*, 320–343. [CrossRef]
22. Vujaskovic, Z.; Song, C.W. Physiological mechanisms underlying heat-induced radiosensitization. *Int. J. Hyperth.* **2004**, *20*, 163–174. [CrossRef]
23. Vaupel, P. Tumor Hypoxia: Causative Factors, Compensatory Mechanisms, and Cellular Response. *Oncol.* **2004**, *9*, 4–9. [CrossRef]
24. Horsman, M.R.; Mortensen, L.S.; Petersen, J.B.; Busk, M.; Overgaard, J. Imaging hypoxia to improve radiotherapy outcome. *Nat. Rev. Clin. Oncol.* **2012**, *9*, 674–687. [CrossRef]
25. Overgaard, J.; Horsman, M.R. Horsman Modification of Hypoxia-Induced Radioresistance in Tumors by the Use of Oxygen and Sensitizers. In *Seminars in radiation oncology*; WB Saunders: Philadelphia, PA, USA, 1996; Volume 6, pp. 10–21. [CrossRef]

26. Overgaard, J. Hypoxic modification of radiotherapy in squamous cell carcinoma of the head and neck – A systematic review and meta-analysis. *Radiother. Oncol.* **2011**, *100*, 22–32. [CrossRef]
27. Minassian, L.M.; Cotechini, T.; Huitema, E.; Graham, C.H. Hypoxia-Induced Resistance to Chemotherapy in Cancer. In *Hypoxia and Cancer Metastasis*; Gilkes, D.M., Ed.; Advances in Experimental Medicine and Biology; Springer: Cham, Switzerland, 2019; Volume 1136, pp. 123–139.
28. Zhang, X.; Ashcraft, K.A.; Warner, A.B.; Nair, S.K.; Dewhirst, M.W. Can Exercise-Induced Modulation of the Tumor Physiologic Microenvironment Improve Antitumor Immunity? *Cancer Res.* **2019**, *79*, 2447–2456. [CrossRef]
29. Brizel, D.; Scully, S.P.; Harrelson, J.M.; Layfield, L.J.; Bean, J.M.; Prosnitz, L.R.; Dewhirst, M.W. Tumor oxygenation predicts for the likelihood of distant metastases in human soft tissue sarcoma. *Cancer Res.* **1996**, *56*.
30. Chan, D.A.; Giaccia, A.J. Hypoxia, gene expression, and metastasis. *Cancer Metastasis Rev.* **2007**, *26*, 333–339. [CrossRef]
31. Hockel, M.; Schlenger, K.; Aral, B.; Mitze, M.; Schaffer, U.; Vaupel, P. Association between tumor hypoxia and malignant progression in advanced cancer of the uterine cervix. *Cancer Res.* **1996**, *56*.
32. Wilson, W.R.; Hay, M.P. Targeting hypoxia in cancer therapy. *Nat. Rev. Cancer* **2011**, *11*, 393–410. [CrossRef]
33. Zhong, H.; De Marzo, A.M.; Laughner, E.; Lim, M.; Hilton, D.A.; Zagzag, D.; Buechler, P.; Isaacs, W.B.; Semenza, G.L.; Simons, J.W. Overexpression of hypoxia-inducible factor 1alpha in common human cancers and their metastases. *Cancer Res.* **1999**, *59*, 5830–5835.
34. Rich, L.; Damasco, J.; Bulmahn, J.; Kutscher, H.; Prasad, P.; Seshadri, M. Photoacoustic and Magnetic Resonance Imaging of Hybrid Manganese Dioxide-Coated Ultra-small NaGdF$_4$ Nanoparticles for Spatiotemporal Modulation of Hypoxia in Head and Neck Cancer. *Cancers* **2020**, *12*, 3294. [CrossRef]
35. Bader, S.B.; Dewhirst, M.W.; Hammond, E.M. Cyclic Hypoxia: An Update on Its Characteristics, Methods to Measure It and Biological Implications in Cancer. *Cancers* **2020**, *13*, 23. [CrossRef]
36. Frost, J.; Frost, M.; Batie, M.; Jiang, H.; Rocha, S. Roles of HIF and 2-Oxoglutarate-Dependent Dioxygenases in Controlling Gene Expression in Hypoxia. *Cancers* **2021**, *13*, 350. [CrossRef]
37. Hompland, T.; Fjeldbo, C.S.; Lyng, H. Tumor Hypoxia as a Barrier in Cancer Therapy: Why Levels Matter. *Cancers* **2021**, *13*, 499. [CrossRef]
38. Benyahia, Z.; Blackman, M.; Hamelin, L.; Zampieri, L.; Capeloa, T.; Bedin, M.; Vazeille, T.; Schakman, O.; Sonveaux, P. In Vitro and In Vivo Characterization of MCT1 Inhibitor AZD3965 Confirms Preclinical Safety Compatible with Breast Cancer Treatment. *Cancers* **2021**, *13*, 569. [CrossRef]
39. Cheung, S.; Jain, P.; So, J.; Shahidi, S.; Chung, S.; Koritzinsky, M. p38 MAPK Inhibition Mitigates Hypoxia-Induced AR Signaling in Castration-Resistant Prostate Cancer. *Cancers* **2021**, *13*, 831. [CrossRef]
40. Kabakov, A.E.; Yakimova, A.O. Hypoxia-Induced Cancer Cell Responses Driving Radioresistance of Hypoxic Tumors: Approaches to Targeting and Radiosensitizing. *Cancers* **2021**, *13*, 1102. [CrossRef]
41. Benej, M.; Wu, J.; Kreamer, M.; Kery, M.; Corrales-Guerrero, S.; Papandreou, I.; Williams, T.; Li, Z.; Graves, E.; Selmic, L.; et al. Pharmacological Regulation of Tumor Hypoxia in Model Murine Tumors and Spontaneous Canine Tumors. *Cancers* **2021**, *13*, 1696. [CrossRef]
42. Xu, J.; Yu, T.; Zois, C.; Cheng, J.-X.; Tang, Y.; Harris, A.; Huang, W. Unveiling Cancer Metabolism through Spontaneous and Coherent Raman Spectroscopy and Stable Isotope Probing. *Cancers* **2021**, *13*, 1718. [CrossRef]
43. Elming, P.; Wittenborn, T.; Busk, M.; Sørensen, B.; Thomsen, M.; Strandgaard, T.; Dyrskjøt, L.; Nielsen, S.; Horsman, M. Refinement of an Established Procedure and Its Application for Identification of Hypoxia in Prostate Cancer Xenografts. *Cancers* **2021**, *13*, 2602. [CrossRef]
44. Uva, P.; Bosco, M.; Eva, A.; Conte, M.; Garaventa, A.; Amoroso, L.; Cangelosi, D. Connectivity Map Analysis Indicates PI3K/Akt/mTOR Inhibitors as Potential Anti-Hypoxia Drugs in Neuroblastoma. *Cancers* **2021**, *13*, 2809. [CrossRef]
45. Zhang, Y.; Coleman, M.; Brekken, R. Perspectives on Hypoxia Signaling in Tumor Stroma. *Cancers* **2021**, *13*, 3070. [CrossRef]
46. Ancel, J.; Perotin, J.-M.; Dewolf, M.; Launois, C.; Mulette, P.; Nawrocki-Raby, B.; Dalstein, V.; Gilles, C.; Deslée, G.; Polette, M.; et al. Hypoxia in Lung Cancer Management: A Translational Approach. *Cancers* **2021**, *13*, 3421. [CrossRef]
47. Birindelli, G.; Drobnjakovic, M.; Morath, V.; Steiger, K.; D'Alessandria, C.; Gourni, E.; Afshar-Oromieh, A.; Weber, W.; Rominger, A.; Eiber, M.; et al. Is Hypoxia a Factor Influencing PSMA-Directed Radioligand Therapy?—An In Silico Study on the Role of Chronic Hypoxia in Prostate Cancer. *Cancers* **2021**, *13*, 3429. [CrossRef]
48. Carles, M.; Fechter, T.; Grosu, A.; Sörensen, A.; Thomann, B.; Stoian, R.; Wiedenmann, N.; Rühle, A.; Zamboglou, C.; Ruf, J.; et al. ^{18}F-FMISO-PET Hypoxia Monitoring for Head-and-Neck Cancer Patients: Radiomics Analyses Predict the Outcome of Chemo-Radiotherapy. *Cancers* **2021**, *13*, 3449. [CrossRef]
49. Song, C.W.; Shakil, A.; Osborn, J.L.; Iwata, K. Tumour oxygenation is increased by hyperthermia at mild temperatures. *Int. J. Hyperth.* **1996**, *12*, 367–373. [CrossRef]
50. Vaupel, P.; Horsman, M.R. Tumour perfusion and associated physiology: Characterization and significance for hyperthermia. *Int. J. Hyperth.* **2010**, *26*, 209–210. [CrossRef]
51. Vaupel, P.; Mueller-Klieser, W.; Ott, J.; Manz, R. Impact of various thermal doses on the oxygenation and blood flow in malignant tumors upon localized hyperthermia. In *Oxygen Transport to Tissue*; Lubbers, D.W., Acker, H., Leniger-Follert, E., Goldstick, T.K., Eds.; Plenum Publishing Corp.: New York, NY, USA, 1984; Volume V, pp. 621–629.

52. Herman, T.S.; Stickney, D.G.; Gerner, E.W. DIFFERENTIAL RATES OF HEATING INFLUENCE HYPERTHERMIA INDUCED CYTOTOXICITY IN NORMAL AND TRANSFORMED-CELLS INVITRO. *Proc. Am. Assoc. Cancer Res.* **1979**, *20*, 165.
53. Dewhirst, M.; Gross, J.; Sim, D.; Arnold, P.; Boyer, D. The effect of rate of heating or cooling prior to heating on tumor and normal tissue microcirculatory blood flow. *Biorheology* **1984**, *21*, 539–558. [CrossRef] [PubMed]
54. Hasegawa, T.; Gu, Y.H.; Takahashi, T.; Haswgawa, T.; Yamamoto, I.Y. Enhancement of hyperthermic effects using rapid hyperthermia. In *Theoretical and Experimental Basasxcdis of Hyperthermia: Thermotherapy for Neoplasia, Inflammation and Pain*; Kosaka, M., Sugahara, T., Schmidt, K.L., Eds.; Springer: Tokyo, Japan, 2003; pp. 439–444.
55. Vaupel, P.; Mullerklieser, W.; Otte, J.; Manz, R.; Kallinowski, F. Blood-Flow, Tissue Oxygenation, and Ph-Distribution in Malignant-Tumors Upon Localized Hyperthermia—Basic Pathophysiological Aspects and the Role of Various Thermal Doses. *Strahlentherapie* **1983**, *159*, 73–81. [PubMed]
56. Kong, G.; Braun, R.D.; Dewhirst, M.W. Characterization of the effect of hyperthermia on nanoparticle extravasation from tumor vasculature. *Cancer Res.* **2001**, *61*, 3027–3032. [PubMed]
57. Moon, E.J.; Sonveaux, P.; Porporato, P.E.; Danhier, P.; Gallez, B.; Batinic-Haberle, I.; Nien, Y.-C.; Schroeder, T.; Dewhirst, M.W. NADPH oxidase-mediated reactive oxygen species production activates hypoxia-inducible factor-1 (HIF-1) via the ERK pathway after hyperthermia treatment. *Proc. Natl. Acad. Sci. USA* **2010**, *107*, 20477–20482. [CrossRef]
58. Bordonaro, M.; Shirasawa, S.; Lazarova, D.L. In Hyperthermia Increased ERK and WNT Signaling Suppress Colorectal Cancer Cell Growth. *Cancers* **2016**, *8*, 49. [CrossRef]
59. Hildebrandt, B.; Wust, P.; Ahlers, O.; Dieing, A.; Sreenivasa, G.; Kerner, T.; Felix, R.; Riess, H. The cellular and molecular basis of hyperthermia. *Crit. Rev. Oncol. Hematol.* **2002**, *43*, 33–56. [CrossRef]
60. Oei, A.L.; Van Leeuwen, C.M.; Cate, R.T.; Rodermond, H.M.; Buist, M.R.; Stalpers, L.J.A.; Crezee, J.; Kok, H.; Medema, J.P.; Franken, N.A.P. Hyperthermia Selectively Targets Human Papillomavirus in Cervical Tumors via p53-Dependent Apoptosis. *Cancer Res.* **2015**, *75*, 5120–5129. [CrossRef]
61. Sapareto, S.A.; Dewey, W.C. Thermal dose determination in cancer therapy. *Int. J. Radiat. Oncol. Biol. Phys.* **1984**, *10*, 787–800. [CrossRef]
62. Vujaskovic, Z.; Poulson, J.M.; Gaskin, A.A.; Thrall, D.E.; Page, R.L.; Charles, H.C.; MacFall, J.R.; Brizel, D.M.; Meyer, R.E.; Prescott, D.M.; et al. Temperature-dependent changes in physiologic parameters of spontaneous canine soft tissue sarcomas after combined radiotherapy and hyperthermia treatment. *Int. J. Radiat. Oncol. Biol. Phys.* **2000**, *46*, 179–185. [CrossRef]
63. Thrall, D.E.; Maccarini, P.; Stauffer, P.; MacFall, J.; Hauck, M.; Snyder, S.; Case, B.; Linder, K.; Lan, L.; McCall, L.; et al. Thermal dose fractionation affects tumour physiological response. *Int. J. Hyperth.* **2012**, *28*, 431–440. [CrossRef]
64. Hannon, G.; Tansi, F.L.; Hilger, I.; Prina-Mello, A. The Effects of Localized Heat on the Hallmarks of Cancer. *Adv. Ther.* **2021**, *4*, 2000267. [CrossRef]
65. Dewhirst, M.W.; Cao, Y.; Moeller, B. Cycling hypoxia and free radicals regulate angiogenesis and radiotherapy response. *Nat. Cancer* **2008**, *8*, 425–437. [CrossRef] [PubMed]
66. Secomb, T.; Hsu, R.; Ong, E.T.; Gross, J.F.; Dewhirst, M.W. Analysis of the Effects of Oxygen Supply and Demand on Hypoxic Fraction in Tumors. *Acta Oncol.* **1995**, *34*, 313–316. [CrossRef] [PubMed]
67. Secomb, T.W.; Hsu, R.; Park, E.Y.H.; Dewhirst, M.W. Green's Function Methods for Analysis of Oxygen Delivery to Tissue by Microvascular Networks. *Ann. Biomed. Eng.* **2004**, *32*, 1519–1529. [CrossRef] [PubMed]
68. Secomb, T.W.; Hsu, R.; Dewhirst, M.W. Synergistic effects of hyperoxic gas breathing and reduced oxygen consumption on tumor oxygenation: A theoretical model. *Int. J. Radiat. Oncol.* **2004**, *59*, 572–578. [CrossRef]
69. Snyder, S.A.; Lanzen, J.L.; Braun, R.D.; Rosner, G.; Secomb, T.; Biaglow, J.; Brizel, D.; Dewhirst, M.W. Simultaneous administration of glucose and hyperoxic gas achieves greater improvement in tumor oxygenation than hyperoxic gas alone. *Int. J. Radiat. Oncol.* **2001**, *51*, 494–506. [CrossRef]
70. Griffin, R.; Okajima, K.; Barrios, B.; Song, C.W. Mild temperature hyperthermia combined with carbogen breathing increases tumor partial pressure of oxygen (pO2) and radiosensitivity. *Cancer Res.* **1996**, *56*.
71. Griffin, R.J.; Okajima, K.; Ogawa, A.; Song, C.W. Radiosensitization of two murine rumours with mild temperature hyperthermia and carbogen breathing. *Int. J. Radiat. Oncol. Biol. Phys.* **1999**, *75*, 1299–1306.
72. Ohara, M.D.; Hetzel, F.W.; Frinak, S. Thermal Distributions in a Water Bath Heated Mouse-Tumor. *Int. J. Radiat. Oncol. Biol. Phys.* **1985**, *11*, 817–822. [CrossRef]
73. Oleson, J.; Dewhirst, M.; Harrelson, J.; Leopold, K.; Samulski, T.; Tso, C. Tumor temperature distributions predict hyperthermia effect. *Int. J. Radiat. Oncol.* **1989**, *16*, 559–570. [CrossRef]
74. Bakker, J.F.; Paulides, M.M.; Obdeijn, I.M.; Van Rhoon, G.C.; A Van Dongen, K.W. An ultrasound cylindrical phased array for deep heating in the breast: Theoretical design using heterogeneous models. *Phys. Med. Biol.* **2009**, *54*, 3201–3215. [CrossRef] [PubMed]
75. Cappiello, G.; Paulides, M.M.; Drizdal, T.; O'Loughlin, D.; O'Halloran, M.; Glavin, M.; Van Rhoon, G.; Jones, E. Robustness of Time-Multiplexed Hyperthermia to Temperature Dependent Thermal Tissue Properties. *IEEE J. Electromagn. RF Microwaves Med. Biol.* **2019**, *4*, 126–132. [CrossRef]
76. Verhaart, R.F.; Rijnen, Z.; Fortunati, V.; Verduijn, G.M.; Van Walsum, T.; Veenland, J.F.; Paulides, M.M. Temperature simulations in hyperthermia treatment planning of the head and neck region. *Strahlenther. und Onkol.* **2014**, *190*, 1117–1124. [CrossRef] [PubMed]

77. Paulides, M.M.; Rodrigues, D.B.; Bellizzi, G.G.; Sumser, K.; Curto, S.; Neufeld, E.; Montanaro, H.; Kok, H.P.; Trefna, H.D. ESHO benchmarks for computational modeling and optimization in hyperthermia therapy. *Int. J. Hyperth.* **2021**, *38*, 1425–1442. [CrossRef]
78. Gavazzi, S.; van Lier, A.L.H.M.W.; Zachiu, C.; Jansen, E.; Lagendijk, J.J.W.; A Stalpers, L.J.; Crezee, H.; Kok, H.P. Advanced patient-specific hyperthermia treatment planning. *Int. J. Hyperth.* **2020**, *37*, 992–1007. [CrossRef]
79. Lüdemann, L.; Wlodarczyk, W.; Nadobny, J.; Weihrauch, M.; Gellermann, J.; Wust, P. Non-invasive magnetic resonance thermography during regional hyperthermia. *Int. J. Hyperth.* **2010**, *26*, 273–282. [CrossRef]
80. Craciunescu, O.I.; Das, S.K.; McCauley, R.L.; MacFall, J.R.; Samulski, T.V. 3D numerical reconstruction of the hyperthermia induced temperature distribution in human sarcomas using DE-MRI measured tissue perfusion: Validation against non-invasive MR temperature measurements. *Int. J. Hyperth.* **2001**, *17*, 221–239. [CrossRef]
81. Li, Z.; Vogel, M.; Maccarini, P.F.; Stakhursky, V.; Soher, B.J.; Craciunescu, O.I.; Das, S.; Arabe, O.A.; Joines, W.T.; Stauffer, P.R. Improved hyperthermia treatment control using SAR/temperature simulation and PRFS magnetic resonance thermal imaging. *Int. J. Hyperth.* **2010**, *27*, 86–99. [CrossRef]
82. DeWhirst, M.; Phillips, T.; Samulski, T.; Stauffer, P.; Shrivastava, P.; Paliwal, B.; Pajak, T.; Gillim, M.; Sapozink, M.; Myerson, R.; et al. RTOG quality assurance guidelines for clinical trials using hyperthermia. *Int. J. Radiat. Oncol.* **1990**, *18*, 1249–1259. [CrossRef]
83. Daniel, R.M.; Danson, M.J. Temperature and the catalytic activity of enzymes: A fresh understanding. *FEBS Lett.* **2013**, *587*, 2738–2743. [CrossRef]
84. Kelleher, D.K.; Engel, T.; Vaupel, P.W. Changes in microregional perfusion, oxygenation, ATP and lactate distribution in subcutaneous rat tumours upon water-filtered IR-A hyperthermia. *Int. J. Hyperth.* **1995**, *11*, 241–255. [CrossRef] [PubMed]
85. Vaupel, P.; Schaefer, C.; Okunieff, P. Intracellular acidosis in murine fibrosarcomas coincides with ATP depletion, hypoxia, and high levels of lactate and total Pi. *NMR Biomed.* **1994**, *7*, 128–136. [CrossRef] [PubMed]
86. Sijens, P.E.; Bovee, W.M.M.J.; Koole, P.; Schipper, J. Phosphorus NMR study of the response of a murine tumour to hyperthermia as a function of treatment time and temperature. *Int. J. Hyperth.* **1989**, *5*, 351–357. [CrossRef] [PubMed]
87. Prescott, D.M.; Charles, H.C.; Sostman, H.D.; Dodge, R.K.; Thrall, D.E.; Page, R.L.; Tucker, J.A.; Harrelson, J.M.; Leopold, K.A.; Oleson, J.R.; et al. Therapy monitoring in human and canine soft tissue sarcomas using magnetic resonance imaging and spectroscopy. *Int. J. Radiat. Oncol.* **1994**, *28*, 415–423. [CrossRef]
88. Maguire, P.D.; Samulski, T.V.; Prosnitz, L.R.; Jones, E.L.; Rosner, G.L.; Powers, B.; Layfield, L.W.; Brizel, D.M.; Scully, S.P.; Harrelson, J.M.; et al. A phase II trial testing the thermal dose parameter CEM43° T90 as a predictor of response in soft tissue sarcomas treated with pre-operative thermoradiotherapy. *Int. J. Hyperth.* **2001**, *17*, 283–290. [CrossRef] [PubMed]
89. Dewhirst, M.W.; Poulson, J.M.; Yu, D.; Sanders, L.; Lora-Michiels, M.; Vujaskovic, Z.; Jones, E.L.; Samulski, T.V.; Powers, B.E.; Brizel, D.M.; et al. Relation between pO2, 31P magnetic resonance spectroscopy parameters and treatment outcome in patients with high-grade soft tissue sarcomas treated with thermoradiotherapy. *Int. J. Radiat. Oncol.* **2005**, *61*, 480–491. [CrossRef]
90. Moeller, B.J.; Cao, Y.; Li, C.Y.; Dewhirst, M.W. Radiation activates HIF-1 to regulate vascular radiosensitivity in tumors: Role of reoxygenation, free radicals, and stress granules. *Cancer Cell* **2004**, *5*, 429–441. [CrossRef]
91. Li, F.; Sonveaux, P.; Rabbani, Z.N.; Liu, S.; Yan, B.; Huang, Q.; Vujaskovic, Z.; Dewhirst, M.W.; Li, C.-Y. Regulation of HIF-1α Stability through S-Nitrosylation. *Mol. Cell* **2007**, *26*, 63–74. [CrossRef]
92. Kim, W.; Kim, M.-S.; Kim, H.-J.; Lee, E.; Jeong, J.-H.; Park, I.; Jeong, Y.K.; Jang, W.I. Role of HIF-1α in response of tumors to a combination of hyperthermia and radiation in vivo. *Int. J. Hyperth.* **2017**, *34*, 276–283. [CrossRef]
93. Westerterp, M.; Omloo, J.M.T.; Sloof, G.W.; Hulshof, M.C.C.M.; Hoekstra, O.S.; Crezee, H.; Boellaard, R.; Vervenne, W.L.; Kate, F.J.W.T.; Van Lanschot, J.J.B. Monitoring of response to pre-operative chemoradiation in combination with hyperthermia in oesophageal cancer by FDG-PET. *Int. J. Hyperth.* **2006**, *22*, 149–160. [CrossRef]
94. Murata, H.; Okamoto, M.; Takahashi, T.; Motegi, M.; Ogoshi, K.; Shoji, H.; Onishi, M.; Takakusagi, Y.; Okonogi, N.; Kawamura, H.; et al. SUVmax-based Parameters of FDG-PET/CT Reliably Predict Pathologic Complete Response After Preoperative Hyperthermo-chemoradiotherapy in Rectal Cancer. *Anticancer Res.* **2018**, *38*, 5909–5916. [CrossRef] [PubMed]
95. Fendler, W.P.; Lehmann, M.; Todica, A.; Herrmann, K.; Knösel, T.; Angele, M.K.; Dürr, H.R.; Rauch, J.; Bartenstein, P.; Cyran, C.C.; et al. PET Response Criteria in Solid Tumors Predicts Progression-Free Survival and Time to Local or Distant Progression After Chemotherapy with Regional Hyperthermia for Soft-Tissue Sarcoma. *J. Nucl. Med.* **2015**, *56*, 530–537. [CrossRef] [PubMed]
96. Dewhirst, M.W.; Viglianti, B.L.; Lora-Michiels, M.; Hanson, M.; Hoopes, P.J. Basic principles of thermal dosimetry and thermal thresholds for tissue damage from hyperthermia. *Int. J. Hyperth.* **2003**, *19*, 267–294. [CrossRef] [PubMed]
97. Rosner, G.L.; Clegg, S.T.; Prescott, D.M.; Dewhirst, M.W. Estimation of cell survival in tumours heated to nonuniform temperature distributions. *Int. J. Hyperth.* **1996**, *12*, 223–239. [CrossRef] [PubMed]
98. Shakil, A.; Osborn, J.L.; Song, C.W. Changes in oxygenation status and blood flow in a rat tumor model by mild temperature hyperthermia. *Int. J. Radiat. Oncol.* **1999**, *43*, 859–865. [CrossRef]
99. Iwata, K.; Shakil, A.; Hur, W.J.; Makepeace, C.M.; Griffin, R.J.; Song, C.W. Tumour pO(2) can be increased markedly by mild hyperthermia. *Br. J. Cancer* **1996**, *74*, S217–S221.
100. Song, C.W.; Park, H.; Griffin, R.J. Improvement of Tumor Oxygenation by Mild Hyperthermia. *Radiat. Res.* **2001**, *155*, 515–528. [CrossRef]

101. Oleson, J.R. Eugene Robertson Special Lecture Hyperthermia from the clinic to the laboratory: A hypothesis. *Int. J. Hyperth.* **1995**, *11*, 315–322. [CrossRef]
102. Okajima, K.; Griffin, R.J.; Iwata, K.; Shakil, A.; Song, C.W. Tumor oxygenation after mild-temperature hyperthermia in combination with carbogen breathing: Dependence on heat dose and tumor type. *Radiat. Res.* **1998**, *149*, 294. [CrossRef]
103. Brizel, D.M.; Scully, S.P.; Harrelson, J.M.; Layfield, L.J.; Dodge, R.K.; Charles, H.C.; Samulski, T.V.; Prosnitz, L.R.; Dewhirst, M.W. Radiation therapy and hyperthermia improve the oxygenation of human soft tissue sarcomas. *Cancer Res.* **1996**, *56*, 5347–5350.
104. Vujaskovic, Z.; Rosen, E.L.; Blackwell, K.L.; Jones, E.L.; Brizel, D.M.; Prosnitz, L.R.; Samulski, T.V.; Dewhirst, M.W. Ultrasound guided pO 2 measurement of breast cancer reoxygenation after neoadjuvant chemotherapy and hyperthermia treatment. *Int. J. Hyperth.* **2003**, *19*, 498–506. [CrossRef] [PubMed]
105. Kong, G.; Braun, R.D.; Dewhirst, M.W. Hyperthermia enables tumor-specific nanoparticle delivery: Effect of particle size. *Cancer Res.* **2000**, *60*, 4440–4445. [PubMed]
106. Matteucci, M.L.; Anyarambhatla, G.; Rosner, G.; Azuma, C.; E Fisher, P.; Dewhirst, M.W.; Needham, D.; E Thrall, D. Hyperthermia increases accumulation of technetium-99m-labeled liposomes in feline sarcomas. *Clin. Cancer Res.* **2000**, *6*, 3748–3755. [PubMed]
107. Jones, E.L.; Prosnitz, L.R.; Dewhirst, M.W.; Marcom, P.K.; Hardenbergh, P.H.; Marks, L.B.; Brizel, D.M.; Vujaskovic, Z. Thermochemoradiotherapy Improves Oxygenation in Locally Advanced Breast Cancer. *Clin. Cancer Res.* **2004**, *10*, 4287–4293. [CrossRef]
108. Thrall, D.E.; LaRue, S.M.; Yu, D.; Samulski, T.; Sanders, L.; Case, B.; Rosner, G.; Azuma, C.; Poulson, J.; Pruitt, A.F.; et al. Thermal Dose Is Related to Duration of Local Control in Canine Sarcomas Treated with Thermoradiotherapy. *Clin. Cancer Res.* **2005**, *11*, 5206–5214. [CrossRef]
109. Lora-Michiels, M.; Yu, D.; Sanders, L.; Poulson, J.M.; Azuma, C.; Case, B.; Vujaskovic, Z.; Thrall, D.E.; Charles, H.C.; Dewhirst, M.W. Extracellular pH and P-31 Magnetic Resonance Spectroscopic Variables are Related to Outcome in Canine Soft Tissue Sarcomas Treated with Thermoradiotherapy. *Clin. Cancer Res.* **2006**, *12*, 5733–5740. [CrossRef]
110. Cline, J.; Rosner, G.L.; Raleigh, J.A.; Thrall, D.E. Quantification of CCI-103F labeling heterogeneity in canine solid tumors. *Int. J. Radiat. Oncol.* **1997**, *37*, 655–662. [CrossRef]
111. Cline, J.M.; Thrall, D.E.; Rosner, G.; Raleigh, J.A. DISTRIBUTION OF THE HYPOXIA MARKER CCI-103F IN CANINE TUMORS. *Int. J. Radiat. Oncol. Biol. Phys.* **1994**, *28*, 921–933. [CrossRef]
112. Chi, J.-T.; Thrall, D.E.; Jiang, C.; Snyder, S.; Fels, D.; Landon, C.; McCall, L.; Lan, L.; Hauck, M.; MacFall, J.R.; et al. Comparison of Genomics and Functional Imaging from Canine Sarcomas Treated with Thermoradiotherapy Predicts Therapeutic Response and Identifies Combination Therapeutics. *Clin. Cancer Res.* **2011**, *17*, 2549–2560. [CrossRef]
113. Li, Y.; Lin, D.; Weng, Y.; Weng, S.; Yan, C.; Xu, X.; Chen, J.; Ye, R.; Hong, J. Early Diffusion-Weighted Imaging and Proton Magnetic Resonance Spectroscopy Features of Liver Transplanted Tumors Treated with Radiation in Rabbits: Correlation with Histopathology. *Radiat. Res.* **2018**, *191*, 52–59. [CrossRef]
114. Morse, D.L.; Galons, J.-P.; Payne, C.M.; Jennings, D.L.; Day, S.; Xia, G.; Gillies, R.J. MRI-measured water mobility increases in response to chemotherapy via multiple cell-death mechanisms. *NMR Biomed.* **2007**, *20*, 602–614. [CrossRef] [PubMed]
115. Cheung, J.S.; Fan, S.J.; Gao, D.S.; Chow, A.M.; Man, K.; Wu, E.X. Diffusion tensor imaging of liver fibrosis in an experimental model. *J. Magn. Reson. Imaging* **2010**, *32*, 1141–1148. [CrossRef] [PubMed]
116. Huang, B.; Geng, D.; Zhan, S.; Li, H.; Xu, X.; Yi, C. Magnetic resonance imaging characteristics of hepatocyte apoptosis (induced by right portal vein ligation) and necrosis (induced by combined right portal vein and right hepatic artery ligation) in rats. *J. Int. Med. Res.* **2014**, *43*, 80–92. [CrossRef] [PubMed]
117. Dewhirst, M.W.; Thrall, D. Data obtained during conduct of Thermal Dose Equivalence Trial, studying companion canine patients with soft tissue sarcomas. 2010. Unpublished work.
118. Moeller, B.J.; Dreher, M.R.; Rabbani, Z.; Schroeder, T.; Cao, Y.; Li, C.Y.; Dewhirst, M.W. Pleiotropic effects of HIF-1 blockade on tumor radiosensitivity. *Cancer Cell* **2005**, *8*, 99–110. [CrossRef] [PubMed]
119. Thrall, D.E.; LaRue, S.M.; Pruitt, A.F.; Case, B.; Dewhirst, M.W. Changes in tumour oxygenation during fractionated hyperthermia and radiation therapy in spontaneous canine sarcomas. *Int. J. Hyperth.* **2006**, *22*, 365–373. [CrossRef] [PubMed]
120. Viglianti, B.L.; Lora-Michiels, M.; Poulson, J.M.; Plantenga, J.P.; Yu, D.; Sanders, L.L.; I Craciunescu, O.; Vujaskovic, Z.; Thrall, D.E.; MacFall, J.R.; et al. Dynamic Contrast-enhanced Magnetic Resonance Imaging as a Predictor of Clinical Outcome in Canine Spontaneous Soft Tissue Sarcomas Treated with Thermoradiotherapy. *Clin. Cancer Res.* **2009**, *15*, 4993–5001. [CrossRef]
121. Leopold, K.A.; Dewhirst, M.; Samulski, T.; Harrelson, J.; Tucker, J.A.; George, S.L.; Dodge, R.K.; Grant, W.; Clegg, S.; Prosnitz, L.R.; et al. Relationships among Tumor Temperature, Treatment Time, and Histopathological Outcome Using Preoperative Hyperthermia with Radiation in Soft-Tissue Sarcomas. *Int. J. Radiat. Oncol. Biol. Phys.* **1992**, *22*, 989–998. [CrossRef]
122. Dewhirst, M.W.; A Sim, D.; Sapareto, S.; Connor, W.G. Importance of minimum tumor temperature in determining early and long-term responses of spontaneous canine and feline tumors to heat and radiation. *Cancer Res.* **1984**, *44*.
123. Thomsen, A.R.; Saalmann, M.A.; Nicolay, N.H.; Grosu, A.-L.; Vaupel, P. Improved oxygenation of human skin, subcutis and superficial cancers upon mild hyperthermia delivered by wIRA-irradiation. *Adv. Exp. Med. Biol.* **2021**, in press.
124. Waterman, F.M.; Nerlinger, R.E.; Moylan, D.J., 3rd; Leeper, D.B. Response of human tumor blood flow to local hyperthermia. *Int. J. Radiat. Oncol. Biol. Phys.* **1987**, *13*, 75–82. [CrossRef]
125. Yuan, H.; Schroeder, T.; E Bowsher, J.; Hedlund, L.W.; Wong, T.; Dewhirst, M.W. Intertumoral differences in hypoxia selectivity of the PET imaging agent 64Cu(II)-diacetyl-bis(N4-methylthiosemicarbazone). *J. Nucl. Med.* **2006**, *47*, 989–998. [PubMed]

126. Hoogsteen, I.J.; Lok, J.; Marres, H.A.; Takes, R.P.; Rijken, P.F.; van der Kogel, A.J.; Kaanders, J.H. Hypoxia in larynx carcinomas assessed by pimonidazole binding and the value of CA-IX and vascularity as surrogate markers of hypoxia. *Eur. J. Cancer* **2009**, *45*, 2906–2914. [CrossRef] [PubMed]
127. E Hansen, A.; Kristensen, A.T.; Jørgensen, J.T.; McEvoy, F.J.; Busk, M.; Van Der Kogel, A.J.; Bussink, J.; A Engelholm, S.; Kjær, A. 64Cu-ATSM and 18FDG PET uptake and 64Cu-ATSM autoradiography in spontaneous canine tumors: Comparison with pimonidazole hypoxia immunohistochemistry. *Radiat. Oncol.* **2012**, *7*, 89. [CrossRef] [PubMed]
128. Dewhirst, M.W.; Secomb, T.W. Transport of drugs from blood vessels to tumour tissue. *Nat. Cancer* **2017**, *17*, 738–750. [CrossRef]
129. Vaishnavi, S.N.; Vlassenko, A.G.; Rundle, M.M.; Snyder, A.Z.; Mintun, M.A.; Raichle, M.E. Regional aerobic glycolysis in the human brain. *Proc. Natl. Acad. Sci.* **2010**, *107*, 17757–17762. [CrossRef]
130. Abramovitch, R.; Dafni, H.; Smouha, E.; E Benjamin, L.; Neeman, M. In vivo prediction of vascular susceptibility to vascular susceptibility endothelial growth factor withdrawal: Magnetic resonance imaging of C6 rat glioma in nude mice. *Cancer Res.* **1999**, *59*, 5012–5016.
131. Huhnt, W. Growth, microvessel density and tumor cell invasion of human colon adenocarcinoma under repeated treatment with hyperthermia and serotonin. *J. Cancer Res. Clin. Oncol.* **1995**, *121*, 423–428. [CrossRef]
132. Li, K.; Shen, S.-Q.; Xiong, C.-L. Microvessel Damage May Play an Important Role in Tumoricidal Effect for Murine H22 Hepatoma Cells with Hyperthermia In Vivo. *J. Surg. Res.* **2008**, *145*, 97–104. [CrossRef]
133. Ting, Z.; Dan, Z.; Luo, Q.M.; Yang, W. Dynamics of blood flow in normal tissue and tumor during local hyperthermia. In Proceedings of the 3rd International Conference on Photonics and Imaging in Biology and Medicine, Wuhan, China, 8–11 June 2003; pp. 484–491.
134. Shan, S.; Rosner, G.; Braun, R.; Hahn, J.; Pearce, C.; Dewhirst, M. Effects of diethylamine/nitric oxide on blood perfusion and oxygenation in the R3230Ac mammary carcinoma. *Br. J. Cancer* **1997**, *76*, 429–437. [CrossRef]
135. Zlotecki, R.A.; Baxter, L.T.; Boucher, Y.; Jain, R.K. Pharmacologic Modification of Tumor Blood Flow and Interstitial Fluid Pressure in a Human Tumor Xenograft: Network Analysis and Mechanistic Interpretation. *Microvasc. Res.* **1995**, *50*, 429–443. [CrossRef]
136. Lüdemann, L.; Sreenivasa, G.; Amthauer, H.; Michel, R.; Gellermann, J.; Wust, P. Use of H215O-PET for investigating perfusion changes in pelvic tumors due to regional hyperthermia. *Int. J. Hyperth.* **2009**, *25*, 299–308. [CrossRef] [PubMed]
137. Ngwa, W.; Irabor, O.C.; Schoenfeld, J.D.; Hesser, J.; Demaria, S.; Formenti, S.C. Using immunotherapy to boost the abscopal effect. *Nat. Cancer* **2018**, *18*, 313–322. [CrossRef] [PubMed]
138. Rickard, A.G.; Palmer, G.M.; Dewhirst, M.W. Clinical and Pre-clinical Methods for Quantifying Tumor Hypoxia. In *Hypoxia and Cancer Metastasis*; Springer: Cham, Switzerland, 2019; Volume 1136, pp. 19–41. [CrossRef]
139. Loshek, D.D.; Orr, J.S.; Solomonidis, E. Interaction of hyperthermia and radiation: The survival surface. *Br. J. Radiol.* **1977**, *50*, 893–901. [CrossRef] [PubMed]
140. Hamilton, S.N.; Tran, E.; Berthelet, E.; Wu, J.; Olson, R. Early (90-day) mortality after radical radiotherapy for head and neck squamous cell carcinoma: A population-based analysis. *Head Neck* **2018**, *40*, 2432–2440. [CrossRef]
141. Munira, A.; Fang, C.Z. MANAGEMENT AND PROGNOSTIC FACTORS OF SQUAMOUS CELL CARCINOMA AND ADENO-CARCINOMA OF THE UTERINE CERVIX. *Int. J. Pharm. Sci. Rev. Res.* **2019**, *6*, 10281–10287. [CrossRef]
142. Lassen, P.; Huang, S.H.; Su, J.; O'Sullivan, B.; Waldron, J.; Andersen, M.; Primdahl, H.; Johansen, J.; Kristensen, C.; Andersen, E.; et al. Impact of tobacco smoking on radiotherapy outcomes in 1875 HPV-positive oropharynx cancer patients. *J. Clin. Oncol.* **2019**, *37*, 6047. [CrossRef]
143. Lapuz, C.; Kondalsamy-Chennakesavan, S.; Bernshaw, D.; Khaw, P.; Narayan, K. Stage IB cervix cancer with nodal involvement treated with primary surgery or primary radiotherapy: Patterns of failure and outcomes in a contemporary population. *J. Med. Imaging Radiat. Oncol.* **2015**, *60*, 274–282. [CrossRef]
144. Dressman, H.K.; Hans, C.; Bild, A.; Olson, J.A.; Rosen, E.; Marcom, P.K.; Liotcheva, V.B.; Jones, E.L.; Vujaskovic, Z.; Marks, J.; et al. Gene Expression Profiles of Multiple Breast Cancer Phenotypes and Response to Neoadjuvant Chemotherapy. *Clin. Cancer Res.* **2006**, *12*, 819–826. [CrossRef]
145. Jentsch, M.; Snyder, P.; Sheng, C.; Cristiano, E.; Loewer, A. p53 dynamics in single cells are temperature-sensitive. *Sci. Rep.* **2020**, *10*, 1481. [CrossRef]
146. Ahmed, K.; Tabuchi, Y.; Kondo, T. Hyperthermia: An effective strategy to induce apoptosis in cancer cells. *Apoptosis* **2015**, *20*, 1411–1419. [CrossRef] [PubMed]
147. Qin, S.; Xu, C.; Li, S.; Wang, X.; Sun, X.; Wang, P.; Zhang, B.; Ren, H. Hyperthermia induces apoptosis by targeting Survivin in esophageal cancer. *Oncol. Rep.* **2015**, *34*, 2656–2664. [CrossRef] [PubMed]
148. Palmer, G.M.; Boruta, R.J.; Viglianti, B.L.; Lan, L.; Spasojevic, I.; Dewhirst, M.W. Non-invasive monitoring of intra-tumor drug concentration and therapeutic response using optical spectroscopy. *J. Control. Release* **2010**, *142*, 457–464. [CrossRef]
149. Lee, C.-T.; Boss, M.-K.; Dewhirst, M.W. Imaging Tumor Hypoxia to Advance Radiation Oncology. *Antioxidants Redox Signal.* **2014**, *21*, 313–337. [CrossRef]

Article

The Effect of Hyperthermia and Radiotherapy Sequence on Cancer Cell Death and the Immune Phenotype of Breast Cancer Cells

Azzaya Sengedorj [1,2,3], Michael Hader [1,2,3], Lukas Heger [4], Benjamin Frey [1,2,3,5,6], Diana Dudziak [4,5,6], Rainer Fietkau [2,3,5,6], Oliver J. Ott [2,3,5], Stephan Scheidegger [7], Sergio Mingo Barba [7,8], Udo S. Gaipl [1,2,3,5,6,*,†] and Michael Rückert [1,2,3,†]

1. Translational Radiobiology, Department of Radiation Oncology, Universitätsklinikum Erlangen, 91054 Erlangen, Germany; azzaya.sengedorj@uk-erlangen.de (A.S.); michael.hader@uni-bayreuth.de (M.H.); benjamin.frey@uk-erlangen.de (B.F.); michael.rueckert@uk-erlangen.de (M.R.)
2. Department of Radiation Oncology, Universitätsklinikum Erlangen, 91054 Erlangen, Germany; rainer.fietkau@uk-erlangen.de (R.F.); oliver.ott@uk-erlangen.de (O.J.O.)
3. Comprehensive Cancer Center Erlangen-EMN (CCC ER-EMN), 91054 Erlangen, Germany
4. Laboratory of Dendritic Cell Biology, Department of Dermatology, Universitätsklinikum Erlangen, Friedrich-Alexander-Universität Erlangen-Nürnberg, 91054 Erlangen, Germany; lukas.heger@uk-erlangen.de (L.H.); diana.dudziak@uk-erlangen.de (D.D.)
5. Deutsche Zentrum Immuntherapie, 91054 Erlangen, Germany
6. Medical Immunology Campus, 91054 Erlangen, Germany
7. ZHAW School of Engineering, Zurich University of Applied Sciences, 8401 Winterthur, Switzerland; scst@zhaw.ch (S.S.); semingo@ucm.es (S.M.B.)
8. Faculty of Science and Medicine, University of Fribourg, 1700 Fribourg, Switzerland
* Correspondence: udo.gaipl@uk-erlangen.de; Tel.: +49-(0)9131-85-44258
† These authors contributed equally to this work.

Simple Summary: Hyperthermia (HT) is a cancer treatment which locally heats the tumor to supraphysiological temperature, and it is an effective sensitizer for radiotherapy (RT) and chemotherapy. HT is further capable of modulating the immune system. Thus, a better understanding of its effect on the immune phenotype of tumor cells, and particularly when combined with RT, would help to optimize combined anti-cancer treatments. Since in clinics, no standards about the sequence of RT and HT exist, we analyzed whether this differently affects the cell death and immunological phenotype of human breast cancer cells. We revealed that the sequence of HT and RT does not strongly matter from the immunological point of view, however, when HT is combined with RT, it changes the immunophenotype of breast cancer cells and also upregulates immune suppressive immune checkpoint molecules. Thus, the additional application of immune checkpoint inhibitors with RT and HT should be beneficial in clinics.

Abstract: Hyperthermia (HT) is an accepted treatment for recurrent breast cancer which locally heats the tumor to 39–44 °C, and it is a very potent sensitizer for radiotherapy (RT) and chemotherapy. However, currently little is known about how HT with a distinct temperature, and particularly, how the sequence of HT and RT changes the immune phenotype of breast cancer cells. Therefore, human MDA-MB-231 and MCF-7 breast cancer cells were treated with HT of different temperatures (39, 41 and 44 °C), alone and in combination with RT (2 × 5 Gy) in different sequences, with either RT or HT first, followed by the other. Tumor cell death forms and the expression of immune checkpoint molecules (ICMs) were analyzed by multicolor flow cytometry. Human monocyte-derived dendritic cells (moDCs) were differentiated and co-cultured with the treated cancer cells. In both cell lines, RT was the main stressor for cell death induction, with apoptosis being the prominent cell death form in MCF-7 cells and both apoptosis and necrosis in MDA-MB-231 cells. Here, the sequence of the combined treatments, either RT or HT, did not have a significant impact on the final outcome. The expression of all of the three examined immune suppressive ICMs, namely PD-L1, PD-L2 and HVEM, was significantly increased on MCF-7 cells 120 h after the treatment of RT with HT of any temperature. Of special interest for MDA-MB-231 cells is that only combinations of RT with HT of both 41 and

44 °C induced a significantly increased expression of PD-L2 at all examined time points (24, 48, 72, and 120 h). Generally, high dynamics of ICM expression can be observed after combined RT and HT treatments. There was no significant difference between the different sequences of treatments (either HT + RT or RT + HT) in case of the upregulation of ICMs. Furthermore, the co-culture of moDCs with tumor cells of any treatment had no impact on the expression of activation markers. We conclude that the sequence of HT and RT does not strongly affect the immune phenotype of breast cancer cells. However, when HT is combined with RT, it results in an increased expression of distinct immune suppressive ICMs that should be considered by including immune checkpoint inhibitors in multimodal tumor treatments with RT and HT. Further, combined RT and HT affects the immune system in the effector phase rather than in the priming phase.

Keywords: hyperthermia; radiotherapy; immune phenotype; hyperthermia treatment sequence; breast cancer; immune checkpoint molecules; dendritic cell activation

1. Introduction

Breast cancer is the most commonly diagnosed cancer amongst women with 23% of total cancer cases and 14% of cancer-related deaths, which makes it the leading cause of cancer-related deaths in women [1]. About 30% of those who are diagnosed with early-stage breast cancer develop distant metastasis later on [2]. Therefore, the goal of anti-cancer therapy should be local tumor control as well as a focus on systemic effects to detain the cancer cells and avoid metastasis. This can be achieved by combining standard cancer therapies, namely radiotherapy (RT) and chemotherapy (CT), with further immune modulators. Immune checkpoint inhibitors (ICIs) have shown some effectiveness in triple negative breast cancers here [3].

In recent years it has become obvious that hyperthermia (HT) is also capable of modulating the immune system [4]. HT is commonly used as an adjuvant therapy with standard cancer treatments like RT and CT [5–9]. HT causes increased blood flow and oxygenation of the tissue, and it affects the cellular repair of DNA damage caused by irradiation, making it one of the most potent radiosensitizers [10,11]. Besides its radio- and chemo-sensitizing properties, HT can create favorable conditions for anti-tumor immune responses that can be further improved by immunotherapies [12]. It has further been shown that HT selectively induces apoptosis in hypoxic cancer cells and increases the cytotoxicity of immune cells against target cancer cells, making it less harmful to normal tissue [13].

One can conclude that HT has both direct effects on the tumor cells and systemic effects, which are mainly immune-mediated. A key focus has been set on the activation of dendritic cells (DCs) by HT- and/or RT-treated tumor cells. Danger-associated molecular patterns (DAMPs), such as high mobility group box 1 protein (HMGB1) and heat shock proteins (HSPs), activate immune cells when being released by the cancer cells after HT [14–18]. Tumor antigens that are bound to HSPs are taken up by antigen presenting cells (APCs) such as DCs, which further cross-present them to CD8$^+$ T-cells, ideally leading to their activation and subsequent T cell-mediated eradication of tumor cells [18,19]. Furthermore, natural killer cells are also activated by HSPs [20]. HT induces not only the release of HSPs but also cytokines and chemokines, resulting in an improved trafficking of immune cells into the tumor and an increased cytotoxicity of immune cells [18,21]. Together, these HT-induced modulations have been preclinically shown to contribute to tumor regressions [15,22].

However, these beneficial local and systemic effects of HT highly depend on numerous factors such as temperature level, timing, and time interval between treatments [23]. Although there are several publications that have suggested standardization of thermal dosing and timing of the HT application [24,25], this is still lacking for HT. In some studies, HT was performed once or twice a week, but the frequency of HT was not the same for all patients, and the total number of the HT treatment session differed in each patient [23]. According to the quality assurance guidelines for HT [26,27], the general duration time of the HT treatment should be 30–60 min with a goal temperature of 40–44 °C, and the interval between HT and RT usually ranges from some minutes to 4 h [28]. However, most of these suggestions have until now not been evaluated for the immune effects of HT and, particularly, the influence of the sequence of HT and RT application on the immune phenotype of tumor cells is still unknown.

The combination of HT and RT has been studied in clinical trials for different cancer entities and showed positive results compared to RT alone [29–33]. Even though there are several preclinical studies and some clinical trials [34] that evaluated immune alterations after HT and RT, the optimal sequence of HT and RT and its effects on the immunophenotype of the cancer cells need more investigation. When HT is applied before RT, it is believed that HT sensitizes tumor cells for RT, and when HT is applied after RT, it exacerbates irradiation-induced damage to the tumor [13,19].

Reirradiation and hyperthermia for recurrent breast cancer in previously irradiated areas is performed with dose concepts such as 8×4 Gy or 10×3 Gy [35]. Clinical studies with thermography-controlled, water-filtered infrared-A achieving good results have focused on 5×4 Gy as the RT schedule, in combination with HT [36]. Furthermore, extreme hypofractionated RT protocols are currently evaluated for breast cancer [37]. For translational biological research, the optimal RT dose has not been established by now [38]. We decided to use 2×5 Gy, as this is a well-accepted hypofractionation RT schedule in preclinical studies which was shown to be particularly effective when combined with HT [39].

Some preclinical studies suggest that applying HT after irradiation achieves better results [40,41]. However, the effect of the treatment sequences varies depending on the readout system and the tumor entity [11,42]. Thus, whether HT should be applied before or after RT is still controversial [13,42]. Furthermore, the impact of distinct temperatures clinically used in HT on the immunological effects in these settings needs further investigation.

Thus, the aim of this work was to evaluate whether the sequence of HT with 39, 41 or 44 °C and hypo-fractionated RT affects the immunophenotype of breast cancer cells differently, and whether this plays a role in the initiation of an immune response, namely in the activation of DCs. Therefore, two human breast cancer cell lines were treated in different sequences of HT with different temperatures and RT. Afterwards, tumor cell death and the expression of prominent ICMs on the cancer cells was analyzed. Finally, co-culture experiments with human monocyte-derived DCs (moDCs) were performed. Our findings indicate for the first time that when HT is combined with RT, it modulates the expression of several immune checkpoint molecules, but the sequence of application has only a minor influence on it. Further, the combination of HT with RT of the examined breast cancer cells rather modulates the immune system in the effector phase, and not in the priming phase, as the co-incubation of the treated tumor cells with moDCs did not significantly alter the activation state of these central APCs.

2. Materials and Methods

2.1. Ex Vivo Heating System for Hyperthermia Treatment of Tumor Cells

The heat treatment of the tumor cells was performed in a self-designed heating chamber under sterile conditions. The heating chamber was designed and built in collaboration with the Keylab Glass Technology (fabrication in the workshop of the Faculty of Engineering) of the University of Bayreuth. The heating chamber consists of the temperature control unit type TS125 (H-Tronic GmbH, Hirschau, Germany), a heating wire type HST 2.0 m 50 W (Horst GmbH, Lorsch, Germany), a junction box for the resistance heating wire (Horst GmbH, Lorsch, Germany) and a temperature sensor (H-Tronic GmbH, Hirschau, Germany). During the 60 min heating session, the temperature was constantly set to distinct temperatures (39 °C, 41 °C, and 44 °C) and automatically controlled, with no more than ± 0.1 °C deviation from the target temperature. In the electric heating chamber, the temperature inside the system was measured and monitored by a surface temperature gauge. We checked the temperature accuracy in our cell culture flasks using dummy flasks by positioning several temperature sensors on the contact surface to the heating chamber as well as into the cell culture medium. It was shown that the measured temperatures were very homogeneous and had very small deviations (±0.2 °C) from the specified temperature in the heating chamber. A graphical illustration of the electrical heating chamber is shown in Figure 1.

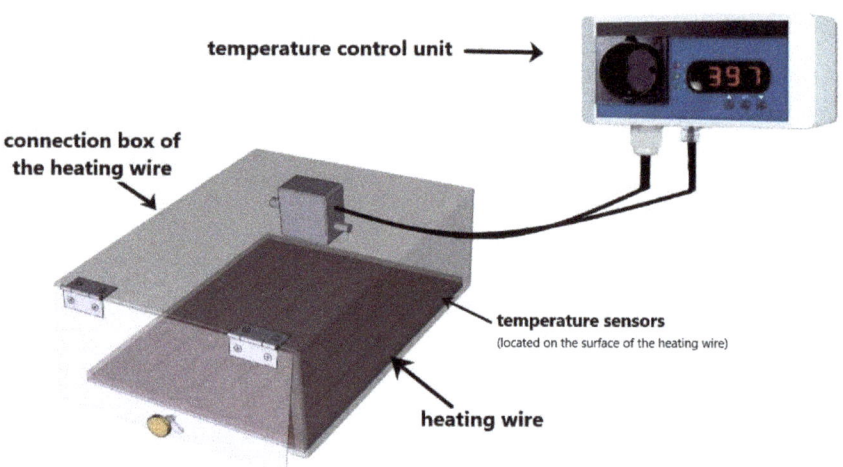

Figure 1. Graphical illustration of the heating device. The heating device was mostly made of stainless steel. The device consists of a temperature control unit, heating wire, temperature sensor, and the connection box for the heating wire. The heating chamber is automatically self-controlled and the target temperature was set to 39 °C, 41 °C, or 44 °C. The temperature deviation was not more than ±0.1 °C.

2.2. Cell Lines and Cell Culture

The two human breast cancer cell lines MCF-7 (Merck KGaA, Darmstadt, Germany) and MDA-MB-231 (Merck KGaA, Darmstadt, Germany) were cultivated at 37 °C in 5% CO_2 and 90% humidity under sterile conditions. Both cell lines were grown in Dulbecco's modified Eagle's serum (DMEM, PAN-Biotech GmbH, Aidenbach, Germany) supplemented with 10% fetal bovine serum (FBS, Biochrome AG, Berlin, Germany) and 1% Penicillin-Streptomycin (PenStrep, Gibco, Carlsbad, CA, USA). The cell lines were tested to be free of mycoplasma.

2.3. Treatments and Sampling

As shown in Figure 2, on the day before treatment, cells of the respective cell lines were seeded in 25 cm^2 cell culture flasks. The confluency of the cells did not exceed 90%. On the treatment day (day 0), each flask was handled as follows: hyperthermia treatment for 60 min was conducted using an electrical heating chamber with three different clinically relevant temperatures (39 °C, 41 °C, and 44 °C). Irradiation of the cells was performed with hypofractionation of 2 times 5 Gy (120 kV, 21.5 mA for 0.7 min) using an X-ray chamber (Isovolt Titan series, GE Technologies, Hürth, Germany). The interval between the irradiation and hyperthermia treatment was within 1–2 h. This treatment schedule was adopted from the clinical hyperthermia guidelines that indicate that the time interval between the radiation therapy and hyperthermia treatments should be close to each other, and that the time interval is mostly around 1 h and less than 4 h [43].

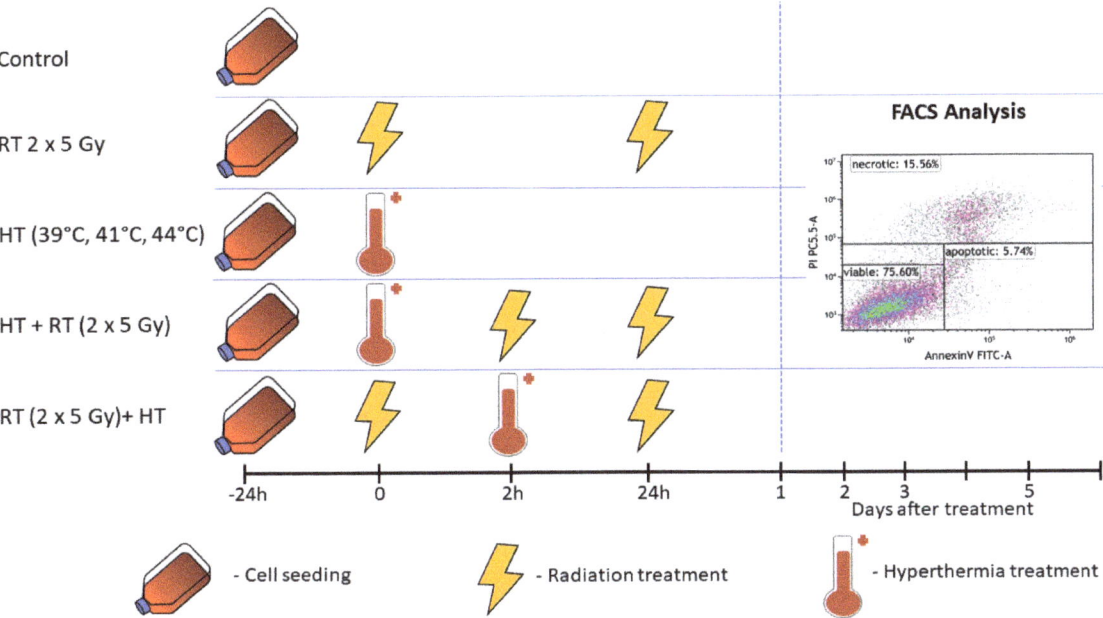

Figure 2. Treatment set-up. On the day before the start of the treatment, the cells of the respective cell line (either MDA-MB-231 or MCF-7) were seeded (displayed with the cell culture flasks). In hyperthermia-only treatment (HT), or HT followed by radiotherapy (HT + RT), HT treatment was performed on day 0 in the heating chamber system for 60 min with three different respective temperatures (39 °C, 41 °C, and 44 °C). After the HT treatment, irradiation was performed at the latest within 2 h for HT + RT. For RT + HT, the respective treatments were performed in the same manner but in reverse order. RT was performed in clinically relevant doses of 2 × 5 Gy. Irradiation in the respective RT + HT arms was always performed 2 h after the initial treatment at the latest. Sampling in all arms was performed on day 1 (24 h), d2 (48 h), d3 (72 h) and d5 (120 h) after the last irradiation.

2.4. Detection of Tumor Cell Death Forms by Annexin V/PI Staining

The cell death forms of tumor cells after irradiation and hyperthermia treatment were analyzed by multicolor flow cytometry, using Annexin V/propidium-iodide (PI) staining [39]: 100,000 cells/well resuspended in Ringer's solution (B. Braun, Melsungen, Germany) were stained with 1 µg/mL of PI (Sigma Aldrich, Munich, Germany) and 0.5 µg/mL FITC-labeled AnnexinV (Geneart, Life Technologies, Regensburg, Germany), incubated for 30 min, at 4 °C, in the dark. The cells were analyzed on a Cytoflex S flow cytometer (Beckman Coulter, Krefeld, Germany). The gating strategy for the detection of cell death forms using Annexin V/PI staining is illustrated in Figure 3.

2.5. Detection of Immune Checkpoint Molecules by Multicolor Flow Cytometry

After the treatments at respective time points, the tumor cells were harvested and 1×10^5 tumor cells per well of a 96-well plate were incubated for 30 min at 4 °C, with no light exposure, with 100 µL of the staining solution (Table 1) in a FACS buffer (PBS, Dulbecco's Phosphate Buffered Saline (Sigma-Aldrich, Munich, Germany), 2% FBS and 2 mM EDTA (Carl Roth, Karlsruhe, Germany)). For an autofluorescence control, only Zombie NIR was put into the FACS buffer. The mean fluorescence intensity (ΔMFI) was calculated by subtracting the fluorescence intensity of autofluorescence control samples from fully stained samples. The samples were measured on a Cytoflex S flow cytometer (Beckman Coulter, Krefeld, Germany) and analyzed using Kaluza 2.0 (Beckman Coulter, Brea, CA, USA).

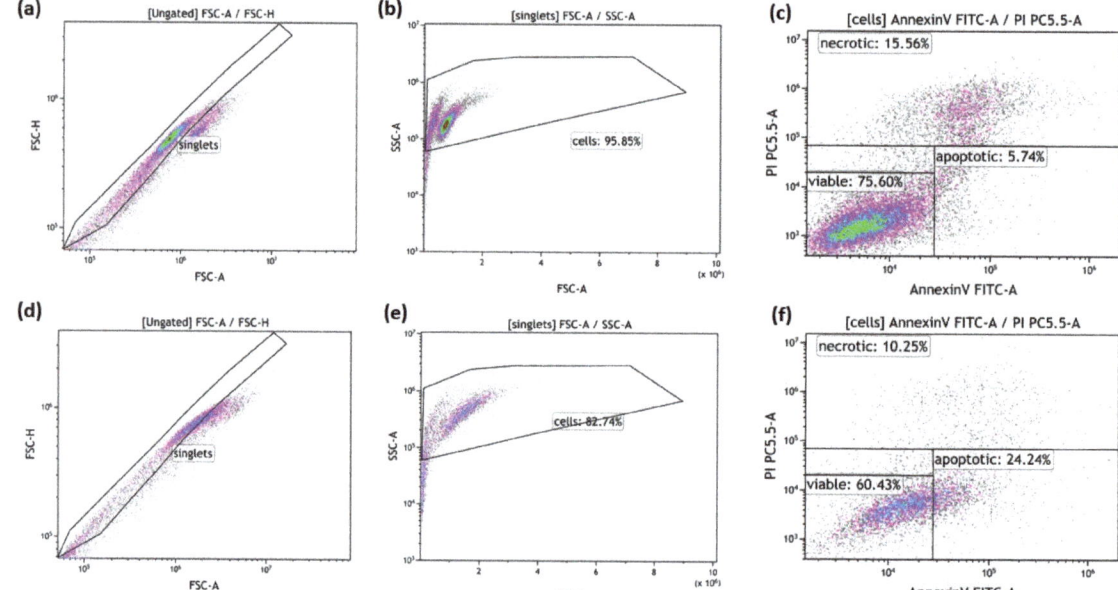

Figure 3. Gating strategy for the detection of cell death forms by AnnexinV/PI staining. Exemplarily shown are data of MCF-7 breast cancer cells. The cells were first gated on singlets (**a**,**d**) by FSC-A vs. FSC-H gating, followed by the exclusion of debris in the FSC/SSC plot (**b**,**e**). Viable cells were defined as Annexin negative/PI negative, apoptotic cells as Annexin positive/PI negative and necrotic cells as Annexin positive/PI positive (**c**,**f**). Data of cultured control samples (**a**–**c**) and of 2 × 5 Gy irradiated cells (**d**–**f**) are shown exemplarily.

Table 1. List of antibodies and dyes for the immune checkpoint molecule analysis on the surface of tumor cells via multicolor flow cytometry.

Marker	Fluorochrome	Manufacturer
PD-L1 (CD274)	BV 605	Biolegend
PD-L2 (CD273)	APC	Biolegend
ICOS-L (CD275)	BV 421	BD Horizon
HVEM (CD270)	APC	Biolegend
TNFRSF9 (CD137-L)	BV 421	Biolegend
OX40-L (CD252)	PE	Biolegend
Live/Dead	Zombie NIR	Biolegend

2.6. Isolation of Human Peripheral Blood Mononuclear Cells (PBMCs), Monocyte Enrichment and Differentiation into Immature Dendritic Cells (imm. moDCs)

Peripheral blood mononuclear cells (PBMC) were isolated from leukoreduction system chambers (LRSC) of healthy, anonymous donors having undergone a strict health check by the Transfusion Medicine and Hemostaseology Department of the Universitätsklinikum Erlangen, Germany. The permission to use these LRSCs was given by the ethics committee of the Friedrich-Alexander-Universität Erlangen-Nürnberg (ethical approval no. 180_13 B and 48_19 B), according to the rules of the Declaration of Helsinki in its current form.

Mononuclear cells were separated by using density gradient solution Lymphoflot (Bio-Rad Medical Diagnostics GmbH, Dreieich, Germany) and centrifugation in Sepmate PBMC isolation tubes (Sepmate™, Stemcell Technologies Inc., Vancouver, BC, Canada). Afterwards, the cell suspension was washed several times at 4 °C (2 times with PBS and 2 times with RPMI-1640 medium) and in-between, the centrifugation was performed from high force to low force; this way, cells that are larger and lighter than mononuclear cells would be eliminated by centrifugation. For imm. moDC differentiation, an optimized protocol was used according to Lühr and colleagues [44]: 30×10^6 monocytes were seeded in IgG (Human IgG, Sigma Aldrich, Taufkirchen, Germany)-precoated cell culture dishes with 10 mL of moDC medium (RPMI-1640 (Merck, Darmstadt, Germany)) supplemented with 1% Pen/Strep (Gibco, Carlsbad, CA, USA), 1% L-Glutamine (Gibco, Carlsbad, CA, USA), 1% Hepes buffer 1M (Biochrom GmbH, Berlin, Germany) and 1% heat-inactivated human serum (Gibco, Carlsbad, CA, USA). After 1 h of incubation, cells that did not attach at the bottom of the plates were rinsed away. Therefore, mainly monocytes which are able to bind to the plate-bound IgG via FcγRs remained, and 10 mL of fresh, pre-warmed moDC medium was added. For the differentiation of monocytes into moDCs, on day 1, old culture medium was removed and 10 mL of fresh moDC medium was added to each cell culture dish containing the following cytokines: 800 U/mL of GM-CSF (MACS Miltenyi Biotec, Bergisch Gladbach, Germany) and 500 U/mL of IL-4 (ImmunoTools, Friesoythe, Germany). On day 3, 4 mL of moDC medium containing the same concentration of cytokines was added. On day 5, 4 mL of moDC medium with half of the previously used concentration of GM-CSF (400 U/mL) and IL-4 (250 U/mL) was added.

2.7. Co-Culture of moDCs with Treated and Untreated MCF-7 Cancer Cells and Detection of DC Activation Markers on the Surface of moDCs

On day 6, the obtained moDCs were harvested from the cell culture dish mechanically by using a serological pipette. After counting the harvested cells, 1×10^5 moDCs were seeded in 6-well plates. For the co-culture, 2×10^5 of differently treated MCF-7 cancer cells were added to the moDCs with 2 mL of moDC medium and 2 mL supernatant of the treated cancer cells. As a positive control, 2 mL of moDC medium with a maturation cocktail containing 13.16 ng/mL of IL-1β (ImmunoTools, Friesoythe, Germany), 1000 U/mL of IL-6 (ImmunoTools, Friesoythe, Germany), 10 ng/mL of TNF-α (ImmunoTools, Friesoythe, Germany) and 1 µg/mL of PGE-2 (Pfizer, Berlin, Germany) were added to the moDCs to generate mature moDCs.

After 24 h and 48 h of co-incubation with untreated and treated MCF-7 cancer cells, the expression of co-stimulatory molecules and activation markers was analyzed on moDCs by using multicolor flow cytometry (Figure 4). Therefore, moDCs in suspension were harvested mechanically using a serological pipette. Then, each condition of moDCs was divided into 2 duplicates, one stained with staining solution (Table 2), while the other duplicate served as an autofluorescence control with only Zombie Yellow in the FACS Buffer.

The cells were gated according to Figure 4. The mean fluorescence intensity (ΔMFI) was calculated by subtracting the fluorescence intensity of autofluorescence control samples from the fully stained samples. The samples were measured on a Cytoflex S flow cytometer (Beckman Coulter, Krefeld, Germany) and analyzed using Kaluza 2.0 (Beckman Coultier, Brea, CA, USA).

2.8. Statistical Analysis

For statistical analysis, the software Prism 7 (Graph Pad, San Diego, CA, USA) was used. Separate Kruskal–Wallis tests with Dunn's correction for multiple testing were used to compare the treatments within one HT temperature to the untreated control. Further, the combinatorial treatments were compared to RT only with a Kruskal–Wallis test with Dunn's correction for multiple testing. To compare the sequence of the combined treatments of one HT temperature (RT + HT vs. HT + RT), a Mann–Whitney U test was used. Results were considered statistically significant for * $p < 0.1$, ** $p < 0.01$, *** $p < 0.001$.

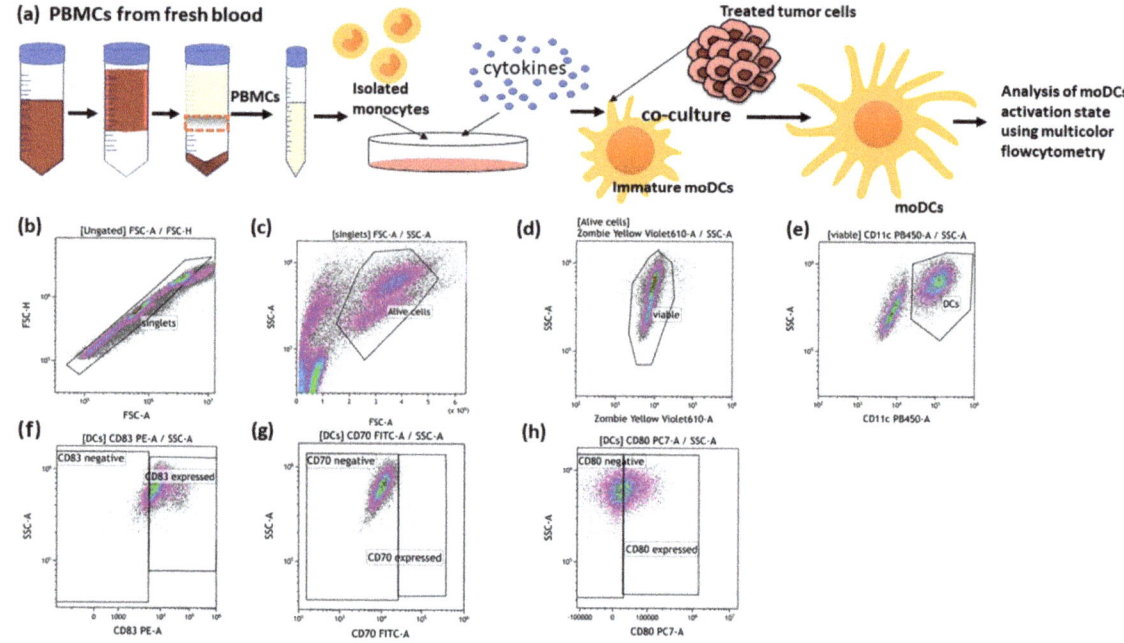

Figure 4. Generation of human monocyte-derived DCs (moDCs) from PBMCs and the detection of DC activation markers after co-incubation with treated cancer cells. (**a**) PBMCs were isolated from buffy coat and seeded into an IgG pre-coated cell culture dish. On day 6 after differentiation, moDCs were co-cultured with differently treated MCF-7 breast cancer cells. After 24 h and 48 h of co-incubation, the activation markers of the moDCs were analysed using multicolor flow cytometry. The gating strategies for flow cytometry are shown (**b**–**h**). (**b**) After pre-gating on the singlets, the viable cells were detected (**c**,**d**). Then, gating on CD11c positive cells identified moDCs (**e**). Dot plots of CD83 (**f**), CD70 (**g**) and CD80 (**h**) expression on the cell surface of moDCs are exemplarily presented.

Table 2. List of antibodies and dyes used to analyze the expression of various activation markers on the surface of moDCs via multicolor flow cytometry.

Marker	Fluorochrome	Manufacturer
CD70	FITC	Biolegend
CD83	PE-Cy7	eBioscience
CD80	APC	Miltenyi Biotec (MACS)
Live/Dead	Zombie Yellow	Biolegend
CD11c	V450	Biolegend

3. Results

3.1. Radiotherapy in Combination with Hyperthermia Significantly Induces Apoptosis in MCF-7 Cells Andboth Apoptosis and Necrosis in MDA-MB-231 Breast Cancer Cells

In order to elucidate the effect of HT on the immune phenotype of human breast cancer cells, three different clinically relevant HT temperatures were used (39 °C, 41 °C, 44 °C). MCF-7 and MDA-MB-231 cells were treated with either HT or RT alone, and in a combinational setting in different sequences with either HT followed by RT (HT + RT), or RT followed by HT (RT + HT).

3.1.1. Radiotherapy in Combination with Hyperthermia Regardless of the Treatment Sequence Significantly Induces Apoptosis in MCF-7 Breast Cancer Cells

Necrosis and apoptosis of MCF-7 cells were determined 24 h, 48 h, 72 h, and 120 h after the respective treatment (Figure 5).

As shown in Figure 5, in MCF-7 cells at an early time point (24 h) after the treatment, a slight increase of necrotic cells was observed, particularly after combinations of RT with HT. However, at later time points, the cancer cell death is dominantly in the form of apoptosis. The key inductor of apoptosis was RT alone (Figure 5e–h). In contrast, neither necrosis nor apoptosis was induced in MCF-7 breast cancer cells by HT as a single treatment, even with up to 44 °C.

As observed for RT alone, a combination of HT and RT induced significantly more apoptosis regardless of the treatment sequence (Figure 5e–h). HT of 44 °C significantly induced apoptotic cancer cell death at all time points when it was combined with radiation therapy (Figure 5e–h). In contrast, 39 °C HT with RT resulted in a slight decrease of apoptosis compared to RT alone.

In any case, the sequences of the combined treatments, either RT or HT first, were not significantly different from each other in the induction of cancer cell death, with the exception of a tendency for less apoptosis when HT of 41 °C was given before RT, as compared to afterwards.

3.1.2. Radiotherapy in Combination with Hyperthermia Regardless of the Treatment Sequence Significantly Induce Apoptosis and Necrosis in MDA-MB-231 Breast Cancer Cells

MDA-MB-231 cells were treated with the respective treatments similar to MCF-7 cells, and afterwards cell death forms were analyzed (Figure 6).

In contrast to MCF-7 breast cancer cells, RT alone could significantly induce apoptosis and necrosis of MDA-MB-231 cells (Figure 6a–d,f–h), but again, HT alone did not induce significantly increased apoptosis or necrosis at all of the examined timepoints.

Again, the percentages of apoptotic cells were slightly lower when HT of 39 °C was combined with RT, compared to 41 °C and 44 °C. The highest induction of necrosis was observed when RT was combined with HT of 44 °C (Figure 6d).

Again, the sequences of the combined treatments, either RT or HT first, were similar in the induction of breast cancer cell death.

3.2. Hyperthermia in Combination with Radiotherapy Affects the Expression of Immune Checkpoint Molecules on Breast Cancer Cells

Next, we investigated the impact of HT, RT, and HT in combination with RT on the expression of immune inhibitory ICMs (PD-L1, PD-L2, HVEM) and on one immune stimulatory ICM (OX40-L) on MCF-7 and MDA-MB-231 breast cancer cells.

3.2.1. Hyperthermia in Combination with Radiotherapy Upregulates the Expression of Several Inhibitory Immune Checkpoint Molecules on MCF-7 Breast Cancer Cells

Regarding RT alone, the well-known inhibitory ICM PD-L1 was significantly upregulated up to 72 h after treatment. (Figure 7a–c). However, PD-L2 and HVEM were also increased following RT (Figure 7e–l).

When adding HT to RT, the time point 120 h is particularly of interest here: all of the three immune suppressive ICMs examined, namely PD-L1, PD-L2 and HVEM, were significantly increased when RT was combined with HT of any temperature. At this time, some of the observed increased expressions of ICMs were significantly enhanced even when compared to RT-only treatment (Figure 7d,h,l).

Generally, a high dynamic of ICM expression can be observed after combined RT and HT treatments. There was no significant difference between the different sequences of treatments (either HT + RT or RT + HT) in case of the upregulation of inhibitory ICMs.

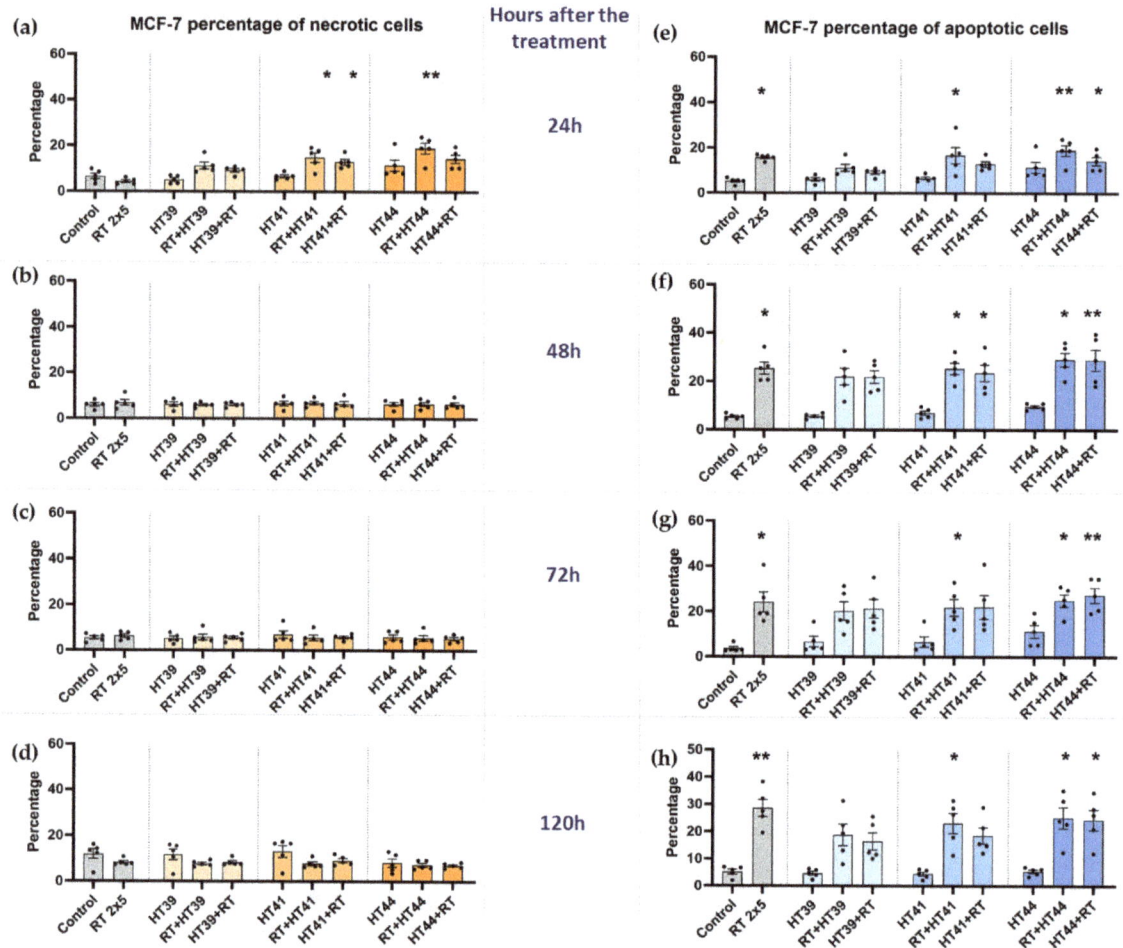

Figure 5. Radiotherapy alone and in combination with hyperthermia regardless of the treatment sequence induces apoptosis in MCF-7 breast cancer cells. The percentage of necrotic MCF-7 cells are shown in graphs (**a**) 24 h, (**b**) 48 h, (**c**) 72 h and (**d**) 120 h after the treatment. The percentage of apoptotic MCF-7 cells is shown in graphs (**e**) 24 h, (**f**) 48 h, (**g**) 72 h and (**h**) 120 h after the treatment. MCF-7 cells were irradiated 2 times with 5 Gy (RT) or treated with HT of different temperatures (39 °C, 41 °C, 44 °C) and combinations of both, either HT followed by RT (HT (39 °C, 41 °C, 44 °C) + RT) or vice versa (RT + HT (39 °C, 41 °C, 44 °C)). The time interval between HT and RT was less than 2 h. The cell death forms were analyzed by AnxV/PI staining using multicolor flow cytometry. Mean ± SD are presented from at least five independent experiments. Statistical significance is calculated by using a Kruskal–Wallis test with Dunn's correction to compare the percentage of necrotic and apoptotic cells of each group of a respective temperature to the untreated control, and a Mann–Whitney U test to compare the different sequences of HT and RT. * ($p < 0.1$), ** ($p < 0.01$) for Kruskal–Wallis test with Dunn's correction.

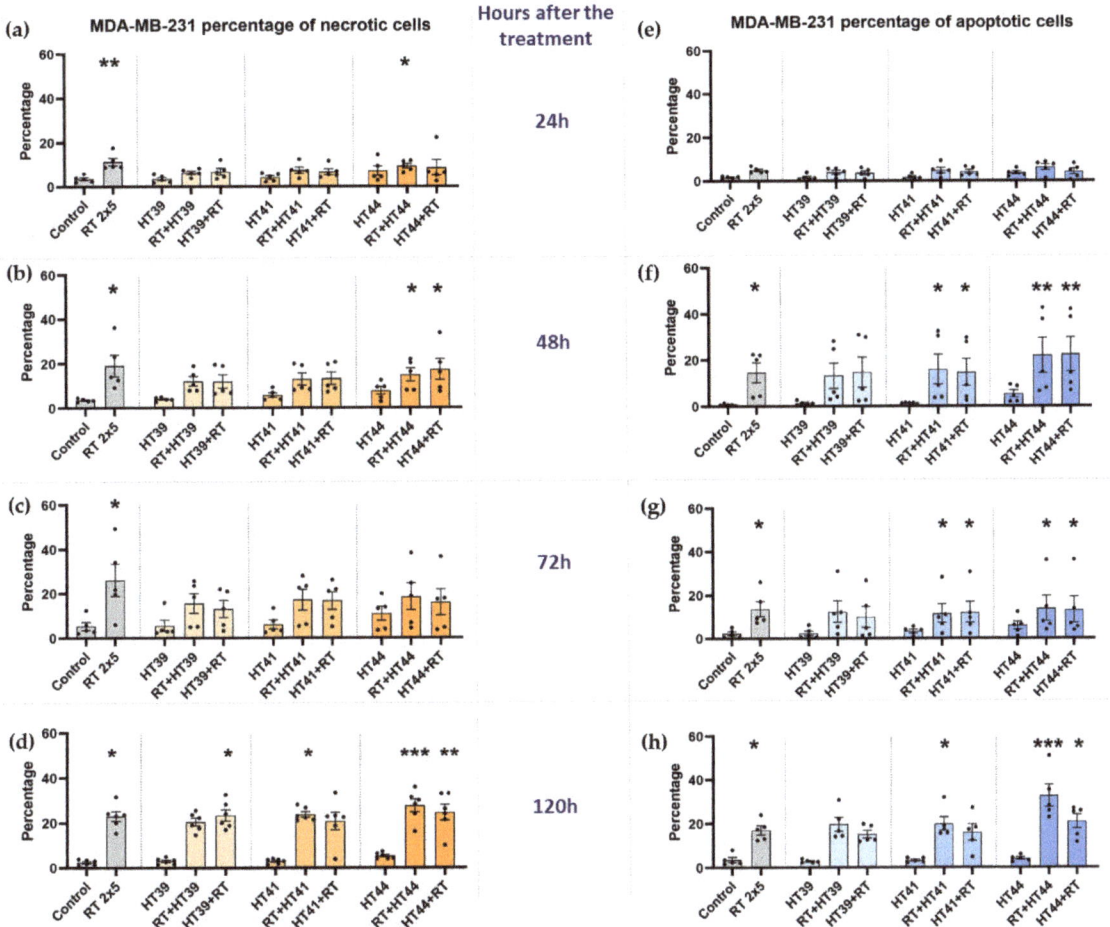

Figure 6. Radiotherapy alone and in combination with hyperthermia regardless of the treatment sequence significantly induces apoptosis and necrosis in MDA-MB-231 breast cancer cells. The percentage of necrotic MDA-MB-231 cells are shown in graphs (**a**) 24 h, (**b**) 48 h, (**c**) 72 h and (**d**) 120 h after the treatment. The percentage of apoptotic MDA-MB-231 cells is shown in graphs (**e**) 24 h, (**f**) 48 h, (**g**) 72 h and (**h**) 120 h after the treatment. MDA-MB-231 breast cancer cells were irradiated 2 times with 5 Gy (RT) or treated with HT of different temperatures (39 °C, 41 °C, 44 °C) and combinations of both, either HT followed by RT (HT (39 °C, 41 °C, 44 °C) + RT) or vice versa (RT + HT (39 °C, 41 °C, 44 °C)). Mean ± SD are presented from at least five independent experiments. Statistical significance was calculated by using a Kruskal–Wallis test with Dunn's correction to compare the percentage of necrotic and apoptotic cells of each group of a respective temperature to the untreated control, and a Mann–Whitney U test to compare the different sequences of HT and RT. * ($p < 0.1$), ** ($p < 0.01$), *** ($p < 0.001$) for Kruskal–Wallis test with Dunn's correction.

3.2.2. Hyperthermia in Combination with Radiotherapy Upregulates the Expression of Several Inhibitory Immune Checkpoint Molecules on MDA-MB-231 Breast Cancer Cells

In contrast to MCF-7 cells, RT alone did not significantly increase the expression of PD-L1 on MDA-MB-231 cells. However, the combination of RT with HT at 44 °C in particular significantly increased PD-L1 expression at earlier time points after treatment (Figure 8a,b). This increase was even significantly higher when compared to RT alone when

RT was given before HT. As for PD-L1, the expression of PD-L2 and HVEM was also not significantly increased by RT only.

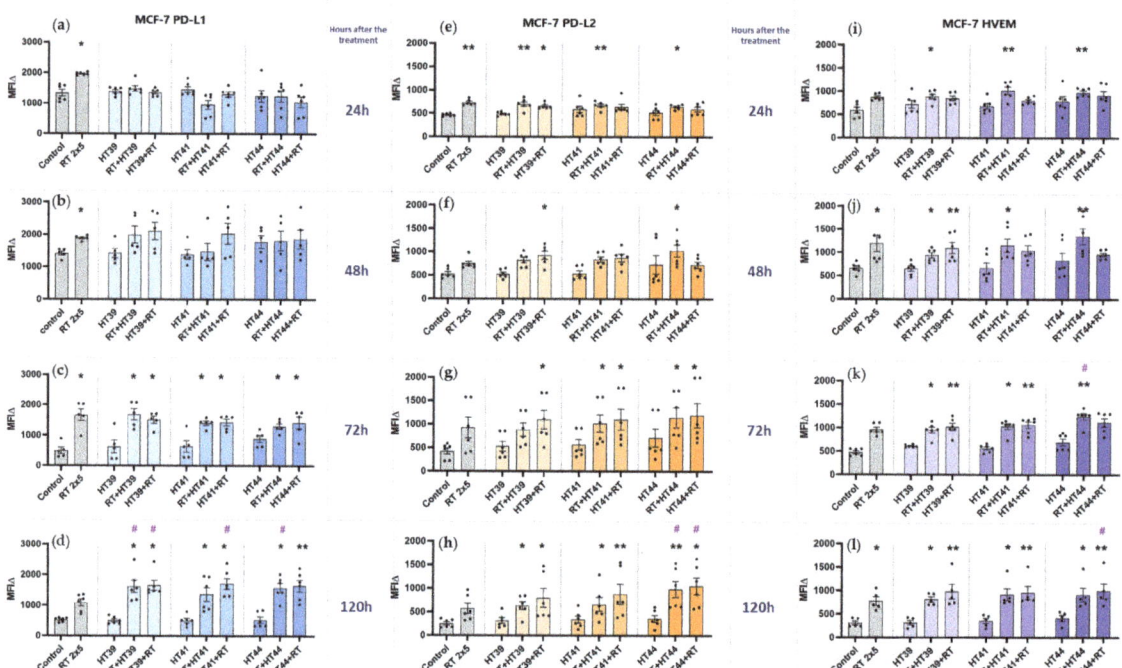

Figure 7. Hyperthermia in combination with radiotherapy affects the expression of inhibitory immune checkpoint molecules (PD-L1, PD-L2, and HVEM) on MCF-7 breast cancer cells. MCF-7 cells were irradiated 2 times with 5 Gy (RT) or treated with HT of different temperatures (39 °C, 41 °C, 44 °C) and combination of both, either HT followed by RT (HT (39 °C, 41 °C, 44 °C) + RT) or vice versa (RT + HT (39 °C, 41 °C, 44 °C)). The time interval between HT and RT was less than 2 h. The expression of ICMs ((a–d): PD-L1, (e–h): PD-L2 and (i–l): HVEM) were analyzed by multicolor flow cytometry. The mean fluorescence intensity (∆MFI) was calculated by subtracting the fluorescence intensity of unstained samples from stained samples. Mean ± SD are presented from at least five independent experiments. Statistical significance is calculated by using Kruskal–Wallis tests with Dunn's correction by comparing the ∆MFI of cells after the treatment to untreated control of the corresponding timepoint, and Mann–Whitney U tests to compare the ∆MFI of different sequences of HT and RT. * ($p < 0.1$), ** ($p < 0.01$). Further, RT alone was compared with combinational treatments (HT + RT and RT + HT); # ($p < 0.1$).

Of special interest for MDA-MB-231 cells is that only the combinations of RT with HT of both 41 and 44 °C induced a significant increased expression of PD-L2 at all examined time points (Figure 8e–h), while the expression of HVEM was only slightly altered at earlier time points, but again with combinations of RT with HT of 41 or 44 °C (Figure 8i,j). At later time points, its expression was even slightly decreased after RT or a combination of RT with HT of 39 or 41 °C (Figure 8l).

Generally, as for MCF-7 cells, a high dynamicity of ICM expression can be observed after combined RT and HT treatments. There was again no significant difference between the tested sequences of treatments (either HT + RT or RT + HT) in case of the upregulation of inhibitory ICMs.

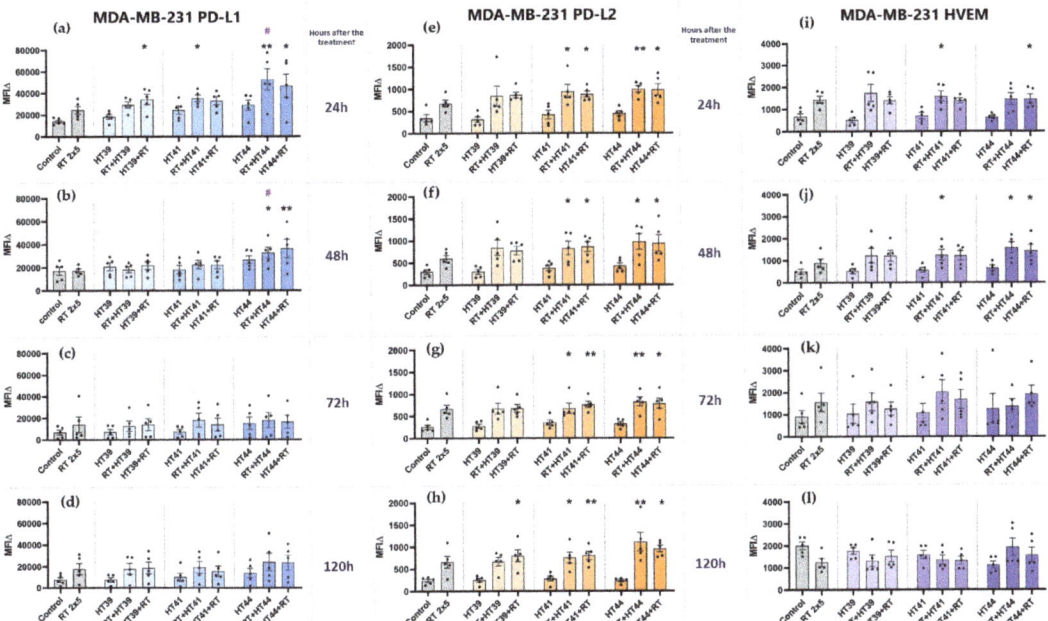

Figure 8. Hyperthermia in combination with radiotherapy affects the expression of inhibitory immune checkpoint molecules (PD-L1, PD-L2, and HVEM) on MDA-MB-231 breast cancer cells. MDA-MB-231 cells were irradiated 2 times with 5 Gy (RT) or treated with HT of different temperatures (39 °C, 41 °C, 44 °C) and a combination of both, either HT followed by RT (HT (39 °C, 41 °C, 44 °C) +RT) or vice versa (RT + HT (39 °C, 41 °C, 44 °C)). The time interval between HT and RT was less than 2 h. The expression of ICMs ((**a–d**): PD-L1, (**e–h**): PD-L2 and (**i–l**): HVEM) was analyzed by multicolor flow cytometry. The mean fluorescence intensity (ΔMFI) was calculated by subtracting the fluorescence intensity of unstained samples from stained samples. Mean ± SD are presented from at least five independent experiments. Statistical significance is calculated by using Kruskal–Wallis tests with Dunn's correction by comparing the ΔMFI of cells after the treatment to untreated control of the corresponding timepoint, and Mann–Whitney U tests to compare the ΔMFI of different sequences of HT and RT. * ($p < 0.1$), ** ($p < 0.01$). RT alone was compared with combinational treatments (HT + RT and RT + HT); # ($p < 0.1$).

3.2.3. Hyperthermia in Combination with Radiotherapy Only Slightly Affects the Expression of Stimulatory Immune Checkpoint Molecules on MCF-7 and MDA-MB-231 Breast Cancer Cells

The expression of the immune stimulatory ICMs ICOS-L, CD27-L, CD137-L (not shown) and of OX40-L (Figure 9) was determined on MCF-7 and MDA-MB-231 breast cancer cells.

In both cell lines, HT alone at any temperature did not significantly affect the expression of OX40-L, and RT increased it only slightly.

The combination of HT with RT led to a significantly increased expression of this immune-stimulatory ICM particularly at 120 h after the treatment (Figure 9d,h). There was no significant difference observed with regard to different combinational treatment sequences (whether RT or HT came first).

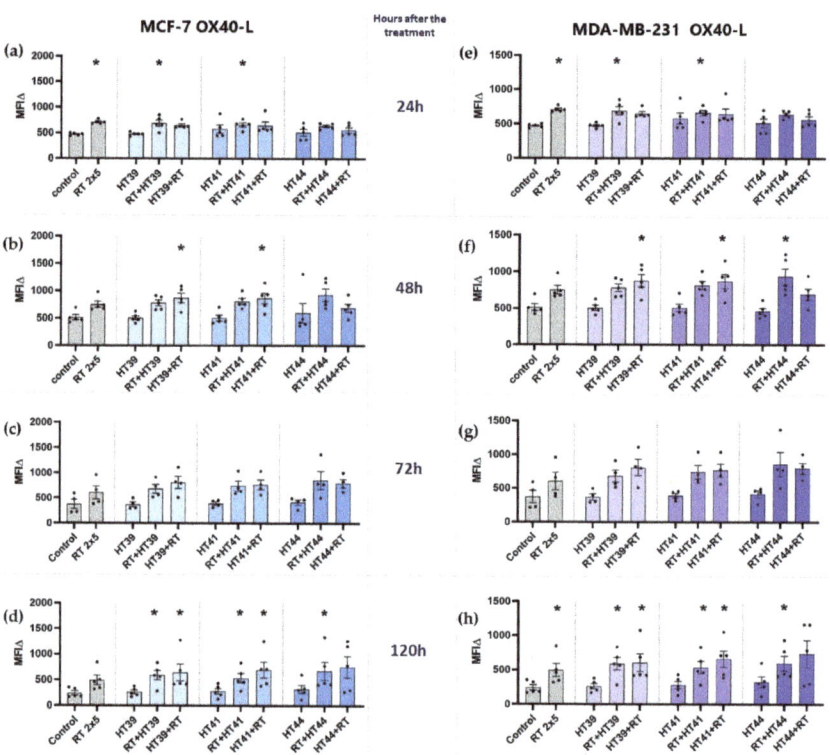

Figure 9. Expression of the immune stimulatory ICM OX40-L on MCF-7 and MDA-MB-231 cells at different timepoints after the treatment. (**a–d**) MCF-7 and (**e–h**) MDA-MB-231 cells were irradiated 2 times with 5 Gy (RT) or treated with HT of different temperatures (39 °C, 41 °C, 44 °C) and combinations of both, either HT followed by RT (HT (39 °C, 41 °C, 44 °C) + RT) or vice versa (RT + HT (39 °C, 41 °C, 44 °C)). The time interval between HT and RT was less than 2 h. The expression of OX40-L was analyzed by multicolor flow cytometry (**a,e**) 24 h, (**b,f**) 48 h, (**c,g**) 72 h, or (**d,h**) 120 h later. The mean fluorescence intensity (ΔMFI) was calculated by subtracting the fluorescence intensity of unstained samples from stained samples. Mean ± SD are presented from at least five independent experiments. Statistical significance is calculated by using Kruskal–Wallis tests with Dunn's correction by comparing the ΔMFI of cells after the treatment to untreated control of the corresponding timepoint, and Mann–Whitney U tests to compare the ΔMFI of different sequences of HT and RT. * ($p < 0.1$).

3.3. The Impact of HT- and RT-Treated Breast Cancer Cells on the Activation State of moDCs

To get first hints whether the immune phenotype characterized by ICM expression of treated breast cancer cells affects the activation state of moDCs, MCF-7 breast cancer cells treated with different sequence of HT and RT were co-cultured with immature moDCs. For this, HT of 44 °C was chosen, alone and in combination with RT, as the most prominent alterations were observed here (Figure 7). The DC activation markers, CD80, CD83 and CD70, were analyzed using multicolor flow cytometry (Figure 10).

As expected, the incubation of immature moDCs with a maturation cocktail induced upregulation of all of the DC activation markers analyzed after 24 h (Figure 10a–c) and 48 h (Figure 10d–f), respectively. Only immature moDCs which were incubated with tumor cells treated with HT of 44 °C significantly upregulated CD70 at 24 h (Figure 10b). Otherwise, moDCs co-incubated with treated breast cancer cells did not show any significant upregulation of their activation markers. Only the expression of CD80 (Figure 10c,f) tended to be higher, when DCs co-cultured with tumor cells are compared to the DCs without the maturation cocktail. However, this was irrespective of the treatment of the breast cancer cells.

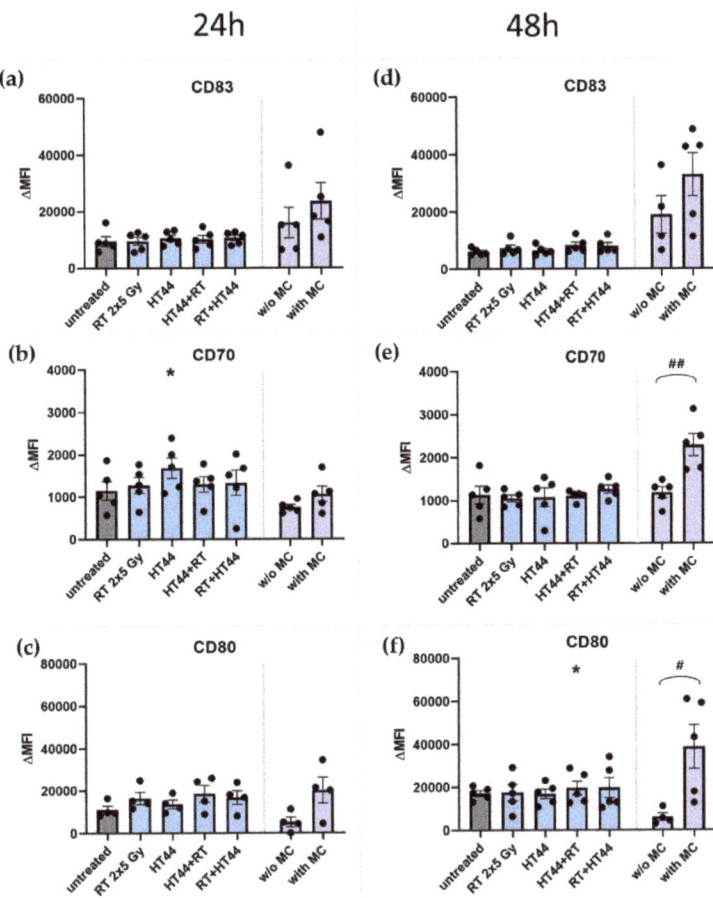

Figure 10. Expression of activation markers on moDCs after contact with hyperthermia- and radiotherapy treated MCF-7 breast cancer cells. Displayed is the expression of DC activation markers after 24 h (**a**)—CD83, (**b**)—CD70, (**c**)—CD80, and 48 h (**d**)—CD83, (**e**)—CD70, (**f**)—CD80 after co-incubation of immature moDCs with untreated MCF-7 tumor cells or with differently treated MCF-7 tumor cells. The tumor cells were treated with 2 × 5 Gy RT, HT of 44 °C, and first HT of 44 °C and then RT or RT followed by HT of 44 °C. As a positive control, immature moDCs were activated with the standard maturation cocktail (MC), and as negative control, immature moDCs were kept in moDC medium without the maturation cocktail (w/o MC). The expression of DC activation markers was analyzed by multicolor flow cytometry. The mean fluorescence intensity (ΔMFI) was calculated by subtracting the fluorescence intensity of unstained samples from stained samples. Mean ± SD are presented from at least four independent experiments. Statistical significance is calculated by using Kruskal–Wallis tests with Dunn's correction by comparing the ΔMFI of the treatments to untreated controls at the corresponding timepoint, and Mann–Whitney U tests to compare the ΔMFI of different sequence of HT and RT. * ($p < 0.1$). The arm without maturation cocktail was compared to the arm with maturation cocktail with a Mann–Whitney U test # ($p < 0.1$), ## ($p < 0.01$).

4. Discussion

4.1. In Human Breast Cancer Cells, Radiotherapy Rather Than Moderate Hyperthermia Is the Key Trigger for Cell Death Induction

RT has been used as a standard anticancer therapy for decades and its effect on the immune system has been studied extensively in recent years. It has become obvious that besides its local killing effects on cancer cells, ionizing radiation also has a strong impact on the immune system [45]. Furthermore, it has been recognized that HT can modulate the immune system and thereby affect the anti-tumor immune response, mostly in combination with RT [46]. This may result in both local and systemic anti-tumor immune responses, also in breast cancer [47]. Combinations of RT with HT [8,48,49], with or without immunotherapy such as ICIs [50,51], are promising multimodal treatments for breast cancer, which however need further optimization. It is still not clear which treatment sequence would have a better effect. Thus, in our preclinical approach, we investigated whether it is better to use HT first and then RT, or RT followed by HT, regarding breast cancer cell death induction, immune checkpoint molecule expression and the activation of DCs after co-incubation with the treated tumor cells.

Immunogenic cancer cell death (ICD) is one of the key triggers that has been reported by several studies to induce anti-tumor immune responses [52]. Indeed, ICD can be induced by a combination of RT with, e.g., graphene-induced HT [53], but also with conventional heat application, as shown, e.g., for colorectal cancer cells [17]. ICD mainly triggers the activation of DCs via the release of danger signals and consecutive cytotoxic T cell priming [54]. However, knowledge about HT-induced immune alterations independently of ICD is scarce, and theoretical evaluations even suggest that HT rather boosts the RT-induced cell killing, but does not fundamentally change the anti-tumor immune response [55].

Our in vitro examinations indicate that RT is the key trigger for cell death induction in breast cancer cells, with apoptosis being prominent in MCF-7 cells and both apoptosis and necrosis in MDA-MB-231 cells. The co-culture experiment with immature moDCs further showed that HT in combination with RT did not induce enough ICD to mature moDCs with the examined breast cancer cells. We therefore conclude that, besides ICD with danger signal release, the immune phenotype of the tumor cell surface plays an additional role in triggering RT-plus-HT-induced anti-tumor immune responses, mainly in the effector phase [56]. Furthermore, with regard to inducing breast cancer cell death, there was no significant difference between HT and RT combinational sequences, i.e., whether to apply HT first or RT first. This finding confirms the analyses by Mei et al. [57] who report no significant difference in the case of cell death induction regarding whether HT is used before or after RT. One has to stress that in these analyses, the focus was set on the temperature effects of HT alone and in combination with RT. However, different heating methods can have different outcomes, as we have recently shown that microwave heating more effectively induced cell death compared to conventional warm bath heating systems [39]. In the current study, we intentionally focused on conventional heating to set the focus on HT-induced immune alterations on the tumor cell surface, rather than on sole ICD induction. However, in addition to performing similar analyses in the future with microwave-based heating for further elucidating synergistic effects of RT plus HT treatments, preclinical in vivo models will have to be used for ICM expression and tumor cell death analyses with a setting closely resembling the clinical situation. This has already been performed for the analyses of the immunogenicity of B16 melanoma tumors following combined RT and HT treatment [19].

4.2. The Combination of Hyperthermia and Radiotherapy Affects Particularly the Expression of Immune Suppressive Immune Checkpoint Molecules of Breast Cancer Cells, but Independently of the Treatment Sequence

Identifying ICM expression profiles of cancer cells is crucial, because ICMs are responsible for tumor evasion from the immune system and strongly regulate the effector phase of the immune response. A high expression of immune inhibitory ICMs is linked to worse clinical outcomes, and ICIs are becoming more and more promising approaches in anti-cancer treatment, either alone or in combination with other treatments like RT and HT [58,59].

It has already become obvious that RT enhances the expression of PD-L1 [60,61], either alone or in combination with other treatments [61,62]. How RT and its combination with HT affect the expression of other ICMs, specifically, which sequence of HT and RT treatment alters the ICMs, is not clear yet. We revealed that the expression of ICMs follows a high dynamic which is strongly time-dependent: in MCF-7 breast cancer cells, not earlier than 72 h after treatment and most pronouncedly after 120 h, three immunosuppressive ICMs, namely PD-L1, PD-L2 and HVEM, were upregulated in their expression following combined RT plus HT treatments, independently of the temperature. This calls for an inhibition of the PD-1 receptor which binds both PD-L1 and PD-L2, rather than sole PD-L1 inhibition, in breast cancer immunotherapies. Further, the inhibition of HVEM should be considered too, as it has already been shown that breast cancer patients have a worse prognosis when low amounts of tumor-infiltrating lymphocytes are present and HVEM is expressed by the tumor cells [63]. Future preclinical in vivo experiments will have to elucidate the best combination of RT, HT and immune checkpoint inhibition. Recent preclinical data of the combination regimens of hyperthermia and ICIs have already demonstrated their combined efficacy [51]. Our in vitro data suggest that the sequence of RT and HT has a minor role in this, as HT in combination with RT, regardless of the sequence, induced the upregulation of inhibitory ICMs, unlike HT alone. It would be of additional interest to examine the effects on immune checkpoints in normal epithelial cells and whether these effects will impact the cytotoxic effects of ICIs in normal breast epithelial cells.

Besides the factor "time after treatment", the characteristics of suppressive ICMs are important. In MDA-MB-231 cells, PD-L2 was upregulated at all examined times when HT of 41 °C or 44 °C was combined with RT. This calls again for targeting the PD-1 receptor in multimodal RT- and HT-based tumor therapies, rather than only PD-L1, as, additionally, the utility of PD-L1 as a predictive biomarker in most of the breast cancer subtypes remains elusive [64].

It has to be further considered that the upregulation of PD-L1 differed in MDA-MB-231 and MCF-7 cells in a time-dependent manner. MCF-7 cells showed an increased expression of PD-L1 at later timepoints (72–120 h), while on the surface of MDA-MB-231 cells, it occurred earlier (24–48 h) after treatments with RT plus HT. This should be also considered for the design of multimodal breast cancer therapies. For lung cancer, it has already been proven in preclinical and clinical studies that the timing of ICI affects the clinical outcome [65,66]. Once again, instead of focusing on one ICM, several other ICMs also should be monitored at different timepoints. Similarly to the findings of Hader et al. [39], we also detected that combinations of RT with HT induced higher expressions of immune-suppressive ICMs compared to HT or RT alone. Li et al. stressed that HT can create a tumor microenvironment with high PD-L1 expression and lymphocyte infiltration, making the tumor more likely to respond to anti-PD1 therapy [51].

Not only inhibitory ICMs were changed, but also the immune-stimulatory ICM OX40-L was significantly upregulated particularly at 120 h after the treatment with RT plus HT. This might offer an opportunity to strengthen the immunostimulatory properties of HT at distinct time points during therapy with OX40-L-agonistic antibodies. The latter has already been used preclinically in combination with other anti-cancer treatments and has shown promising results [67]. However, besides OX40-L, the other immune-activating ICMs (ICOS-L, CD27-L, CD137-L) examined were not strongly affected by RT and HT (not shown). This is in contrast to other tumor entities, such as, e.g., head and neck cancer, where ICOS-L is upregulated on HPV-positive cancer cells after RT [68].

We conclude that in the area of multimodal tumor therapies, the temporal expression of several ICMs should be monitored closely, and personalized therapy approaches will become more and more important. Here, HT will find a new place as an immunomodulator and as a combination partner with RT and ICIs. Even though cell death induction tends to be higher when HT of 44 °C is combined with RT, the expression of ICMs is modulated by even lower temperatures, such as 41 °C and 39 °C. This highlights that the immunomodulating effects of HT are manifold, and besides focusing on the level of temperature with regard to tumor cell death induction [69], the immunomodulating phenotype of tumor cells has to be considered in a timely manner after treatment. Nevertheless, precise monitoring of the temperature in the tumor during the treatment will not only improve the efficacy of the local treatment, but also gives a chance to predict the changes in immune phenotype of the cancer cells. Besides monitoring of local immune alterations inside and around the treated tumor, systemic effects should be complementarily considered in the future to increase knowledge about immune modulations induced by RT alone and in combination with HT and ICIs [70,71].

Even though the sequence of application might affect several cellular processes [28,72], it does not significantly impact on the immune phenotype of the surface of breast cancer cells. In addition to the sequence, different time intervals between RT and HT should be analyzed in the future in vitro and particularly in vivo, also taking into account the oxygenation status of the tissues [73]. In clinics, still no consensus regarding the sequence of application of RT with HT has been reached, and at least from the immunological points of view that were analyzed in this work, it does not matter very much. However, immune factors have to be included in considerations of thermometric parameters to guide HT in the future and to finally validate them in prospective clinical trials [74].

4.3. The Co-Incubation of RT- and HT-Treated Breast Cancer Cells Does Not Affect the Activation State of Dendritic Cells

An immune response consists of a priming and an effector phase. In the priming phase, antigens are taken up by DCs, which have to additionally be stimulated by adjuvants such as danger signals. The latter can be released by stressed tumor cells and mostly in connection with ICD [54]. However, anti-tumor immune responses are not only triggered by the initial priming of T cells against the tumor, but also by restoring anti-tumor immunity in the effector phase. Both modes of action have already been proven to be involved in RT-induced anti-tumor immune responses [75].

Our data now show for the first time that the combination of RT and HT in breast cancer treatment affects the expression of several ICMs in a time-dependent manner. However, there was no significant difference between the different treatments and sequences in regard to the upregulation of activation markers on moDCs. Matsumoto et al. observed that treatment of tumor cells with HT and consecutive co-incubation with murine bone marrow DCs also did not induce activation of these APCs. In order to improve this, they suggest to additionally expose the DCs themselves to mild HT [76]. Thus, future research should analyze this with in vivo systems, but taking both the priming and effector phases of the anti-tumor immune response into consideration [77].

5. Conclusions

The Combination of HT of 39 °C, 41 °C and 44 °C with hypofractionated RT particularly affects the surface immune phenotype of human breast cancer cells. Mainly, immune suppressive ICMs are upregulated following combined treatments, in dependence of the tumor cells, the time after treatment and the nature of the ICM. Besides PD-L1, further suppressive ICMs such as PD-L2 and HVEM should be considered for clinicians when treating breast cancer patients in multimodal settings including RT and HT.

One has to stress that the sequence of the application of RT and HT has no significant impact on the breast cancer cell immune phenotype, and from the immunological point of view, it does not matter very much how this is currently handled in distinct clinics/institutes. For the first time it was shown here, at least preclinically, that rather the immune effector than the immune priming phase is modulated by combination treatments of RT with HT. Besides the induction of ICD, the modulation of the cancer cell's surface immune phenotype has to be considered for the design of innovative prospective clinical trials for breast cancer, including HT. In multimodal treatment settings it might be beneficial to add distinct ICIs in the combinational therapy of HT and RT.

Author Contributions: The structure and the content of the manuscript was conceptualized by U.S.G., M.R., M.H. and A.S. A.S. performed most of the experiments with support of L.H. and D.D. regarding the dendritic cell experiments. The drafts of the manuscripts were written by A.S., M.H., U.S.G. and B.F. The final manuscript was written by A.S., M.R., U.S.G., B.F., M.H., R.F., O.J.O., S.S. and S.M.B. All authors have read and agreed to the published version of the manuscript.

Funding: This research has been funded by the European Union's Horizon 2020 research and innovation programme under the Marie Skłodowska-Curie grant agreement No. 955625, Hyperboost. Further funding was awarded by the Deutsche Forschungsgemeinschaft (DFG, German Research Foundation)—RTG2599 (421758891) to D.D. (P1) and U.G. (P10) and the SFB TRR 305—B05 to D.D.

Institutional Review Board Statement: Peripheral blood mononuclear cells (PBMC) were isolated from leukoreduction system chambers (LRSC) of healthy, anonymous donors having undergone a strict health check by the Transfusion Medicine and Hemostaseology Department of the Universitätsklinikum Erlangen, Germany. The permission to use these LRSCs was given by the ethics committee of the Friedrich-Alexander-Universität Erlangen-Nürnberg (ethical approval no. 180_13 B and 48_19 B), according to the rules of the Declaration of Helsinki in its current form.

Informed Consent Statement: Not applicable.

Data Availability Statement: The data presented in this study are available on reasonable request from the corresponding author.

Acknowledgments: We thank the staff and particularly Erwin Strasser of the Transfusion Medicine and Hemostaseology Department of the Universitätsklinikum Erlangen, Germany, for co-operation in the generation of primary immune cells from biomaterial of leukoreduction system chambers (LRSC) of healthy, anonymous donors. We further acknowledge the support by the German Research Foundation and the Friedrich-Alexander-Universität Erlangen-Nürnberg within the funding program Open Access Publishing. This work has been supported by the European Union's Horizon 2020 research and innovation programme under the Marie Skłodowska-Curie grant agreement No 955625, Hyperboost.

Conflicts of Interest: The authors declare no conflict of interest with regard to the work presented here.

References

1. Jemal, A.; Bray, F.; Center, M.M.; Ferlay, J.; Ward, E.; Forman, D. Global cancer statistics. *CA Cancer J. Clin.* **2011**, *61*, 69–90. [CrossRef]
2. O'Shaughnessy, J. Extending Survival with Chemotherapy in Metastatic Breast Cancer. *Oncologist* **2005**, *10*, 20–29. [CrossRef]
3. Villacampa, G.; Tolosa, P.; Salvador, F.; Sánchez-Bayona, R.; Villanueva, L.; Dienstmann, R.; Ciruelos, E.; Pascual, T. Addition of immune checkpoint inhibitors to chemotherapy versus chemotherapy alone in first-line metastatic triple-negative breast cancer: A systematic review and meta-analysis. *Cancer Treat. Rev.* **2022**, *104*, 102352. [CrossRef]
4. Frey, B.; Rückert, M.; Deloch, L.; Rühle, P.F.; Derer, A.; Fietkau, R.; Gaipl, U.S. Immunomodulation by ionizing radiation-impact for design of radio-immunotherapies and for treatment of inflammatory diseases. *Immunol. Rev.* **2017**, *280*, 231–248. [CrossRef]
5. Issels, R.; Kampmann, E.; Kanaar, R.; Lindner, L. Hallmarks of hyperthermia in driving the future of clinical hyperthermia as targeted therapy: Translation into clinical application. *Int. J. Hyperth.* **2016**, *32*, 89–95. [CrossRef]
6. Hurwitz, M.; Stauffer, P. Hyperthermia, Radiation and Chemotherapy: The Role of Heat in Multidisciplinary Cancer Care. *Semin. Oncol.* **2014**, *41*, 714–729. [CrossRef]
7. Issels, R.D. Hyperthermia adds to chemotherapy. *Eur. J. Cancer* **2008**, *44*, 2546–2554. [CrossRef]
8. De-Colle, C.; Weidner, N.; Heinrich, V.; Brucker, S.; Hahn, M.; Macmillan, K.; Lamprecht, U.; Gaupp, S.; Voigt, O.; Zips, D. Hyperthermic chest wall re-irradiation in recurrent breast cancer: A prospective observational study. *Strahlenther. Onkol.* **2019**, *195*, 318–326. [CrossRef]
9. Oldenborg, S.; Rasch, C.R.N.; Van Os, R.; Kusumanto, Y.H.; Oei, B.S.; Venselaar, J.L.; Heymans, M.; Vörding, P.J.Z.V.S.; Crezee, J.; Van Tienhoven, G. Reirradiation + hyperthermia for recurrent breast cancer en cuirasse. *Strahlenther. Onkol.* **2017**, *194*, 206–214. [CrossRef]
10. Song, C.W.; Shakil, A.; Osborn, J.L.; Iwata, K. Tumour oxygenation is increased by hyperthermia at mild temperatures. *Int. J. Hyperth.* **2009**, *12*, 367–373. [CrossRef]

11. Horsman, M.R.; Overgaard, J. Hyperthermia: A Potent Enhancer of Radiotherapy. *Clin. Oncol.* **2007**, *19*, 418–426. [CrossRef] [PubMed]
12. Tsang, Y.-W.; Huang, C.-C.; Yang, K.-L.; Chi, M.-S.; Chiang, H.-C.; Wang, Y.-S.; Andocs, G.; Szasz, A.; Li, W.-T.; Chi, K.-H. Improving immunological tumor microenvironment using electro-hyperthermia followed by dendritic cell immunotherapy. *BMC Cancer* **2015**, *15*, 708. [CrossRef]
13. Rao, W.; Deng, Z.-S.; Liu, J. A Review of Hyperthermia Combined With Radiotherapy/Chemotherapy on Malignant Tumors. *Crit. Rev. Biomed. Eng.* **2010**, *38*, 101–116. [CrossRef]
14. Chen, T.; Guo, J.; Han, C.; Yang, M.; Cao, X. Heat shock protein 70, released from heat-stressed tumor cells, initiates antitumor immunity by inducing tumor cell chemokine production and activating dendritic cells via TLR4 pathway. *J. Immunol.* **2009**, *182*, 1449–1459. [CrossRef]
15. Datta, N.R.; Gómez Ordóñez, S.; Gaipl, U.S.; Paulides, M.M.; Crezee, H.; Gellermann, J.; Marder, D.; Puric, E.; Bodis, S. Local hyperthermia combined with radiotherapy and-/or chemotherapy: Recent advances and promises for the future. *Cancer Treat. Rev.* **2015**, *41*, 742–753. [CrossRef]
16. Schildkopf, P.; Frey, B.; Mantel, F.; Ott, O.J.; Weiss, E.-M.; Sieber, R.; Janko, C.; Sauer, R.; Fietkau, R.; Gaipl, U.S. Application of hyperthermia in addition to ionizing irradiation fosters necrotic cell death and HMGB1 release of colorectal tumor cells. *Biochem. Biophys. Res. Commun.* **2010**, *391*, 1014–1020. [CrossRef]
17. Schildkopf, P.; Frey, B.; Ott, O.J.; Rubner, Y.; Multhoff, G.; Sauer, R.; Fietkau, R.; Gaipl, U.S. Radiation combined with hyperthermia induces HSP70-dependent maturation of dendritic cells and release of pro-inflammatory cytokines by dendritic cells and macrophages. *Radiother. Oncol.* **2011**, *101*, 109–115. [CrossRef]
18. Skitzki, J.J.; A Repasky, E.; Evans, S.S. Hyperthermia as an immunotherapy strategy for cancer. *Curr. Opin. Investig. Drugs* **2009**, *10*, 550–558.
19. Werthmöller, N.; Frey, B.; Rückert, M.; Lotter, M.; Fietkau, R.; Gaipl, U.S. Combination of ionising radiation with hyperthermia increases the immunogenic potential of B16-F10 melanoma cells in vitro and in vivo. *Int. J. Hyperth.* **2016**, *32*, 23–30. [CrossRef]
20. Schmid, T.E.; Multhoff, G. Radiation-induced stress proteins—The role of heat shock proteins (HSP) in anti-tumor responses. *Curr. Med. Chem.* **2012**, *19*, 1765–1770. [CrossRef]
21. Peer, A.J.; Grimm, M.J.; Zynda, E.R.; Repasky, E.A. Diverse immune mechanisms may contribute to the survival benefit seen in cancer patients receiving hyperthermia. *Immunol. Res.* **2009**, *46*, 137–154. [CrossRef]
22. Knippertz, I.; Stein, M.F.; Dörrie, J.; Schaft, N.; Müller, I.; Deinzer, A.; Steinkasserer, A.; Nettelbeck, D.M. Mild hyperthermia enhances human monocyte-derived dendritic cell functions and offers potential for applications in vaccination strategies. *Int. J. Hyperth.* **2011**, *27*, 591–603. [CrossRef] [PubMed]
23. Crezee, J.; Oei, A.L.; Franken, N.A.P.; Stalpers, L.J.A.; Kok, H.P. Response: Commentary: The Impact of the Time Interval between Radiation and Hyperthermia on Clinical Outcome in Patients with Locally Advanced Cervical Cancer. *Front. Oncol.* **2020**, *10*, 10. [CrossRef] [PubMed]
24. Bakker, A.; Van Der Zee, J.; Van Tienhoven, G.; Kok, H.P.; Rasch, C.R.N.; Crezee, H. Temperature and thermal dose during radiotherapy and hyperthermia for recurrent breast cancer are related to clinical outcome and thermal toxicity: A systematic review. *Int. J. Hyperth.* **2019**, *36*, 1024–1039. [CrossRef] [PubMed]
25. Crezee, H.; Kok, H.P.; Oei, A.L.; Franken, N.A.P.; Stalpers, L.J.A. The Impact of the Time Interval between Radiation and Hyperthermia on Clinical Outcome in Patients with Locally Advanced Cervical Cancer. *Front. Oncol.* **2019**, *9*, 412. [CrossRef]
26. Dobšíček Trefná, H.; Schmidt, M.; van Rhoon, G.C.; Kok, H.P.; Gordeyev, S.S.; Lamprecht, U.; Marder, D.; Nadobny, J.; Ghadjar, P.; Abdel-Rahman, S.; et al. Quality assurance guidelines for interstitial hyperthermia. *Int. J. Hyperth.* **2019**, *36*, 276–293. [CrossRef] [PubMed]
27. Lagendijk, J.J.W.; Van Rhoon, G.C.; Hornsleth, S.N.; Wust, P.; De Leeuw, A.C.C.; Schneider, C.J.; Van Ddk, J.D.P.; Van Der Zee, J.; Van Heek-Romanowski, R.; Rahman, S.A.; et al. Esho Quality Assurance Guidelines for Regional Hyperthermia. *Int. J. Hyperth.* **2009**, *14*, 125–133. [CrossRef]
28. Elming, P.B.; Sørensen, B.S.; Oei, A.L.; Franken, N.A.P.; Crezee, J.; Overgaard, J.; Horsman, M.R. Hyperthermia: The Optimal Treatment to Overcome Radiation Resistant Hypoxia. *Cancers* **2019**, *11*, 60. [CrossRef]
29. Vernon, C.C.; Hand, J.W.; Field, S.B.; Machin, B.; Whaley, J.B.; van der Zee, J.; van Putten, W.L.; van Rhoon, G.C.; van Dijk, J.D.; González González, D.; et al. Radiotherapy with or without hyperthermia in the treatment of superficial localized breast cancer: Results from five randomized controlled trials. *Int. J. Radiat. Oncol. Biol. Phys.* **1996**, *35*, 731–744.
30. Overgaard, J.; Bentzen, S.M.; Overgaard, J.; Gonzalez, D.G.; Hulshof, M.C.C.M.; Arcangeli, G.; Dahl, O.; Mella, O. Randomised trial of hyperthermia as adjuvant to radiotherapy for recurrent or metastatic malignant melanoma. *Lancet* **1995**, *345*, 540–543. [CrossRef]
31. Van Der Zee, J.; González, D.G. The Dutch Deep Hyperthermia Trial: Results in cervical cancer. *Int. J. Hyperth.* **2009**, *18*, 1–12. [CrossRef]
32. van der Zee, J.; González, D.; van Rhoon, G.C.; van Dijk, J.D.; van Putten, W.L.; Hart, A.A. Comparison of radiotherapy alone with radiotherapy plus hyperthermia in locally advanced pelvic tumours: A prospective, randomised, multicentre trial. *Lancet* **2000**, *355*, 1119–1125. [CrossRef]

33. Ott, O.J.; Schmidt, M.; Semrau, S.; Strnad, V.; Matzel, K.E.; Schneider, I.; Raptis, D.; Uter, W.; Grützmann, R.; Fietkau, R. Chemoradiotherapy with and without deep regional hyperthermia for squamous cell carcinoma of the anus. *Strahlenther. Onkol.* **2018**, *195*, 607–614. [CrossRef] [PubMed]
34. Issels, R.D.; Noessner, E.; Lindner, L.H.; Schmidt, M.; Albertsmeier, M.; Blay, J.-Y.; Stutz, E.; Xu, Y.; Bueckelin, V.; Altendorf-Hofmann, A.; et al. Immune infiltrates in patients with localised high-risk soft tissue sarcoma treated with neoadjuvant chemotherapy without or with regional hyperthermia: A translational research program of the EORTC 62961-ESHO 95 randomised clinical trial. *Eur. J. Cancer* **2021**, *158*, 123–132. [CrossRef]
35. Schouten, D.; van Os, R.; Westermann, A.M.; Crezee, H.; van Tienhoven, G.; Kolff, M.W.; Bins, A.D. A randomized phase-II study of reirradiation and hyperthermia versus reirradiation and hyperthermia plus chemotherapy for locally recurrent breast cancer in previously irradiated area. *Acta Oncol.* **2022**, 441–448. [CrossRef] [PubMed]
36. Notter, M.; Stutz, E.; Thomsen, A.R.; Vaupel, P. Radiation-Associated Angiosarcoma of the Breast and Chest Wall Treated with Thermography-Controlled, Contactless wIRA-Hyperthermia and Hypofractionated Re-Irradiation. *Cancers* **2021**, *13*, 3911. [CrossRef]
37. Murray Brunt, A.; Haviland, J.S.; Wheatley, D.A.; Sydenham, M.A.; Alhasso, A.; Bloomfield, D.J.; Chan, C.; Churn, M.; Cleator, S.; Coles, C.E.; et al. Hypofractionated breast radiotherapy for 1 week versus 3 weeks (FAST-Forward): 5-year efficacy and late normal tissue effects results from a multicentre, non-inferiority, randomised, phase 3 trial. *Lancet* **2020**, *395*, 1613–1626. [CrossRef]
38. Demaria, S.; Guha, C.; Schoenfeld, J.; Morris, Z.; Monjazeb, A.; Sikora, A.; Crittenden, M.; Shiao, S.; Khleif, S.; Gupta, S.; et al. Radiation dose and fraction in immunotherapy: One-size regimen does not fit all settings, so how does one choose? *J. Immunother. Cancer* **2021**, *9*, e002038. [CrossRef]
39. Hader, M.; Savcigil, D.P.; Rosin, A.; Ponfick, P.; Gekle, S.; Wadepohl, M.; Bekeschus, S.; Fietkau, R.; Frey, B.; Schlücker, E.; et al. Differences of the Immune Phenotype of Breast Cancer Cells after Ex Vivo Hyperthermia by Warm-Water or Microwave Radiation in a Closed-Loop System Alone or in Combination with Radiotherapy. *Cancers* **2020**, *12*, 1082. [CrossRef]
40. Gillette, E.L.; Ensley, B.A. Effect of heating order on radiation response of mouse tumor and skin. *Int. J. Radiat. Oncol.* **1979**, *5*, 209–213. [CrossRef]
41. Hill, S.A.; Denekamp, J. The response of six mouse tumours to combined heat and X rays: Implications for therapy. *Br. J. Radiol.* **1979**, *52*, 209–218. [CrossRef] [PubMed]
42. van der Zee, J.; de Bruijne, M.; van Rhoon, G.C. Thermal medicine, heat shock proteins and cancer. *Int. J. Hyperth.* **2006**, *22*, 433–437; author reply 437–447.
43. Trefná, H.D.; Crezee, H.; Schmidt, M.; Marder, D.; Lamprecht, U.; Ehmann, M.; Hartmann, J.; Nadobny, J.; Gellermann, J.; Van Holthe, N.; et al. Quality assurance guidelines for superficial hyperthermia clinical trials: I. Clinical requirements. *Int. J. Hyperth.* **2017**, *33*, 471–482. [CrossRef] [PubMed]
44. Lühr, J.J.; Alex, N.; Amon, L.; Kräter, M.; Kubánková, M.; Sezgin, E.; Lehmann, C.H.K.; Heger, L.; Heidkamp, G.F.; Smith, A.-S.; et al. Maturation of Monocyte-Derived DCs Leads to Increased Cellular Stiffness, Higher Membrane Fluidity, and Changed Lipid Composition. *Front. Immunol.* **2020**, *11*, 11. [CrossRef] [PubMed]
45. Rückert, M.; Deloch, L.; Fietkau, R.; Frey, B.; Hecht, M.; Gaipl, U.S. Immune modulatory effects of radiotherapy as basis for well-reasoned radioimmunotherapies. *Strahlenther. Onkol.* **2018**, *194*, 509–519. [CrossRef]
46. Hader, M.; Frey, B.; Fietkau, R.; Hecht, M.; Gaipl, U.S. Immune biological rationales for the design of combined radio- and immunotherapies. *Cancer Immunol. Immunother.* **2020**, *69*, 293–306. [CrossRef]
47. Kolberg, H.C.; Hoffmann, O.; Baumann, R. The Abscopal Effect: Could a Phenomenon Described Decades Ago Become Key to Enhancing the Response to Immune Therapies in Breast Cancer? *Breast Care* **2020**, *15*, 443–449. [CrossRef]
48. Zagar, T.M.; Oleson, J.R.; Vujaskovic, Z.; Dewhirst, M.W.; Craciunescu, O.I.; Blackwell, K.L.; Prosnitz, L.R.; Jones, E.L. Hyperthermia combined with radiation therapy for superficial breast cancer and chest wall recurrence: A review of the randomised data. *Int. J. Hyperth.* **2010**, *26*, 612–617. [CrossRef]
49. Arslan, S.A.; Ozdemir, N.; Sendur, M.A.; Eren, T.; Ozturk, H.F.; Aral, I.P.; Soykut, E.D.; Inan, G.A. Hyperthermia and radiotherapy combination for locoregional recurrences of breast cancer: A review. *Breast Cancer Manag.* **2017**, *6*, 117–126. [CrossRef]
50. Ho, A.Y.; Barker, C.A.; Arnold, B.B.; Powell, S.N.; Hu, Z.I.; Gucalp, A.; Lebron-Zapata, L.; Wen, H.Y.; Kallman, C.; D'Agnolo, A.; et al. A phase 2 clinical trial assessing the efficacy and safety of pembrolizumab and radiotherapy in patients with metastatic triple-negative breast cancer. *Cancer* **2020**, *126*, 850–860. [CrossRef]
51. Li, Z.; Deng, J.; Sun, J.; Ma, Y. Hyperthermia Targeting the Tumor Microenvironment Facilitates Immune Checkpoint Inhibitors. *Front. Immunol.* **2020**, *11*, 11. [CrossRef] [PubMed]
52. Kroemer, G.; Galassi, C.; Zitvogel, L.; Galluzzi, L. Immunogenic cell stress and death. *Nat. Immunol.* **2022**, *23*, 487–500. [CrossRef] [PubMed]
53. Podolska, M.J.; Shan, X.; Janko, C.; Boukherroub, R.; Gaipl, U.S.; Szunerits, S.; Frey, B.; Muñoz, L.E. Graphene-Induced Hyperthermia (GIHT) Combined with Radiotherapy Fosters Immunogenic Cell Death. *Front. Oncol.* **2021**, *11*, 664615. [CrossRef] [PubMed]
54. Galluzzi, L.; Vitale, I.; Warren, S.; Adjemian, S.; Agostinis, P.; Martinez, A.B.; Chan, T.A.; Coukos, G.; Demaria, S.; Deutsch, E.; et al. Consensus guidelines for the definition, detection and interpretation of immunogenic cell death. *J. Immunother. Cancer* **2020**, *8*, e000337. [CrossRef]

55. Scheidegger, S.; Barba, S.M.; Gaipl, U.S. Theoretical Evaluation of the Impact of Hyperthermia in Combination with Radiation Therapy in an Artificial Immune—Tumor-Ecosystem. *Cancers* **2021**, *13*, 5764. [CrossRef]
56. Andersen, M.H. The Balance Players of the Adaptive Immune System. *Cancer Res.* **2018**, *78*, 1379–1382. [CrossRef]
57. Mei, X.; Ten Cate, R.; Van Leeuwen, C.M.; Rodermond, H.M.; De Leeuw, L.; Dimitrakopoulou, D.; Stalpers, L.J.A.; Crezee, J.; Kok, H.P.; Franken, N.A.P.; et al. Radiosensitization by hyperthermia: The effects of temperature, sequence, and time interval in cervical cell lines. *Cancers* **2020**, *12*, 582. [CrossRef]
58. Mondini, M.; Levy, A.; Meziani, L.; Milliat, F.; Deutsch, E. Radiotherapy–immunotherapy combinations—Perspectives and challenges. *Mol. Oncol.* **2020**, *14*, 1529–1537. [CrossRef]
59. Ibuki, Y.; Takahashi, Y.; Tamari, K.; Minami, K.; Seo, Y.; Isohashi, F.; Koizumi, M.; Ogawa, K. Local hyperthermia combined with CTLA-4 blockade induces both local and abscopal effects in a murine breast cancer model. *Int. J. Hyperth.* **2021**, *38*, 363–371. [CrossRef]
60. Kordbacheh, T.; Honeychurch, J.; Blackhall, F.; Faivre-Finn, C.; Illidge, T. Radiotherapy and anti-PD-1/PD-L1 combinations in lung cancer: Building better translational research platforms. *Ann. Oncol.* **2018**, *29*, 301–310. [CrossRef]
61. Derer, A.; Spiljar, M.; Bäumler, M.; Hecht, M.; Fietkau, R.; Frey, B.; Gaipl, U.S. Chemoradiation Increases PD-L1 Expression in Certain Melanoma and Glioblastoma Cells. *Front. Immunol.* **2016**, *7*, 610. [CrossRef] [PubMed]
62. Lim, Y.J.; Koh, J.; Kim, S.; Jeon, S.-R.; Chie, E.K.; Kim, K.; Kang, G.H.; Han, S.-W.; Kim, T.-Y.; Jeong, S.-Y.; et al. Chemoradiation-Induced Alteration of Programmed Death-Ligand 1 and CD8 + Tumor-Infiltrating Lymphocytes Identified Patients With Poor Prognosis in Rectal Cancer: A Matched Comparison Analysis. *Int. J. Radiat. Oncol.* **2017**, *99*, 1216–1224. [CrossRef] [PubMed]
63. Tsang, J.Y.S.; Chan, K.-W.; Ni, Y.-B.; Hlaing, T.; Hu, J.; Cheung, S.-Y.; Tse, G.M. Expression and Clinical Significance of Herpes Virus Entry Mediator (HVEM) in Breast Cancer. *Ann. Surg. Oncol.* **2017**, *24*, 4042–4050. [CrossRef] [PubMed]
64. Abad, M.N.; Calabuig-Fariñas, S.; de Mena, M.L.; Torres-Martínez, S.; González, C.G.; García, J.; Ángel, G.; González-Cruz, V.I.; Herrero, C.C. Programmed Death-Ligand 1 (PD-L1) as Immunotherapy Biomarker in Breast Cancer. *Cancers* **2022**, *14*, 307. [CrossRef] [PubMed]
65. Breen, W.G.; Leventakos, K.; Dong, H.; Merrell, K.W. Radiation and immunotherapy: Emerging mechanisms of synergy. *J. Thorac. Dis.* **2020**, *12*, 7011–7023. [CrossRef] [PubMed]
66. Zhao, X.; Li, J.; Zheng, L.; Yang, Q.; Chen, X.; Chen, X.; Yu, Y.; Li, F.; Cui, J.; Sun, J. Immune Response on Optimal Timing and Fractionation Dose for Hypofractionated Radiotherapy in Non–Small-Cell Lung Cancer. *Front. Mol. Biosci.* **2022**, *9*, 786864. [CrossRef]
67. Aspeslagh, S.; Postel-Vinay, S.; Rusakiewicz, S.; Soria, J.-C.; Zitvogel, L.; Marabelle, A. Rationale for anti-OX40 cancer immunotherapy. *Eur. J. Cancer* **2016**, *52*, 50–66. [CrossRef]
68. Wimmer, S.; Deloch, L.; Hader, M.; Derer, A.; Grottker, F.; Weissmann, T.; Hecht, M.; Gostian, A.-O.; Fietkau, R.; Frey, B.; et al. Hypofractionated Radiotherapy Upregulates Several Immune Checkpoint Molecules in Head and Neck Squamous Cell Carcinoma Cells Independently of the HPV Status While ICOS-L Is Upregulated Only on HPV-Positive Cells. *Int. J. Mol. Sci.* **2021**, *22*, 9114. [CrossRef]
69. Kok, H.P.; Wust, P.; Stauffer, P.R.; Bardati, F.; van Rhoon, G.C.; Crezee, J. Current state of the art of regional hyperthermia treatment planning: A review. *Radiat. Oncol.* **2015**, *10*, 196. [CrossRef]
70. Frey, B.; Mika, J.; Jelonek, K.; Cruz-Garcia, L.; Roelants, C.; Testard, I.; Cherradi, N.; Lumniczky, K.; Polozov, S.; Napieralska, A.; et al. Systemic modulation of stress and immune parameters in patients treated for prostate adenocarcinoma by intensity-modulated radiation therapy or stereotactic ablative body radiotherapy. *Strahlenther. Onkol.* **2020**, *196*, 1018–1033. [CrossRef]
71. Zhou, J.-G.; Donaubauer, A.-J.; Frey, B.; Becker, I.; Rutzner, S.; Eckstein, M.; Sun, R.; Ma, H.; Schubert, P.; Schweizer, C.; et al. Prospective development and validation of a liquid immune profile-based signature (LIPS) to predict response of patients with recurrent/metastatic cancer to immune checkpoint inhibitors. *J. Immunother. Cancer* **2021**, *9*, e001845. [CrossRef] [PubMed]
72. Oei, A.; Kok, H.; Oei, S.; Horsman, M.; Stalpers, L.; Franken, N.; Crezee, J. Molecular and biological rationale of hyperthermia as radio- and chemosensitizer. *Adv. Drug Deliv. Rev.* **2020**, *163–164*, 84–97. [CrossRef] [PubMed]
73. Overgaard, J.; Grau, C.; Lindegaard, J.; Horsman, M. The potential of using hyperthermia to eliminate radioresistant hypoxic cells. *Radiother. Oncol.* **1991**, *20*, 113–116. [CrossRef]
74. Ademaj, A.; Veltsista, D.P.; Ghadjar, P.; Marder, D.; Oberacker, E.; Ott, O.J.; Wust, P.; Puric, E.; Hälg, R.A.; Rogers, S.; et al. Clinical Evidence for Thermometric Parameters to Guide Hyperthermia Treatment. *Cancers* **2022**, *14*, 625. [CrossRef]
75. Demaria, S.; Golden, E.B.; Formenti, S.C. Role of Local Radiation Therapy in Cancer Immunotherapy. *JAMA Oncol.* **2015**, *1*, 1325–1332. [CrossRef]
76. Yamamoto, N.; Matsumoto, K.; Hagiwara, S.; Saito, M.; Furue, H.; Shigetomi, T.; Narita, Y.; Mitsudo, K.; Tohnai, I.; Kobayashi, T.; et al. Optimization of hyperthermia and dendritic cell immunotherapy for squamous cell carcinoma. *Oncol. Rep.* **2011**, *25*, 1525–1532. [CrossRef]
77. Rückert, M.; Flohr, A.-S.; Hecht, M.; Gaipl, U.S. Radiotherapy and the immune system: More than just immune suppression. *Stem Cells* **2021**, *39*, 1155–1165. [CrossRef]

Review

Hyperthermia: A Potential Game-Changer in the Management of Cancers in Low-Middle-Income Group Countries

Niloy R. Datta [1,*], Bharati M. Jain [1], Zatin Mathi [1], Sneha Datta [2], Satyendra Johari [3], Ashok R. Singh [1], Pallavi Kalbande [1], Pournima Kale [1], Vitaladevuni Shivkumar [4], and Stephan Bodis [5,6]

[1] Department of Radiotherapy, Mahatma Gandhi Institute of Medical Sciences, Sevagram, Wardha 442012, India; bharati@mgims.ac.in (B.M.J.); zatinmathi@gmail.com (Z.M.); ashoksingh@mgims.ac.in (A.R.S.); pallavikalbande@mgims.ac.in (P.K.); pournimakale@mgims.ac.in (P.K.)
[2] Animal Production and Health Laboratory, Joint FAO/IAEA Division of Nuclear Techniques in Food and Agriculture, Department of Nuclear Sciences and Applications, International Atomic Energy Agency (IAEA), P.O. Box 100, 1400 Vienna, Austria; S.Datta@iaea.org
[3] Johari Digital Healthcare Limited, Jodhpur 342012, India; sjohari@joharidigital.com
[4] Department of Pathology, Mahatma Gandhi Institute of Medical Sciences, Sevagram, Wardha 442012, India; shivkumar@mgims.ac.in
[5] Foundation for Research on Information Technologies in Society (IT'IS), 8004 Zurich, Switzerland; s.bodis@bluewin.ch
[6] Department of Radiation Oncology, University Hospital Zurich, 8091 Zurich, Switzerland
* Correspondence: niloydatta@mgims.ac.in

Simple Summary: As per the Global Cancer Observatory, in 2020, 59% of all cancers globally have been reported from the low-middle-income group countries (LMICs). Cancers of the breast, cervix and head and neck constitute around one-third of the cancers in the LMICs. Most of them are in advanced stages and thus deemed inoperable. Chemoradiotherapy is usually advocated for treatment of these cases with limited success. Moderate hyperthermia at 40–44 °C is a multifaceted therapeutic modality. It is a potent radiosensitizer, chemosensitizer and enforces immunomodulation akin to "in situ tumour vaccination". The safety and benefit of addition of hyperthermia to radiotherapy and/or chemotherapy in these sites have been well documented in various phase III randomized clinical trials and meta-analysis. Thus, including hyperthermia in the therapeutic armamentarium of clinical care, especially in the LMICs could be a potential game-changer and provide a cost-effective addendum to the existing therapeutic options, especially for these tumour sites.

Abstract: Loco-regional hyperthermia at 40–44 °C is a multifaceted therapeutic modality with the distinct triple advantage of being a potent radiosensitizer, a chemosensitizer and an immunomodulator. Risk difference estimates from pairwise meta-analysis have shown that the local tumour control could be improved by 22.3% ($p < 0.001$), 22.1% ($p < 0.001$) and 25.5% ($p < 0.001$) in recurrent breast cancers, locally advanced cervix cancer (LACC) and locally advanced head and neck cancers, respectively by adding hyperthermia to radiotherapy over radiotherapy alone. Furthermore, thermochemoradiotherapy in LACC have shown to reduce the local failure rates by 10.1% ($p = 0.03$) and decrease deaths by 5.6% (95% CI: 0.6–11.8%) over chemoradiotherapy alone. As around one-third of the cancer cases in low-middle-income group countries belong to breast, cervix and head and neck regions, hyperthermia could be a potential game-changer and expected to augment the clinical outcomes of these patients in conjunction with radiotherapy and/or chemotherapy. Further, hyperthermia could also be a cost-effective therapeutic modality as the capital costs for setting up a hyperthermia facility is relatively low. Thus, the positive outcomes evident from various phase III randomized trials and meta-analysis with thermoradiotherapy or thermochemoradiotherapy justifies the integration of hyperthermia in the therapeutic armamentarium of clinical management of cancer, especially in low-middle-income group countries.

Keywords: low-middle-income group countries; cancer; hyperthermia; radiotherapy; chemotherapy; recurrent breast cancers; cervical cancer; head and neck cancers; cost-effective; meta-analysis

1. Introduction

1.1. Cancer Status in Low-Middle-Income Group Countries

According to the Global Cancer Observatory of the World Health Organization (WHO), the total cancer incidence estimated in 2020 was 19.3 M and is expected to rise to 24.1 M in 2030 [1]. In 2020, 11.4 M (59%) of these cases were reported in the low-middle-income countries (LMICs) where the cancer burden is projected to escalate to 14.6 M (+28.2%) and 17.9 M (+56.8%) by 2030 and 2040, respectively. Of the 11.4 M cancer cases in LMICs, presently, cancers of breast, cervix and head and neck regions combined constitutes around 3 M (26.2%) of cases. Furthermore, the cancers in these sites in LMICs constitute 61.1%, 88.1% and 71.8% of the global cancers, respectively (Table 1). In view of the advanced stages of their presentation, most of these cases are inoperable. Thus, radiotherapy (RT) and/or chemotherapy (CT) forms the mainstay of their treatment, resulting in a %mortality/incidence at 36%, 58.7% and 38.2% in cancers of the breast, cervix and head and neck, respectively in LMICs (Figure 1, Table 1). Certainly, there is a need to explore other cost-effective options to improve these treatment outcomes in LMICs [2].

Table 1. Estimated number of cancer cases and deaths as per the Global Cancer Observatory in ages (0–85+ years) pertaining to breast, cervix and head and neck region globally and in low-middle-income countries (LMICs) in 2020 [1]. Countries classified in various income groups based on the World Bank classification.

Cancer Sites	Cancer Incidence			Cancer Mortality			% Mortality/Incidence in LMICs
	All Countries	LMICs Only	Proportion in LMICs (%)	All Countries	LMICs Only	Proportion in LMICs (%)	
All sites	19,292,789	11,441,886	59.3	9,958,133	7,063,070	70.9	61.7
Breast	2,261,419	1,381,539	61.1	684,996	497,496	72.6	36.0
Cervix	604,127	532,239	88.1	341,831	312,373	91.4	58.7
Head and neck #	1,518,133	1,090,262	71.8	510,771	416,206	81.5	38.2

includes cancers of lip, oral cavity, nasopharynx, oropharynx, hypopharynx, larynx, salivary glands and thyroid; Data as on 12 September 2021 [1].

1.2. Hyperthermia as a "Potential Game-Changer"

Loco-regional hyperthermia (HT) or thermotherapy, at 40–44 °C, has been shown to be a potent radiosensitizer, a chemosensitizer and an immunomodulator with no significantly added side effects [3–5]. HT sensitizes the hypoxic tumour cells and inhibits the repair of RT- and/or CT-induced DNA damage. In addition, cells in radioresistant "S" phase are heat sensitive [3]. Furthermore, thermoradiobiologically, HT has been shown to impart high LET properties to low LET proton or photon beams [6]. The addition of HT to photons creates a radiobiological advantage in tumours akin to fast beam neutrons. The physiological vasodilation at temperatures of 39–45 °C allows rapid heat dissipation from normal tissues, thereby sparing the normal tissues from HT-induced morbidity. On the contrary, the chaotic and relatively rigid tumour vasculature results in heat retention leading to higher intratumoural temperatures. Consequently, the high LET attributes of HT with photon radiations are mostly limited to the confines of the heated tumour, while the normothermic normal tissues get irradiated with low LET photons. HT thereby augments photon therapy by conferring therapeutic advantages of high LET radiations to the tumours akin to neutrons, while the 'heat-sink' effect spares the normal tissues from thermal radiosensitization. Thus, photon thermoradiotherapy imparts radiobiological advantages selectively to tumours analogous to neutrons without exaggerating normal tissue morbidities.

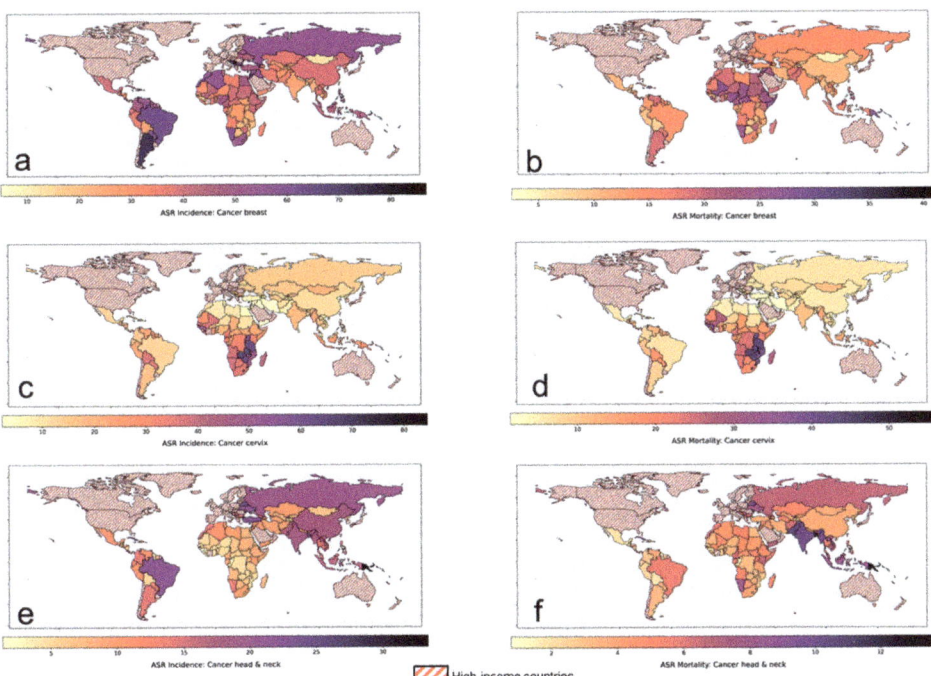

Figure 1. Age-standardized rates of (ASR) for incidence and mortality for (**a,b**) breast cancer (**c,d**) cervical cancer and (**e,f**) head and neck cancers, respectively in low-middle-income group countries. Based on data from Global Cancer Observatory [1].

Accordingly, HT could be an effective therapeutic modality in conjunction with RT and/or CT. Moderate HT, as defined by the Kadota Forum in 2008, is elevation of the tumour temperature between 39 °C and 45 °C [7]. The biological and physiological mechanisms involved in HT at 38–45 °C has been very aptly summarized by van Rhoon [8]. The thermodynamic changes are initiated at around 38 °C and results in a gradual increase in tumour blood flow and subsequent oxygenation while the thermoradiobiological mechanisms lead to direct cell kill, thermal sensitization and inhibition of DNA repair between 39 °C and 45 °C. Thus, at the usual clinically achievable temperature of 40–42 °C, HT could lead to appreciable radiosensitization, chemosensitization and immunomodulation along with RT ± CT.

Incorporating HT along with the standard therapeutic modalities, namely RT and/or CT, could thus be expected to augment therapeutic outcomes through the multifaceted actions of HT [3,4]. In LMICs, most patients present in relatively locally advanced stages, thereby limiting the role of primary surgical option. Thus, RT and/or CT forms the mainstay of management of these locally advanced tumours—namely of head and neck, cervix and breast. The treatment needs to be tolerable as patients usually have compromised nutritional status, especially in LMICs. In addition, due to limited health insurance coverage, most patients may have to bear the cost of their treatment through out-of-pocket resources. All these factors, enforces one to consider cost-effective strategies that are also tolerable with low acute and late morbidities. HT, a safe modality, with limited toxicities, and a known potentiator of RT and CT could thus be a possible therapeutic addendum in clinical settings in LMICs. The present report summarizes the available clinical evidence to justify the inclusion of HT in the management of these common cancers in LMICs along with RT ± CT. As evident, HT could indeed emerge as a potential game-changer by improving the therapeutic outcome in the common cancers prevalent in LMICs.

2. Locally Advanced Breast Cancers: Scope for Improvement with Hyperthermia

Locally advanced breast cancers (LABC) are a fairly common problem in LMICs. Most patients present in an advanced stage where primary surgical intervention is usually not feasible. Thus, patients are usually subjected to neoadjuvant chemotherapy (NACT) to enable tumour downstaging followed by mastectomy. Most CT drugs exhibit thermal synergism by (a) increasing the cellular uptake of drugs, (b) increased oxygen radical production, (c) increasing DNA damage, and (d) inhibiting chemotherapeutic-induced DNA damage [9–11]. HT inflicts oxidative damage and/or strand cross links, as well as single or double strand DNA breaks, along with CT agents, namely adriamycin, cyclophosphamide, 5-flurouracil and taxanes commonly used as NACT agents for LABC. Further, HT also interferes with the various DNA repair process involving excision repair, non-homologous end joining and/or homologous recombination [9,11].

Clinical Outcomes with Hyperthermia in Locally Advanced Breast Cancers

In a recently reported randomized clinical trial in stages IIB-IIIA breast cancers, patients treated with NACT (adriamycin, cyclophosphamide, 5-flurouracil) with loco-regional HT using 27.1 MHz, experienced a significant reduction in both primary tumour (+15.9%, $p = 0.034$) and axillary lymph nodes (+14.1%, $p = 0.011$) compared to those treated with NACT alone [12]. Further, a higher proportion of patients underwent breast conservative surgery (+13.6%) with NACT + HT following appreciable tumour regression. A significantly improved overall survival at 10-year was also evident in patients treated with NACT + HT ($p = 0.009$).

In a phase I/II study, Vujaskovic et al. [13], evaluated the safety and efficacy of a NACT with paclitaxel, liposomal doxorubicin and HT in LABC. A combined response rate of 72% was reported at the end of NACT with four of the 43 patients achieving a complete response (CR). A 4-year disease-free and overall survival rate of 63% and 75% were attained, respectively.

HT has been reported to increase the systolic blood flow in breast tumours by about 3.5 times compared to pre-HT blood flow [12].

Thus, NACT + HT could be a viable option for LABC and the consequence of its effects on the key outcomes need to be examined systematically in future studies. These should also incorporate a detailed histopathological evaluation to explore HT-induced immunomodulation.

3. Recurrent Breast Cancers and Other Cancers: Scope for Improvement with Hyperthermia

Locoregional recurrence in breast cancers has been reported in one-third of the patients with 80% of these recurrences evident within the first 5 years of primary treatment [14]. Although surgery is the preferred initial option, its role is restricted mostly to operable lesions. The efficacy of CT is yet to be established as evident from a Cochrane review [15]. In an open label randomized study, the efficacy of chemotherapy was limited only to resected oestrogen receptor negative local recurrences [16]. RT alone has been tried in several studies. However, in patients with previously irradiated chest wall, reirradiation (ReRT) with high ReRT doses could lead to a higher risk of radiation-induced normal tissue morbidity depending on the organs at risk, previous dose of irradiation, total RT dose, dose/fraction and the time interval between the first and proposed ReRT.

Clinical Outcomes with Hyperthermia in Recurrent Breast Cancers

HT, being a potent radiosensitizer, has been used in various clinical studies along with RT as thermoradiotherapy (HTRT) [14]. These include both phase II single arm and phase III randomized control studies. Variable RT doses (24–60 Gy), dose/fraction (1.8–4 Gy/fr) have been explored. HT has been delivered with either microwaves or radiofrequencies (8–2450 MHz) as one to two weekly sessions (total number of sessions, mean: 6.3 ± 2.7) with variable sequences of HT and RT (both before and after RT), based on the institutional protocols and availability of HT equipment. An average temperature of 42.5 °C was attained with HT of 30–90 min duration.

Oldenberg et al. [17] recently reported the efficacy of ReRT with HT in 196 patients of unresectable locoregional recurrent breast cancer en cuirasse who had received a prior RT of 50 Gy. ReRT was delivered as 8 fractions of 4 Gy each or 12 fractions of 3 Gy each along with locoregional HT once or twice a week. An overall clinical response of 72% with a CR of 30% was reported.

A meta-analysis evaluated the efficacy of HTRT over RT alone in recurrent breast cancers [14]. This included 34 studies of which eight were 2-arm comparative trials (n = 627 patients) while 26 pertained to single arm studies (n = 1483 patients). In the 2-arm studies, a CR of 60.2% vs. 38.1% was evident with HTRT vs. RT alone (odds ratio: 2.64, p < 0.001). The risk difference in favour of HTRT was 0.22 (p < 0.001) (Figure 2). In the 26 single arm studies, 63.4% attained CR with HTRT. Further, even in 779 patients who had been previously irradiated, a 66.6% CR was documented with a mean ReRT dose of 36.7 Gy (SD: ±7.7 Gy). Mean acute and late grade III/IV toxicities were reported as 14.4% and 5.2%, respectively.

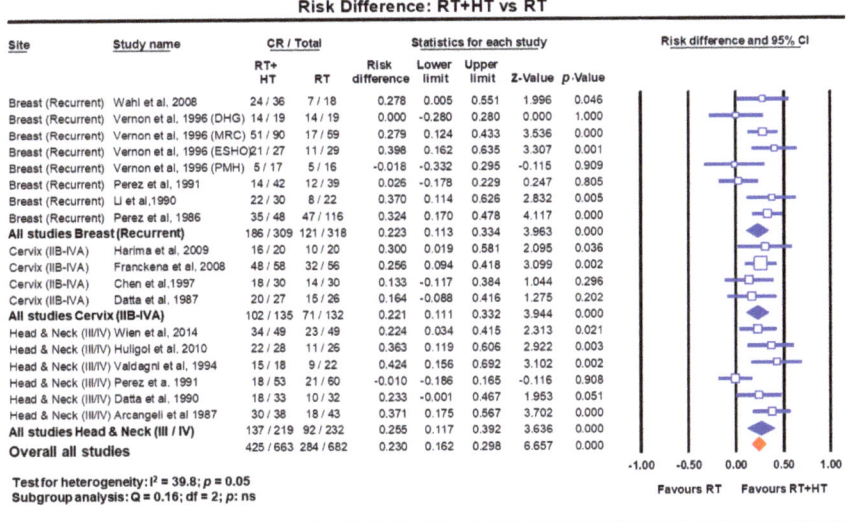

Figure 2. Forest plots depicting the risk difference for complete response with radiotherapy (RT) with hyperthermia (HT) versus RT alone in recurrent breast cancers, locally advanced cervical cancer (stages IIB-IVA) and locally advanced head and neck cancers (stages III/IV). Data extracted from Datta et al. [14,18,19] and replotted. Addition of hyperthermia to radiotherapy favours the outcome compared to radiotherapy alone in all sites with a risk difference of 23% (p < 0.001). (Q test: test for heterogeneity; df: degree of freedom and ns: not significant). For citations of the studies listed, please refer to [14,18,19].

Thus, based on the randomized studies and meta-analysis, HT along with RT appears to be an effective and safe palliative modality in recurrent breast cancers. One could expect a CR with HTRT in nearly two-third of the patients. This is around 22% higher than that with RT alone.

In line with the evidence of role of HT along with RT in recurrent breast cancers, this could be also extended to recurrent tumours of head and neck, cervix and other sites, especially those which have been preirradiated. As seen in recurrent breast tumours, a moderate dose of RT along with a few fractions of HT could be systematically investigated for recurrent tumours in other sites.

4. Locally Advanced Cervical Cancer: Scope for Improvement with Hyperthermia

Of all the cervical cancer reported globally in 2020, LMICs account for 88.1% of all cases and 91.4% of all mortalities [1] (Figure 1, Table 1). Thus, the %mortality/incidence in LMICs is estimated at 58.7%. This could be attributed to presentation in most patients in LMICs as locally advanced cervical cancer (LACC). Following the National Cancer Institute guidelines in 1992 [20], chemoradiotherapy (CTRT) using cisplatin as single or in combination is the most common therapeutic intervention in LACC. In a meta-analysis from 14 randomized clinical trials which included 2445 patients, CTRT has been shown to improve the CR (+10.2%, $p = 0.027$), locoregional control (+8.4%, $p < 0.001$) and overall survival (+7.5%, $p < 0.001$) over RT alone [21]. Thus, even though CTRT has shown to improve outcomes over RT alone, it appears that there could still be scope to explore for a possible improvement.

Clinical Outcomes with Hyperthermia in Locally Advanced Cervical Cancer

HT has also been used along with RT in several randomized clinical trials in LACC. The outcomes as evident on meta-analysis between HTRT vs. RT, shows a distinct improvement with HTRT in terms of CR at the end of treatment and loco-regional control of 22% ($p < 0.001$) and 23% ($p < 0.001$), respectively (Figure 3) [18]. A non-significant survival advantage of 8.4% with HTRT was also noted without any significant escalation of acute or late morbidities with HT added to RT. Even when HT was used with CTRT, the risk difference from three randomized clinical trials (total patients = 738) for local control and overall survival showed an advantage with HTCTRT over CTRT by 10.1% ($p = 0.03$) and 5.6% (p: ns), respectively [22,23] (Figure 3).

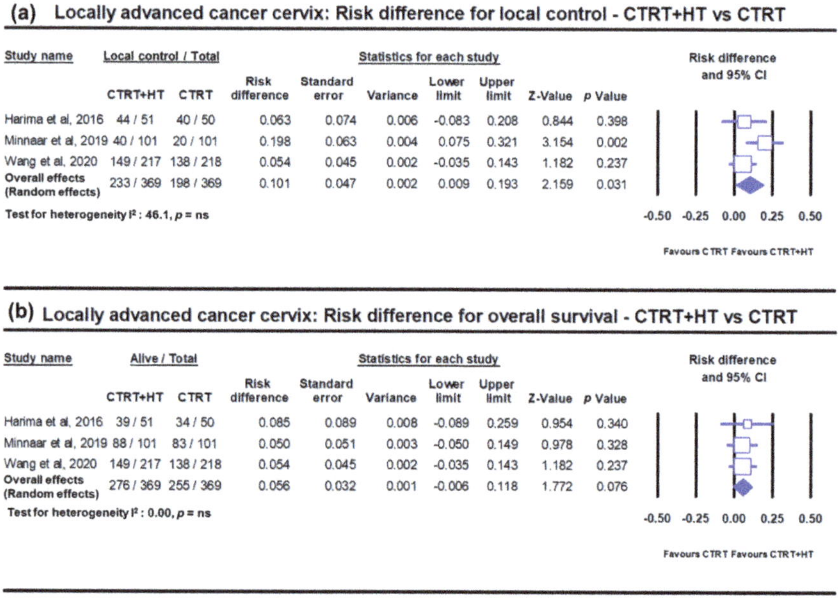

(a) Locally advanced cancer cervix: Risk difference for local control - CTRT+HT vs CTRT

Study name	Local control / Total		Risk difference	Standard error	Variance	Lower limit	Upper limit	Z-Value	p Value
	CTRT+HT	CTRT							
Harima et al, 2016	44 / 51	40 / 50	0.063	0.074	0.006	−0.083	0.208	0.844	0.398
Minnaar et al, 2019	40 / 101	20 / 101	0.198	0.063	0.004	0.075	0.321	3.154	0.002
Wang et al, 2020	149 / 217	138 / 218	0.054	0.045	0.002	−0.035	0.143	1.182	0.237
Overall effects (Random effects)	233 / 369	198 / 369	0.101	0.047	0.002	0.009	0.193	2.159	0.031

Test for heterogeneity I² : 46.1, p = ns

Favours CTRT   Favours CTRT+HT

(b) Locally advanced cancer cervix: Risk difference for overall survival - CTRT+HT vs CTRT

Study name	Alive / Total		Risk difference	Standard error	Variance	Lower limit	Upper limit	Z-Value	p Value
	CTRT+HT	CTRT							
Harima et al, 2016	39 / 51	34 / 50	0.085	0.089	0.008	−0.089	0.259	0.954	0.340
Minnaar et al, 2019	88 / 101	83 / 101	0.050	0.051	0.003	−0.050	0.149	0.978	0.328
Wang et al, 2020	149 / 217	138 / 218	0.054	0.045	0.002	−0.035	0.143	1.182	0.237
Overall effects (Random effects)	276 / 369	255 / 369	0.056	0.032	0.001	−0.006	0.118	1.772	0.076

Test for heterogeneity I² : 0.00, p = ns

Favours CTRT   Favours CTRT+HT

Figure 3. Forest plots depicting the risk difference in locally advanced cancer cervix for (**a**) local disease control and (**b**) overall survival with chemoradiotherapy (CTRT) with hyperthermia (HT) versus CTRT alone. Data from Minnaar et al. [23] has been added to the meta-analysis from Yea et al. [22] and replotted. The risk difference for local failure with HT added to CTRT reduces by 10.1% ($p = 0.03$) while the overall survival improves by 5.6% ($p = 0.07$). (ns: not significant). For citations of the studies listed, please refer to [22,23].

Network meta-analysis, which provides the highest level of clinical evidence, was reported in LACC, in which all the 13 different therapeutic approaches were evaluated from 49 clinical trials totalling 9894 patients [24]. The surface under cumulative ranking curve (SUCRA) estimates provide an objective assessment and ranking of the locoregional control, overall survival, acute and late morbidity. The SUCRA values ranked all the 13 different strategies used in randomized clinical trial settings. Incidentally, the top two approaches evident on SUCRA values were HTRT and HTCTRT in LACC (Figure 4).

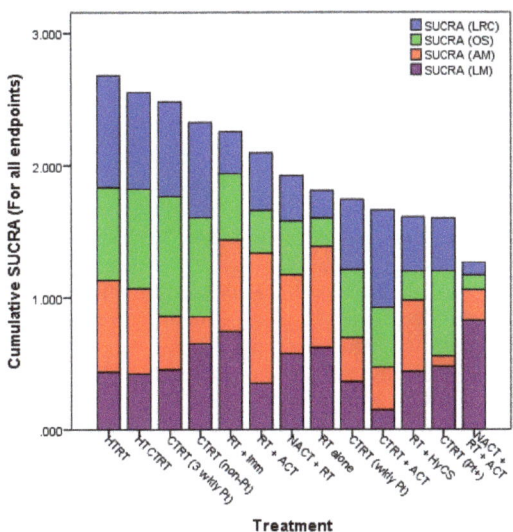

Figure 4. Surface under the cumulative ranking curve (SUCRA) values for endpoints from all studies (1974–2018) in locally advanced cancer cervix. LRC = loco-regional control; OS = overall survival; AM = acute morbidity (grade ≥ 3); LM = late morbidity (grade ≥ 3) (Reproduced with permission from Datta et al. [24]).

Thus, based on the highest levels of clinical evidence obtained through both conventional pairwise and network meta-analysis, HT with either RT or CTRT appears to provide a superior therapeutic benefit even when compared to the standard practice of CTRT in LACC. Moreover, HT has been shown to be safe with no significant additional acute or late morbidity to RT or CTRT. It would therefore be pertinent to incorporate HT in the routine clinical management of LACC along with RT or CTRT. This may help to mitigate the high %mortality/incidence seen in cervical cancer in LMICs.

5. Locally Advanced Head and Neck Cancers: Scope of Improvement with Hyperthermia

In 2020, 71.8% and 81.5% of all global incidence and mortalities in head and neck cancers were reported in the LMICs [1]. The %mortality/incidence in LMICs for these cancers are estimated at 38.2% (Figure 1, Table 1). As in the cervix, most patients present as locally advanced head and neck cancers (LAHNC), CTRT has been the mainstay of their treatment. CTRT has been shown to improve outcomes in successive reports of the Meta-analysis of Chemotherapy in Head and Neck (MACH-NC) collaborative group. In their latest update of 107 randomized trials with 19,085 patients published in 2021, a 6.5% absolute benefit at 5 years was demonstrated (hazard ratio: 0.83; 95% CI: 0.79–0.86) [25]. However, this benefit reduced with increasing patient age and poor performance status.

Clinical Outcomes with Hyperthermia in Locally Advanced Head and Neck Cancer

In LMICs, patients with LAHNC are often in poor performance status due to inadequate nutritional intake. This could have a bearing on the outcomes with CTRT. HT has been used with RT and outcomes compared with RT alone. In a meta-analysis of six clinical trials comprising 451 cases of LAHNC, HTRT improved the overall CR by 25.5% over RT alone ($p < 0.0001$) [19] (Figure 2). Acute and late morbidities appear similar.

The positive outcomes of HTCTRT in LACC, which also share a similar histology with LAHNC, should encourage patients to be recruited for phase III randomized trial with HTCTRT vs. CTRT alone. However, one of limitations could be lack of a proper HT unit for head and neck region that would allow adequate heating and monitoring of HT during individual treatment session. A dedicated HT delivery system working at 433 MHz–the HYPERCollar (Sensius, Rotterdam, The Netherlands) fills in the long-standing gap for a site-specific HT for LAHNC [26–32]. The system initially had 12 antennas, which was later upgraded to 20 antennas. Presently, an MR-compatible version of this applicator is being used within a 1.5 T MR system. This would allow online monitoring of the temperature using non-invasive thermometry with the proton resonance frequency shift method [33,34]. In addition, model-based and other new MR-thermometry temperature reconstruction methods are emerging which are quite promising [35–37]. The unit is currently being validated in clinics for HT delivery in head and neck regions [38].

Thus, LAHNC provides yet another common site in which HT, along with RT or CTRT, could be expected to improve therapeutic outcomes without any significant added toxicities. It is therefore highly desirable that HT should be evaluated systematically in LAHNC. As LMICs harbour more than two-thirds of global head and neck cancers, these patients need to be included in single/multicentric clinical trials for evaluating HTCTRT vs. CTRT alone.

6. Setting Up a Hyperthermia Treatment Facility in Low-Middle-Income Countries

6.1. Choice of Hyperthermia Unit for LMICs

Local HT treatments could be delivered by a host of methods—external HT (radiative or capacitive), local invasive (intraluminal and interstitial), regional perfusion or water-filtered infra-red [7,39]. Clinical HT is usually delivered using radiofrequency (radiative or capacitive), microwaves (434–915 MHz), ultrasound or infrared (>300 GHz) devices. A detailed technical description of each of these methods is beyond the scope of this manuscript. Readers may like to refer to the European Society for Hyperthermia Oncology (ESHO) guidelines that also gives a detailed descriptions of these devices for use in clinics [40–43]. However, due to different heating patterns in depth, the choice of equipment, especially in a resource constraint situation, should preferably be based on the type of common tumours prevalent in the geographical area to be catered by the institution. Even the instrument design and the choice of frequencies of the radiative or capitative systems would need to be selected based on the tumour site and its depth that would be commonly treated by a centre [44]. In addition, the availability of trained personnel for HT treatment delivery, thermometry systems for online temperature monitoring, and the resources allocated, need to be considered before planning to set up such a facility. Presently, HT is not available in most LMICs, and therefore, all these factors would have to be carefully weighed before one launches into such a programme.

Radiofrequency capacitive systems operating at 27.1 MHz are cheap and are commonly used in most of the physiotherapy centres in LMICs as a short-wave diathermy. These units are based on plane-wave matching, in which the antenna's plane-parallel plates are tuned as per the standard antenna-tuning method [45]. The target tissue placed between the condenser plates act as a capacitor to store electrical charge, resulting in local heating of the tissue. Heat is induced by the resulting currents and is directed toward the smallest electrode [44,46]. Capacitive heating creates high power densities around the bolus edges, but one needs to be careful due to its preferential heating in the subcutaneous fat layer. This may be of special relevance to obese patients with considerable subcutaneous fat.

Thus, these units need a circulatory water bolus to have adequate skin cooling. The operation of the unit is relatively simple and technical staff can be easily trained on these units compared to the other state-of-the-art commercially available HT units that are based on radiative/microwave technologies, some of which could also be compatible with MRI thermometry. However, fibreoptic single or multi-sensor radiofrequency immune thermometry probes or thermocouples are required for continuous temperature monitoring. Additional components for thermal simulation and treatment planning supported by quality assurance needs to be introduced for a better temperature assessment in the heated volumes. It should be reasonably feasible to treat the common tumour sites in LMICs–LAHNC, LABC and LACC using 27.1 MHz, after incorporating a circulatory water bolus for surface skin cooling and thermometry for temperature monitoring. However, the 27.1 MHz capacitive heating device would not allow non-invasive thermometry as feasible with some of the MR-compatible versions of HT delivery currently available commercially (HYPERCollar from Sensius and BSD-2000 3D/MR from Pyrexar Medical, Salt Lake City, UT, USA).

Capacitive heating using 27.1 MHz radiofrequency has been used clinically for HT in some clinical studies [12,47] with satisfactory outcomes. As discussed earlier, the recently reported randomized phase III trial NACT + HT vs. HT in stages IIA-IIIB was conducted using 27.1 MHz in 200 patients [12]. This had resulted in a significant favourable outcome for patients treated with NACT + HT in terms of the objective response rate, the proportion of women eligible for breast-conserving and reconstructive surgery and the 10-year overall survival rates compared with NACT alone. The objective response at the primary site was reported to be higher by 15.9% with HT + NACT compared to NACT alone ($p = 0.034$). Correspondingly in the lymph nodes, the response was higher by 14.1% ($p = 0.011$). Computer-assisted planning helped to select a personalized distribution of the magnetic, electric and thermal fields generated by the unit.

6.2. Cost Computations and Its Implications for a Hyperthermia Setup in LMICs

HT units cost a fraction of the RT units and is a one-time investment with minimal recurring costs. These usually have a working life of 10 years. Unlike RT, the daily patient throughput is lower as each treatment may take around 90 min. In an 8 h working day, four to five patients can be treated/day/unit, that is, 20–25 patients/week, as HT is usually delivered once or twice a week. Thus, 170–325 patients/year could be treated with HT, if delivered once a week for 4–6 weeks. This may go down to 85–162 patients, if twice a week HT treatment scheduled is adopted by a department [3].

Thus, a centre may need to compute the break-even point (BEP) and % return on investment (%ROI) following capital investment to set up a HT facility. Assuming, the capital cost to set up a HT unit is "C" USD, number of patients treated with HT per year as "N" and user cost as "U" USD, the BEP would be

$$\text{BEP} = \frac{C}{NU} \text{ (in years)}. \tag{1}$$

Assuming that the HT unit has a working life of 10 years, the income generated in the post-BEP period would be estimated as,

$$\text{Income generated in the post} - \text{BEP period} = \left(10 - \frac{C}{NU}\right) \times NU. \tag{2}$$

Thus,

$$\% \text{ ROI} = \frac{\text{Income generated in the post} - \text{BEP period} - \text{Cost of investment}}{\text{Cost of investment}} \times 100 = \frac{10NU - 2C}{C} \times 100. \tag{3}$$

Using the above expressions, any department in any country can work out the optimal BEP and %ROI based on the planned capital investment, number of patients estimated to be treated per year and the user cost. The investment for HT unit could vary and depend on the availability of resources–both financial and human. The corresponding returns would hinge on the patient load, treatment charges, working schedule and departmental policy of weekly or biweekly HT treatments. Cost computations and the %returns on investment (%ROI) need to be computed by individual countries, taking into consideration the above factors, as this may vary from country to country. A cost of EUR 6800 was computed for a series of five treatments in the Dutch Deep Hyperthermia Trial, of which half of the amount was for personnel and one-third for equipment [7]. This is likely to be much lower in LMICs and hence higher returns could be expected. HT could contribute to just a minimal fraction of the cost to the primary treatment in comparison to most standard CT regimes and also immunotherapies, which are being increasingly advocated in many tumour sites. This would not only help to bring down the treatment cost, but also make it more affordable, tolerable and by virtue of improving the therapeutic outcomes, could also improve the quality of life with least morbidity.

7. Conclusions

Apart from being a cost-effective option, HT provides several tangible and nontangible gains and should be explored in LMICs. The tangible gains would comprise cost of treatment, cost efficacy, response rates, survival, etc. while the nontangible would be more subjective and include wellbeing of the patients, reporting back to work early, supporting their families, etc. It is perhaps time to integrate HT in the therapeutic management of cancers, especially the locally advanced and recurrent tumours as seen in LMICs. Though the efficacy of HT has been discussed in three specific sites of LAHNC, LACC, LABC and recurrent breast cancers which are common in LMICs, the benefit of HT with RT ± CT has been documented in various sites, namely superficial tumours, melanoma, choroidal melanoma, brain tumours, malignant germ cell tumours, soft tissue sarcoma, bone metastases, oesophagus, lung, pancreas, urinary bladder, prostate, rectum, anus and others [3,4,48–50]. Clinical evidence indicates a steady benefit of integrating HT with the standard treatments in most sites.

Thus, based on the above thermoradiobiological rationale and clinical evidence, HT could certainly prove to be a "potential game-changer" when integrated in the therapeutic strategies for various malignancies, especially those with locally advanced tumours as prevalent in LMICs. HT is a cost-effective and a unique multifaceted treatment modality and deserves to be incorporated in the present-day clinical oncology practice and management.

Author Contributions: Conceptualization—N.R.D.; methodology—N.R.D., B.M.J., Z.M., S.J. and V.S.; data analysis—N.R.D. and S.D.; writing—original draft preparation, N.R.D., B.M.J., A.R.S., P.K. (Pallavi Kalbande), S.D. and V.S.; review and editing, N.R.D., B.M.J., Z.M., S.D., S.J., A.R.S., P.K. (Pallavi Kalbande), P.K. (Pournima Kale), V.S. and S.B.; clinical perspective, N.R.D., B.M.J., Z.M., A.R.S., P.K. (Pallavi Kalbande), P.K. (Pournima Kale), V.S. and S.B.; supervision and funding, N.R.D. and S.B. All authors have read and agreed to the published version of the manuscript.

Funding: This research received no external funding.

Conflicts of Interest: The authors declare no conflict of interest.

References

1. Ferlay, J.; Ervik, M.; Lam, F.; Colombet, M.; Mery, L.; Piñeros, M.; Znaor, A.; Soerjomataram, I.; Bray, F. Global cancer observatory: Cancer Today. In *Book Global Cancer Observatory: Cancer Today*; International Agency for Research on Cancer: Lyon, France, 2020.
2. Sankaranarayanan, R.; Swaminathan, R.; Jayant, K.; Brenner, H. An overview of cancer survival in Africa, Asia, Caribbean and Central America. In *Cancer Survival in Africa, Asia, the Caribbean and Central America*; Sankaranarayanan, R., Swaminathan, R., Lucas, E., Eds.; IARC Scientific Publication: Lyon, France, 2011; pp. 257–291.
3. Datta, N.R.; Kok, H.P.; Crezee, H.; Gaipl, U.S.; Bodis, S. Integrating loco-regional hyperthermia into the current oncology practice: SWOT and TOWS analyses. *Front. Oncol.* **2020**, *10*, 819. [CrossRef]
4. Datta, N.R.; Ordonez, S.G.; Gaipl, U.S.; Paulides, M.M.; Crezee, H.; Gellermann, J.; Marder, D.; Puric, E.; Bodis, S. Local hyperthermia combined with radiotherapy and-/or chemotherapy: Recent advances and promises for the future. *Cancer Treat. Rev.* **2015**, *41*, 742–753. [CrossRef]

5. Frey, B.; Weiss, E.M.; Rubner, Y.; Wunderlich, R.; Ott, O.J.; Sauer, R.; Fietkau, R.; Gaipl, U.S. Old and new facts about hyperthermia-induced modulations of the immune system. *Int. J. Hyperth.* **2012**, *28*, 528–542. [CrossRef] [PubMed]
6. Datta, N.R.; Bodis, S. Hyperthermia with photon radiotherapy is thermo-radiobiologically analogous to neutrons for tumours without enhanced normal tissue toxicity. *Int. J. Hyperth.* **2019**, *36*, 1073–1078. [CrossRef] [PubMed]
7. Van der Zee, J.; Vujaskovic, Z.; Kondo, M.; Sugahara, T. The Kadota Fund International Forum 2004–clinical group consensus. *Int. J. Hyperth.* **2008**, *24*, 111–122. [CrossRef] [PubMed]
8. Van Rhoon, G.C. Is CEM43 still a relevant thermal dose parameter for hyperthermia treatment monitoring? *Int. J. Hyperth.* **2016**, *32*, 50–62. [CrossRef]
9. Issels, R.D. Hyperthermia adds to chemotherapy. *Eur. J. Cancer* **2008**, *44*, 2546–2554. [CrossRef]
10. Issels, R. Hyperthermia combined with chemotherapy—Biological rationale, clinical application, and treatment results. *Oncol. Res. Treat.* **1999**, *22*, 374–381. [CrossRef]
11. Oei, A.L.; Vriend, L.E.; Crezee, J.; Franken, N.A.; Krawczyk, P.M. Effects of hyperthermia on DNA repair pathways: One treatment to inhibit them all. *Radiat. Oncol.* **2015**, *10*, 165. [CrossRef] [PubMed]
12. Loboda, A.; Smolanka, I., Sr.; Orel, V.E.; Syvak, L.; Golovko, T.; Dosenko, I.; Lyashenko, A.; Smolanka, I., Jr.; Dasyukevich, O.; Tarasenko, T.; et al. Efficacy of combination neoadjuvant chemotherapy and regional inductive moderate hyperthermia in the treatment of patients With locally advanced breast cancer. *Technol. Cancer Res. Treat.* **2020**, *19*, 1533033820963599. [CrossRef] [PubMed]
13. Vujaskovic, Z.; Kim, D.W.; Jones, E.; Lan, L.; McCall, L.; Dewhirst, M.W.; Craciunescu, O.; Stauffer, P.; Liotcheva, V.; Betof, A.; et al. A phase I/II study of neoadjuvant liposomal doxorubicin, paclitaxel, and hyperthermia in locally advanced breast cancer. *Int. J. Hyperth.* **2010**, *26*, 514–521. [CrossRef] [PubMed]
14. Datta, N.R.; Puric, E.; Klingbiel, D.; Gomez, S.; Bodis, S. Hyperthermia and radiation therapy in locoregional recurrent breast cancers: A systematic review and meta-analysis. *Int. J. Radiat. Oncol. Biol. Phys.* **2016**, *94*, 1073–1087. [CrossRef] [PubMed]
15. Rauschecker, H.; Clarke, M.; Gatzemeier, W.; Recht, A. Systemic therapy for treating locoregional recurrence in women with breast cancer. *Cochrane Database Syst. Rev.* **2001**, *2021*, CD002195. [CrossRef]
16. Wapnir, I.L.; Price, K.N.; Anderson, S.J.; Robidoux, A.; Martín, M.; Nortier, J.W.R.; Paterson, A.H.G.; Rimawi, M.F.; Láng, I.; Baena-Cañada, J.M.; et al. Efficacy of chemotherapy for ER-negative and ER-positive isolated locoregional recurrence of breast cancer: Final analysis of the CALOR trial. *J. Clin. Oncol.* **2018**, *36*, 1073–1079. [CrossRef] [PubMed]
17. Oldenborg, S.; Rasch, C.R.N.; van Os, R.; Kusumanto, Y.H.; Oei, B.S.; Venselaar, J.L.; Heymans, M.W.; Zum Vörde Sive Vörding, P.J.; Crezee, H.; van Tienhoven, G. Reirradiation + hyperthermia for recurrent breast cancer en cuirasse. *Strahlenther. Onkol.* **2018**, *194*, 206–214. [CrossRef] [PubMed]
18. Datta, N.R.; Rogers, S.; Klingbiel, D.; Gomez, S.; Puric, E.; Bodis, S. Hyperthermia and radiotherapy with or without chemotherapy in locally advanced cervical cancer: A systematic review with conventional and network meta-analyses. *Int. J. Hyperth.* **2016**, *32*, 809–821. [CrossRef] [PubMed]
19. Datta, N.R.; Rogers, S.; Ordonez, S.G.; Puric, E.; Bodis, S. Hyperthermia and radiotherapy in the management of head and neck cancers: A systematic review and meta-analysis. *Int. J. Hyperth.* **2016**, *32*, 31–40. [CrossRef]
20. National Institute of Health; National Cancer Institute (NCI). NCI Issues Clinical Announcement on Cervical Cancer: Chemotherapy Plus Radiation Improves Survival. Chemotherapy Plus Radiation Improves Survival, 1999. Published 1999. Available online: http://www3.scienceblog.com/community/older/archives/B/nih478.html (accessed on 15 December 2017).
21. Datta, N.R.; Stutz, E.; Liu, M.; Rogers, S.; Klingbiel, D.; Siebenhuner, A.; Singh, S.; Bodis, S. Concurrent chemoradiotherapy vs. radiotherapy alone in locally advanced cervix cancer: A systematic review and meta-analysis. *Gynecol. Oncol.* **2017**, *145*, 374–385. [CrossRef] [PubMed]
22. Yea, J.W.; Park, J.W.; Oh, S.A.; Park, J. Chemoradiotherapy with hyperthermia versus chemoradiotherapy alone in locally advanced cervical cancer: A systematic review and meta-analysis. *Int. J. Hyperth.* **2021**, *38*, 1333–1340. [CrossRef]
23. Minnaar, C.A.; Kotzen, J.A.; Ayeni, O.A.; Naidoo, T.; Tunmer, M.; Sharma, V.; Vangu, M.D.; Baeyens, A. The effect of modulated electro-hyperthermia on local disease control in HIV-positive and -negative cervical cancer women in South Africa: Early results from a phase III randomised controlled trial. *PLoS ONE* **2019**, *14*, e0217894. [CrossRef]
24. Datta, N.R.; Stutz, E.; Gomez, S.; Bodis, S. Efficacy and safety evaluation of the various therapeutic options in locally advanced cervix cancer: A systematic review and network meta-analysis of randomized clinical trials. *Int. J. Radiat. Oncol. Biol. Phys.* **2019**, *103*, 411–437. [CrossRef]
25. Lacas, B.; Carmel, A.; Landais, C.; Wong, S.J.; Licitra, L.; Tobias, J.S.; Burtness, B.; Ghi, M.G.; Cohen, E.E.W.; Grau, C.; et al. Meta-analysis of chemotherapy in head and neck cancer (MACH-NC): An update on 107 randomized trials and 19,805 patients, on behalf of MACH-NC Group. *Radiother. Oncol.* **2021**, *156*, 281–293. [CrossRef]
26. Paulides, M.M.; Bakker, J.F.; Neufeld, E.; van der Zee, J.; Jansen, P.P.; Levendag, P.C.; van Rhoon, G.C. The HYPERcollar: A novel applicator for hyperthermia in the head and neck. *Int. J. Hyperth.* **2007**, *23*, 567–576. [CrossRef] [PubMed]
27. Paulides, M.M.; Bakker, J.F.; Zwamborn, A.P.; Van Rhoon, G.C. A head and neck hyperthermia applicator: Theoretical antenna array design. *Int. J. Hyperth.* **2007**, *23*, 59–67. [CrossRef] [PubMed]
28. Paulides, M.M.; Dobsicek Trefna, H.; Curto, S.; Rodrigues, D.B. Recent technological advancements in radiofrequency- and microwave-mediated hyperthermia for enhancing drug delivery. *Adv. Drug Deliv. Rev.* **2020**, *163*, 3–18. [CrossRef] [PubMed]

29. Paulides, M.M.; Verduijn, G.M.; Van Holthe, N. Status quo and directions in deep head and neck hyperthermia. *Radiat. Oncol.* **2016**, *11*, 21. [CrossRef] [PubMed]
30. Drizdal, T.; Paulides, M.M.; van Holthe, N.; van Rhoon, G.C. Hyperthermia treatment planning guided applicator selection for sub-superficial head and neck tumors heating. *Int. J. Hyperth.* **2018**, *34*, 704–713. [CrossRef]
31. Verduijn, G.M.; de Wee, E.M.; Rijnen, Z.; Togni, P.; Hardillo, J.A.U.; Ten Hove, I.; Franckena, M.; van Rhoon, G.C.; Paulides, M.M. Deep hyperthermia with the HYPERcollar system combined with irradiation for advanced head and neck carcinoma—A feasibility study. *Int. J. Hyperth.* **2018**, *34*, 994–1001. [CrossRef]
32. Verhaart, R.F.; Rijnen, Z.; Fortunati, V.; Verduijn, G.M.; van Walsum, T.; Veenland, J.F.; Paulides, M.M. Temperature simulations in hyperthermia treatment planning of the head and neck region: Rigorous optimization of tissue properties. *Strahlenther. Onkol.* **2014**, *190*, 1117–1124. [CrossRef]
33. Gellermann, J.; Hildebrandt, B.; Issels, R.; Ganter, H.; Wlodarczyk, W.; Budach, V.; Felix, R.; Tunn, P.U.; Reichardt, P.; Wust, P. Noninvasive magnetic resonance thermography of soft tissue sarcomas during regional hyperthermia: Correlation with response and direct thermometry. *Cancer* **2006**, *107*, 1373–1382. [CrossRef]
34. Craciunescu, O.I.; Stauffer, P.R.; Soher, B.J.; Wyatt, C.R.; Arabe, O.; Maccarini, P.; Das, S.K.; Cheng, K.S.; Wong, T.Z.; Jones, E.L.; et al. Accuracy of real time noninvasive temperature measurements using magnetic resonance thermal imaging in patients treated for high grade extremity soft tissue sarcomas. *Med. Phys.* **2009**, *36*, 4848–4858. [CrossRef] [PubMed]
35. Poorman, M.E.; Braskute, I.; Bartels, L.W.; Grissom, W.A. Multi-echo MR thermometry using iterative separation of baseline water and fat images. *Magn. Reson. Med.* **2019**, *81*, 2385–2398. [CrossRef] [PubMed]
36. Zhang, L.; Armstrong, T.; Li, X.; Wu, H.H. A variable flip angle golden-angle-ordered 3D stack-of-radial MRI technique for simultaneous proton resonant frequency shift and T1-based thermometry. *Magn. Reson. Med.* **2019**, *82*, 2062–2076. [CrossRef]
37. Tan, J.; Mougenot, C.; Pichardo, S.; Drake, J.M.; Waspe, A.C. Motion compensation using principal component analysis and projection onto dipole fields for abdominal magnetic resonance thermometry. *Magn. Reson. Med.* **2019**, *81*, 195–207. [CrossRef]
38. Sumser, K.; Drizdal, T.; Bellizzi, G.G.; Hernandez-Tamames, J.A.; van Rhoon, G.C.; Paulides, M.M. Experimental validation of the MRcollar: An MR compatible applicator for deep heating in the head and neck region. *Cancers* **2021**, *13*, 5617. [CrossRef]
39. Notter, M.; Piazena, H.; Vaupel, P. Hypofractionated re-irradiation of large-sized recurrent breast cancer with thermography-controlled, contact-free water-filtered infra-red-A hyperthermia: A retrospective study of 73 patients. *Int. J. Hyperth.* **2017**, *33*, 227–236. [CrossRef]
40. Trefna, H.D.; Crezee, H.; Schmidt, M.; Marder, D.; Lamprecht, U.; Ehmann, M.; Hartmann, J.; Nadobny, J.; Gellermann, J.; van Holthe, N.; et al. Quality assurance guidelines for superficial hyperthermia clinical trials: I. clinical requirements. *Int. J. Hyperth.* **2017**, *33*, 471–482. [CrossRef] [PubMed]
41. Trefna, H.D.; Crezee, J.; Schmidt, M.; Marder, D.; Lamprecht, U.; Ehmann, M.; Nadobny, J.; Hartmann, J.; Lomax, N.; Abdel-Rahman, S.; et al. Quality assurance guidelines for superficial hyperthermia clinical trials: II. technical requirements for heating devices. *Strahlenther. Onkol.* **2017**, *193*, 351–366. [CrossRef]
42. Lagendijk, J.J.; Van Rhoon, G.C.; Hornsleth, S.N.; Wust, P.; De Leeuw, A.C.; Schneider, C.J.; Van Dijk, J.D.; Van Der Zee, J.; Van Heek-Romanowski, R.; Rahman, S.A.; et al. ESHO quality assurance guidelines for regional hyperthermia. *Int. J. Hyperth.* **1998**, *14*, 125–133. [CrossRef]
43. Bruggmoser, G.; Bauchowitz, S.; Canters, R.; Crezee, H.; Ehmann, M.; Gellermann, J.; Lamprecht, U.; Lomax, N.; Messmer, M.B.; Ott, O.; et al. Quality assurance for clinical studies in regional deep hyperthermia. *Strahlenther. Onkol.* **2011**, *187*, 605–610. [CrossRef] [PubMed]
44. Kok, H.P.; Crezee, J. A comparison of the heating characteristics of capacitive and radiative superficial hyperthermia. *Int. J. Hyperth.* **2017**, *33*, 378–386. [CrossRef] [PubMed]
45. Szasz, A. The capacitative coupling modalities for oncological hyperthermia. *Open J. Biophys.* **2021**, *11*, 252–313. [CrossRef]
46. Abe, M.; Hiraoka, M.; Takahashi, M.; Egawa, S.; Matsuda, C.; Onoyama, Y.; Morita, K.; Kakehi, M.; Sugahara, T. Multi-institutional studies on hyperthermia using an 8-MHz radiofrequency capacitive heating device (Thermotron RF-8) in combination with radiation for cancer therapy. *Cancer* **1986**, *58*, 1589–1595. [CrossRef]
47. Reddy, N.M.; Maithreyan, V.; Vasanthan, A.; Balakrishnan, I.S.; Bhaskar, B.K.; Jayaraman, R.; Shanta, V.; Krishnamurthi, S. Local RF capacitive hyperthermia: Thermal profiles and tumour response. *Int. J. Hyperth.* **1987**, *3*, 379–387. [CrossRef]
48. Datta, N.R.; Schneider, R.; Puric, E.; Ahlhelm, F.J.; Marder, D.; Bodis, S.; Weber, D.C. Proton irradiation with hyperthermia in unresectable soft tissue sarcoma. *Int. J. Part. Ther.* **2016**, *3*, 327–336. [CrossRef]
49. Datta, N.R.; Stutz, E.; Puric, E.; Eberle, B.; Meister, A.; Marder, D.; Timm, O.; Rogers, S.; Wyler, S.; Bodis, S. A pilot study of radiotherapy and local hyperthermia in elderly patients with muscle-invasive bladder cancers unfit for definitive surgery or chemoradiotherapy. *Front. Oncol.* **2019**, *9*, 889. [CrossRef] [PubMed]
50. Rogers, S.J.; Datta, N.R.; Puric, E.; Timm, O.; Marder, D.; Khan, S.; Mamot, C.; Knuchel, J.; Siebenhuner, A.; Pestalozzi, B.; et al. The addition of deep hyperthermia to gemcitabine-based chemoradiation may achieve enhanced survival in unresectable locally advanced adenocarcinoma of the pancreas. *Clin. Transl. Radiat. Oncol.* **2021**, *27*, 109–113. [CrossRef]

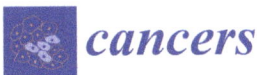

Review

Clinical Evidence for Thermometric Parameters to Guide Hyperthermia Treatment

Adela Ademaj [1,2], Danai P. Veltsista [3], Pirus Ghadjar [3], Dietmar Marder [1], Eva Oberacker [3], Oliver J. Ott [4,5], Peter Wust [3], Emsad Puric [1], Roger A. Hälg [1,6], Susanne Rogers [1], Stephan Bodis [1,7], Rainer Fietkau [4,5], Hans Crezee [8] and Oliver Riesterer [1,*]

1. Center for Radiation Oncology KSA-KSB, Cantonal Hospital Aarau, 5001 Aarau, Switzerland; adela.ademaj@ksa.ch (A.A.); dietmar.marder@ksa.ch (D.M.); emsad.puric@ksa.ch (E.P.); roger.haelg@ksa.ch (R.A.H.); susanne.rogers@ksa.ch (S.R.); s.bodis@bluewin.ch (S.B.)
2. Doctoral Clinical Science Program, Medical Faculty, University of Zurich, 8032 Zürich, Switzerland
3. Department Radiation Oncology, Charité-Universitätsmedizin Berlin, Corporate Member of Freie Universität Berlin and Humboldt-Universität zu Berlin, 13353 Berlin, Germany; paraskevi-danai.veltsista@charite.de (D.P.V.); pirus.ghadjar@charite.de (P.G.); eva.oberacker@charite.de (E.O.); peter.wust@charite.de (P.W.)
4. Department of Radiation Oncology, Universitätsklinikum Erlangen, 91054 Erlangen, Germany; oliver.ott@uk-erlangen.de (O.J.O.); rainer.fietkau@uk-erlangen.de (R.F.)
5. Comprehensive Cancer Center Erlangen-EMN, 91054 Erlangen, Germany
6. Institute of Physics, Science Faculty, University of Zurich, 8057 Zurich, Switzerland
7. Department of Radiation Oncology, University Hospital Zurich, University of Zurich, 8091 Zurich, Switzerland
8. Department of Radiation Oncology, Amsterdam UMC, University of Amsterdam, Cancer Center Amsterdam, 1105 AZ Amsterdam, The Netherlands; h.crezee@amsterdamumc.nl
* Correspondence: oliver.riesterer@ksa.ch; Tel.: +41-62838-4249

Simple Summary: Hyperthermia (HT) is a promising therapeutic option for multiple cancer entities as it has the potential to increase the cytotoxicity of radiotherapy (RT) and chemotherapy (CT). Thermometric parameters of HT are considered to have potential as predictive factors of treatment response. So far, only limited data about the prognostic and predictive role of thermometric parameters are available. In this review, we investigate the existing clinical evidence regarding the correlation of thermometric parameters and cancer response in clinical studies in which patients were treated with HT in combination with RT and/or CT. Some studies show that thermometric parameters correlate with treatment response, indicating their potential significance for treatment guidance. Thus, the establishment of specific thermometric parameters might pave the way towards a better standardization of HT treatment protocols.

Abstract: Hyperthermia (HT) is a cancer treatment modality which targets malignant tissues by heating to 40–43 °C. In addition to its direct antitumor effects, HT potently sensitizes the tumor to radiotherapy (RT) and chemotherapy (CT), thereby enabling complete eradication of some tumor entities as shown in randomized clinical trials. Despite the proven efficacy of HT in combination with classic cancer treatments, there are limited international standards for the delivery of HT in the clinical setting. Consequently, there is a large variability in reported data on thermometric parameters, including the temperature obtained from multiple reference points, heating duration, thermal dose, time interval, and sequence between HT and other treatment modalities. Evidence from some clinical trials indicates that thermal dose, which correlates with heating time and temperature achieved, could be used as a predictive marker for treatment efficacy in future studies. Similarly, other thermometric parameters when chosen optimally are associated with increased antitumor efficacy. This review summarizes the existing clinical evidence for the prognostic and predictive role of the most important thermometric parameters to guide the combined treatment of RT and CT with HT. In conclusion, we call for the standardization of thermometric parameters and stress the importance for their validation in future prospective clinical studies.

Citation: Ademaj, A.; Veltsista, D.P.; Ghadjar, P.; Marder, D.; Oberacker, E.; Ott, O.J.; Wust, P.; Puric, E.; Hälg, R.A.; Rogers, S.; et al. Clinical Evidence for Thermometric Parameters to Guide Hyperthermia Treatment. *Cancers* 2022, 14, 625. https://doi.org/10.3390/cancers14030625

Academic Editor: David Wong

Received: 30 November 2021
Accepted: 19 January 2022
Published: 26 January 2022

Publisher's Note: MDPI stays neutral with regard to jurisdictional claims in published maps and institutional affiliations.

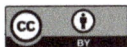

Copyright: © 2022 by the authors. Licensee MDPI, Basel, Switzerland. This article is an open access article distributed under the terms and conditions of the Creative Commons Attribution (CC BY) license (https://creativecommons.org/licenses/by/4.0/).

Keywords: hyperthermia; thermometric parameters; preclinical data; clinical evidence

1. Introduction

Hyperthermia (HT) is a clinical treatment for cancer which extraneously and intrinsically heats malignant cells to a temperature of 40–43 °C for a suitable period of time [1,2]. Heat delivered to tumor tissues can act as a cytotoxic or sensitizing agent to enhance their remission or at least regression by utilizing several biological mechanisms and pleiotropic effects when combined with other conventional cancer treatment techniques, such as radiotherapy (RT) and/or chemotherapy (CT).

The biological effects of HT, which all favor its use in combination with RT and CT, include direct cytotoxicity, radiosensitization, chemosensitization, and immune modulation. HT-induced cell lethality is predominantly a result of conformational changes and the destabilization of macromolecule structures including the disruptions in cell metabolism, inhibition of DNA repair, and triggering of cellular apoptotic pathways [3–6]. The direct HT-induced cell lethality is known to be intrinsically tumor-selective for hypoxic cells [7]. During heating, enhanced blood perfusion in tumor tissues influences the radiosensitizing and chemosensitizing effects of HT by increasing the tumor oxygenation level and local concentration of CT drugs respectively [4,8,9]. Radiosensitization and chemosensitization effects, as well as the inhibition of DNA synthesis and repair, on the molecular level depend on the aggregation of proteins produced by HT-induced denaturation [10]. Moreover, protein unfolding and the intracellular accumulation of proteins trigger molecular chaperones including the heat shock proteins (HSPs) [11]. The release of HSPs and other "immune activating signals" underly the inflammatory and immunogenic responses to HT in combination with RT and/or CT and can promote anti-tumor immunity [12–14]. Exploiting molecular and physiological mechanisms evoked by HT can improve the efficacy of RT and CT. Therefore, HT in cancer treatment is used mainly within the framework of multimodal treatment strategies [3,8].

Multiple preclinical studies have been designed to unravel the relationship between biological mechanisms induced by HT and thermometric parameters as predictors of tumor response [15–20]. The parameters investigated in these studies include the temperature achieved during HT [6,15], heating duration, thermal dose [21], time interval between HT and the other treatment modality [15,22,23], the number of HT sessions [24], and the sequence of treatment modality [15,25,26]. All of these parameters were shown to influence the extent to which HT enhances the effect of RT or CT using cellular assays and in vivo models. In addition to thermometric parameters, the treatment parameters of RT and CT, such as total radiation dose, number of RT fractions, type of chemotherapeutic drug and the number of CT cycles, prescribed for a specific clinical indication, also play a significant role in attaining a therapeutic window with synergistic effects when combined with HT [25,27,28].

The effectiveness of HT combined with RT and/or CT has been investigated in many clinical studies with different tumor types. Unfortunately, to date, there is no consensus on HT delivery when combined with these cancer treatment modalities, resulting in substantial heterogeneity of the HT treatment protocols applied. Any comparison of these studies in terms of outcome should be made with caution in view of this heterogeneity in HT protocols. A good understanding of thermometric parameters and their interpretation is mandatory in this regard. However, there is inconclusive clinical evidence about the relationship of thermometric parameters with both tumor and normal tissue responses to HT in combination with RT and/or CT. The reason for this is that thermometric parameters are inconsistently reported or analyzed in prospective clinical studies and the retrospective analyses are conflicting. For instance, minimum tumor temperature was identified as a prognostic factor in a few studies [29–31]. However, another study showed that different metrics such as temperature achieved in 90% (T_{90}), 50% (T_{50}), and 10% (T_{10}) in the target volume were more strongly correlated with cancer response than minimum achieved temperature [32]. Furthermore, a short time interval between HT and RT was shown to significantly predict treatment outcome in retrospective analyses of cervical cancer patients [22]. However, conflicting results have been also reported [33] which may be attributed to differences in time interval and tumor temperature achieved, and in patient population [34]. Thermal dose has been successfully tested in several clinical trials as a predictor of tumor response to combined RT and HT treatment [35–42]. These did not result in established thresholds for thermal dose for treating different cancer sites, even though European Society for Hyperthermic Oncology (ESHO) guidelines recommend superficial HT maintains $T_{50} \geq 41\ °C$ and $T_{90} \geq 40\ °C$ [43]. The concept of a relationship between thermometric parameters with treatment outcome is highly attractive because it could improve the understanding of tumor-specific mechanisms of interaction between HT and RT and/or CT. Defining thermometric parameters is therefore important for a meaningful clinical evaluation of HT treatment outcomes when combined with RT and/or CT.

A limited amount of clinical information is available about the effect of thermometric parameters on treatment response. Increasing awareness of the importance of such parameters on the efficacy of HT combined with other cancer treatments is important, and thus these parameters should be evaluated and reported routinely. Achieving the defined thermometric parameters during HT treatment would further increase the effectiveness of biological mechanisms when combined with RT and/or CT. Future prospective clinical studies should include description of all relevant thermometric parameters to pave the way towards the proper analysis and standardization of thermometric parameters for each clinical indication treated with HT in combination with RT and/or CT.

This work summarizes the evidence underlying thermometric parameters as predictors of treatment outcomes as reported in clinical studies using HT in combination with RT and/or CT for treating different cancer types and emphasizes the need for reference thermometric parameters to improve HT efficacy. For completeness, the findings pertaining to thermometric parameters from preclinical studies are also discussed, to provide comprehensive information about their significance and underlying mechanisms.

2. Materials and Methods

2.1. Data Sources and Search Strategies

The literature search included databases of clinicaltrials.gov and pubmed.ncbi.nlm.nih.gov from March to September 2021 and randomized prospective and retrospective clinical studies with specific criteria were identified. The search terms were hyperthermia, cancer treatment, randomized clinical studies, prospective clinical studies, and retrospective clinical studies. Those terms were used mainly to search for the title and abstract. We also found articles which were recommended, suggested, or sent to us on the internet. Additionally, we handsearched the reference lists of the most relevant clinical studies and review articles.

2.2. Inclusion and Exclusion Criteria of Clinical Studies

This non-systematic review included randomized, prospective, and retrospective clinical studies that recruited patients with cancer who were treated with HT and RT and/or CT. The data from randomized trials are only from the patient group which received HT in combination with either RT and/or CT. Data from the non-HT arm were not extracted.

The main inclusion criteria was the use of either electromagnetic, radiative, or capacitive HT systems, independent of cancer type. Another criterion was more than 10 patients recruited in prospective and retrospective studies. Retrospective studies were only included if analysis of thermometric parameters for HT in combination with RT had been performed.

Clinical studies which used the thermal ablation technique, interstitial-based/modulated electro HT techniques, interstitial RT techniques, high intensity focused ultrasound (HIFU) HT, whole body HT, and studies in pediatric patients were not included in this review. Pilot and feasibility studies were also excluded.

2.3. Data Extraction and List of Variables Included

The data extracted from the clinical studies contained the following information:
- First author of the study
- Study design: prospective or retrospective
- RT treatment data: total dose, number of fractionations
- CT treatment data: drug and concentration prescribed, number of cycles
- Thermometric parameters
- Reported clinical endpoints
- Reported relationship between thermometric parameters and clinical endpoint

2.4. A Summary of HT Techniques

The clinical studies included in this review administered HT using externally applied power with electromagnetic–based techniques, such as radiofrequency, microwave, or infrared. These techniques differ with regard to their application to treat superficial or deep-seated tumors, as summarized elsewhere [44].

For superficial tumors, the electromagnetic radiative and capacitive systems are the those used in the clinical trials included in this review. The superficial HT techniques and their application are explained in detail elsewhere [43]. The radiative and capacitive systems differ in the way they are applied in the clinic. A study showed that for superficial cancers, the radiative HT system performs better than capacitive systems in terms of temperature distribution [45]. The commercially available radiative superficial systems are the BSD-500 device (Pyrexar Medical, Salt Lake, UT, USA), the ALBA ON4000 (Alba Hyperthermia, Rome, Italy) and contact flexible microwave applicators (SRPC Istok, Fryazino, Moscow region, Russia). Thermotron RF8 (Yamamoto Vinita Co, Osaka, Japan), Oncotherm (Oncotherm Kft., Budapest, Hungary) and Celsius TCS (Celsius42 GmbH, Cologne, Germany) are examples of commercial capacitive systems used for superficial tumors.

Different HT techniques with unique specifications, characteristics, and limitations are used to treat deep-seated tumors [46]. The ESHO guidelines provide information as to how and when a specific particular HT device should be used to treat deep-seated tumors [46,47]. The radiative HT systems for deep-seated tumors used in clinical trials are the BSD-2000 device (Pyrexar Medical, Salt Lake, UT, USA), the ALBA 4D (Alba Hyperthermia, Rome, Italy), and the Synergo RITE (Medical Enterprises Europe B.V., Amstelveen, The Netherlands), and capacitive systems are Oncotherm (Oncotherm Kft., Budapest, Hungary), Celsius TCS (Celsius 42 GmbH, Cologne, Germany), and Thermotron RF8 (Yamamoto Vinita Co, Osaka, Japan). Another simulation study showed a difference in heating patterns between radiative and capacitive HT for deep-seated tumors [48]. The radiative technique yields more favorable simulated temperature distributions for deep-seated tumors than the capacitive technique.

2.5. Definition of Thermometric Parameters

In this work, the thermometric parameters were extracted from the selected perspective and retrospective clinical studies. The definitions of these parameters are listed in Table 1.

Table 1. Definition of thermometric parameters.

Thermometric Parameters	Definitions
Heating Temperature	
T_{min}	Minimum temperature achieved in target volume (°C).
T_{max}	Maximum temperature achieved in target volume (°C).
T_{avg}	Average temperature achieved in target volume (°C).
T_{10}	Temperature achieved in 10% of the target volume (°C).
T_{20}	Temperature achieved in 20% of the target volume (°C).
T_{50}	Temperature achieved in 50% of the target volume (°C).
T_{80}	Temperature achieved in 80% of the target volume (°C).
T_{90}	Temperature achieved in 90% of the target volume (°C).
Heating duration	
t_{pre}	Warm-up period is the time required to achieve the desired treatment temperature and therapeutic time (min).
t_{treat}	Treatment period is the time during which a constant temperature in the tumor (≥ 41 °C) is maintained (min).
Thermal Dose	
CEM43°CT_{90}	Cumulative equivalent minutes at 43 °C when the measured temperature is T_{90} (min).
CEM43°CT_{50}	Cumulative equivalent minutes at 43 °C when the measured temperature is T_{50} (min).
CEM43°CT_{10}	Cumulative equivalent minutes at 43 °C when the measured temperature is T_{10} (min).
TRISE	T_{50} values above 37 °C multiplied by the duration of all heating sessions normalized to a duration of 450 min (°C) [36].
AUC	Actual time-temperature plots by computing the area under the curve (AUC) for T > 37 °C and T $\geq$ 39 °C (°C-min) [49].
HT sessions	
N_{week}	Number of HT sessions per week.
N_{total}	Total number of HT sessions during the treatment course.
Time interval	
t_{int}	The time interval between HT and RT and/or CT.
Sequencing	The scheduling order of HT with RT and/or CT.

Temperature measurements in the target volume or surrounding tissue are crucial for assessing treatment quality and are represented by temperature metrics. During a HT session, the temperature is usually monitored and recorded using high resistance thermistor probes, fiber optic temperature probes or thermocouples by invasively placing the probes in the target volume or in the vicinity of the target volume [43,46,50]. The ESHO guidelines recommend that after the definition of the tumor volume as a planning target volume, a target point should be defined where the probe is positioned intraluminally or intratumorally [46]. In addition, the guidelines strongly suggest keeping a record of thermometry measurement points within or close to the tumor sites [43]. After completion of the HT session, recorded temperature data during t_{treat} are evaluated by computing temperature metrics. For instance, T_{max} is calculated as the maximum temperature value recorded in the target volume (Table 1). T_{10}, another maximum temperature metric, is computed as the temperature value received by 10% of the target volume [32]. Similarly, the other temperature metrics listed in Table 1 are computed. In current practice, the thermometric parameters and thermal dose are computed by software integrated in the HT systems or using thermal analysis tools such as RHyThM [51].

To illustrate how temperature, t_{pre} and t_{treat} terms are measured in clinical practice, Figure 1 shows the temperature and heating duration parameters of a patient treated with HT in the radiation oncology center at Cantonal Hospital Aarau (KSA) using BSD-500 system (BSD Medical Corporation, Salt Lake City, UT, USA).

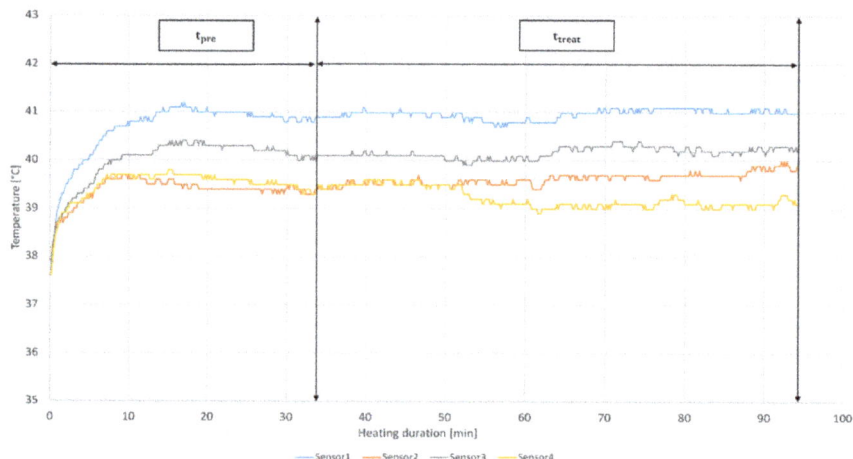

Figure 1. Recorded treatment data of a single HT session for a breast cancer patient. Temperature in °C and heating duration in minutes are measured non-invasively using four sensors located in close proximity to the tumor tissue. t_{pre} and t_{treat} of 33 and 60 min respectively according to the KSA clinical protocol are indicated.

The temperature metrics and thermal doses can be also computed by using the data from Figure 1. A decade ago, a new thermal dose entitled "TRISE" was proposed by Franckena et al. [36]. However, this parameter has not yet been evaluated in experimental studies. Another newly proposed thermal dose parameter is the area under the curve (AUC) [49]. In contrast to CEM43°C and TRISE, AUC is computed without any prior assumptions by summating AUC for the entire treatment session, including t_{pre} and t_{treat}. Similarly to TRISE, AUC has not yet been investigated in preclinical studies. Another parameter related to HT used in this review is thermal enhancement ratio (TER), defined as 'the ratio between RT dose required to achieve a specific endpoint and RT dose to achieve the same endpoint in combination with HT' [52].

3. Evidence for Predictive Values of Thermometric Parameters in Preclinical Studies
3.1. Heating Temperature

The responsiveness of a tumor to HT is determined by different heat-induced mechanisms at the cellular level. The oxygenation rate is affected by temperature, as a higher rate was reported at 41–41.5 °C in comparison to higher temperature (at 43 °C) in rodent tumors, human tumor xenografts, canine, and human tumors [53]. Heating at 40 °C potentiated the cytotoxicity of CT drugs in human maxillary carcinoma cells [28], and the cytotoxicity was further increased on heating to 43.5–44 °C [54]. In contrast, another preclinical study showed no such dependency at 41–43.5 °C [55]. An in vitro study showed that apoptosis in human keratinocytes occurred at temperatures of 39 °C and above [56]. However, the majority of studies show synergistic actions of HT with RT and CT at temperatures above 41 °C [5,57], leading to the inhibition of DNA repair and chromosomal aberrations, induction of DNA breaks by RT and CT, and protein damage as an underlying molecular event of heat treatment [5,58,59]. To benefit from additive and synergistic effects of HT when combined with RT and/or CT, uniform temperature in the target volume should be delivered during the whole treatment course.

The temperature metrics are used to present the heating temperature achieved during treatment, not only in the target volume, which encompasses the tumor, but also for adjacent healthy tissue. T_{90}, T_{80}, T_{50}, T_{20}, and T_{10} are considered to be less sensitive than T_{min}, T_{avg} and T_{max}, due to the number and arbitrary positioning of sensors in the tissue.

Such temperature metrics can be used to understand the response to heat of various cancer types for a specific duration and, at the same time, the heat-induced effects on surrounding normal tissues. However, except for T_{min} and T_{max}, most descriptive metrics of temperature have no specific reference values yet (Table 2).

Table 2. Reference temperature metrics.

Temperature Metrics	Reference Value (°C)
T_{min}	39
T_{max}	44
T_{avg}	Undefined
T_{10}	Undefined
T_{20}	Undefined
T_{50}	≥ 41 *
T_{80}	Undefined
T_{90}	≥ 40 *

* According to ESHO guidelines for superficial HT [43].

T_{50} and T_{90} reference values are defined according to ESHO guidelines for treatment with superficial HT, but not for the deep HT technique. No reference values for temperature metrics are based on experimental data (Table 2), even though temperature distributions can be better controlled in preclinical than in clinical studies. In an in vivo study, no temperature variations were observed in tumors as they were recorded intratumorally [15]. Temperature at a reference value with minor variations (± 0.05 °C) was reported in a vitro study [60]. In contrast, the temperature data recorded in patients are limited for various reasons. For example, thermistor probes inserted in deep-seated tumors in patients have the potential to cause complications or sometimes are impractical to insert intraluminally or intratumorally [61]. The value of the lowest temperature achieved during HT treatment is shown to have a prognostic role in describing the biological effects of HT. According to an in vivo study, T_{90} was a predictive parameter of reoxygenation and radiosensitization effects [62]. An in vitro experiment which investigated the difference in thermal sensitivity between hypoxic and oxic cells demonstrated that direct cytotoxicity induced by HT is more selective to the hypoxic cells [7]. Thus, temperatures required to achieve comparable thermal enhancement effect of HT vary depending on tissue type and characteristics.

3.2. Heating Duration

Temperature fluctuations, such as a decrease by 0.5 °C, have been shown to have a strong effect on the extent of cell kill, which was compensated by doubling the heating duration [6,63]. Therapeutic ratio, defined as the ratio of thermosensitive liposomal doxorubicin delivered to the heated tumor increased from 1.9-fold with 10 min heating to 4.4-fold with 40 min heating [64]. In an in vivo study, TER for mouse mammary adenocarcinoma (C3H) increased with respect to heating exposure longer than 30 min at 41.5 °C [15]. A study used mouse leukemia, human cervical carcinoma (HeLa), and Chinese hamster ovary (CHO) cells to demonstrate that the time required to kill 90% of the cells at 43 °C varied according to type [65]. The survival data from different tissues were analyzed using the Arrhenius equation to understand the effect of t_{treat} for different cell types [66]. These analyses showed that the reference t_{treat} value is set at 60 min when heating constantly at reference temperature (Table 3).

Table 3. Reference heating duration parameters for HT.

Heating Duration Parameters	Reference Value (min)
t_{pre}	undefined
t_{treat}	60 [1]

[1] According to the Arrhenius plot [66].

Heating for longer than 60 min is restricted by thermotolerance, which was observed after 20 min while heating at 43.5 °C [67]. In addition, the surviving fraction of asynchronous CHO cells heated to 41.5 °C was decreased with increasing t_{treat}, until the thermotolerance effect appeared [21]. Thermotolerance is activated by different forms of stress including heat exposure for a specific time [68], which depends on the temperature and the amount of HT damage induced [69]. In an experimental study, the effect of thermotolerance was observed using the human tumor cell line (HTB-66) and CHO cells after 4 h of heating at 42.5 °C and 3 h of heating at either 42.5 or 43 °C [70]. The degree of thermotolerance is determined by cell type, heating temperature, and time of heating including the interval between successive heat treatments [71].

3.3. Thermal Dose

The relationship between temperature and t_{treat} was demonstrated experimentally in two preclinical studies, which showed that the same thermal enhancement of ionizing radiation in cells lines was achieved by heating for 7–11 min at 45 °C or for 120 min at 42 °C [26,72]. It was also shown that different survival rates were obtained when heating asynchronous CHO cells to different temperatures for varying t_{treat} [66]. These preclinical data showed that heating temperature and t_{treat} influence thermal damage. The relationship of temperature and t_{treat} to the biological effects induced by HT is described using the Arrhenius equation, which models the relationship of the inactivation rate in a biological system [21]. This led to the discovery that the relationship between temperature and t_{treat} depends on the activation energy required to induce a particular HT-induced biological event, such as protein denaturation [59,66]. The thermal dose concept, CEM43°C, was established to account for the biological effects induced by HT in terms of both temperature and t_{treat} [21]. More specifically, CEM43°C calculates the equivalent time of a HT treatment session by correlating temperature, t_{treat} and inactivation rate of a biological effect induced by heat based on the Arrhenius equation. The reference temperature of 43 °C was shown as a breakpoint in the Arrhenius plot with a steeper slope between 41.5 and 43 °C in comparison to 43–57 °C [66]. The threshold values of CEM43°C for tissue damage differ for specific tissues as identified in in vivo studies and are reviewed elsewhere [70,73,74]. In addition, these data underline that CEM43°C is an important parameter that has biological validity to assess the thermal damage in tissues. CEM43°CT_{90} is one of the most frequently used thermal dose descriptors at T_{90}, not only in clinical, but also in experimental settings. In an in vivo study, Thrall et al. [75] showed a relationship between CEM43°CT_{90} and local control in canine sarcomas, but not with CEM43°CT_{50} and CEM43°CT_{10}. Another in vivo study using breast (MDA-MB-231) and pancreatic cancer (BxPC-3) xenografts showed that at relatively low values of CEM43°CT_{90}, tumor volumes could be reduced by exposure to heat alone [76]. However, none of the preclinical studies proposed reference values for clinical validation, as shown in Table 4.

Table 4. Reference thermal dose parameters for HT.

Thermal Dose Parameters	Reference Value
CEM43°CT_{10}	Undefined (min)
CEM43°CT_{50}	Undefined (min)
CEM43°CT_{90}	Undefined (min)
TRISE	Undefined (°C)
AUC	Undefined (°C-min)

Although there is no reference threshold value for the CEM43°C, its efficacy to predict tumor response and local control has been experimentally proven [75,77]. CEM43°C is considered as a thermal dose parameter with few weaknesses which have been discussed elsewhere [78].

3.4. Number of HT Sessions

Thermotolerance is an undesirable side effect of HT which renders tumor cells insensitive to heat treatment for 48 to 72 h [79]. Thermotolerance consists of an induction phase, a development phase, and a decay phase. Each of these components may have its own temperature dependence as well as dependence on other factors, such as pH and presence of nutrients [80]. Thermotolerance plays an important role on how HT sessions are scheduled during the treatment course. An in vivo study using C3H mouse mammary carcinoma confirmed that preheating for 30 min at 43.5 °C induced thermotolerance for the next heating session [81]. Twice weekly heating to 43 °C for 60 min in combination with RT at 3 Gray (Gy) per fraction for 4 weeks was shown to result in a steady state decline in oxygenation level suggesting vascular thermotolerance [82]. In comparison, Nah et al. reported that heating at 42.5 °C for 60 min could render the tumor blood vessels resistant to the next heating session after an interval of 72 h [83]. It has also been shown that when HT was delivered daily with RT 5 days a week, no significant thermal enhancement could be detected in comparison to one single HT session, even when heat was delivered simultaneously or sequentially [84]. With the agreement of these findings, N_{week} is defined as 1 or 2 sessions separated by at least 72 h (Table 5).

Table 5. Reference HT treatment session parameters. N: positive constant value.

Heating Session Parameter	Reference Value (N)
N_{total}	Defined [1]
N_{week}	1–2 [2]

[1] Depending on RT and CT schedules; [2] Depending on cancer site.

In summary, HT should be delivered once or twice weekly, taking into account the type of cancer, RT fractionation and CT drug scheduling. Due to logistical reasons, the N_{total} usually depends on, the treatment plan for different cancer sites, number of RT fractions or number of CT cycles (Table 5).

3.5. Time Interval Parameter between HT and RT and/or CT

The t_{int} between HT and RT and/or CT treatment is another parameter that affects sensitization due to time-dependent biological effects and its contribution to thermotolerance.

Recently, an in vitro study of human papillomavirus (HPV)-positive (HPV16$^+$, HPV18+) and HPV-negative cell lines that were treated with HT either 0, 2 and 4 h before and after RT showed that the shortest t_{int} resulted in lower cell survival fractions and decreased DNA damage repair [85]. The influence of t_{int} has been investigated in an in vivo study, which reported that TER is greatest when heat and radiation are delivered simultaneously [15]. Unfortunately, simultaneous delivery is currently technically impossible in clinical routine and therefore heat and radiation are usually delivered sequentially. A very short t_{int} of approximately five min is considered as an almost simultaneous application [86]. Dewey et al. concluded that HT should be applied simultaneously or within 5–10 min either side of radiation to benefit maximally from the radiosensitizing effect of heat [6]. TER is decreased faster for the normal cells than for cancerous cells when $t_{int} \leq 4$ h between HT and RT [15]. Thus, it can be argued that a slightly longer t_{int} could ensure the sparing of normal tissue from radiosensitization before or after RT. A t_{int} longer than 4 h, no sensitization effects induced by HT were observed [15,85]. The wide range of acceptable t_{int} values reported in experimental studies is from 0 (when CT is delivered during HT) to 4 h (Table 6).

Table 6. Reference t_{int} parameter for HT in combination with RT or CT.

Time Interval Parameter	Reference Value (min)
t_{int}	0–240

In contrast to RT, CT can be given simultaneously or immediately after or before HT [87]. A preclinical study, in which cisplatin and heat were used to treat C3H xenografts, showed that a higher additive effect can be obtained when cisplatin was given 15 min before HT in comparison with an interval longer than 4 h [55].

Furthermore, HT has been shown to sensitize the effects of gemcitabine at 43 °C when the drug was given 24 h after heating [88], whereas another study showed an optimal effect when the drug was given 24–48 h before heating [89]. The type of CT agent and its interaction with heat are factors which determine the t_{int} between HT and CT (Table 6).

3.6. Sequencing of HT in Combination with and RT and/or CT

An additional predictive parameter for the effectiveness of radiosensitization and chemosensitization is the sequencing of heat prior to or after the application of RT or CT. Usually, HT and RT are delivered sequentially but there is no consensus as to the optimal sequence. An in vivo study by Overgaard investigated the impact of sequence and interval between the two modalities on local tumor control and normal tissue damage in a murine breast cancer model and found that the sequence did not have any significant effect on the thermal enhancement in tumor tissues [15]. However, an experimental study using Chinese hamster ovary (HA-1) and mouse mammary sarcoma (EMT-6) cell lines showed that sequencing of radiation and heat altered radiosensitivity for these two cancer cell types [90]. HT before RT showed more thermal enhancement in synchronous HA-1 cell lines and the opposite sequence increased the thermal enhancement in EMT-6 cell lines. Other experimental studies reported no impact of the sequence of RT and HT in V79 cells on thermal enhancement [26,72]. In line with these results, an experimental study with HPV cell lines showed no difference in radiosensitization or cell death when heat was delivered prior or after radiation [85]. Due to conflicting results with regard to the treatment sequencing of HT and RT, additional preclinical mechanistic studies on different cell types are required.

An in vivo study where heat was combined with cisplatin CT showed that simultaneous application of both treatments resulted in prolonged tumor growth delay in comparison with administration of cisplatin after HT [55]. Another study found that simultaneous exposure of human colorectal cancer (HCT116) cells to HT and doxorubicin was more effective than sequential administration because of higher intercellular drug concentrations at 42 °C [91]. In conclusion, better insight into the interaction of various CT drugs with HT and RT is required to define the optimal sequencing of specific drugs and RT dose.

4. Evidence for the Predictive Values of Thermometric Parameters in Clinical Studies Combining HT with RT

Numerous prospective and retrospective clinical studies have been conducted to assess the efficacy of HT in combination with RT for treating superficial and deep-seated tumors. The design of most clinical studies was based on the translation of experimental findings aiming to reproduce benefit of HT when combined with RT.

Tables 7 and 8 show the results of the most important clinical studies. The prospective clinical studies in Table 7 reported improved clinical results, apart from the study by Mitsumori et al. which did not show a significant difference in the primary clinical endpoint of local tumor control between two treatment arms [92]. The underlying reason could have been differences in RT dose prescriptions and missing patient treatment data. Although the study showed a significant difference in progression free survival, this was judged to be not a substantial benefit. The authors stressed the need for internationally standardized treatment protocols for the combination of HT and RT.

In reality, temperature and thermal dose are usually reported as post-treatment data recordings (Tables 2 and 4) to account for temperature homogeneity or sensitivity. Even though temperature cannot always be measured invasively, depending on the location of the tumor, a strong correlation was reported between intratumoral and intraluminal temperatures, suggesting that intraluminal temperature measurements are a good surrogate for pelvic tumor measurements [50,93]. In addition, retrospective studies showed that a higher intra-esophageal temperature (>41 °C) predicts longer overall survival, improved local control and metastasis-free rate [94,95]. The difficulty of performing invasive measurements was illustrated by a randomized phase III study by Chi et al. [96] in which only 3 out of 29 patients with bone metastases had directly measured intratumoral temperature. In the study by Nishimura et al. [97], the HT session was defined as effective if an intratumoral temperature exceeded 42 °C for more than 20 min. However, according to the Arrhenius relationship, this is not considered long enough to induce a significant biological effect [21].

Another obstacle during HT is the non-standardized methodology for describing the temporal and spatial variance of temperature fields. Several groups have investigated the correlation between various temperature metrics. The study by Oleson et al. showed that T_{min}, tumor volume, radiation dose, and heating technique play significant roles in predicting treatment response for patients treated with RT in combination with HT [29]. In contrast, Leopold et al. reported that the more robust parameters T_{90}, T_{50}, and T_{10} are better temperature descriptors and predictors of histopathologic outcome than T_{min} and T_{max} [32]. The median T_{min}, T_{min} during the first heat treatment and tumor volume were reported to be factors predictive for the duration of cancer response (Table 7) [98], even though it is considered that skin surface temperature is not representative for superficial tumors and cannot be associated with clinical outcomes [42]. For deep-seated tumors, Tilly et al. reported that T_{max} was a predictive treatment parameter for prostate-specific antigen (PSA) control [99]. The relationship of high ($T_{avg} \geq 41.5$ °C) and low ($T_{avg} < 41.5$ °C) tumor temperature with clinical response has been analyzed in a study by Masunaga et al. [100]. They showed that heating the tumor to temperatures of $T_{avg} \geq 41.5$ °C for a duration of 15–40 min achieved better tumor down-staging and better tumor degeneration rates [100]. This finding supports the concept that direct cytotoxic effects of HT are enhanced at temperatures higher than 41 °C, as suggested in preclinical studies [5,57]. A higher response rate was also reported when tumors were heated with $T_{avg} > 42$ °C for 3–5 HT sessions [97]. In contrast, a study showed no difference in clinical outcome when patients were treated with mean $T_{min} = 40.2$ °C, $T_{max} = 44.8$ °C or $T_{avg} = 42.5$ °C for N_{total} of 2 or 6 [24]. Other studies also reported no impact of N_{total} and N_{week} on clinical outcome [40,101]. The contradictory results derived from clinical studies with regard to the predictive power of temperature descriptors and N_{total} are why we did not list reference values for these descriptors in Table 5.

The predictive role of thermal dose has been investigated in both prospective and retrospective clinical studies (Tables 7 and 8). However, there is still no conclusion about the values for thermal dose that should be obtained during HT treatment for maximal enhancement effect. In prospective studies (Table 7), the correlation between thermal dose and treatment outcome is rarely reported. Retrospective studies reported that thermal dose, CEM43°C, is an adequate predictor of treatment response and its best prognostic descriptor is CEM43°CT_{90} [32,33,36–38,102].

Table 7. Prospective clinical studies using RT in combination with HT.

Author(s)	Cancer Site, n	RT Dose (Gy) /Fractions	Temperature Metrics (°C)	HT Session	t_{treat} (min)	Thermal Dose (min)	t_{int} (min)	Sequence	Clinical Outcome (Comment)
Chi et al. [96]	Bone metastases, n = 29	30.0/10	T_{max}†: 41.9 ± 1.2	N_{total}: 4 N_{week}: 2	40	n.r.	120	HT after RT	• Increased 3-months radiologic CR[1] and PR[2] rate: 37.9% (11/29) and 66.7% (10/15), respectively. No grade III toxicity was reported. • HT increased pain control rate, no progression of pain achieved after 29 days. (correlation of thermometric parameters with clinical outcome not presented)
Valdagni et al. [103]	Head & neck, n = 18	64.0–70.0 /32–35	T_{max}†: 43.3 ± 0.2 T_{min}†: 40.4 ± 0.2 T_{50}: 41.8 ± 0.2 T_{90}: 39.8 ± 0.02	N_{total}: 6 N_{week}: 2	n.r.	max CEM42.5°C[5]: 83.84 ± 9.4min CEM42.5°C: 12.8–2.1	20–25	HT after RT	• 3-month CR: 83.3% (15/18), PR: 5.56% (1/18), PD[3] rate of 11.1% (2/18), overall improved LC[4]. • 5-year nodal control rate: 68.6% with TER: 2.83. • N_{total} of two or six yielded similar results (80% CR with 6 sessions vs. 87%, with 2 sessions). • No enhanced acute or late toxicities were reported. Extensive thermal analysis performed: no relation between thermometric parameters and response or toxicity.

Table 7. Cont.

Author(s)	Cancer Site, n	RT Dose (Gy) /Fractions	Temperature Metrics (°C)	HT Session	t_{treat} (min)	Thermal Dose (min)	t_{int} (min)	Sequence	Clinical Outcome (Comment)
Jones et al. [35]	Superficial cancers, n = 56	30.0–66.0 /15–33 when previously unirradiated 60.0–70.0 /30–35	n.r.	N_{total}: 4–10 N_{week}: 2	60 min	CEM43°CT_{90} [†]: 14.3 (0.57–36.21)	n.r.	n.r.	• CR: 66.1%, LC for pre-irradiated tumors: 48%. • CEM43°CT_{90} associated with CR rate. • Greater than 10 CEM43°CT_{90} showed a significant LC benefit. • The improvement in LC was most pronounced for patients who were previously irradiated. • No significant toxicity or survival benefit was reported.
van der Zee et al. [104]	Locally advanced pelvic tumors, n = 182	Bladder: 66.0–70.0 /33–35 Cervix: 40.0–50.0 /23–28 with HDR-IRT [23] (^{192}Ir): 14.0 or LDR-IRT [24] (^{192}Ir): 20.0–30.0 Rectum: 46.0–50.0 /20–22	n.r.	N_{total}: 5 N_{week}: 1	60	n.r.	60–240	HT after RT	• CR for all patients: 55%, bladder: 73%, cervical: 83%, rectal: 21%. • 3-year LC for all patients: 38%, for bladder: 42% for cervical: 61%, for rectal: 16%. • 3-year OS^6 rate for all patients: 30%, for bladder: 28%, for cervical: 51%, for rectal: 22%. • 2.2% had grade III-IV HT-related toxicity. (correlation of thermometric parameters with clinical outcome not presented)

Table 7. Cont.

Author(s)	Cancer Site, n	RT Dose (Gy) /Fractions	Temperature Metrics (°C)	HT Session	t_{treat} (min)	Thermal Dose (min)	t_{int} (min)	Sequence	Clinical Outcome (Comment)
Harina et al. [105]	Cervix cancer, $n = 20$	52.2/29 with HDR-IRT (^{192}Ir): 30.0/4	T_{max} †: 41.8 ± 1.1 T_{avg} †: 40.6 ± 1.0 T_{min} †: 39.6 ± 0.9	N_{total}: 3 N_{week}: 1	60	n.r.	30	HT after RT	• CR: 80% (16/20), PR: 15% (3/20), NC [7]: 5% (1/20). 3-year local LRFS [8], DFS [9] and OS: 79.7%, 63.6% and 58.2%, respectively. • Acute toxicity, grade III: 2 patients. • Late toxicity, grade III: 1 patient. (correlation of thermometric parameters with clinical outcome not presented)
Mitsumori et al. [92]	Locally advanced non-small cell lung cancers, $n = 40$	66.0–70.0 /33–38	T_{max} †: 41.3 (37.7–44.0) T_{min} †: 39.5 (35.5–41.7) T_{avg} †: 40.3 (37.0–42.7)	N_{total}: 7 N_{week}: 1	60	n.r.	n.r.	n.r.	• RR [10]: 45.0%. • 1-year LRFS and OS: 67.5% and 43%, respectively. • Acute toxicity, grade II: 4 patients and grade III: 2 patients. • Late toxicity, grade II: 3 patients and no grade III. (correlation of thermometric parameters with clinical outcome not presented)
Masunaga et al. [100]	Urinary bladder cancer, $n = 28$	24.0/6	T_{avg} †: 41.5 ± 1.1 (39–44)	N_{total}: 4 N_{week}: 2	15–40	n.r.	n.r.	HT after RT	• $T_{avg} \geq 41.5$ °C achieved better results: 83.3% (10/12) tumor down-staging and degeneration, 0% local recurrence, 33% distant metastasis, in contrast with $T_{avg} < 41.5$ °C. • Survival rate was higher if $T_{avg} \geq 41.5$ °C than $T_{avg} < 41.5$ °C. • The toxicity associated with HT: pain during treatment.

Table 7. Cont.

Author(s)	Cancer Site, n	RT Dose (Gy) /Fractions	Temperature Metrics (°C)	HT Session	t_{treat} (min)	Thermal Dose (min)	t_{int} (min)	Sequence	Clinical Outcome (Comment)
Berdov et al. [106]	Advanced rectal cancer, $n = 56$	40.0/10	n.r.	N_{total}: 4–5 N_{week}: n.r.	60	n.r.	10	HT before RT	• 1-,2-,3-,4-, and 5-year survival: $61.8 \pm 6.6\%$, $48.1 \pm 6.7\%$, $43.9 \pm 6.7\%$, $35.6 \pm 6.4\%$, and $35.6 \pm 6.4\%$. • The mean for CR rate (>50%): 53.6% (30/56) and for CR rate (<50%): 23.3% (13/56). (correlation of thermometric parameters with clinical outcome not presented)
Maluta et al. [107]	Locally advanced high risk prostate cancer, $n = 144$	70.0–76.0 /35–38	Rectum T_{max} †: 42.7 T_{90} †: 40.2 (38.4–42.0) Bladder T_{90} †: 41.3 (39.5–42.3)	N_{total}: 4 N_{week}: 1	n.r.	CEM40 °CT_{90} †: 24.4 (14.4–34.4)	15–30	HT before RT	• 5-year OS: 87% and 5-year biochemical progression-free survival: 49%. • No late grade III toxicity or significant acute HT-correlated toxicity. (correlation of thermometric parameters with clinical outcome not presented)
Leopold et al. [40]	Superficial cancers, $n = 111$	24.0–70.0 /7–28	n.r.	N_{total} †:4.5(1–6) for N_{week}=1 and 7 (2–13) for N_{week}=2 N_{week}: 1–2	60	n.r.	30–90	HT after RT	• CR: 46%, PR: 34%, OS: 80%. • T_{90} was significantly related to CR. • Cumulative minutes of T_{90} ≥ 40 °C and logarithm of RT dose were predictive of both CR and OS. • T_{min}, N_{week} and N_{total} were not significantly related to either end points. • Toxicity, grade IV: 1 patient and grade III: 7 patients.

Table 7. *Cont.*

Author(s)	Cancer Site, n	RT Dose (Gy) /Fractions	Temperature Metrics (°C)	HT Session	t_{treat} (min)	Thermal Dose (min)	t_{int} (min)	Sequence	Clinical Outcome (Comment)
Nishimura et al. [97]	Colorectal cancer, $n = 33$	40.0–70.0 /25–35	Abdominal wall & hip: T_{max} †: 44.2 ± 2.1 T_{avg} †: 42.6 ± 1.3 T_{min} †: 40.5 ± 0.7 Perineum: T_{max} †: 43.1 ± 1.7 T_{avg} †: 42.2 ± 1.2 T_{min} †: 40.5 ± 1.1 Pelvis: T_{max} †: 42.1 ± 1.5 T_{avg} †: 41.2 ± 1.5 T_{min} †: 40.1 ± 1.1	N_{total}: 2–14 N_{week}: 1–2	40–60	n.r.	10–30	HT after RT	• 6- and 12-months LC: 59% (17/29) and 31% (8/21), respectively. • CR rate: 11% (4/35) and PR: 43% (15/35). Better treatment response of unresectable colorectal cancers than recurrent tumors. • Higher response rate of 67% reported when tumors heated with T_{avg} † > 42 °C for N_{total} = 3–5. • N_{total} ≥ 5–14 showed not to increase the response rate.
Anscher et al. [108]	Prostate cancer, $n = 21$	65–70 /32–35	Intraprostate median T_{90} †: 39.3 ± 0.9 T_{50} †: 40.4 ± 0.8	N_{total}: 5–10 N_{week}: 1–2	60	CEM43°CT_{90} †: 2.34 ± 3.23	60–154	HT after RT	• Rectal temperatures were not predictive of prostate temperatures. • The mean cumulative minutes with T_{90} of > 40 °C was 12 min in the prostate versus 28 min in the rectal lumen. • 3-year DFS: 25% and 12 patients (67%) had relapsed. • No higher complication of Grade III. • T_{90}, T_{50}, and log(CEM43°CT_{90}) were not significantly associated with time to relapse.

Table 7. Cont.

Author(s)	Cancer Site, n	RT Dose (Gy) /Fractions	Temperature Metrics (°C)	HT Session	t_{treat} (min)	Thermal Dose (min)	t_{int} (min)	Sequence	Clinical Outcome (Comment)
Gabriele et al. [109]	Inoperable or recurrent parotid carcinoma, n = 13	Inoperable: 70.0/35 Recurrent: 30.0/15	T_{min} ‡: 40.28 ± 0.83 T_{max} ‡: 42.83 ± 1.32	N_{total}: 4–10 N_{week}: 2	30–45	n.r.	n.r.	n.r.	• CR: 80% (16/20), PR: 20% (4/20), LR [11]: 20% (16/20), 5-year actuarial LC: 62.3 ± 13.2%. • Higher maximum temperatures correlated with acute toxicity and maximum tumor diameter but without statistical significance. • Major acute toxicities included three patients (15%) with superficial necrosis, 2/3 healed spontaneously within 4 to 6 months. • No correlation between T_{min} and T_{max} and early or long term response was found.
Maguire et al. [110]	Soft tissue sarcomas, n = 35	50.0/25–27	n.r.	N_{total}: 10 N_{week}: 2	60	CEM43°CT_{90} ‡: 38 (0.1–601)	n.r.	n.r.	• 14% (5/35) of patients had non-heatable tumors. • pCR [12]: 52% (15/29), LF [13]: 10% (3/29) with heatable tumors. • DM [14]: 14/30 patients with heatable tumors and 2/5 with non-heatable tumors. • Thermal goal of CEM43°CT_{90} ≥ 10 reached for 25 out of 30 patients. • Treatment-induced toxicity: 10/30 patients with heatable tumors. • No correlation of thermal dose with histologic response was observed.

Table 7. Cont.

Author(s)	Cancer Site, n	RT Dose (Gy) /Fractions	Temperature Metrics (°C)	HT Session	t_{treat} (min)	Thermal Dose (min)	t_{int} (min)	Sequence	Clinical Outcome (Comment)
Tilly et al. [99]	Recurrent or locally advanced prostate cancer, n = 22	68.4/38	Primary cancer: T_{90} †: 40.7 ± 0.3 T_{max} †: 41.4 ± 0.4 Recurrent cancer: T_{90} †: 40.6 ± 0.8 T_{max} †: 41.0 ± 0.7	N_{total}: 5–6 N_{week}: 1	0–30	n.r.	30	HT before RT or HT after RT	• 6-year OS: 95% and 6-year RrR [15]: 60%. • Severe acute grade III toxicity: 8 patients and grade II: 2 patients. Late toxicity, grade III: 1 patient and grade II: 2 patients. • No correlation between thermal parameters and toxicity. • The thermal parameters were correlated with clinical endpoints: toxicity, PSA [16] control. T_{max} was the only relevant predictive factor for PSA control.
Lutgens et al. [111]	Locally advanced cervical cancer, n = 42	50.0/25 with HDR-IRT (^{192}Ir): 21.0/3 weekly or LDR: 32.0/1–2 or MDR: 29.0/1–2	n.r.	N_{total}: 5 N_{week}: 1	60	n.r.	60–240	HT after RT	• Treatment failure in the pelvis: 19% (8/42). • OS: comparable between RT + CT and RT + HT groups. • Toxicity of grade ≥III: 5 patients. (correlation of thermometric parameters with clinical outcome not reported)
Hurwitz et al. [112]	Locally advanced prostate cancer, n = 37	66.60–70.0 /33–37	T_{min} †: 40.1 (37.5–41.8) T_{max} †: 42.5 (40.5–45.9) T_{avg} †: 41.2 (39.2–42.8)	N_{total}: 2 N_{week}: 1	60	CEM43°CT_{90} †: 8.4	60	HT before RT	• 7-year OS: 94% and failure free: 61%. • 2-year DFS: 84% compared with a rate of 64% for similar patients on 4-month androgen suppression. The difference in median CEM43°CT_{90} between these patient groups who achieved 2.8 min and 10.5 min, respectively, was significant ($p = 0.004$). • A small difference in DFS in favor of patients treated with higher temperatures.

Table 7. Cont.

Authors(s)	Cancer Site, n	RT Dose (Gy) /Fractions	Temperature Metrics (°C)	HT Session	t$_{treat}$ (min)	Thermal Dose (min)	t$_{int}$ (min)	Sequence	Clinical Outcome (Comment)
Vernon et al. [113]	Localized superficial breast cancer, n = 306	DHG [17] (p): 32.0/16 DHG (r): 40.5–50.0/25 + boost: 10.0–20.0 MRC [18] BrR (p): 28.8/8 MRC BrI(r) + MRC BrR(r): 50.0/25 + boost: 15.0/5 ESHO [19]: 32.0/8 PMH [20](p): 32.0/18 PMH(r): 50.0/25	DHG: T$_{90}$†: 39.0 T$_{50}$†: 40.7 T$_{max}$†: 43.5 MRC BrR: T$_{90}$†: 40.7 T$_{50}$†: 42.5 T$_{max}$†: 45.6 MRC BrI: T$_{90}$†: 40.4 T$_{50}$†: 42.3 T$_{max}$†: 45.1 ESHO: T$_{90}$†: 39.5 T$_{50}$†: 41.1 T$_{max}$†: 43.3 PMH: T$_{90}$†: 40.7 T$_{50}$†: 42.2 T$_{max}$†: 44.6	n.r.	DHG: 60 (55–61) MRC BrR: 60 (30–60) MRC BrI: 60 (17–65) ESHO: 60 (60–60) PMH: 60	DGH: maximum of CEM42 °C†: 0 (0–69.5) CEM43°C†: 3.95 (0–122) MRC: maximum of CEM42 °C†: 9 (0–60) CEM43°C†: 7.5 (0.1–87.7) ESHO: maximum of CEM42 °C†: 5 (0–59) CEM43°C†: 8.4 (0.2–74) PMH: maximum of CEM42 °C†: 0 (0–32.8) CEM43°C†: 1.5 (0–25) data from Sherar et al. [39]	n.r.	n.r.	• Total CR: 59%, DHG: 73.6% (14/19), MRC BrI: 55.5% (10/18), MRC BrR: 56.67% (51/90), ESHO: 77.77% (21/27), PMH: 29.41% (5/17). • CR rate of previously non-irradiated: 61% and CR rate of previously irradiated tumor: 46%. • 2-year actuarial survival rate for all patients: 40%. • Two largest studies (ESHO and MRC BrR) showed a statistically significant (p = 0.004 and 0.001, respectively) advantage for the addition of HT, whereas the other three trials do not show a benefit (ORs < 1). • CR rate show dependency on size of tumor, the depth of the lesion, and on a history or presence of metastatic dis-ease outside the target area (univariate analysis). • OS did not differ markedly but patients receiving HT has a marginally inferior survival. • Sherar et al. [39]: initial CR rate is significantly correlated with thermal dose and no correlation between N$_{total}$ and initial CR rate.

Table 7. Cont.

Author(s)	Cancer Site, n	RT Dose (Gy) /Fractions	Temperature Metrics (°C)	HT Session	t_{treat} (min)	Thermal Dose (min)	t_{int} (min)	Sequence	Clinical Outcome (Comment)
Datta et al. [114]	Head & neck cancer, n = 33	50.0 /25	n.r.	N_{total}: 8–10 N_{week}: 2	n.r.	n.r.	n.r.	HT before RT	• RR: 76%, CR: 55%, PR: 21% and DFS: 33%. • Particularly significant effect in patients with advanced disease. (correlation of thermometric parameters with clinical outcome not presented)
Overgaard et al. [115]	Recurrent or metastatic malignant melanoma, n = 63	24.0–27.0 /3	n.r.	N_{total}: 3 N_{week}: 1	60	CEM43°C †: 9 (0–219) data from Overgaard et al. [116]	30	HT after RT	• HT did not significantly increase acute or late radiation reactions. • 5-year survival rate was 19% and was 38% for the patients for with control of all known disease. • RR: 80%, initial CR rate: 62%, PR: 32%, NR: 20%, 2-year actuarial LC: 37%. • The response rate was higher receiving 27 Gy than those receiving a lower dose. • Both acute and late adverse effects were deemed acceptable. • Overgaard et al. [116]: there is a significance of thermal dose relationship with the heat effect but no correlation between N_{total} and the outcome of treatment.

Table 7. Cont.

Author(s)	Cancer Site, n	RT Dose (Gy) /Fractions	Temperature Metrics (°C)	HT Session	t_{treat} (min)	Thermal Dose (min)	t_{int} (min)	Sequence	Clinical Outcome (Comment)
Dinges et al. [41]	Uterine cervix carcinomas, n = 18	50.4/28 with HDR-IRT (^{192}Ir): 20.0/4	T_{20} †: 41.7 (40.3–43.2) T_{50} †: 41.1 (39.2–42.5) T_{90} †: 39.9 (37.7–41.9)	N_{total}: 4 N_{week}: 2	60	CEM43°CT_{20} †: 48.2 (5.9–600.5) CEM43°CT_{50} †: 15.2 (0.6–54.0) CEM43°CT_{90} †: 6.8 (0.4–23.0)	n.r.	n.r.	• CR: 13/18, PR: 4/18 and NR [21]: 1/18. • 2-year LC rate: 48.1%, development of distant metastases: 48.5% and DSS [22]: 31.8%. • CEM43°CT_{90} was a significant parameter in terms of local tumor control for N_{tot} = 4 (univariate analysis), but had no impact in terms of metastatic spread. • T_{20}, T_{50}, T_{90}, cumulative minutes of T_{90} > 40 °C, CEM43°CT_{20} and CEM43°CT_{50} were not significant in terms of local tumor control and DSS. • No acute toxicity, grade III or IV. • Late toxicity, grade III and IV: 3 patients.
Kim et al. [117]	Inoperable hepatoma, n = 30	30.6/17	n.r.	N_{total}: 6 N_{week}: 2	30–60	n.r.	30	n.r.	• Subjective response rate: 78.6%, PR: 40%, stable disease: 46.7%, PD: 13.3%. • 1-year survival values for all patients and for the partial responders were 34% and 50%, respectively. (correlation of thermometric parameters with clinical outcome not presented)

Table 7. Cont.

Author(s)	Cancer Site, n	RT Dose (Gy) /Fractions	Temperature Metrics (°C)	HT Session	t_{treat} (min)	Thermal Dose (min)	t_{int} (min)	Sequence	Clinical Outcome (Comment)
Engin et al. [98]	Superficial tumors, n = 50	60.0–70.0 /30–35 when previously irradiated: 40.0/10	Group A: T_{min} ‡: 39.6 ± 0.2 Group B: T_{min} ‡: 39.3 ± 0.2	Group A: N_{total}: 4 N_{week}: 1 Group B: N_{total}: 8 N_{week}: 2	60	Group A: CEM 43°C ‡: 12.1 ± 3.9 Group B: CEM43°C ‡: 15.0 ± 5.1	15–30	HT after RT	• Group A patients treated with once-weekly HT session had CR: 59% (12/22), PR: 36% (8/22), NR: 5% (1/22). • Group B patients treated with twice-weekly HT sessions had CR: 55% (12/22), PR: 45% (10/22). • T_{min} did not influence response between Group A and Group B. • Neither tumor response, duration of LC nor occurrence of skin reactions were significantly affected by N_{week}.

n: number of patients assigned to be treated with HT in combination with RT; †: mean value (±standard deviation) or mean value (range); ‡: median (range); n.r.: not reported; [1] CR: complete response; [2] PR: partial response; [3] PD: progressive disease; [4] LC: local control; [5] CEM42.5 °C: cumulative equivalent minutes at reference temperature 42.5 °C; [6] OS: overall survival; [7] NC: no change; [8] LRFS: local relapse-free survival; [9] DFS: disease free survival; [10] RR: responserate; [11] LR: local response; [12] pCR: pathological CR; [13] LF: local failure; [14] DM: distant metastasis; [15] RrR: recurrence rate; [16] PSA: prostate specific antigen; [17] DHG: Daniel den Hoed Cancer Center in Rotterdam; [18] MRC: Medical Research Council at the Hammersmith Hospital; [19] ESHO: European Society of Hyperthermic Oncology; [20] PMH: Princess Margaret Hospital/Ontario Cancer Institute; [21] NR: no response; [22] DSS: disease specific survival; [23] HDR-IRT: high dose rate interventional radiotherapy; [24] LDR-IRT: low dose rate interventional radiotherapy.

In a phase III study of the International Collaborative Hyperthermia Group, led by Vernon et al. [113], thermal dose was associated with complete response (CR) in patients treated for superficial recurrences of breast cancer [39]. Another randomized study showed that the best tumor control probability was dependent on thermal dose [106]. Further, retrospective analyses indicate that thermal dose is a significant predictor of different clinical endpoints (Table 8) [33,36]. A few studies did not find such significant relationships between clinical endpoints and thermal dose [103,109,110]. For example, in the prospective study of Maguire et al., a total CEM43°CT$_{90}$ with a threshold above 10 min did not show a significant effect on CR [110]. However, the association of CEM43°CT$_{90}$ with CR was later reported for patients treated with superficial malignant cancers [35]. Similar to the study by Maguire et al., the minimum effective thermal dose was set as 10 CEM43°CT$_{90}$. In addition, a test HT session was performed to verify if the tumor was heatable, and a thermal dose of higher than 0.5 CEM43°CT$_{90}$ could be achieved [35,110]. The objective of the study by Hurwitz et al. was to achieve a CEM 43 °CT$_{90}$ of 10 min, yet the resulting mean of thermal dose for all 37 patients was only 8.4 min [112]. The cumulative minutes T$_{90}$ > 40.5 °C, defined as 'the time in minutes with T$_{90}$ > 40.5 °C for the whole N$_{total}$', with a mean of 179 ± 92 min, together with T$_{90}$ and T$_{max}$ were reported to correlate with toxicity and prostate specific antigen clinical endpoints [99]. Similarly, Leopold et al. showed that cumulative minutes of T$_{90}$ > 40 °C is a predictor of treatment endpoints [40]. In retrospective studies, TRISE thermal dose concepts [36] were shown to have a predictive role in treatment response. These retrospective analyses showed that TRISE had a significant effect on local control for a cohort of patients with cervical cancer [33].

The effect of the t$_{int}$ parameter has been only analyzed with respect to treatment endpoints in retrospective studies. The study by van Leeuwen et al. reported that a t$_{int}$ less than 79.2 min between RT and reaching 41 °C during HT was associated with a lower risk of in-field recurrences (IFR) and a better overall survival (OS) in comparison to a longer t$_{int}$ [22]. In contrast, another retrospective study showed that neither a shorter t$_{int}$ of 30–74 min nor a longer t$_{int}$ of 75–220 min between RT and the start of HT were significant predictors of local control (LC), disease free survival (DFS), disease specific survival (DSS) or OS [33]. Thus, the optimal t$_{int}$ between HT and RT to achieve a maximal effect on the tumor remains unknown.

Apart from heat-related parameters, the total dose of ionizing radiation and its fractionation in combination with HT has an impact on clinical treatment response [118,119]. Valdagni et al. [103] reported that increasing the total dose of RT appeared to improve clinical response as 71% (5/7) and 90% (9/10) CR rates were observed for patients with nodal metastases of head and neck cancers who received total doses of 64–66 Gy or 66.1–70 Gy, respectively. In addition, it was reported that previously irradiated tumors, which are typically more resistant to ionizing radiation, achieved higher CR rates when treated with combined RT and HT in comparison with RT alone [35].

Furthermore, RT technique has been reported to have a beneficial effect on combined RT and HT treatment outcomes [29]. For example, technological advance such as MRI-guided brachytherapy were shown to improve the treatment outcome when RT is combined with HT [36].

The weak, and in part contradictory, evidence from clinical studies clearly shows that further analyses of thermometric parameters are required to define reference values for clinical use. The reported values for thermometric parameters from prospective and retrospective clinical studies (Tables 7 and 8) can be translated into standard references after being tested and validated in prospective clinical trials.

Table 8. Retrospective clinical studies using RT in combination with HT.

Author(s)	Cancer Site, n	RT Dose (Gy)/Fractions	Temperature Metrics (°C)	HT Session	t_{treat} (min)	Thermal Dose (min)	t_{int} (min)	Sequence	Clinical Outcome (Comment)
Franckena et al. [36]	Locally advanced cervix cancer, n = 420	46.0–50.4 /23–28 with HDR-IRT [11] (^{192}Ir): 17.0/2 weekly or LDR-IRT [12]: 18.0/3 weekly or LDR: 30 Gy in 60 h	n.r.	N_{total}: 5 N_{week}: 1	60	CEM43°CT$_{90}$ [†]: 5.05 ± 4.18 min	n.r.	n.r.	• CR [1]: 78%, PR [2]: 16%, SD [3]: 3%, PD [4]: 1%. • 1-year PTC [5]: 65% (95% CI: 60–70%), 5-year PTC: 53% (95% CI: 47–58%). • 1 year DSS [6]: 75% (95% CI: 71–79%) and 5-year DSS: 47% (95% CI: 41–53%). • Toxicity of grade I: 51% (80/153), grade II: 39% (60/153), grade III: 9% (16/153) and grade IV: 0.6% (1/153). • Tumor stage, performance status, radiotherapy dose and tumor size, CEM43°CT$_{90}$ and TRISE emerged as significant predictors of the various end-points.
Kroesen et al. [33]	Locally advanced cervix cancer, n = 400	46.0–50.4 /23–28 with HDR-IRT (^{192}Ir): 17.0/2 or MRI-IRT 7.0/3–4	n.r.	N_{total}: 5 N_{week}: 1	60	CEM43°CT$_{90}$ [†]: 3.40 (1.89–5.83) TRISE [†]: 3.46 (2.93–3.86)	30–230	HT after RT	• TRISE and CEM43T$_{90}$ had a significant effect on LC (univariate and multivariate analyses). • TRISE, and IGBT showed a significant effect on DFS [7], DSS, and OS [8] (univariate analyses). • t_{int} grouped based on median value in short t_{int} (30–74 min) and long t_{int} (75–220 min) were not significant predictor of LC, DFS, DSS and OS. • The incidence of late grade III toxicity did not differ between low or high TRISE or low or high t_{int} patients.

Table 8. Cont.

Author(s)	Cancer Site, n	RT Dose (Gy) /Fractions	Temperature Metrics (°C)	HT Session	t_{treat} (min)	Thermal Dose (min)	t_{int} (min)	Sequence	Clinical Outcome (Comment)
van Leeuwen et al. [22]	Locally advanced cervix cancer, $n = 58$	46.0–50.4 /23–28 with PDR: 24	n.r.	N_{total}: 4–5 N_{week}: 1	60	n.r.	33.8– 125.2 †	HT after RT	• 3-year IFR [9]: 18% (0–35%) in the short t_{int} (≤ 79.2 min) group and 53% (18–82%) in the long t_{int} (>79.2 min) group. • 5-year OS: 52% (35–77%). • OS ‡: 61 months (38–83 months) in the short t_{int} group and 19 months (13–26 months) in the long t_{int} group. No difference in toxicity was observed between short and long t_{int} group.
Franckena et al. [120]	Locally advanced cervix cancer, $n = 378$	46.0–50.4 /23–28 with HDR-IRT (^{192}Ir): 17.0/2 or 18.0–21.0/3 or 20.0–24.0/1 or HDR: 30.0/1	T_{avg} †: 40.6	N_{total}: 5 N_{week}: 1	60	n.r.	30–240	HT after RT	• CR: 77%. • 5-year PTC: 53% for all patients (95% CI, 48–59) and 5-year DSS: 47% (95% CI, 41–53). • N_{total} significant influence on CR, DSS and OS (univariate analysis) and on CR and DSS (multivariate analysis).

Table 8. Cont.

Author(s)	Cancer Site, n	RT Dose (Gy) /Fractions	Temperature Metrics (°C)	HT Session	t_{treat} (min)	Thermal Dose (min)	t_{int} (min)	Sequence	Clinical Outcome (Comment)
Oldenborg et al. [121]	Recurrent breast cancer, n = 78	32.0/8	T_{90} †: 41.1 (37.7–42.4) T_{50} †: 42.2 (39.0–43.4) T_{10} †: 43.2 (41.0–44.5)	N_{total}: 4 N_{week}: 1	60	CEM43°CT_{90} †: 22.3 (1.5–107.7) CEM43°CT_{50} †: 37.3 (3.3–96.0)	60	HT after RT	• 3- and 5-year OS: 66% and 49%, respectively. • 3- and 5-year LC: 78% and 65%, respectively. • The only significant prognostic factor: time between primary and recurrent disease (multivariate analyses) • CEM43°CT_{90} was not analyzed because skin temperature measurements are poor indicators of tumor temperature.
Datta et al. [49]	Muscle invasive bladder cancer, n = 18	unifocal cancer: 48.0/16 multifocal cancer: 50.0/20	T_{avg} †: 40.5 ± 0.5 T_{min} †: 36.7 ± 0.3 T_{max} †: 42.0 ± 0.6	N_{total}: 4 N_{week}: 1	60	CEM43°C: 59.8 ± 45.6	15–20	HT before RT	• 16/21 patients were free from local recurrence until their last follow-up or death. • Temperature attained during t_{treat} was significantly lower in patients with local failure. • AUC > 37 °C and AUC ≥ 39 °C were significantly lower in patients who had a local relapse. • N_{week} and N_{total}, no significant differences between CEM43°C and CEM43°C for T > 37 °C. • T_{avg}: significantly greater in patients with no local bladder failure for both individual and N_{total}.

Table 8. Cont.

Author(s)	Cancer Site, n	RT Dose (Gy) /Fractions	Temperature Metrics (°C)	HT Session	t_{treat} (min)	Thermal Dose (min)	t_{int} (min)	Sequence	Clinical Outcome (Comment)
Leopold et al. [32]	Soft tissue sarcoma, n = 45	50.0–50.4 /25–28	T_{90} ‡: 39.5 T_{50} ‡: 41.6 T_{10} ‡: 43.0 T_{min} ‡: 37.7 T_{max} ‡: 44.0	Group A: N_{total}: 5 N_{week}: 1 Group B: N_{total}: 10 N_{week}: 2	60	n.r.	30–60	HT after RT	• Strongest predictive value for cumulative minimum T_{90}, average min T_{90}, cumulative minutes of T_{50}, and average minutes T_{50}: 40.5 °C, 40.5 °C, 41.5 °C, and 41.5 °C, respectively. • N_{week}: 2 were superior to N_{week}: 1 with respect to the degree of histopathologic changes, but not predictive. • T_{50} and T_{90} are substantially temperature distribution descriptors.
Ohguri et al. [94]	Non-small cell lung cancer, n = 35	45.0–80.0 /23–30	T_{max} ‡: 43.2 (38.9–48.1) T_{avg} ‡: 42.6 (38.8–47.0) T_{min} ‡: 41.7 (38.6–45.6)	N_{total} ‡: 11 (3–17) N_{week}: 1–2	40–70	n.r.	15	HT after RT	• CR: 2%, PR: 66%, and NC [10]: 14%. • Median OS, local recurrence-free, and distant metastasis-free survival times: 14.1, 7.7, and 6.1 months, respectively. • Acute toxicity: 14% and late toxicity: 17%. • All thermal parameters, T_{min}, T_{avg} and T_{max} of intraesophageal temperature significantly correlated with median radiofrequency-output power.

n: number of patients assigned to be treated with HT in combination with RT; †: mean value (±standard deviation) or mean value (range); n.r.: not reported; [1] CR: complete response; [2] PR: partial response; [3] SD: stable disease; [4] PD: progressive disease; [5] PTC: pelvic tumor control; [6] DSS: disease specific survival; [7] DFS: disease free survival; [8] OS: overall survival; [9] IFR: in-field recurrence; [10] NC: no change; [11] HDR-IRT: high dose rate interventional radiotherapy; [12] LDR-IRT: low dose rate interventional radiotherapy.

5. Evidence for Predictive Values of Thermometric Parameters in Clinical Studies Combining HT and CT

The added value of combining CT with HT has been established, not only in in vitro and in vivo studies, but also in clinical studies. Randomized clinical studies, which demonstrate that the combination of CT and HT results in improved clinical outcome in comparison with single modality treatment [122–125], confirm the preclinical findings [126]. The positive prospective and retrospective clinical studies are summarized in Tables 9 and 10 respectively, with a focus on thermometric parameters.

The effectiveness of CT drugs has been enhanced by HT in a variety of clinical situations, such as localized, irradiated, recurrent, and advanced cancers, but only few indications are really promising. Long term outcome data, e.g., regarding the combination of CT with HT for bladder cancer, underline the clinical efficacy of this treatment strategy [125]. Chemosensitization by HT is induced by specifics biological interactions between CT drugs and heat. The increased blood flow and the increased fluidity of the cytoplasmic membrane of the cells induced by HT increase the concentration of CT drugs within malignant tissues. Interestingly, Zagar et al. performed a joint analysis of two different clinical trials and reported no significant correlation between drug concentration and combined treatment effect of CT and HT [127]. However, only a few CT drugs with specific properties (Tables 9 and 10) are good candidates to use with HT. Alkylating agents, nitrosureas, platinum drugs, and some antibiotic classes show synergism with HT, whereas only additive effects are reported with pyrimidine antagonists and vinca alkaloids [59]. For example, heat increases the cytotoxicity of cisplatin, as shown by in vitro and in vivo studies [28,55]. Cisplatin concentration increases linearly with temperatures above 38 °C when applied simultaneously [28,128]. Synergy between HT and CT could be obtained at temperatures below 43.5 °C in a preclinical study [55]. Similarly, enhanced toxicity has been demonstrated for bleomycin [126,129], liposomal doxorubicin [130], and mitomycin-C [131]. Based on the summary of preclinical data, van Rhoon et al. suggested a CEM43°C of 1–15 min from heating to 40–42 °C for 30–60 min for any free CT drug, including thermos-sensitive liposomal drugs [132].

Lower temperatures might increase the therapeutic window by differential chemosensitization of cancer and normal tissues. In the prospective study of Rietbroek et al. [133] in patients with recurrent cervical cancer treated with weekly cisplatin and HT, three temperature descriptors, T_{20}, T_{50}, and T_{90}, including the time in minutes in which 50% of the measured tumor sites were above 41 °C, indicated a significant difference in these parameters between patients who did and who did not exhibit a CR after treatment. However, there was neither a difference in T_{max} between responders and non-responders in a cohort of patients with recurrent soft tissue sarcomas treated with CT and HT [134], nor in a cohort of patients with recurrent cervical cancer [135].

In a prospective study of patients treated with CT and HT for recurrent ovarian cancer, no significant relationship of T_{90} and T_{50} and CEM43°CT_{90} and CEM43°CT_{50} with clinical outcome was found [136]. Similarly, the independency of T_{90} and CEM43°CT_{90} was also demonstrated in a retrospective study in soft tissue sarcoma [137]. Although a relationship of thermal dose with treatment response has been reported by Vujaskovic et al. [138], the parameters CEM43°CT_{50} and CEM43°CT_{90} were not statistically different between patients who did or did not respond to the treatment. The low mean value of T_{90} = 39.7 (33.5–39.8) °C reported in this study might be the reason for the non-significant relationship of thermal dose with the clinical endpoint in addition to other factors such as hypoxia and vascularization level of the tumor. The first randomized phase III study that assessed the safety and efficacy of CT in combination with HT also recorded a low ($\leq$40 °C) mean value of T_{90} = 39.2 °C (38.5–39.8 °C). However, the thermometric data were not analyzed or reported in correlation with treatment response [123]. Further investigations are required to understand which temperature is needed to achieve a maximum therapeutic effect, according to the type of CT drug and its concentration.

Table 9. Prospective clinical studies using CT in combination with HT.

Author(s)	Cancer Site, n	CT Drug(s) (mg/m^2) × Cycles	Temperature Metrics (°C)	HT Session	t_{treat} (min)	Thermal Dose	t_{int} (min)	Sequence	Clinical Outcome (Comment)
Issels et al. [123]	Localised high-risk soft-tissue sarcoma, $n = 104$	125 etoposide twice weekly × 4 1500 ifosfamide four times weekly × 4 50 doxorubicin once weekly × 4	T_{max} ‡: 41.8 (IQR: 41.1–43.2) T_{20} ‡: 40.8 (IQR: 40.1–42.3) T_{50} ‡: 40.3 (IQR: 39.5–41.0) T_{90} ‡: 39.2 (IQR: 38.5–39.8)	N_{total}: 8 N_{week}: 2	60	n.r.	n.r.	n.r.	• The proportion of patients who underwent amputation was 6.7% (7/104). • After surgery, 108 patients received mean dose of 53.3 ± 8.9 Gy. • 2-year and 4-year LPFS [1]: 58% (51–66%) and 42% (35–51%), respectively; • 2-year and 4-year OS [2]: 78% (72–84%) and 59% (51–67%), respectively; • CR [3], PR [4], SD [5], PD [6] rates were 2.5%, 26.3%, 55.9%, 6.8%, 8.5%, respectively. • The most frequent nonhaematological adverse events, grade III or IV: 23 patients. (correlation of thermometric parameters with clinical outcome not presented)

Table 9. Cont.

Author(s)	Cancer Site, n	CT Drug(s) (mg/m^2) × Cycles	Temperature Metrics (°C)	HT Session	t_{treat} (min)	Thermal Dose	t_{int} (min)	Sequence	Clinical Outcome (Comment)
Alvarez Secord et al. [136]	Refractory ovarian cancer, $n = 30$	40 doxil once weekly × 6	T_{90} [†]: 39.78 ± 0.59 T_{50} [†]: 40.47 ± 0.56	N_{total}: 6	60	CEM43°CT_{90} [†]: 5.84 ± 5.66 CEM43°CT_{50} [†]: 13.00 ± 11.25	0–60	HT after CT	• PR: 10% (3/30), SD: 27% (8/30), PD: 63% (19/30). • Median of PFS [7]: 3.4 and OS: 10.8 months, respectively. • Toxicity due to HT, grade III: one patient. • No significant differences between the T_{90}, T_{50}, CEM43°CT_{90} or CEM43°CT_{50} and those patients who had PD compared to SD or PR. • No significant change in overall QoL was found between baseline and after treatment.
Fiegl et al. [134]	Advanced soft tissue sarcoma, $n = 20$	1500 ifosfamide four times weekly × 7 100 carboplatin four times weekly × 7 150 etoposide four times weekly × 7	T_{max} [†]: 40.6 (39.1–42.2)	N_{total}: 8 N_{week}: 2	60	n.r.	n.r.	n.r.	• Time [‡] to progression: 6 and to OS: 14.6 months. • 3- and 6-months PFR [8] estimates: 60% and 45%, respectively. • Grade III/IV haematological toxicities during CT: 70%. • Objective RR [9]: 20% PR: 20% (4/20), PD: 45% (9/20); • No difference in T_{max} between responders or non-responders.

Table 9. Cont.

Author(s)	Cancer Site, n	CT Drug(s) (mg/m^2) × Cycles	Temperature Metrics (°C)	HT Session	t_{treat} (min)	Thermal Dose	t_{int} (min)	Sequence	Clinical Outcome (Comment)
Rietbroek et al. [133]	Irradiated recurrent cervical cancer, $n = 23$	50 cisplatin once weekly × 12	T_{20} †: 41.9 ± 0.9 °C T_{50} †: 41.3 ± 0.8 °C T_{90} †: 40.5 ± 0.7 °C	N_{total}: 12 N_{week}: 1	60	n.r.	30	HT after CT	• RR: 52% observed after a median number of 8 cycles of treatment. • OS ‡ rate: 8 months, specifically for responders: 12 months. • T_{20}, T_{50}, T_{90} values were higher for responders than non-responders but it did not show a statistical significance.
Zagar et al. [127]	Recurrent breast cancer, $n_{trial\,1} = 18$ $n_{trial\,2} = 11$	Trial A: 20–60 LTDL [13] every 21–35 days × 6 Trial B: 40–50 LTDL every 21–35 days × 6	max T_{90}: 42.6 min T_{90}: 36.0	N_{total}: 6	60 min	n.r.	30–60	HT after CT	• Combined trials (A and B), CR: 17.2% (5/29) and PR: 31% (9/29). • Patients with at least one or 20% of HT sessions with a T_{90} of target below 39 °C had similar local objective RR. • Toxicity, grade IV: three patients (10.3%) and grade III: six patients (20.7%). • No drug dose response relationship was observed between trial A and B. (correlation of thermometric parameters with clinical outcome not presented)

201

Table 9. Cont.

Author(s)	Cancer Site, n	CT Drug(s) (mg/m^2) × Cycles	Temperature Metrics (°C)	HT Session	t_{treat} (min)	Thermal Dose	t_{int} (min)	Sequence	Clinical Outcome (Comment)
Ishikawa et al. [139]	Locally advanced or metastatic pancreatic cancer, $n = 18$	1000 gemcitabine once weekly × 12	n.r.	N_{total}: 20 N_{week}: 1	40	n.r.	0–1440	HT before CT	• Major grade III-IV adverse events were neutropenia and anemia, no sepsis. • Objective RR and disease control rates were 11.1% and 61.1%, respectively. • OS †: 8 months, and the 1-year survival rate was 33.3%. (correlation of thermometric parameters with clinical outcome not presented)
Vujaskovic et al. [138]	Locally advanced breast cancer, $n = 43$	30–75 LTDL × 4 100–175 paclitaxel × 4	T_{90} †: 39.7(37.7–41.8)	N_{total}: 4 N_{week}: 2	60	CEM43°CT$_{90}$ †: 11.5 (1.5–159.3)	60	HT after CT	• CR: 9% (4/43) and pathological CR: 60% (26/43); • 4-year DFS [10] and OS: 63% and 75%, respectively. • CEM43°CT$_{90}$ † in responders was significantly greater than non-responders, 28.6 and 10.3 min, respectively. • Patients had grade III and IV toxicity • No statistical difference in the CEM43°CT$_{50}$ and CEM43°CT$_{90}$ between treatment responders and non-responders.

Table 9. Cont.

Author(s)	Cancer Site, n	CT Drug(s) (mg/m^2) × Cycles	Temperature Metrics (°C)	HT Session	t_{treat} (min)	Thermal Dose	t_{int} (min)	Sequence	Clinical Outcome (Comment)
de Wit et al. [135]	Recurrent uterine cervical carcinoma, $n = 19$	60, 70, 80 cisplatin once weekly × 6	T_{max} †: 41.6 ± 0.7 (39.7–43.6)	N_{total}: 6 N_{week}: 1	60	n.r.	0	HT after CT	• No dose limiting toxicity at the 80 mg/m^2 dose level of cisplatin. • CR: 1 patient (dose level 80 mg/m^2), PR: 18 patients, SD: 18 patients and PD: 3 patients (dose level: 60–80 mg/m^2) and OS ‡: 54%. • The improvement rate in QoL [11]: 82.5%. • No differences between responders and non-responders for tumor: contact temperatures, indicative temperatures, tumor volume, oral temperature increase or total power applied.
Sugimach et al. [124]	Oesophageal carcinoma, $n = 20$	30 * bleomycin twice weekly × 3 50 * cisplatin once weekly × 3	n.r.	N_{total}: 6 N_{week}: 2	30	n.r.	n.r.	HT after CT	• CR: 5%, PR: 25%, minimal response: 20%, NC [12]: 50% and decrease of tumor size in comparison to CT treatment only. (correlation of thermometric parameters with clinical outcome not presented)

n: number of patients assigned to be treated with HT in combination with CT; †: mean value (±standard deviation) or mean value (range); ‡: median (range); n.r.: not reported; *: in mg unit only; [1] LPFS: local progression free survival; [2] OS: overall survival; [3] CR: complete response; [4] PR: partial response; [5] SD: stable disease; [6] PD: progressive disease; [7] PFS: progression free survival; [8] PFR: progression free rate; [9] RR: response rate; [10] DFS: disease free survival; [11] QoL: quality of life; [12] NC: no change; [13] LTDL: low temperature liposomal doxorubicin.

Table 10. Retrospective clinical trial studies using CT in combination with HT.

Author(s)	Cancer Site, n	CT Drug(s) (mg/m^2) × Cycles	Temperature Metrics (°C)	HT Session	t_{treat} (min)	Thermal Dose	t_{int} (min)	Sequence	Clinical Outcome (Comment)
Yang et al. [140]	Advanced non-small cell lung cancer, $n = 48$	1000 gemcitabine twice weekly × 6; 75 cisplatin twice weekly × 6	n.r.	N_{total}: 8; N_{week}: 2	40–60	n.r.	n.r.	HT after CT or HT before CT	• No CR [1] reported, PR [2]: 37.5% (18/23), SD [3]: 33.3% (16/23), PD [4]: 29.2% (14/23). • ORR [5]: 37.5% and DCR [6]: 70.8%. • 1- and 2-year survival rates: 14% and 1.3%, respectively. • Toxicity, grade III: 14 patients and grade IV: no patients. (correlation of thermometric parameters with clinical outcome not presented)
Tschoep-Lechner et al. [141]	Advanced pancreatic cancer, $n = 23$	1000 gemcitabine once weekly × 8; 25 cisplatin twice weekly × 8	T_{max} ‡: 42.1 (40.9–44.1)	N_{week}: 2; N_{total} ‡: 8	60	n.r.	0	simultaneously	• PR: 4.34% (1/23), SD: 30.4% (7/23), PD: 34.7% (8/23); • OS [7]‡: 12.9 months (CI: 9.9–15.9 months). • Mild (grade 1 and 2) position-related pain during HT treatment. (correlation of thermometric parameters with clinical outcome not presented)

Table 10. *Cont.*

Author(s)	Cancer Site, n	CT Drug(s) (mg/m^2) × Cycles	Temperature Metrics (°C)	HT Session	t_{treat} (min)	Thermal Dose	t_{int} (min)	Sequence	Clinical Outcome (Comment)
Stahl et al. [137]	Soft tissue sarcomas, n = 46	250 etoposide × 4 6000 ifosfamide × 4 50 adriamycin × 4	T_{90} ‡: 39.90 ± 0.74 (good responders) and T_{90} ‡: 39.42 ± 1.78 (bad responders)	N_{week}: 2 N_{total} ‡: 8	60	CEM43°CT$_{90}$ ‡: 17.96 ± 7.16 (good responders) CEM43°CT$_{90}$ ‡: 11.07 ± 5.58 (good responders)	0	simultaneously	• PR: 31.6% (6/19 in the good responder group for RECIST[8]) to 37% (10/27 in the poor responder group for RECIST). • SD: 63.2% (12/19 for the good responder group in WHO[9] and volume) to 70.3% (19/27 in the poor responder group for volume). • T_{90} and CEM43°CT$_{90}$ parameters did not differ significantly between the groups.

n: number of patients assigned to be treated with HT in combination with CT; †: mean value (±standard deviation) or mean value (range); ‡: median (range); [1] CR: complete response; [2] PR: partial response; [3] SD: stable disease; [4] PD: progression disease; [5] ORR: objective response rate; [6] DCR: disease control rate; [7] OS: overall survival; [8] RECIST: Response Evaluation Criteria in Solid Tumors; [9] WHO: world health organization.

Based on preclinical studies, the delivery of simultaneous CT and HT is recommended to achieve the greatest chemosensitization effect by HT [55,142]. However, in contrast to experimental results [20,55], most of the prospective studies listed in Table 9 were designed to deliver heat sequentially, and in most studies the CT drugs were administered prior to HT. Despite the fact that a considerable supra-additive or synergistic effect can be achieved by the simultaneous delivery of CT and RT, the sequential application of CT and HT may protect normal tissues from chemosensitization. The cell killing of hypoxic and oxygenated tumor cells can still be obtained with sequential delivery of CT drugs and HT [54]. In clinical studies, the t_{int} between modalities is usually kept under an hour [122,127,133,136,138]. Of note, the study of Ishikawa et al. showed a different scheduling of gemcitabine and HT for the treatment of locally advanced or metastatic pancreatic cancer [139]. Patients enrolled in this clinical study were treated with HT prior to CT with a t_{int} of 0–24 h. This unique flexible relationship of gemcitabine cytotoxicity with the t_{int} and sequence was revealed in an in vitro study [143]. The specific properties of CT drugs are main factors in determining the most efficient treatment sequence between CT and HT for each class of drugs.

That treatment protocols might require individualized standards for HT thermometric parameters as has recently been illustrated by an interim analysis of cisplatin and etoposide given concurrently with HT for treatment of patients with esophageal carcinoma. This analysis showed a relationship between tumor location and temperature reporting, i.e., higher temperatures were achieved in distal tumors [144]. Similar treatment site-dependent analysis of thermometric parameters should be performed in future trials. Although the biology underlying the interaction between CT drugs and heat in cancer and normal tissues is largely unknown, thermometric parameters have been shown to predict outcome when HT is combined with CT. Therefore, as discussed above, no definitive conclusions can be drawn regarding the optimal thermometric parameters for an enhanced effect of HT with CT.

6. Evidence for Predictive Values of Thermometric Parameters in Clinical Studies Using RT and CT in Combination with HT

Clinical malignancies, in particular advanced and inoperable tumors, can be treated using triplet therapy consisting of CT, RT and HT as a maximal treatment approach. The number of prospective and retrospective clinical studies investigating this approach is limited, the most important of which are listed in Tables 11 and 12, respectively. These studies have already reported the feasibility of this trimodal approach for cervical cancer, rectal cancer, and pancreatic cancer.

The optimal combination of CT, RT, and HT in a single framework is complex, be-cause so many biological processes underly the interactions between the three modalities. In addition, clinical factors often influence the optimal combination of RT and CT. A template with fundamental specifications for designing a clinical study with the trimodal treatment is proposed by Herman et al. [145].

Even though there is no consensus as to the optimal scheduling of trimodal treatment, clinical studies to date integrate HT in combination with daily RT and CT drugs based on the concept that CT should interact with both RT and HT. Scheduling CT weekly is most feasible in terms of maintaining an optimal t_{int} between HT sessions, drug administration, and RT fraction [145].

The reason why cisplatin is most frequently used in trimodality regimens is less based on a specific interaction with heat, but rather on extensive evidence from phase III randomized trials showing that cisplatin potently improves the antitumor efficacy of radiotherapy, albeit at the cost of increased toxicity. Drug concentration has been shown to affect treatment response [146], as proven experimentally [147]. A phase I-II study reported that a higher cisplatin dose (50 mg/m^2) in comparison with a lower dose (20–40 mg/m^2) combined with RT and HT was positively correlated with CR [146]. Interestingly, overall survival between patients treated with two different CT regimes in combination with RT and HT did not differ [148]. However, the study was limited by the small size of the patient cohort. With reference to Table 11, clinical studies using trimodality treatment usually used conventional fractionation schemes with 1.8–2.0 Gy per fractions, leaving it largely unknown whether other schedules such as hypofractionation (>10 Gy per week or large single fractions) might be biologically more favorable. The total dose varied according to cancer type. In the case of cervical cancer, brachytherapy at high dose rate (HDR) or low dose rate (LDR) was applied to deliver the boost dose [149,150]. Furthermore, high or low total RT dose was reported to have an influence on CR rate when combined with 5-FU, leucovorin and HT [151]. In contrast to CT and RT treatment parameters, HT treatment parameters were frequently not reported. Thermometric parameters, such as temperature and thermal dose including t_{int}, are reported but not set as fixed treatment requirements as there are no accepted reference values.

Disregarding the Arrhenius relationship of heating temperature and t_{treat}, Amichetti et al. [152] reported a short t_{treat} of 30 min with mean temperature range values of T_{max} = 43.2 °C (41.5–44.5 °C) and T_{min} = 40.1 °C (37–42 °C). This might explain why this study did not result in a higher CR rate in comparison to the previous study by Valdagni et al. [103]. A correlation of achieved temperature with treatment response such as disease-free interval to local relapse (DFILR) was reported in the study by Kouloulias et al. [153]. This study showed that the DFILR rate was greater in patients who achieved heating temperature T_{90} > 44 °C for longer than 16 min during HT treatment. No significant correlation of DFILR with mean values of temperature descriptor T_{min} was confirmed. Referring to the last row in Tables 7–12, the clinical endpoints among studies differ, which adds another level of complexity to generalizing the thermometric parameter correlations reported in studies.

Thermal dose was reported less frequently than temperature measurements, hence there is a lack of information about its predictive role for treatment response. In one study, thermal dose was directly and proportionally associated with CR, as patients who exhibited CR after treatment with a measured CEM43°CT_{90} of 4.6 min in comparison with patients with a PR and a CEM43°CT_{90} of only 2.0 min [146]. Recently, a prospective phase II study investigating neoadjuvant triplet therapy in patients with rectal cancer showed that patients achieving good local tumor regression had received a high thermal dose [154]. However, no threshold, only the mean of CEM 43 °C, was reported. The retrospective analysis of thermometric parameters of the prospective study by Harima et al. [149] showed that >1 min CEM43°CT_{90} is the threshold value which significantly correlates with treatment response (CR and disease-free survival rates). It also confirmed that CEM43°CT_{90} below 1 min are insufficient to achieve enhancement of RT and CT [155]. Unfortunately, no further analyses of the relationship between HT treatment parameters with clinical outcomes in studies using triplet therapy were reported.

Furthermore, the optimal interval between heat, radiation and anticancer drugs is still unclear. With reference to preclinical and clinical outcomes, t_{int} affects the thermal enhancement effect of HT on both ionizing radiation and CT drugs. A particular interaction between HT and CT in terms of t_{int} was reported according to properties of the CT drugs. A short t_{int} between sequential HT and doxorubicin resulted in more rapid treatment response [153]. However, it is not clear whether the CT drug interacts primarily with RT only when administered on the same day or also during an extended time period. In the first scenario, CT and HT could typically be administered within a range of 1–6 h prior to RT to optimally exploit the biological interaction.

Table 11. Prospective clinical studies using RT and CT in combination with HT.

Author(s)	Cancer Site, n	CT Drug(s) (mg/m^2) × Cycles	RT Dose (Gy) /Fractions	Temperature Metrics (°C)	Session	t_{treat} (min)	Thermal Dose (min)	t_{int} (min)	Sequence	Clinical Outcome (Comment)
Amichetti et al. [152]	Locally advanced head & neck cancer, n = 18	20 cisplatin once weekly × 7	70.0/35	T_{max} ‡: 43.2 (41.5–44.5) T_{min} ‡: 40.1 (37–42) T_{90} ‡: 40.4 (38.7–42.2)	N_{total}: 2 N_{week}: 2	30	CEM42.5 °C T_{min} ‡: 4.36 (0–27) CEM42.5 °C T_{max} ‡: 88 (31.8–174)	20	HT after RT & CT	• CR^1: 72.2% (13/18), PR^2: 16.6% (3/18); NC^3: 11.1% (2/18). • OS^4: 88.8%, 3-year actuarial survival and probability of remaining free of nodal disease: 50.3% and 53.3%, respectively. • No temperature metrics correlated with an increased acute side effects and the amount of skin toxicity.
Maluta et al. [156]	Primary or recurrent locally advanced pancreatic cancer, n = 40	1000 gemcitabine × 1–2 30 cisplatin ×	30.0–66.0 /10–33	T_{90} ‡: 40.5 (95% CI: 39.8–41) T_{max} ‡: 41.1 (95% CI: 40.2–42.5)	N_{total}: 3–10 N_{week}: 2	60	n.r.	n.r.	CT before HT & RT	• OS ‡: 15 (6–20) months • The most common hematological toxicity was grade 2 anemia. Toxicity, grade III: 5 patients. (correlation of thermometric parameters with clinical outcome not presented)

Table 11. Cont.

Author(s)	Cancer Site, n	CT Drug(s) (mg/m^2) × Cycles	RT Dose (Gy) /Fractions	Temperature Metrics (°C)	Session	t_{treat} (min)	Thermal Dose (min)	t_{int} (min)	Sequence	Clinical Outcome (Comment)
Asao et al. [151]	Locally advanced rectal cancer, n = 29	250 5-fluorouracil for 5 days × 2 25 for 5 days × 2	40.0–50.0 /20–25	T_{max} †: 40.3 ± 0.89 (38.6–41.9)	N_{total}: 3 N_{week}: 1	60	n.r.	n.r.	HT after RT during CT	• Toxicity, grade III: 2 patients. • CR: 55.5% in patients with a total radiation dose of 50 Gy, which was significantly higher compared to patients treated with 40 Gy. • 41.4% of patients had significant downstaging. (correlation of thermometric parameters with clinical outcome not reported)
Westermann et al. [150]	Cervix cancer, n = 68	40 cisplatin once weekly × 35	45.0–50.4 with LDR-IRT [7] and HDR-IRT [7] (^{192}Ir)	T_{90} †: 39.4 T_{50} †: 40.7	N_{total}: 8–10 N_{week}: 1	60	n.r.	n.r.	HT & CT after/before RT	• CR: 90%, 2-year DFS [5] and OS: 71.6% and 78.5%, respectively. • A significant difference in DFS between Netherlands and US clinical centers. • Specific toxicity associated with HT was mild. (correlation of thermometric parameters with clinical outcome not reported)

Table 11. Cont.

Author(s)	Cancer Site, n	CT Drug(s) (mg/m^2) × Cycles	RT Dose (Gy) /Fractions	Temperature Metrics (°C)	Session	t_{treat} (min)	Thermal Dose (min)	t_{int} (min)	Sequence	Clinical Outcome (Comment)
Harima et al. [149]	Locally advanced cervical cancer, $n = 51$	30–40 cisplatin once weekly × 3–5	30.0–50.0 /15–25 with LDR-IRT7 (192 Ir): 5.0–6.0 /3–5	T_{max} †: 42.2 (40.1–44.6) T_{avg} †: 41.1 (39.6–42.5) Data from Ohguri et al. [155] T_{90} ‡: 38.9 (37.7–42.2) T_{50} ‡: 39.9 (38.4–42.4)	N_{total}: 4–6 N_{week}: 1	60	CEM43°CT_{90} †: 3.8 (0.1–46.6)	20	HT after RT&CT	• CR: 88% (44/50). • 5-year OS, DFS, and LPFS ^{6} were 77.8%, 70.8% and 80.1%, respectively. • It was well tolerated and caused no additional acute or long term toxicity. • Ohguri et al. [155]: CEM43°CT_{90} ≥ 1 min tended to predict better DFS and CR.
Kouloulias et al. [153]	Recurrent breast cancer, $n = 15$	40–60 liposomal doxorubicin once monthly × 6	30.6/17	T_{max} †: 43.2 (41.5–44.5) T_{min} †: 45.0 (44.2–45.7)	N_{total}: 6 $N_{monthly}$: 1	60	n.r.	180–240	HT after CT&RT	• CR: 2% (3/15), PR: 80% (12/15); • CR or PR obtained more quickly with a shorter t_{int} between HT and CT. • DFILR ^{7} was better for $T_{90} > 44$ °C of ≥16 min compared with those for whom $T_{90} > 44$ °C of <16 min. • DFILR was significantly correlated with T_{min} † but not with T_{max} †.

Table 11. *Cont.*

Author(s)	Cancer Site, n	CT Drug(s) (mg/m^2) × Cycles	RT Dose (Gy) /Fractions	Temperature Metrics (°C)	Session	t_{treat} (min)	Thermal Dose (min)	t_{int} (min)	Sequence	Clinical Outcome (Comment)
Herman et al. [146]	Locally advanced malignancies, n = 24	20–50 cisplatin once weekly × 6	60.0–66.0 /30-33 or 24.0–36.0 /12–18	T_{max} †: 43.7 ± 2.6 T_{min} †: 38.2 ± 2.0 T_{avg} †: 40.8 ± 1.9	N_{total}: 6 N_{week}: 1	60	CEM42°CT$_{90}$ †: 11.2 ± 21.3 CEM43°CT$_{90}$ †: 3.1 ± 5.4	n.r.	HT before CT&RT	• CR: 50% (12/24), PR: 50% (12/24); • No grade III acute toxicity. • Late toxicity, grade IV: only 1 patient. • With thermal dose of CEM43°CT$_{90}$ † = 4.6 min, 50% of patients achieved CR and with CEM43°CT$_{90}$ † = 2.0 min, 50% patients achieved PR. • Cisplatin concentration amount correlated with CR.
Barsukov et al. [157]	Locally advanced rectal cancer, n = 68	650 capecitabine on days 1–22 × 6–8 50 oxaliplatin on days 3, 10 and 17 after × 6–8 10 metronidazole on days 8 and 15	40.0/10	n.r.	N_{total}: 4 N_{week}: 2	60	n.r.	60	n.r.	• 2-year OS: 91%, DFS: 83% and local RR: 13.6% • R0 resection was achieved in 59 (92.2%). only five (7.8%) untreated patients remained inoperable. • 12 (18.7%) and 1 (1.6%) patients had grade III and IV toxicity, respectively. (correlation of thermometric parameters with clinical outcome not presented)

Table 11. Cont.

Author(s)	Cancer Site, n	CT Drug(s) (mg/m²) × Cycles	RT Dose (Gy) /Fractions	Temperature Metrics (°C)	Session	t_{treat} (min)	Thermal Dose (min)	t_{int} (min)	Sequence	Clinical Outcome (Comment)
Ott et al. [158]	Locally advanced or recurrent rectal cancer, n = 105	250 5-fluorouracil on days 1–14 and 22–35 or 1650 capecitabine on days 1–14 and 22–35 50 oxaliplatin × 4	LARC 50.4/28 LCC 45/25	n.r.	N_{total} ‡: 10 N_{week}: 2	60	LARC [19] CEM43°C †: 6.4 ± 5.2 LCC [20] CEM43°C †: 6.4 ± 4.9	n.r.	HT before RT	• 11% (2/19) and 27% (16/59) DLT [8] criteria, corresponding to FR [9]: 90% and 73%, respectively. • Pathological CR: 20% (19/95), CTR [10]: 28% (18/64) and 38% (3/8) in patients with LARC and LRRC, respectively. 5-year OS: 75% for the whole group. • No grade 4–5 adverse events. (correlation of thermometric parameters with clinical outcome not presented)
Gani et al. [154]	Locally advanced rectal cancer, n = 78	1000 5-fluorouracil × 4	50.4/28	T_{90} ‡: 39.5 (IQR: 39.1–39.9)	N_{total}: 8 N_{week}: 2	60	CEM43°C ‡: 4.5 (IQR: 2.2–8.2)	n.r.	n.r.	• 19/78 (24%) patients: died or had tumor recurrence. • 3-year OS: 94%, DFS: 81%, LC [11]: 96% and DC: 87%. • Pathological CR: 14% (the threshold not met). • Patients with good tumor regression had higher values for CEM43°C. • Comparable global health status with the data from general population based on EORTC-QLQ-C30 [12].

Table 11. Cont.

Author(s)	Cancer Site, n	CT Drug(s) (mg/m^2) × Cycles	RT Dose (Gy) /Fractions	Temperature Metrics (°C)	Session	t_{treat} (min)	Thermal Dose (min)	t_{int} (min)	Sequence	Clinical Outcome (Comment)
Rau et al. [159]	Locally advanced rectal cancer, n = 37	300–350 5-fluorouracil 50 * mg leucovorin 5 times weekly × 2	45.0–50.0 /25	Data from Rau et al. [160]: T_{90} †: 40.2 ± 1.2 T_{max} †: 41.4 ± 0.6	N_{total} †: 5 N_{week}: 1	60	Data from Rau et al. [160] CEM43°CT$_{90}$ †: 7.7 ± 5.6 CEM43°CT$_{max}$ †: 33.1 ± 28.0	n.r.	RT after concurrent HT&CT	• Grade III toxicity: 16%. • ORR [13]: 89%, and 31 resection specimens had negative margins. RR [14]: 59.4%, CR: 14%, OS: 56%. • Cumulative minutes at $T_{90} \geq 40.5$ °C and T_{90} correlate with the RR but not with long term OS and DFSR [15] [160] but T_{max} showed no significant influence on RR. • RR: 33% when $T_{90} < 40.5$ °C and RR: 75% response, $T_{90} > 40.5$ °C.
Wittlinger et al. [161]	Bladder cancer, n = 45	20 cisplatin 5 times weekly × 2 600 5-fluorouracil 5 times weekly × 2	50.4–55.8/ 28–31	T_{avg} †: 40.8 (95%CI: 40.5–41.6)	N_{total}: 5–7 N_{week}: 1	60	CEM43°C †:57 (95%CI: 40.5–41.6)	60	RT after concurrent CT&HT	• CR: 96%, NC: 4%. • Freedom from any local and distant relapse: 69% and relapse: 16%. • 3-year bladder preservation: 96%, LPFS: 81%, DSS: 88%, DFS: 71%, OS: 80% and MFS [16]. 89%. • One of significant prognostic factors for OS: N_{week}. • Acute toxicity, grades III-IV: 27%. • Late toxicity, grades III-IV: 24%.

Table 11. *Cont.*

Author(s)	Cancer Site, n	CT Drug(s) (mg/m^2) × Cycles	RT Dose (Gy) /Fractions	Temperature Metrics (°C)	Session	t_{treat} (min)	Thermal Dose (min)	t_{int} (min)	Sequence	Clinical Outcome (Comment)
Milani et al. [162]	Recurrent rectal cancer, n = 24	350 5-fluorouracil 5 times weekly × 4 (continuous infusion)	30.0–45.0/ 16–25	T_{90} †: 41.4 T_{50} †: 42.9 T_{20} †: 43.5	N_{total} ‡: 8 N_{week}: 2	60	n.r.	60	HT after concurrent RT&CT	• CR: 0% (0/20), PR: 10% (2/20), NC: 85% (17/20), PD: 5% (1/20). • 1-year OS, DMFS [17], LPFR [18]: 87%, 82%, 61%, respectively. • 2-year OS, DMFS, LPFR: 60%, 52%, 30%, respectively. • 3-year OS, DMFS, LPFR: 30%, 39%, 15%, respectively. • Acute toxicity, grade III: 12.5% of the patients. (correlation of thermometric parameters with clinical outcome not presented)

n: number of patients assigned to be treated with HT in combination with RT and CT; †: mean value (±standard deviation) or mean value (range); ‡: median (range); [1] CR: complete response; [2] PR: partial response; [3] NC: no change; [4] OS: overall survival; [5] DFS: disease free survival; [6] LPFS: local progression free survival; [7] DFILR: disease-free interval to local relapse; [8] DLT: dose limiting toxicities; [9] FR: feasibility rate; [10] CTR: complete tumor regression; [11] LC: local control; [12] EORTC-QLQ: European Organization for research and treatment of cancer-quality of life questionnaire; [13] ORR: objective response rate; [14] RR: response rate; [15] DFSR: disease-free survival rate; [16] MFS: metastasis-free survival; [17] DMFS: distant metastases-free survival; [18] LPFR: local progression-free survival; [19] LARC: locally advanced rectal cancer; [20] LCC: recurrent rectal cancer.

Table 12. Retrospective clinical studies using RT and CT in combination with HT.

Author(s)	Cancer Site, n	CT Drug (s)(mg/m²) × Cycles	RT Dose (Gy) /Fractions	Temperature Metrics (°C)	Session	t_{treat} (min)	Thermal Dose (min)	t_{int} (min)	Sequence	Clinical Outcome (Comment)
Zhu et al. [163]	Locally advanced esophageal cancer, n = 78	450 5-fluorouracil five times weekly × 4–6 25 cisplatin five times weekly × 4–6	60.0–66.0 /30–33	n.r.	N_{total}: 6–12 N_{week}: 2	60	n.r.	120	n.r.	• CR[1]: 39.7% (31/78), PR[2]: 56.4% (43/78), SD[3]: 3.9% (3/78). • 1-, 2- and 3-year LRC[4]: 76.9%, 55.1% and 47.4%, respectively; • 1-, 2- and 3-year DMFS[5]: 67.9%, 38.5% and 30.8% respectively; • 1-, 2- and 3-year OS[6]: 67.9%, 41.0% and 33.3%, respectively (correlation of thermometric parameters with clinical outcome not presented)
Ohguri et al. [148]	Locally advanced pancreatic cancer, n = 20	Group A: 40–50 gemcitabine twice weekly × 4 Group B: 200–500 gemcitabine once weekly × 3	50.4–64.8 /28–36	n.r.	N_{total}: 6 N_{week}: 1	n.r.	n.r.	Group A: Instant Group B: 60–180	HT after CT&RT	• Grade II-IV hematological toxicities: 8 patients. • The objective tumor response, CR for 1 patient, PR for 4, and NC[7] for 15. DM[8]: 13 and LF[9]: 5 patients. • DPFS[10]: 8.8 months, OS[‡]: 18.6 months. • The treatment regimen did not correlate with the survival rates. (correlation of thermometric parameters with clinical outcome not presented)

Table 12. Cont.

Author(s)	Cancer Site, n	CT Drug (s)(mg/m^2) × Cycles	RT Dose (Gy) /Fractions	Temperature Metrics (°C)	Session	t_{treat} (min)	Thermal Dose (min)	t_{int} (min)	Sequence	Clinical Outcome (Comment)
Gani et al. [164]	Locally advanced rectal cancer, n = 60	1000 5-fluorouracil × 4	50.4/28	T_{90} ‡: 39.3 (37.1–40.6)	N_{total} ‡: 4 N_{week}: 1–2	60	CEM43°C ‡: 1.1 (0.0–9.2)	n.r.	n.r.	• 5-year OS, DFS [11], local control and DMFS were 83%, 75%, 93% and 76%, respectively. • No impact of HT on DFS and DMFS. • N_{total} not predictive for OS, DFS, LC, or DMFS. Postoperative nodal stage remained a significant prognosticator for OS, DFS and DMFS (multivariate analysis).
Merten et al. [165]	Bladder cancer, n = 79	20 cisplatin 5 times weekly × 2 600 5-fluorouracil 5 times weekly × 2	50.4–55.8/ 28–31	n.r.	N_{total}: 5–7 N_{week}: 1	60	n.r.	0–60	RT after concurrent CT&HT	• CR: 87% (67/77). • 5- and 10-year OS: 87% and 60%, respectively. • 5- and 10-year DFS to 66% and 46% respectively. • Acute toxicity, grade III: 11% and grade IV: 3%. • Late toxicity, grade III: 1.3%. (correlation of thermometric parameters with clinical outcome not presented)

Table 12. *Cont.*

Author(s)	Cancer Site, n	CT Drug (s)(mg/m²) × Cycles	RT Dose (Gy) /Fractions	Temperature Metrics (°C)	Session	t_{treat} (min)	Thermal Dose (min)	t_{int} (min)	Sequence	Clinical Outcome (Comment)
van Haaren et al. [166]	Esophageal cancer, n = 29	50 paclitaxelonce weekly × 5 and carboplatin (AUC=2) once weekly × 5	41.4/23	T_{90} ‡: 38.6 ± 0.5 T_{50} ‡: 39.2 ± 0.6 T_{10} ‡: 40.1 ± 0.8	N_{total}: 5 N_{week}: 1	60	n.r.	0–60	HT after CT & RT	• CR: 19% (5/29), mPR [12]: 26% (7/29), PR: 33% (9/29) and SD: 22% (6/29). • The dependence of T_{50} on the body size parameters was substantial. (correlation of thermometric parameters with clinical outcome not presented)

n: number of patients assigned to be treated with HT in combination with RT; ‡: mean value (±standard deviation) or mean value (range); ‡: median (range); [1] CR: complete response; [2] PR: partial response; [3] SD: stable disease; [4] LRC:locoregional control, [5] DMFS: distant metastasis-free survival; [6] OS: overall survival; [7] NC: no change; [8] DM: distant metastases; [9] LF: local failure; [10] DPFS: disease progression-free survival; [11] DFS:disease free survival; [12] mPR: partial remission with only residual microscopic tumor foci.

Moreover, the N_{total} was shown to be a prognostic factor for OS for bladder cancer patients treated with combined CT, RT, and HT followed by surgery [161]. In contrast, Gani et al. [164] reported that the number of HT sessions was not predictive for OS, DFS, LC, or distant metastasis-free survival. Neither did the sequencing of CT, HT, and RT in clinical reports follow a specific pattern. Preclinical studies are required to better understand the interaction of CT, RT, and heat and how they should be combined in future clinical trials.

7. Future Prospects

The main limitations of HT as a cancer treatment in current clinical practice are the need for better standardization of treatment protocols, up-to-date quality assurance guidelines that are widely applicable and dedicated planning systems to generate patient treatment plans. The wide variation of thermometric parameters derived from clinical studies indicate that HT treatment is currently delivered according to individual clinical center guidelines. Consequently, the comparison of clinical study outcomes is substantially hampered by the large degree of variation in treatment parameters. Regarding the data summarized in Tables 6–11, apart from thermal dose and temperature measured during treatment, other thermometric parameters reported often include only t_{treat}, t_{int}, or N_{week}.

Monitoring and measuring temperature is one of the main challenges in routine clinical practice and has hindered the clinical expansion of HT. The future of HT in combination with RT and CT requires novel technical developments for the delivery and measurement of homogenous heating of the malignant tissues. Not all studies (Tables 7–12) recorded temperatures in the region of the tumor. The process of inserting temperature probes to monitor and record the HT is considered invasive and uncomfortable, and sometimes the tumor site is inaccessible for the temperature probe. For example, Milani et al. [162] reported that even though the tumors were not deep-seated, intratumoral temperature measurements were only feasible in one of 24 patients, so no representative thermal doses could be reported. One of the non-invasive approaches currently under clinical evaluation is magnetic resonance thermometry (MRT) that provides 3-D temperature measurements. Hybrid MR/HT devices are currently installed in five European clinical centers.

Temperature measurements in anthropomorphic phantoms with MRT are accurate in comparison with thermistor probes [167], but clinical measurements are currently inaccurate in most pelvic and abdominal tumors [168]. The physiological changes in tissue microenvironment, patient movements, magnetic field drift over time, limited sensitivity in fatty tissues, and respiratory motion, including cardiac activity in regions of the pelvis and abdomen, hamper the accurate temperature measurement by MRT [168]. The temperature images from MRT systems contain image distortion, artifacts, and noise, leading to inaccurate temperature measurement, low temporal resolution, and low imaging to signal-to-noise ratio (SNR) [169]. The sources and solutions of image artifacts as a result of additional frequencies were described by Gellermann et al. [170]. Proton-resonance frequency shift (PRFS), apparent diffusion coefficient (ADC), longitudinal relaxation time (T_1), transversal relaxation time (T2), and equilibrium magnetization (M0) are the imaging techniques used to exploit temperature-dependent parameters [170–173]. The PRFS technique is the most frequently used MRT method, even though it was shown that when there is a poor magnetic field homogeneity, ADC or T_1 techniques are preferable [174]. However, the accuracy of temperature measurements was in the range of ± 0.4 to ± 0.5 °C between PRFS method and thermistor probe using a heterogeneous phantom [175]. A stronger correlation between MRT and thermistor probes was found in patients with soft tissue sarcomas of lower extremities and pelvis [176] in comparison with recurrent rectal carcinoma [177]. The successful implementation of MRT in clinical centers, as automated temperature feedback during the HT session, might have a considerable impact on clinical outcomes to deliver the desired heating and conform the heat distribution to spare healthy surrounding tissues. This could substantially help to standardize data collection and the analysis of thermometric parameters. Another experimental approach to monitoring treatment temperature during HT sessions is electrical impedance tomography (EIT) as recently reported in a simulation study by Poni et al. [178]. EIT captures the electrical conductivity of tissues depends on temperature elevation. For example, the multifrequency EIT technique detects the changes in conductivity due to perfusion increase induced by the change in temperature [179]. The accuracy of EIT for temperature measurements was reported to range from 1.5 °C to 5 °C [180]. The potential of EIT to monitor temperature in the cardiac thermal ablation field is being investigated [181]. This technique also holds promise for HT treatment. Both MRT and EIT may allow for improvement of the spatial homogeneity of heat to the cancer tissues.

The technological advances and standardization of international treatment protocols for different cancer types will improve the effectiveness and synergy of HT in combination with RT and/or CT. In line with this, there is a need for clinically accepted processes for the recording and reporting of thermometric data. This will allow for the inclusion of specific thermometric parameters in future clinical studies combining HT with RT and/or CT. For any future prospective study, it should be mandatory that thermometric parameters are recorded and some recommendations are available in the current guidelines [43,46]. The integration of thermometric parameters is one of the objectives of the HYPERBOOST ("Hyperthermia boosting the effect of Radiotherapy") international consortium within the European Horizon 2020 Program MSCA-ITN. The HYPERBOOST network aims to create a novel treatment planning system, including the standardization of thermometric parameters derived from retrospective and prospective clinical trials.

8. Conclusions

In this review, we provide an extensive overview of thermometric parameters reported in prospective and retrospective clinical studies which applied HT in combination with RT and/or CT and their correlation with clinical outcome. It is recognized that there is a wide variety in the practice of HT between clinical centers, and we aimed to elucidate the use and reporting of thermometric parameters in different clinical settings. It emerged that the sequencing of HT and RT varies more than the sequencing of HT and CT. Only a few standards seem to exist with regard to the sequence of HT with RT and CT in a triplet for specific CT drug, RT fractionation and thermal dose. According to the evaluated studies, t_{int} is a critical parameter in clinical routine, but no clinical reference values have been established. Of note, a constant t_{treat} of 60 min throughout the HT treatment course was described in most clinical studies. The most important parameter seems to be temperature itself, which correlates with thermal dose. Revealing the relationship between thermal dose and treatment response for different cancer entities in future clinical studies will lead to the improved application of heat to promote the synergistic actions of HT with RT and CT. We suggest that it become mandatory for new clinical study protocols to include the extensive recording and analysis of thermometric parameters for their validation and overall standardization of HT. This would allow for the definition of thermometric parameters, in particular of thresholds for temperature descriptors and thermal dose.

Author Contributions: Conceptualization, O.R. and P.G.; writing, A.A. and O.R.; writing—review and editing, A.A., O.R., D.P.V., P.G., D.M., H.C., E.O., O.J.O., S.R., P.W., R.A.H., E.P., S.B. and R.F.; visualization, A.A. and O.R.; supervision, H.C., R.F., O.R. and P.G. All authors have read and agreed to the published version of the manuscript.

Funding: This research has received support from the European Union's Horizon 2020 research and innovation programme under the Marie Skłodowska-Curie (MSCA-ITN) grant "Hyperboost" project, no. 955625.

Conflicts of Interest: The authors declare no conflict of interest.

References

1. Wust, P.; Hildebrandt, B.; Sreenivasa, G.; Rau, B.; Gellermann, J.; Riess, H.; Felix, R.; Schlag, P.M. Hyperthermia in combined treatment of cancer. *Lancet Oncol.* **2002**, *3*, 487–497. [CrossRef]
2. Van der Zee, J. Heating the patient: A promising approach? *Ann. Oncol.* **2002**, *13*, 1173–1184. [CrossRef] [PubMed]

3. Horsman, M.R.; Overgaard, J. Hyperthermia: A potent enhancer of radiotherapy. *Clin. Oncol. (R Coll. Radiol.)* **2007**, *19*, 418–426. [CrossRef]
4. Engin, K. Biological rationale and clinical experience with hyperthermia. *Control Clin. Trials* **1996**, *17*, 316–342. [CrossRef]
5. Oei, A.L.; Vriend, L.E.; Crezee, J.; Franken, N.A.; Krawczyk, P.M. Effects of hyperthermia on DNA repair pathways: One treatment to inhibit them all. *Radiat. Oncol.* **2015**, *10*, 165. [CrossRef]
6. Dewey, W.C.; Hopwood, L.E.; Sapareto, S.A.; Gerweck, L.E. Cellular responses to combinations of hyperthermia and radiation. *Radiology* **1977**, *123*, 463–474. [CrossRef]
7. Overgaard, J. Effect of hyperthermia on the hypoxic fraction in an experimental mammary carcinoma in vivo. *Br. J. Radiol.* **1981**, *54*, 245–249. [CrossRef]
8. Oei, A.L.; Kok, H.P.; Oei, S.B.; Horsman, M.R.; Stalpers, L.J.A.; Franken, N.A.P.; Crezee, J. Molecular and biological rationale of hyperthermia as radio- and chemosensitizer. *Adv. Drug Deliv. Rev.* **2020**, *163–164*, 84–97. [CrossRef]
9. Dewhirst, M.W.; Vujaskovic, Z.; Jones, E.; Thrall, D. Re-setting the biologic rationale for thermal therapy. *Int. J. Hyperthermia* **2005**, *21*, 779–790. [CrossRef]
10. Lepock, J.R. Role of nuclear protein denaturation and aggregation in thermal radiosensitization. *Int. J. Hyperthermia* **2004**, *20*, 115–130. [CrossRef]
11. Calderwood, S.K.; Theriault, J.R.; Gong, J. How is the immune response affected by hyperthermia and heat shock proteins? *Int. J. Hyperthermia* **2005**, *21*, 713–716. [CrossRef] [PubMed]
12. Repasky, E.A.; Evans, S.S.; Dewhirst, M.W. Temperature matters! And why it should matter to tumor immunologists. *Cancer Immunol. Res.* **2013**, *1*, 210–216. [CrossRef] [PubMed]
13. Mukhopadhaya, A.; Mendecki, J.; Dong, X.; Liu, L.; Kalnicki, S.; Garg, M.; Alfieri, A.; Guha, C. Localized hyperthermia combined with intratumoral dendritic cells induces systemic antitumor immunity. *Cancer Res.* **2007**, *67*, 7798–7806. [CrossRef] [PubMed]
14. Frey, B.; Weiss, E.M.; Rubner, Y.; Wunderlich, R.; Ott, O.J.; Sauer, R.; Fietkau, R.; Gaipl, U.S. Old and new facts about hyperthermia-induced modulations of the immune system. *Int. J. Hyperthermia* **2012**, *28*, 528–542. [CrossRef] [PubMed]
15. Overgaard, J. Simultaneous and sequential hyperthermia and radiation treatment of an experimental tumor and its surrounding normal tissue in vivo. *Int. J. Radiat. Oncol. Biol. Phys.* **1980**, *6*, 1507–1517. [CrossRef]
16. Henle, K.J.; Leeper, D.B. Interaction of hyperthermia and radiation in CHO cells: Recovery kinetics. *Radiat. Res.* **1976**, *66*, 505–518. [CrossRef]
17. Overgaard, J.; Suit, H.D. Time-temperature relationship th hyperthermic treatment of malignant and normal tissue in vivo. *Cancer Res.* **1979**, *39*, 3248–3253.
18. Nielsen, O.S.; Overgaard, J.; Kamura, T. Influence of thermotolerance on the interaction between hyperthermia and radiation in a solid tumour in vivo. *Br. J. Radiol.* **1983**, *56*, 267–273. [CrossRef]
19. Roizin-Towle, L.; Pirro, J.P. The response of human and rodent cells to hyperthermia. *Int. J. Radiat. Oncol. Biol. Phys.* **1991**, *20*, 751–756. [CrossRef]
20. Dahl, O.; Mella, O. Effect of timing and sequence of hyperthermia and cyclophosphamide on a neurogenic rat tumor (BT4A) in vivo. *Cancer* **1983**, *52*, 983–987. [CrossRef]
21. Sapareto, S.A.; Dewey, W.C. Thermal dose determination in cancer therapy. *Int. J. Radiat. Oncol. Biol. Phys.* **1984**, *10*, 787–800. [CrossRef]
22. Van Leeuwen, C.M.; Oei, A.L.; Chin, K.; Crezee, J.; Bel, A.; Westermann, A.M.; Buist, M.R.; Franken, N.A.P.; Stalpers, L.J.A.; Kok, H.P. A short time interval between radiotherapy and hyperthermia reduces in-field recurrence and mortality in women with advanced cervical cancer. *Radiat. Oncol.* **2017**, *12*, 75. [CrossRef] [PubMed]
23. Overgaard, J. Influence of sequence and interval on the biological response to combined hyperthermia and radiation. *Natl. Cancer Inst. Monogr.* **1982**, *61*, 325–332. [PubMed]
24. Kapp, D.S.; Petersen, I.A.; Cox, R.S.; Hahn, G.M.; Fessenden, P.; Prionas, S.D.; Lee, E.R.; Meyer, J.L.; Samulski, T.V.; Bagshaw, M.A. Two or six hyperthermia treatments as an adjunct to radiation therapy yield similar tumor responses: Results of a randomized trial. *Int. J. Radiat. Oncol. Biol. Phys.* **1990**, *19*, 1481–1495. [CrossRef]
25. Arcangeli, G.; Nervi, C.; Cividalli, A.; Lovisolo, G.A. Problem of sequence and fractionation in the clinical application of combined heat and radiation. *Cancer Res.* **1984**, *44*, 4857s–4863s.
26. Gerweck, L.E.; Gillette, E.L.; Dewey, W.C. Effect of heat and radiation on synchronous Chinese hamster cells: Killing and repair. *Radiat. Res.* **1975**, *64*, 611–623. [CrossRef]
27. Pauwels, B.; Korst, A.E.; Lardon, F.; Vermorken, J.B. Combined modality therapy of gemcitabine and radiation. *Oncologist* **2005**, *10*, 34–51. [CrossRef]
28. Ohtsubo, T.; Saito, H.; Tanaka, N.; Matsumoto, H.; Sugimoto, C.; Saito, T.; Hayashi, S.; Kano, E. Enhancement of cisplatin sensitivity and platinum uptake by 40 degrees C hyperthermia in resistant cells. *Cancer Lett.* **1997**, *119*, 47–52. [CrossRef]
29. Oleson, J.R.; Sim, D.A.; Manning, M.R. Analysis of prognostic variables in hyperthermia treatment of 161 patients. *Int. J. Radiat. Oncol. Biol. Phys.* **1984**, *10*, 2231–2239. [CrossRef]
30. Cox, R.S.; Kapp, D.S. Correlation of thermal parameters with outcome in combined radiation therapy-hyperthermia trials. *Int. J. Hyperthermia* **1992**, *8*, 719–732. [CrossRef]
31. Dewhirst, M.W.; Sim, D.A. The utility of thermal dose as a predictor of tumor and normal tissue responses to combined radiation and hyperthermia. *Cancer Res.* **1984**, *44*, 4772s–4780s. [PubMed]

32. Leopold, K.A.; Dewhirst, M.; Samulski, T.; Harrelson, J.; Tucker, J.A.; George, S.L.; Dodge, R.K.; Grant, W.; Clegg, S.; Prosnitz, L.R.; et al. Relationships among tumor temperature, treatment time, and histopathological outcome using preoperative hyperthermia with radiation in soft tissue sarcomas. *Int. J. Radiat. Oncol. Biol. Phys.* **1992**, *22*, 989–998. [CrossRef]
33. Kroesen, M.; Mulder, H.T.; van Holthe, J.M.L.; Aangeenbrug, A.A.; Mens, J.W.M.; van Doorn, H.C.; Paulides, M.M.; Oomen-de Hoop, E.; Vernhout, R.M.; Lutgens, L.C.; et al. The Effect of the Time Interval Between Radiation and Hyperthermia on Clinical Outcome in 400 Locally Advanced Cervical Carcinoma Patients. *Front. Oncol.* **2019**, *9*, 134. [CrossRef] [PubMed]
34. Crezee, J.; Oei, A.L.; Franken, N.A.P.; Stalpers, L.J.A.; Kok, H.P. Response: Commentary: The Impact of the Time Interval Between Radiation and Hyperthermia on Clinical Outcome in Patients With Locally Advanced Cervical Cancer. *Front. Oncol.* **2020**, *10*, 528. [CrossRef] [PubMed]
35. Jones, E.L.; Oleson, J.R.; Prosnitz, L.R.; Samulski, T.V.; Vujaskovic, Z.; Yu, D.; Sanders, L.L.; Dewhirst, M.W. Randomized trial of hyperthermia and radiation for superficial tumors. *J. Clin. Oncol.* **2005**, *23*, 3079–3085. [CrossRef]
36. Franckena, M.; Fatehi, D.; de Bruijne, M.; Canters, R.A.; van Norden, Y.; Mens, J.W.; van Rhoon, G.C.; van der Zee, J. Hyperthermia dose-effect relationship in 420 patients with cervical cancer treated with combined radiotherapy and hyperthermia. *Eur. J. Cancer* **2009**, *45*, 1969–1978. [CrossRef]
37. Kapp, D.S.; Cox, R.S. Thermal treatment parameters are most predictive of outcome in patients with single tumor nodules per treatment field in recurrent adenocarcinoma of the breast. *Int. J. Radiat. Oncol. Biol. Phys.* **1995**, *33*, 887–899. [CrossRef]
38. Oleson, J.R.; Samulski, T.V.; Leopold, K.A.; Clegg, S.T.; Dewhirst, M.W.; Dodge, R.K.; George, S.L. Sensitivity of hyperthermia trial outcomes to temperature and time: Implications for thermal goals of treatment. *Int. J. Radiat. Oncol. Biol. Phys.* **1993**, *25*, 289–297. [CrossRef]
39. Sherar, M.; Liu, F.F.; Pintilie, M.; Levin, W.; Hunt, J.; Hill, R.; Hand, J.; Vernon, C.; van Rhoon, G.; van der Zee, J.; et al. Relationship between thermal dose and outcome in thermoradiotherapy treatments for superficial recurrences of breast cancer: Data from a phase III trial. *Int. J. Radiat. Oncol. Biol. Phys.* **1997**, *39*, 371–380. [CrossRef]
40. Leopold, K.A.; Dewhirst, M.W.; Samulski, T.V.; Dodge, R.K.; George, S.L.; Blivin, J.L.; Prosnitz, L.R.; Oleson, J.R. Cumulative minutes with T90 greater than Tempindex is predictive of response of superficial malignancies to hyperthermia and radiation. *Int. J. Radiat. Oncol. Biol. Phys.* **1993**, *25*, 841–847. [CrossRef]
41. Dinges, S.; Harder, C.; Wurm, R.; Buchali, A.; Blohmer, J.; Gellermann, J.; Wust, P.; Randow, H.; Budach, V. Combined treatment of inoperable carcinomas of the uterine cervix with radiotherapy and regional hyperthermia. Results of a phase II trial. *Strahlenther. Onkol.* **1998**, *174*, 517–521. [CrossRef] [PubMed]
42. Bakker, A.; van der Zee, J.; van Tienhoven, G.; Kok, H.P.; Rasch, C.R.N.; Crezee, H. Temperature and thermal dose during radiotherapy and hyperthermia for recurrent breast cancer are related to clinical outcome and thermal toxicity: A systematic review. *Int. J. Hyperthermia* **2019**, *36*, 1024–1039. [CrossRef]
43. Trefná, H.D.; Crezee, H.; Schmidt, M.; Marder, D.; Lamprecht, U.; Ehmann, M.; Hartmann, J.; Nadobny, J.; Gellermann, J.; van Holthe, N.; et al. Quality assurance guidelines for superficial hyperthermia clinical trials: I. Clinical requirements. *Int. J. Hyperthermia* **2017**, *33*, 471–482. [CrossRef]
44. Paulides, M.M.; Dobsicek Trefna, H.; Curto, S.; Rodrigues, D.B. Recent technological advancements in radiofrequency- and microwave-mediated hyperthermia for enhancing drug delivery. *Adv. Drug Deliv. Rev.* **2020**, *163–164*, 3–18. [CrossRef] [PubMed]
45. Kok, H.P.; Crezee, J. A comparison of the heating characteristics of capacitive and radiative superficial hyperthermia. *Int. J. Hyperthermia* **2017**, *33*, 378–386. [CrossRef] [PubMed]
46. Bruggmoser, G.; Bauchowitz, S.; Canters, R.; Crezee, H.; Ehmann, M.; Gellermann, J.; Lamprecht, U.; Lomax, N.; Messmer, M.B.; Ott, O.; et al. Guideline for the clinical application, documentation and analysis of clinical studies for regional deep hyperthermia: Quality management in regional deep hyperthermia. *Strahlenther. Onkol.* **2012**, *188* (Suppl. 2), 198–211. [CrossRef]
47. Dobšíček Trefná, H.; Crezee, J.; Schmidt, M.; Marder, D.; Lamprecht, U.; Ehmann, M.; Nadobny, J.; Hartmann, J.; Lomax, N.; Abdel-Rahman, S.; et al. Quality assurance guidelines for superficial hyperthermia clinical trials: II. Technical requirements for heating devices. *Strahlenther. Onkol.* **2017**, *193*, 351–366. [CrossRef]
48. Kroeze, H.; Kokubo, M.; Kamer, J.B.V.D.; Leeuw, A.A.C.D.; Kikuchi, M.; Hiraoka, M.; Lagendijk, J.J.W. Comparison of a Capacitive and a Cavity Slot Radiative Applicator for Regional Hyperthermia. *Therm. Med. (Jpn. J. Hyperthermic Oncol.)* **2002**, *18*, 75–91. [CrossRef]
49. Datta, N.R.; Marder, D.; Datta, S.; Meister, A.; Puric, E.; Stutz, E.; Rogers, S.; Eberle, B.; Timm, O.; Staruch, M.; et al. Quantification of thermal dose in moderate clinical hyperthermia with radiotherapy: A relook using temperature-time area under the curve (AUC). *Int. J. Hyperthermia* **2021**, *38*, 296–307. [CrossRef]
50. Fatehi, D.; van der Zee, J.; Notenboom, A.; van Rhoon, G.C. Comparison of intratumor and intraluminal temperatures during locoregional deep hyperthermia of pelvic tumors. *Strahlenther. Onkol.* **2007**, *183*, 479–486. [CrossRef]
51. Fatehi, D.; de Bruijne, M.; van der Zee, J.; van Rhoon, G.C. RHyThM, a tool for analysis of PDOS formatted hyperthermia treatment data generated by the BSD2000/3D system. *Int. J. Hyperthermia* **2006**, *22*, 173–184. [CrossRef] [PubMed]
52. Overgaard, J. Formula to estimate the thermal enhancement ratio of a single simultaneous hyperthermia and radiation treatment. *Acta Radiol. Oncol.* **1984**, *23*, 135–139. [CrossRef] [PubMed]
53. Song, C.W.; Park, H.; Griffin, R.J. Improvement of tumor oxygenation by mild hyperthermia. *Radiat. Res.* **2001**, *155*, 515–528. [CrossRef]

54. Overgaard, J.; Radacic, M.M.; Grau, C. Interaction of hyperthermia and cis-diamminedichloroplatinum(II) alone or combined with radiation in a C3H mammary carcinoma in vivo. *Cancer Res.* **1991**, *51*, 707–711. [PubMed]
55. Lindegaard, J.C.; Radacic, M.; Khalil, A.A.; Horsman, M.R.; Overgaard, J. Cisplatin and hyperthermia treatment of a C3H mammary carcinoma in vivo. Importance of sequence, interval, drug dose, and temperature. *Acta Oncol.* **1992**, *31*, 347–351. [CrossRef] [PubMed]
56. Hintzsche, H.; Riese, T.; Stopper, H. Hyperthermia-induced micronucleus formation in a human keratinocyte cell line. *Mutat. Res.* **2012**, *738–739*, 71–74. [CrossRef]
57. Urano, M.; Ling, C.C. Thermal enhancement of melphalan and oxaliplatin cytotoxicity in vitro. *Int. J. Hyperthermia* **2002**, *18*, 307–315. [CrossRef]
58. Kampinga, H.H.; Dynlacht, J.R.; Dikomey, E. Mechanism of radiosensitization by hyperthermia (> or = 43 degrees C) as derived from studies with DNA repair defective mutant cell lines. *Int. J. Hyperthermia* **2004**, *20*, 131–139. [CrossRef]
59. Kampinga, H.H. Cell biological effects of hyperthermia alone or combined with radiation or drugs: A short introduction to newcomers in the field. *Int. J. Hyperthermia* **2006**, *22*, 191–196. [CrossRef]
60. Ohtsubo, T.; Chang, S.W.; Tsuji, K.; Picha, P.; Saito, H.; Kano, E. Effects of cis-diamminedichloroplatinum (CDDP) and cis-diammine (1,1-cyclobutanedicarboxylate) platinum (CBDCA) on thermotolerance development and thermosensitivity of the thermotolerant cells. *Int. J. Hyperthermia* **1990**, *6*, 1031–1039. [CrossRef]
61. Van der Zee, J.; Peer-Valstar, J.N.; Rietveld, P.J.; de Graaf-Strukowska, L.; van Rhoon, G.C. Practical limitations of interstitial thermometry during deep hyperthermia. *Int. J. Radiat. Oncol. Biol. Phys.* **1998**, *40*, 1205–1212. [CrossRef]
62. Oleson, J.R. Eugene Robertson Special Lecture. Hyperthermia from the clinic to the laboratory: A hypothesis. *Int. J. Hyperthermia* **1995**, *11*, 315–322. [CrossRef] [PubMed]
63. Sapareto, S.A.; Hopwood, L.E.; Dewey, W.C.; Raju, M.R.; Gray, J.W. Effects of hyperthermia on survival and progression of Chinese hamster ovary cells. *Cancer Res.* **1978**, *38*, 393–400. [PubMed]
64. Bing, C.; Patel, P.; Staruch, R.M.; Shaikh, S.; Nofiele, J.; Wodzak Staruch, M.; Szczepanski, D.; Williams, N.S.; Laetsch, T.; Chopra, R. Longer heating duration increases localized doxorubicin deposition and therapeutic index in Vx2 tumors using MR-HIFU mild hyperthermia and thermosensitive liposomal doxorubicin. *Int. J. Hyperthermia* **2019**, *36*, 196–203. [CrossRef]
65. Bhuyan, B.K.; Day, K.J.; Edgerton, C.E.; Ogunbase, O. Sensitivity of different cell lines and of different phases in the cell cycle to hyperthermia. *Cancer Res.* **1977**, *37*, 3780–3784. [PubMed]
66. Dewey, W.C. Arrhenius relationships from the molecule and cell to the clinic. *Int. J. Hyperthermia* **2009**, *25*, 3–20. [CrossRef]
67. Law, M.P. Induced thermal resistance in the mouse ear: The relationship between heating time and temperature. *Int. J. Radiat. Biol. Relat. Stud. Phys. Chem. Med.* **1979**, *35*, 481–485. [CrossRef]
68. Li, G.C.; Mivechi, N.F.; Weitzel, G. Heat shock proteins, thermotolerance, and their relevance to clinical hyperthermia. *Int. J. Hyperthermia* **1995**, *11*, 459–488. [CrossRef]
69. Field, S.B.; Morris, C.C. The relationship between heating time and temperature: Its relevance to clinical hyperthermia. *Radiother. Oncol.* **1983**, *1*, 179–186. [CrossRef]
70. Dewhirst, M.W.; Viglianti, B.L.; Lora-Michiels, M.; Hanson, M.; Hoopes, P.J. Basic principles of thermal dosimetry and thermal thresholds for tissue damage from hyperthermia. *Int. J. Hyperthermia* **2003**, *19*, 267–294. [CrossRef]
71. Nielsen, O.S. Fractionated hyperthermia and thermotolerance. Experimental studies on heat-induced resistance in tumour cells treated with hyperthermia alone or in combination with radiotherapy. *Dan. Med. Bull.* **1984**, *31*, 376–390. [PubMed]
72. Ben-Hur, E.; Elkind, M.M.; Bronk, B.V. Thermally enhanced radioresponse of cultured Chinese hamster cells: Inhibition of repair of sublethal damage and enhancement of lethal damage. *Radiat. Res.* **1974**, *58*, 38–51. [CrossRef] [PubMed]
73. Van Rhoon, G.C.; Samaras, T.; Yarmolenko, P.S.; Dewhirst, M.W.; Neufeld, E.; Kuster, N. CEM43°C thermal dose thresholds: A potential guide for magnetic resonance radiofrequency exposure levels? *Eur. Radiol.* **2013**, *23*, 2215–2227. [CrossRef] [PubMed]
74. Yarmolenko, P.S.; Moon, E.J.; Landon, C.; Manzoor, A.; Hochman, D.W.; Viglianti, B.L.; Dewhirst, M.W. Thresholds for thermal damage to normal tissues: An update. *Int. J. Hyperthermia* **2011**, *27*, 320–343. [CrossRef]
75. Thrall, D.E.; LaRue, S.M.; Yu, D.; Samulski, T.; Sanders, L.; Case, B.; Rosner, G.; Azuma, C.; Poulson, J.; Pruitt, A.F.; et al. Thermal dose is related to duration of local control in canine sarcomas treated with thermoradiotherapy. *Clin. Cancer Res.* **2005**, *11*, 5206–5214. [CrossRef]
76. Kossatz, S.; Ludwig, R.; Dähring, H.; Ettelt, V.; Rimkus, G.; Marciello, M.; Salas, G.; Patel, V.; Teran, F.J.; Hilger, I. High therapeutic efficiency of magnetic hyperthermia in xenograft models achieved with moderate temperature dosages in the tumor area. *Pharm. Res.* **2014**, *31*, 3274–3288. [CrossRef]
77. Dewhirst, M.W.; Sim, D.A.; Sapareto, S.; Connor, W.G. Importance of minimum tumor temperature in determining early and long-term responses of spontaneous canine and feline tumors to heat and radiation. *Cancer Res.* **1984**, *44*, 43–50.
78. Van Rhoon, G.C. Is CEM43 still a relevant thermal dose parameter for hyperthermia treatment monitoring? *Int. J. Hyperthermia* **2016**, *32*, 50–62. [CrossRef]
79. Gerner, E.W.; Boone, R.; Connor, W.G.; Hicks, J.A.; Boone, M.L. A transient thermotolerant survival response produced by single thermal doses in HeLa cells. *Cancer Res.* **1976**, *36*, 1035–1040.
80. Li, Z.; Sun, Q.; Huang, X.; Zhang, J.; Hao, J.; Li, Y.; Zhang, S. The Efficacy of Radiofrequency Hyperthermia Combined with Chemotherapy in the Treatment of Advanced Ovarian Cancer. *Open Med.* **2018**, *13*, 83–89. [CrossRef]

81. Kamura, T.; Nielsen, O.S.; Overgaard, J.; Andersen, A.H. Development of thermotolerance during fractionated hyperthermia in a solid tumor in vivo. *Cancer Res.* **1982**, *42*, 1744–1748.
82. Zywietz, F.; Reeker, W.; Kochs, E. Changes in tumor oxygenation during a combined treatment with fractionated irradiation and hyperthermia: An experimental study. *Int. J. Radiat. Oncol. Biol. Phys.* **1997**, *37*, 155–162. [CrossRef]
83. Nah, B.S.; Choi, I.B.; Oh, W.Y.; Osborn, J.L.; Song, C.W. Vascular thermal adaptation in tumors and normal tissue in rats. *Int. J. Radiat. Oncol. Biol. Phys.* **1996**, *35*, 95–101. [CrossRef]
84. Overgaard, J.; Nielsen, O.S. The importance of thermotolerance for the clinical treatment with hyperthermia. *Radiother. Oncol.* **1983**, *1*, 167–178. [CrossRef]
85. Mei, X.; Ten Cate, R.; van Leeuwen, C.M.; Rodermond, H.M.; de Leeuw, L.; Dimitrakopoulou, D.; Stalpers, L.J.A.; Crezee, J.; Kok, H.P.; Franken, N.A.P.; et al. Radiosensitization by Hyperthermia: The Effects of Temperature, Sequence, and Time Interval in Cervical Cell Lines. *Cancers* **2020**, *12*, 582. [CrossRef] [PubMed]
86. Notter, M.; Piazena, H.; Vaupel, P. Hypofractionated re-irradiation of large-sized recurrent breast cancer with thermography-controlled, contact-free water-filtered infra-red-A hyperthermia: A retrospective study of 73 patients. *Int. J. Hyperthermia* **2017**, *33*, 227–236. [CrossRef] [PubMed]
87. Hurwitz, M.; Stauffer, P. Hyperthermia, radiation and chemotherapy: The role of heat in multidisciplinary cancer care. *Semin. Oncol.* **2014**, *41*, 714–729. [CrossRef]
88. Joschko, M.A.; Webster, L.K.; Groves, J.; Yuen, K.; Palatsides, M.; Ball, D.L.; Millward, M.J. Enhancement of radiation-induced regrowth delay by gemcitabine in a human tumor xenograft model. *Radiat. Oncol. Investig.* **1997**, *5*, 62–71. [CrossRef]
89. Van Bree, C.; Beumer, C.; Rodermond, H.M.; Haveman, J.; Bakker, P.J. Effectiveness of 2′,2′difluorodeoxycytidine (Gemcitabine) combined with hyperthermia in rat R-1 rhabdomyosarcoma in vitro and in vivo. *Int. J. Hyperthermia* **1999**, *15*, 549–556.
90. Li, G.C.; Kal, H.B. Effect of hyperthermia on the radiation response of two mammalian cell lines. *Eur. J. Cancer* **1977**, *13*, 65–69. [CrossRef]
91. Chen, H.; Ma, G.; Wang, X.; Zhou, W.; Wang, S. Time interval after heat stress plays an important role in the combination therapy of hyperthermia and cancer chemotherapy agents. *Int. J. Hyperthermia* **2020**, *37*, 254–255. [CrossRef] [PubMed]
92. Mitsumori, M.; Zeng, Z.F.; Oliynychenko, P.; Park, J.H.; Choi, I.B.; Tatsuzaki, H.; Tanaka, Y.; Hiraoka, M. Regional hyperthermia combined with radiotherapy for locally advanced non-small cell lung cancers: A multi-institutional prospective randomized trial of the International Atomic Energy Agency. *Int. J. Clin. Oncol.* **2007**, *12*, 192–198. [CrossRef] [PubMed]
93. Wust, P.; Gellermann, J.; Harder, C.; Tilly, W.; Rau, B.; Dinges, S.; Schlag, P.; Budach, V.; Felix, R. Rationale for using invasive thermometry for regional hyperthermia of pelvic tumors. *Int. J. Radiat. Oncol. Biol. Phys.* **1998**, *41*, 1129–1137. [CrossRef]
94. Ohguri, T.; Imada, H.; Yahara, K.; Morioka, T.; Nakano, K.; Terashima, H.; Korogi, Y. Radiotherapy with 8-MHz radiofrequency-capacitive regional hyperthermia for stage III non-small-cell lung cancer: The radiofrequency-output power correlates with the intraesophageal temperature and clinical outcomes. *Int. J. Radiat. Oncol. Biol. Phys.* **2009**, *73*, 128–135. [CrossRef] [PubMed]
95. Ohguri, T.; Yahara, K.; Moon, S.D.; Yamaguchi, S.; Imada, H.; Terashima, H.; Korogi, Y. Deep regional hyperthermia for the whole thoracic region using 8 MHz radiofrequency-capacitive heating device: Relationship between the radiofrequency-output power and the intra-oesophageal temperature and predictive factors for a good heating in 59 patients. *Int. J. Hyperthermia* **2011**, *27*, 20–26. [PubMed]
96. Chi, M.S.; Yang, K.L.; Chang, Y.C.; Ko, H.L.; Lin, Y.H.; Huang, S.C.; Huang, Y.Y.; Liao, K.W.; Kondo, M.; Chi, K.H. Comparing the Effectiveness of Combined External Beam Radiation and Hyperthermia Versus External Beam Radiation Alone in Treating Patients With Painful Bony Metastases: A Phase 3 Prospective, Randomized, Controlled Trial. *Int. J. Radiat. Oncol. Biol. Phys.* **2018**, *100*, 78–87. [CrossRef]
97. Nishimura, Y.; Hiraoka, M.; Akuta, K.; Jo, S.; Nagata, Y.; Masunaga, S.; Takahashi, M.; Abe, M. Hyperthermia combined with radiation therapy for primarily unresectable and recurrent colorectal cancer. *Int. J. Radiat. Oncol. Biol. Phys.* **1992**, *23*, 759–768. [CrossRef]
98. Engin, K.; Tupchong, L.; Moylan, D.J.; Alexander, G.A.; Waterman, F.M.; Komarnicky, L.; Nerlinger, R.E.; Leeper, D.B. Randomized trial of one versus two adjuvant hyperthermia treatments per week in patients with superficial tumours. *Int. J. Hyperthermia* **1993**, *9*, 327–340. [CrossRef]
99. Tilly, W.; Gellermann, J.; Graf, R.; Hildebrandt, B.; Weissbach, L.; Budach, V.; Felix, R.; Wust, P. Regional hyperthermia in conjunction with definitive radiotherapy against recurrent or locally advanced prostate cancer T3 pN0 M0. *Strahlenther. Onkol.* **2005**, *181*, 35–41. [CrossRef]
100. Masunaga, S.I.; Hiraoka, M.; Akuta, K.; Nishimura, Y.; Nagata, Y.; Jo, S.; Takahashi, M.; Abe, M.; Terachi, T.; Oishi, K.; et al. Phase I/II trial of preoperative thermoradiotherapy in the treatment of urinary bladder cancer. *Int. J. Hyperthermia* **1994**, *10*, 31–40. [CrossRef]
101. Valdagni, R.; Liu, F.F.; Kapp, D.S. Important prognostic factors influencing outcome of combined radiation and hyperthermia. *Int. J. Radiat. Oncol. Biol. Phys.* **1988**, *15*, 959–972. [CrossRef]
102. Kroesen, M.; Mulder, H.T.; van Holthe, J.M.L.; Aangeenbrug, A.A.; Mens, J.W.M.; van Doorn, H.C.; Paulides, M.M.; Oomen-de Hoop, E.; Vernhout, R.M.; Lutgens, L.C.; et al. Confirmation of thermal dose as a predictor of local control in cervical carcinoma patients treated with state-of-the-art radiation therapy and hyperthermia. *Radiother. Oncol.* **2019**, *140*, 150–158. [CrossRef] [PubMed]

103. Valdagni, R.; Amichetti, M. Report of long-term follow-up in a randomized trial comparing radiation therapy and radiation therapy plus hyperthermia to metastatic lymph nodes in stage IV head and neck patients. *Int. J. Radiat. Oncol. Biol. Phys.* **1994**, *28*, 163–169. [CrossRef]
104. Van der Zee, J.; González González, D.; van Rhoon, G.C.; van Dijk, J.D.; van Putten, W.L.; Hart, A.A.; Dutch Deep Hyperthermia Group. Comparison of radiotherapy alone with radiotherapy plus hyperthermia in locally advanced pelvic tumours: A prospective, randomised, multicentre trial. *Lancet* **2000**, *355*, 1119–1125. [CrossRef]
105. Harima, Y.; Nagata, K.; Harima, K.; Ostapenko, V.V.; Tanaka, Y.; Sawada, S. A randomized clinical trial of radiation therapy versus thermoradiotherapy in stage IIIB cervical carcinoma. *Int. J. Hyperthermia* **2001**, *17*, 97–105. [CrossRef] [PubMed]
106. Berdov, B.A.; Menteshashvili, G.Z. Thermoradiotherapy of patients with locally advanced carcinoma of the rectum. *Int. J. Hyperthermia* **1990**, *6*, 881–890. [CrossRef]
107. Maluta, S.; Dall'Oglio, S.; Romano, M.; Marciai, N.; Pioli, F.; Giri, M.G.; Benecchi, P.L.; Comunale, L.; Porcaro, A.B. Conformal radiotherapy plus local hyperthermia in patients affected by locally advanced high risk prostate cancer: Preliminary results of a prospective phase II study. *Int. J. Hyperthermia* **2007**, *23*, 451–456. [CrossRef] [PubMed]
108. Anscher, M.S.; Samulski, T.V.; Dodge, R.; Prosnitz, L.R.; Dewhirst, M.W. Combined external beam irradiation and external regional hyperthermia for locally advanced adenocarcinoma of the prostate. *Int. J. Radiat. Oncol. Biol. Phys.* **1997**, *37*, 1059–1065. [CrossRef]
109. Gabriele, P.; Amichetti, M.; Orecchia, R.; Valdagni, R. Hyperthermia and radiation therapy for inoperable or recurrent parotid carcinoma. A phase I/II study. *Cancer* **1995**, *75*, 908–913. [CrossRef]
110. Maguire, P.D.; Samulski, T.V.; Prosnitz, L.R.; Jones, E.L.; Rosner, G.L.; Powers, B.; Layfield, L.W.; Brizel, D.M.; Scully, S.P.; Harrelson, J.M.; et al. A phase II trial testing the thermal dose parameter CEM43 degrees T90 as a predictor of response in soft tissue sarcomas treated with pre-operative thermoradiotherapy. *Int. J. Hyperthermia* **2001**, *17*, 283–290. [CrossRef]
111. Lutgens, L.C.; Koper, P.C.; Jobsen, J.J.; van der Steen-Banasik, E.M.; Creutzberg, C.L.; van den Berg, H.A.; Ottevanger, P.B.; van Rhoon, G.C.; van Doorn, H.C.; Houben, R.; et al. Radiation therapy combined with hyperthermia versus cisplatin for locally advanced cervical cancer: Results of the randomized RADCHOC trial. *Radiother. Oncol.* **2016**, *120*, 378–382. [CrossRef] [PubMed]
112. Hurwitz, M.D.; Hansen, J.L.; Prokopios-Davos, S.; Manola, J.; Wang, Q.; Bornstein, B.A.; Hynynen, K.; Kaplan, I.D. Hyperthermia combined with radiation for the treatment of locally advanced prostate cancer: Long-term results from Dana-Farber Cancer Institute study 94-153. *Cancer* **2011**, *117*, 510–516. [CrossRef] [PubMed]
113. Vernon, C.C.; Hand, J.W.; Field, S.B.; Machin, D.; Whaley, J.B.; van der Zee, J.; van Putten, W.L.; van Rhoon, G.C.; van Dijk, J.D.; González González, D.; et al. Radiotherapy with or without hyperthermia in the treatment of superficial localized breast cancer: Results from five randomized controlled trials. International Collaborative Hyperthermia Group. *Int. J. Radiat. Oncol. Biol. Phys.* **1996**, *35*, 731–744. [PubMed]
114. Datta, N.R.; Bose, A.K.; Kapoor, H.K.; Gupta, S. Head and neck cancers: Results of thermoradiotherapy versus radiotherapy. *Int. J. Hyperthermia* **1990**, *6*, 479–486. [CrossRef]
115. Overgaard, J.; Gonzalez Gonzalez, D.; Hulshof, M.C.; Arcangeli, G.; Dahl, O.; Mella, O.; Bentzen, S.M. Randomised trial of hyperthermia as adjuvant to radiotherapy for recurrent or metastatic malignant melanoma. European Society for Hyperthermic Oncology. *Lancet* **1995**, *345*, 540–543. [CrossRef]
116. Overgaard, J.; Gonzalez Gonzalez, D.; Hulshof, M.C.; Arcangeli, G.; Dahl, O.; Mella, O.; Bentzen, S.M. Hyperthermia as an adjuvant to radiation therapy of recurrent or metastatic malignant melanoma. A multicentre randomized trial by the European Society for Hyperthermic Oncology. *Int. J. Hyperthermia* **1996**, *12*, 3–20. [CrossRef] [PubMed]
117. Kim, B.S.; Chung, H.C.; Seong, J.S.; Suh, C.O.; Kim, G.E. Phase II trial for combined external radiotherapy and hyperthermia for unresectable hepatoma. *Cancer Chemother. Pharmacol.* **1992**, *31*, S119–S127. [CrossRef]
118. Overgaard, J.; Overgaard, M.; Hansen, P.V.; von der Maase, H. Some factors of importance in the radiation treatment of malignant melanoma. *Radiother. Oncol.* **1986**, *5*, 183–192. [CrossRef]
119. Emami, B.; Perez, C.A.; Konefal, J.; Pilepich, M.V.; Leybovich, L.; Straube, W.; VonGerichten, D.; Hederman, M.A. Thermoradiotherapy of malignant melanoma. *Int. J. Hyperthermia* **1988**, *4*, 373–381. [CrossRef]
120. Franckena, M.; Lutgens, L.C.; Koper, P.C.; Kleynen, C.E.; van der Steen-Banasik, E.M.; Jobsen, J.J.; Leer, J.W.; Creutzberg, C.L.; Dielwart, M.F.; van Norden, Y.; et al. Radiotherapy and hyperthermia for treatment of primary locally advanced cervix cancer: Results in 378 patients. *Int. J. Radiat. Oncol. Biol. Phys.* **2009**, *73*, 242–250. [CrossRef]
121. Oldenborg, S.; Van Os, R.M.; Van rij, C.M.; Crezee, J.; Van de Kamer, J.B.; Rutgers, E.J.; Geijsen, E.D.; Zum vörde sive vörding, P.J.; Koning, C.C.; Van tienhoven, G. Elective re-irradiation and hyperthermia following resection of persistent locoregional recurrent breast cancer: A retrospective study. *Int. J. Hyperthermia* **2010**, *26*, 136–144. [CrossRef] [PubMed]
122. Shen, H.; Li, X.D.; Wu, C.P.; Yin, Y.M.; Wang, R.S.; Shu, Y.Q. The regimen of gemcitabine and cisplatin combined with radio frequency hyperthermia for advanced non-small cell lung cancer: A phase II study. *Int. J. Hyperthermia* **2011**, *27*, 27–32. [CrossRef]
123. Issels, R.D.; Lindner, L.H.; Verweij, J.; Wust, P.; Reichardt, P.; Schem, B.C.; Abdel-Rahman, S.; Daugaard, S.; Salat, C.; Wendtner, C.M.; et al. Neo-adjuvant chemotherapy alone or with regional hyperthermia for localised high-risk soft-tissue sarcoma: A randomised phase 3 multicentre study. *Lancet Oncol.* **2010**, *11*, 561–570. [CrossRef]
124. Sugimachi, K.; Kuwano, H.; Ide, H.; Toge, T.; Saku, M.; Oshiumi, Y. Chemotherapy combined with or without hyperthermia for patients with oesophageal carcinoma: A prospective randomized trial. *Int. J. Hyperthermia* **1994**, *10*, 485–493. [CrossRef]

125. Colombo, R.; Salonia, A.; Leib, Z.; Pavone-Macaluso, M.; Engelstein, D. Long-term outcomes of a randomized controlled trial comparing thermochemotherapy with mitomycin-C alone as adjuvant treatment for non-muscle-invasive bladder cancer (NMIBC). *BJU Int.* **2011**, *107*, 912–918. [CrossRef] [PubMed]
126. Braun, J.; Hahn, G.M. Enhanced cell killing by bleomycin and 43 degrees hyperthermia and the inhibition of recovery from potentially lethal damage. *Cancer Res.* **1975**, *35*, 2921–2927.
127. Zagar, T.M.; Vujaskovic, Z.; Formenti, S.; Rugo, H.; Muggia, F.; O'Connor, B.; Myerson, R.; Stauffer, P.; Hsu, I.C.; Diederich, C.; et al. Two phase I dose-escalation/pharmacokinetics studies of low temperature liposomal doxorubicin (LTLD) and mild local hyperthermia in heavily pretreated patients with local regionally recurrent breast cancer. *Int. J. Hyperthermia* **2014**, *30*, 285–294. [CrossRef]
128. Wallner, K.E.; DeGregorio, M.W.; Li, G.C. Hyperthermic potentiation of cis-diamminedichloroplatinum(II) cytotoxicity in Chinese hamster ovary cells resistant to the drug. *Cancer Res.* **1986**, *46*, 6242–6245.
129. Magin, R.L.; Sikic, B.I.; Cysyk, R.L. Enhancement of bleomycin activity against Lewis lung tumors in mice by local hyperthermia. *Cancer Res.* **1979**, *39*, 3792–3795.
130. Kong, G.; Anyarambhatla, G.; Petros, W.P.; Braun, R.D.; Colvin, O.M.; Needham, D.; Dewhirst, M.W. Efficacy of liposomes and hyperthermia in a human tumor xenograft model: Importance of triggered drug release. *Cancer Res.* **2000**, *60*, 6950–6957.
131. Van der Heijden, A.G.; Jansen, C.F.; Verhaegh, G.; O'Donnell M, A.; Schalken, J.A.; Witjes, J.A. The effect of hyperthermia on mitomycin-C induced cytotoxicity in four human bladder cancer cell lines. *Eur. Urol.* **2004**, *46*, 670–674. [CrossRef] [PubMed]
132. Van Rhoon, G.C.; Franckena, M.; Ten Hagen, T.L.M. A moderate thermal dose is sufficient for effective free and TSL based thermochemotherapy. *Adv. Drug Deliv. Rev.* **2020**, *163–164*, 145–156. [CrossRef] [PubMed]
133. Rietbroek, R.C.; Schilthuis, M.S.; Bakker, P.J.; van Dijk, J.D.; Postma, A.J.; González González, D.; Bakker, A.J.; van der Velden, J.; Helmerhorst, T.J.; Veenhof, C.H. Phase II trial of weekly locoregional hyperthermia and cisplatin in patients with a previously irradiated recurrent carcinoma of the uterine cervix. *Cancer* **1997**, *79*, 935–943. [CrossRef]
134. Fiegl, M.; Schlemmer, M.; Wendtner, C.M.; Abdel-Rahman, S.; Fahn, W.; Issels, R.D. Ifosfamide, carboplatin and etoposide (ICE) as second-line regimen alone and in combination with regional hyperthermia is active in chemo-pre-treated advanced soft tissue sarcoma of adults. *Int. J. Hyperthermia* **2004**, *20*, 661–670. [CrossRef] [PubMed]
135. De Wit, R.; van der Zee, J.; van der Burg, M.E.; Kruit, W.H.; Logmans, A.; van Rhoon, G.C.; Verweij, J. A phase I/II study of combined weekly systemic cisplatin and locoregional hyperthermia in patients with previously irradiated recurrent carcinoma of the uterine cervix. *Br. J. Cancer* **1999**, *80*, 1387–1391. [CrossRef]
136. Alvarez Secord, A.; Jones, E.L.; Hahn, C.A.; Petros, W.P.; Yu, D.; Havrilesky, L.J.; Soper, J.T.; Berchuck, A.; Spasojevic, I.; Clarke-Pearson, D.L.; et al. Phase I/II trial of intravenous Doxil and whole abdomen hyperthermia in patients with refractory ovarian cancer. *Int. J. Hyperthermia* **2005**, *21*, 333–347. [CrossRef]
137. Stahl, R.; Wang, T.; Lindner, L.H.; Abdel-Rahman, S.; Santl, M.; Reiser, M.F.; Issels, R.D. Comparison of radiological and pathohistological response to neoadjuvant chemotherapy combined with regional hyperthermia (RHT) and study of response dependence on the applied thermal parameters in patients with soft tissue sarcomas (STS). *Int. J. Hyperthermia* **2009**, *25*, 289–298. [CrossRef]
138. Vujaskovic, Z.; Kim, D.W.; Jones, E.; Lan, L.; McCall, L.; Dewhirst, M.W.; Craciunescu, O.; Stauffer, P.; Liotcheva, V.; Betof, A.; et al. A phase I/II study of neoadjuvant liposomal doxorubicin, paclitaxel, and hyperthermia in locally advanced breast cancer. *Int. J. Hyperthermia* **2010**, *26*, 514–521. [CrossRef]
139. Ishikawa, T.; Kokura, S.; Sakamoto, N.; Ando, T.; Imamoto, E.; Hattori, T.; Oyamada, H.; Yoshinami, N.; Sakamoto, M.; Kitagawa, K.; et al. Phase II trial of combined regional hyperthermia and gemcitabine for locally advanced or metastatic pancreatic cancer. *Int. J. Hyperthermia* **2012**, *28*, 597–604. [CrossRef]
140. Yang, W.H.; Xie, J.; Lai, Z.Y.; Yang, M.D.; Zhang, G.H.; Li, Y.; Mu, J.B.; Xu, J. Radiofrequency deep hyperthermia combined with chemotherapy in the treatment of advanced non-small cell lung cancer. *Chin. Med. J.* **2019**, *132*, 922–927. [CrossRef]
141. Tschoep-Lechner, K.E.; Milani, V.; Berger, F.; Dieterle, N.; Abdel-Rahman, S.; Salat, C.; Issels, R.D. Gemcitabine and cisplatin combined with regional hyperthermia as second-line treatment in patients with gemcitabine-refractory advanced pancreatic cancer. *Int. J. Hyperthermia* **2013**, *29*, 8–16. [CrossRef] [PubMed]
142. Monge, O.R.; Rofstad, E.K.; Kaalhus, O. Thermochemotherapy in vivo of a C3H mouse mammary carcinoma: Single fraction heat and drug treatment. *Eur. J. Cancer Clin. Oncol.* **1988**, *24*, 1661–1669. [CrossRef]
143. Adachi, S.; Kokura, S.; Okayama, T.; Ishikawa, T.; Takagi, T.; Handa, O.; Naito, Y.; Yoshikawa, T. Effect of hyperthermia combined with gemcitabine on apoptotic cell death in cultured human pancreatic cancer cell lines. *Int. J. Hyperthermia* **2009**, *25*, 210–219. [CrossRef] [PubMed]
144. Albregts, M.; Hulshof, M.C.; Zum Vörde Sive Vörding, P.J.; van Lanschot, J.J.; Richel, D.J.; Crezee, H.; Fockens, P.; van Dijk, J.D.; González González, D. A feasibility study in oesophageal carcinoma using deep loco-regional hyperthermia combined with concurrent chemotherapy followed by surgery. *Int. J. Hyperthermia* **2004**, *20*, 647–659. [CrossRef] [PubMed]
145. Herman, T.S.; Teicher, B.A.; Jochelson, M.; Clark, J.; Svensson, G.; Coleman, C.N. Rationale for use of local hyperthermia with radiation therapy and selected anticancer drugs in locally advanced human malignancies. *Int. J. Hyperthermia* **1988**, *4*, 143–158. [CrossRef]

146. Herman, T.S.; Jochelson, M.S.; Teicher, B.A.; Scott, P.J.; Hansen, J.; Clark, J.R.; Pfeffer, M.R.; Gelwan, L.E.; Molnar-Griffin, B.J.; Fraser, S.M.; et al. A phase I-II trial of cisplatin, hyperthermia and radiation in patients with locally advanced malignancies. *Int. J. Radiat. Oncol. Biol. Phys.* **1989**, *17*, 1273–1279. [CrossRef]
147. Herman, T.S.; Teicher, B.A. Sequencing of trimodality therapy[cis-diamminedichloroplatinum(II)/hyperthermia/radiation] as determined by tumor growth delay and tumor cell survival in the FSaIIC fibrosarcoma. *Cancer Res.* **1988**, *48*, 2693–2697.
148. Ohguri, T.; Imada, H.; Yahara, K.; Narisada, H.; Morioka, T.; Nakano, K.; Korogi, Y. Concurrent chemoradiotherapy with gemcitabine plus regional hyperthermia for locally advanced pancreatic carcinoma: Initial experience. *Radiat. Med.* **2008**, *26*, 587–596. [CrossRef]
149. Harima, Y.; Ohguri, T.; Imada, H.; Sakurai, H.; Ohno, T.; Hiraki, Y.; Tuji, K.; Tanaka, M.; Terashima, H. A multicentre randomised clinical trial of chemoradiotherapy plus hyperthermia versus chemoradiotherapy alone in patients with locally advanced cervical cancer. *Int. J. Hyperthermia* **2016**, *32*, 801–808. [CrossRef]
150. Westermann, A.M.; Jones, E.L.; Schem, B.C.; van der Steen-Banasik, E.M.; Koper, P.; Mella, O.; Uitterhoeve, A.L.; de Wit, R.; van der Velden, J.; Burger, C.; et al. First results of triple-modality treatment combining radiotherapy, chemotherapy, and hyperthermia for the treatment of patients with stage IIB, III, and IVA cervical carcinoma. *Cancer* **2005**, *104*, 763–770. [CrossRef]
151. Asao, T.; Sakurai, H.; Harashima, K.; Yamaguchi, S.; Tsutsumi, S.; Nonaka, T.; Shioya, M.; Nakano, T.; Kuwano, H. The synchronization of chemotherapy to circadian rhythms and irradiation in pre-operative chemoradiation therapy with hyperthermia for local advanced rectal cancer. *Int. J. Hyperthermia* **2006**, *22*, 399–406. [CrossRef] [PubMed]
152. Amichetti, M.; Graiff, C.; Fellin, G.; Pani, G.; Bolner, A.; Maluta, S.; Valdagni, R. Cisplatin, hyperthermia, and radiation (trimodal therapy) in patients with locally advanced head and neck tumors: A phase I-II study. *Int. J. Radiat. Oncol. Biol. Phys.* **1993**, *26*, 801–807. [CrossRef]
153. Kouloulias, V.E.; Dardoufas, C.E.; Kouvaris, J.R.; Gennatas, C.S.; Polyzos, A.K.; Gogas, H.J.; Sandilos, P.H.; Uzunoglu, N.K.; Malas, E.G.; Vlahos, L.J. Liposomal doxorubicin in conjunction with reirradiation and local hyperthermia treatment in recurrent breast cancer: A phase I/II trial. *Clin. Cancer Res.* **2002**, *8*, 374–382.
154. Gani, C.; Lamprecht, U.; Ziegler, A.; Moll, M.; Gellermann, J.; Heinrich, V.; Wenz, S.; Fend, F.; Königsrainer, A.; Bitzer, M.; et al. Deep regional hyperthermia with preoperative radiochemotherapy in locally advanced rectal cancer, a prospective phase II trial. *Radiother. Oncol.* **2021**, *159*, 155–160. [CrossRef] [PubMed]
155. Ohguri, T.; Harima, Y.; Imada, H.; Sakurai, H.; Ohno, T.; Hiraki, Y.; Tuji, K.; Tanaka, M.; Terashima, H. Relationships between thermal dose parameters and the efficacy of definitive chemoradiotherapy plus regional hyperthermia in the treatment of locally advanced cervical cancer: Data from a multicentre randomised clinical trial. *Int. J. Hyperthermia* **2018**, *34*, 461–468. [CrossRef]
156. Maluta, S.; Schaffer, M.; Pioli, F.; Dall'oglio, S.; Pasetto, S.; Schaffer, P.M.; Weber, B.; Giri, M.G. Regional hyperthermia combined with chemoradiotherapy in primary or recurrent locally advanced pancreatic cancer: An open-label comparative cohort trial. *Strahlenther. Onkol.* **2011**, *187*, 619–625. [CrossRef]
157. Barsukov, Y.A.; Gordeyev, S.S.; Tkachev, S.I.; Fedyanin, M.Y.; Perevoshikov, A.G. Phase II study of concomitant chemoradiotherapy with local hyperthermia and metronidazole for locally advanced fixed rectal cancer. *Colorectal Dis.* **2013**, *15*, 1107–1114. [CrossRef]
158. Ott, O.J.; Gani, C.; Lindner, L.H.; Schmidt, M.; Lamprecht, U.; Abdel-Rahman, S.; Hinke, A.; Weissmann, T.; Hartmann, A.; Issels, R.D.; et al. Neoadjuvant Chemoradiation Combined with Regional Hyperthermia in Locally Advanced or Recurrent Rectal Cancer. *Cancers* **2021**, *13*, 1279. [CrossRef]
159. Rau, B.; Wust, P.; Hohenberger, P.; Löffel, J.; Hünerbein, M.; Below, C.; Gellermann, J.; Speidel, A.; Vogl, T.; Riess, H.; et al. Preoperative hyperthermia combined with radiochemotherapy in locally advanced rectal cancer: A phase II clinical trial. *Ann. Surg.* **1998**, *227*, 380–389. [CrossRef]
160. Rau, B.; Wust, P.; Tilly, W.; Gellermann, J.; Harder, C.; Riess, H.; Budach, V.; Felix, R.; Schlag, P.M. Preoperative radiochemotherapy in locally advanced or recurrent rectal cancer: Regional radiofrequency hyperthermia correlates with clinical parameters. *Int. J. Radiat. Oncol. Biol. Phys.* **2000**, *48*, 381–391. [CrossRef]
161. Wittlinger, M.; Rödel, C.M.; Weiss, C.; Krause, S.F.; Kühn, R.; Fietkau, R.; Sauer, R.; Ott, O.J. Quadrimodal treatment of high-risk T1 and T2 bladder cancer: Transurethral tumor resection followed by concurrent radiochemotherapy and regional deep hyperthermia. *Radiother. Oncol.* **2009**, *93*, 358–363. [CrossRef] [PubMed]
162. Milani, V.; Pazos, M.; Issels, R.D.; Buecklein, V.; Rahman, S.; Tschoep, K.; Schaffer, P.; Wilkowski, R.; Duehmke, E.; Schaffer, M. Radiochemotherapy in combination with regional hyperthermia in preirradiated patients with recurrent rectal cancer. *Strahlenther. Onkol.* **2008**, *184*, 163–168. [CrossRef] [PubMed]
163. Zhu, H.; Huo, X.; Chen, L.; Wang, H.; Yu, H. Clinical experience with radio-, chemo- and hyperthermotherapy combined trimodality on locally advanced esophageal cancer. *Mol. Clin. Oncol.* **2013**, *1*, 1009–1012. [CrossRef] [PubMed]
164. Gani, C.; Schroeder, C.; Heinrich, V.; Spillner, P.; Lamprecht, U.; Berger, B.; Zips, D. Long-term local control and survival after preoperative radiochemotherapy in combination with deep regional hyperthermia in locally advanced rectal cancer. *Int. J. Hyperthermia* **2016**, *32*, 187–192. [CrossRef] [PubMed]
165. Merten, R.; Ott, O.; Haderlein, M.; Bertz, S.; Hartmann, A.; Wullich, B.; Keck, B.; Kühn, R.; Rödel, C.M.; Weiss, C.; et al. Long-Term Experience of Chemoradiotherapy Combined with Deep Regional Hyperthermia for Organ Preservation in High-Risk Bladder Cancer (Ta, Tis, T1, T2). *Oncologist* **2019**, *24*, e1341–e1350. [CrossRef] [PubMed]

166. Van Haaren, P.M.; Hulshof, M.C.; Kok, H.P.; Oldenborg, S.; Geijsen, E.D.; Van Lanschot, J.J.; Crezee, J. Relation between body size and temperatures during locoregional hyperthermia of oesophageal cancer patients. *Int. J. Hyperthermia* **2008**, *24*, 663–674. [CrossRef]
167. Curto, S.; Aklan, B.; Mulder, T.; Mils, O.; Schmidt, M.; Lamprecht, U.; Peller, M.; Wessalowski, R.; Lindner, L.H.; Fietkau, R.; et al. Quantitative, Multi-institutional Evaluation of MR Thermometry Accuracy for Deep-Pelvic MR-Hyperthermia Systems Operating in Multi-vendor MR-systems Using a New Anthropomorphic Phantom. *Cancers* **2019**, *11*, 1709. [CrossRef]
168. Winter, L.; Oberacker, E.; Paul, K.; Ji, Y.; Oezerdem, C.; Ghadjar, P.; Thieme, A.; Budach, V.; Wust, P.; Niendorf, T. Magnetic resonance thermometry: Methodology, pitfalls and practical solutions. *Int. J. Hyperthermia* **2016**, *32*, 63–75. [CrossRef]
169. Adibzadeh, F.; Sumser, K.; Curto, S.; Yeo, D.T.B.; Shishegar, A.A.; Paulides, M.M. Systematic review of pre-clinical and clinical devices for magnetic resonance-guided radiofrequency hyperthermia. *Int. J. Hyperthermia* **2020**, *37*, 15–27. [CrossRef]
170. Gellermann, J.; Faehling, H.; Mielec, M.; Cho, C.H.; Budach, V.; Wust, P. Image artifacts during MRT hybrid hyperthermia-causes and elimination. *Int. J. Hyperthermia* **2008**, *24*, 327–335. [CrossRef]
171. Ishihara, Y.; Calderon, A.; Watanabe, H.; Okamoto, K.; Suzuki, Y.; Kuroda, K.; Suzuki, Y. A precise and fast temperature mapping using water proton chemical shift. *Magn. Reson. Med.* **1995**, *34*, 814–823. [CrossRef] [PubMed]
172. Le Bihan, D.; Delannoy, J.; Levin, R.L. Temperature mapping with MR imaging of molecular diffusion: Application to hyperthermia. *Radiology* **1989**, *171*, 853–857. [CrossRef] [PubMed]
173. Gellermann, J.; Wlodarczyk, W.; Feussner, A.; Fähling, H.; Nadobny, J.; Hildebrandt, B.; Felix, R.; Wust, P. Methods and potentials of magnetic resonance imaging for monitoring radiofrequency hyperthermia in a hybrid system. *Int. J. Hyperthermia* **2005**, *21*, 497–513. [CrossRef] [PubMed]
174. Lüdemann, L.; Wlodarczyk, W.; Nadobny, J.; Weihrauch, M.; Gellermann, J.; Wust, P. Non-invasive magnetic resonance thermography during regional hyperthermia. *Int. J. Hyperthermia* **2010**, *26*, 273–282. [CrossRef]
175. Gellermann, J.; Wlodarczyk, W.; Ganter, H.; Nadobny, J.; Fähling, H.; Seebass, M.; Felix, R.; Wust, P. A practical approach to thermography in a hyperthermia/magnetic resonance hybrid system: Validation in a heterogeneous phantom. *Int. J. Radiat. Oncol. Biol. Phys.* **2005**, *61*, 267–277. [CrossRef]
176. Gellermann, J.; Hildebrandt, B.; Issels, R.; Ganter, H.; Wlodarczyk, W.; Budach, V.; Felix, R.; Tunn, P.U.; Reichardt, P.; Wust, P. Noninvasive magnetic resonance thermography of soft tissue sarcomas during regional hyperthermia: Correlation with response and direct thermometry. *Cancer* **2006**, *107*, 1373–1382. [CrossRef]
177. Gellermann, J.; Wlodarczyk, W.; Hildebrandt, B.; Ganter, H.; Nicolau, A.; Rau, B.; Tilly, W.; Fähling, H.; Nadobny, J.; Felix, R.; et al. Noninvasive magnetic resonance thermography of recurrent rectal carcinoma in a 1.5 Tesla hybrid system. *Cancer Res.* **2005**, *65*, 5872–5880. [CrossRef]
178. Poni, R.; Neufeld, E.; Capstick, M.; Bodis, S.; Samaras, T.; Kuster, N. Feasibility of Temperature Control by Electrical Impedance Tomography in Hyperthermia. *Cancers* **2021**, *13*, 3297. [CrossRef]
179. Esrick, M.A.; McRae, D.A. The effect of hyperthermia-induced tissue conductivity changes on electrical impedance temperature mapping. *Phys. Med. Biol.* **1994**, *39*, 133–144. [CrossRef]
180. Paulsen, K.D.; Moskowitz, M.J.; Ryan, T.P.; Mitchell, S.E.; Hoopes, P.J. Initial in vivo experience with EIT as a thermal estimator during hyperthermia. *Int. J. Hyperthermia* **1996**, *12*, 573–591. [CrossRef]
181. Nguyen, D.M.; Andersen, T.; Qian, P.; Barry, T.; McEwan, A. Electrical Impedance Tomography for monitoring cardiac radiofrequency ablation: A scoping review of an emerging technology. *Med. Eng. Phys.* **2020**, *84*, 36–50. [CrossRef] [PubMed]

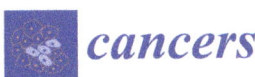

Article

Present Practice of Radiative Deep Hyperthermia in Combination with Radiotherapy in Switzerland

Emanuel Stutz [1,2], Emsad Puric [2], Adela Ademaj [2,3], Arnaud Künzi [4], Reinhardt Krcek [1], Olaf Timm [2], Dietmar Marder [2], Markus Notter [5], Susanne Rogers [2], Stephan Bodis [2,6,7] and Oliver Riesterer [2,*]

1. Department of Radiation Oncology, Inselspital, Bern University Hospital, University of Bern, 3010 Bern, Switzerland; emanuel.stutz@insel.ch (E.S.); reinhardt.krcek@insel.ch (R.K.)
2. Department of Radiation Oncology KSA-KSB, Kantonsspital Aarau, 5001 Aarau, Switzerland; emsad.puric@ksa.ch (E.P.); adela.ademaj@ksa.ch (A.A.); olaf.timm@ksa.ch (O.T.); dietmar.marder@ksa.ch (D.M.); susanne.rogers@ksa.ch (S.R.); s.bodis@bluewin.ch (S.B.)
3. Doctoral Clinical Science Program, Medical Faculty, University of Zürich, 8032 Zürich, Switzerland
4. Clinical Trials Unit, University of Bern, 3010 Bern, Switzerland; arnaud.kuenzi@ctu.unibe.ch
5. Radiation Oncology, Lindenhofspital Bern, 3012 Bern, Switzerland; markus.notter@lindenhofgruppe.ch
6. Department of Radiation Oncology, University Hospital Zurich, 8032 Zürich, Switzerland
7. Foundation for Research on Information Technologies in Society (IT'IS), 8004 Zürich, Switzerland
* Correspondence: oliver.riesterer@ksa.ch; Tel.: +41-62838-4249

Simple Summary: Moderate hyperthermia is a potent radiosensitizer and its efficacy has been proven in randomized clinical trials for specific tumor entities. In spite of this, hyperthermia still lacks general acceptance in the oncological community and implementation of hyperthermia in clinical practice is still low. Reimbursement is one key factor regarding the availability of hyperthermia for deep-seated tumors, with high variability in reimbursement between countries. We report the current reimbursement status and related pattern of care for the use of deep hyperthermia in Switzerland over a time period of 4.5 years. This analysis will provide the basis for the national standardization of deep hyperthermia treatment schedules and quality assurance guidelines, as well as for the expansion of deep hyperthermia indications in the future. This comprehensive insight into deep hyperthermia reimbursement and practice in Switzerland might also be of interest for other national hyperthermia societies.

Abstract: Background: Moderate hyperthermia is a potent and evidence-based radiosensitizer. Several indications are reimbursed for the combination of deep hyperthermia with radiotherapy (dHT+RT). We evaluated the current practice of dHT+RT in Switzerland. Methods: All indications presented to the national hyperthermia tumor board for dHT between January 2017 and June 2021 were evaluated and treatment schedules were analyzed using descriptive statistics. Results: Of 183 patients presented at the hyperthermia tumor board, 71.6% were accepted and 54.1% (99/183) finally received dHT. The most commonly reimbursed dHT indications were "local recurrence and compression" (20%), rectal (14.7%) and bladder (13.7%) cancer, respectively. For 25.3% of patients, an individual request for insurance cover was necessary. 47.4% of patients were treated with curative intent; 36.8% were in-house patients and 63.2% were referred from other hospitals. Conclusions: Approximately two thirds of patients were referred for dHT+RT from external hospitals, indicating a general demand for dHT in Switzerland. The patterns of care were diverse with respect to treatment indication. To the best of our knowledge, this study shows for the first time the pattern of care in a national cohort treated with dHT+RT. This insight will serve as the basis for a national strategy to evaluate and expand the evidence for dHT.

Keywords: moderate hyperthermia; deep hyperthermia; radiative hyperthermia; radiotherapy; patterns of care; reimbursement

Citation: Stutz, E.; Puric, E.; Ademaj, A.; Künzi, A.; Krcek, R.; Timm, O.; Marder, D.; Notter, M.; Rogers, S.; Bodis, S.; et al. Present Practice of Radiative Deep Hyperthermia in Combination with Radiotherapy in Switzerland. *Cancers* 2022, *14*, 1175. https://doi.org/10.3390/cancers14051175

Academic Editor: Girolamo Ranieri

Received: 28 January 2022
Accepted: 18 February 2022
Published: 24 February 2022

Publisher's Note: MDPI stays neutral with regard to jurisdictional claims in published maps and institutional affiliations.

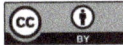

Copyright: © 2022 by the authors. Licensee MDPI, Basel, Switzerland. This article is an open access article distributed under the terms and conditions of the Creative Commons Attribution (CC BY) license (https://creativecommons.org/licenses/by/4.0/).

1. Introduction

Moderate-temperature (39–45 degree Celsius) regional hyperthermia (HT) is concurrently applied with radiotherapy (RT) or chemotherapy [1]. Adding HT to RT improves treatment outcomes such as local tumor control or overall survival in specific tumor entities with a negligible toxicity profile [2,3]. HT can be applied with superficial HT devices for superficial tumors (less than 4 cm depth below the skin) or with deep HT (dHT) devices for tumors located at depth (more than 4 cm from the skin). Several techniques and devices for the clinical application of dHT exist [1,4,5]. Although its effect has been proven in several tumor entities with positive phase III randomized trials and meta-analyses [3], there is no widespread use in Europe. Reasons are multifactorial and have been previously summarized by Van der Zee et al. [1] and Overgaard et al. [6], but are still "hot". Briefly, not only proving that the tumor region was adequately heated but also to heat and sustain a uniform temperature in the tumor region are challenging as the body attempts to maintain temperature homeostasis. Some earlier trials with dHT reported questionable results with worse outcomes with dHT, most probably caused by insufficient heating, missing quality assurance and an imbalance in the patient groups ([7] and discussion in [8]). This confusion resulted in a persistent loss of credibility in the oncological community [6,8,9].

Another reason for the lack of widespread availability is that HT, and especially dHT, is relatively labor-intensive and needs trained staff [1,10]. Furthermore, the use of dHT as a radiosensitizer competes with concurrent chemotherapy. The advantages of chemotherapy include easy administration, a lesser requirement of technical experience and comprehensive availability. The prime example of this is cervical cancer ([11], discussion in [12]). A financial obstacle is the uncertain cost reimbursement of HT treatment in most countries, limiting HT practice to university centers [8,9] and withholding it from the broader target population. Therefore, despite good but aged evidence, only a few dHT indications were incorporated into international oncology treatment guidelines.

HT has a long tradition in Switzerland, starting in 1980 with the first clinical application of superficial HT with RT at the Center for Radiation-Oncology Kantonsspital Aarau. In 1988, the first dHT treatment in combination with RT (dHT+RT) was performed there. Superficial HT was later rolled out to a second hospital in Switzerland and clinical applications, mainly for recurrent breast cancer, were maintained at this site. Thus, prior to 2017, there were only two centers applying HT based on ESHO guidelines [13–16] in Switzerland (Kantonsspital Aarau and Lindenhofspital Bern), with only the Kantonsspital Aarau applying dHT. During this time, for every HT treatment, an individual request to the patients' health insurance for reimbursement was required. The national Swiss Hyperthermia Network (SHN) was founded to synchronize and coordinate HT research activities at the national level, guarantee treatment quality and improve the evidence base for HT. In 2016, the SHN submitted a proposal for the reimbursement of HT+RT for selected evidence-based indications to the Swiss Federal Office of Public Health for superficial HT and dHT. Subsequently, four indications for superficial HT and five indications for dHT were temporarily approved for reimbursement for a period of two years as from 2017 (Table 1). It was stipulated that every patient receiving HT had to be presented to and have the indication confirmed by the national SHN tumor board, which was constituted by HT experts to guarantee the high quality of treatment decisions [17–20]. For patients who were likely to benefit from dHT+RT without a listed reimbursed indication, a specific request for insurance cover was necessary.

Table 1. Indications for deep hyperthermia (dHT) with granted reimbursement in Switzerland [18–20] are stated with specifications and underlying evidence.

Deep HT Indication	Specification	Reimbursement Status per Time Period			Evidence
		2017 2018	2019 2020	2021 2022	
Cervical cancer	- Prior irradiation - Contraindication for ChT	yellow	yellow	green	[12,21–23]
Bladder cancer	- Function preservation - Prior irradiation - Contraindication for ChT	yellow	yellow	red	[24–29]
Rectal cancer	- Function preservation - Local recurrence in pre-irradiated area - Contraindication for ChT	yellow	yellow	red	[27,30–32]
Soft tissue sarcoma	- Function preservation - Contraindication for ChT	yellow	yellow	yellow	[33–35]
Pancreatic cancer	- Locally advanced, initially inoperable tumor	yellow	yellow	red	[36–38]
Local tumor recurrence with compression	- Patients with local tumor recurrence and symptoms due to tumor compression (palliative situation) - Tumor depth > 5 cm	grey	yellow	yellow	[2]
Painful bone metastasis	- Located in the pelvis or vertebral bodies - Tumor depth > 5 cm	grey	yellow	green	[39]

Prerequisites are (i) combination with radiotherapy (RT), (ii) the indication has to be presented and confirmed at the Swiss Hyperthermia Network (SHN) tumor board, (iii) the combined dHT + RT has to be performed at an institution affiliated with the SHN. The reimbursement status is indicated per time period and coded with underlying colors. Green = time-unrestricted reimbursement; yellow = reimbursed indications limited for two further years; red = indications no longer reimbursed; grey = initially not reimbursed indications (request for insurance cover was required). Abbreviations: ChT: chemotherapy, HT: hyperthermia.

At the end of the 2 years, the SHN submitted an update of the current evidence for dHT to the Swiss Federal Office of Public Health. After reevaluation, dHT indications were expanded in 2019 with the indications of "local tumor recurrence and compression" and "painful bone metastasis", making a total of seven reimbursed dHT indications. As of July 2021, the Swiss Federal Office of Public Health granted unrestricted coverage for the dHT indications of "cervical cancer" and "painful bone metastasis". Reimbursement for the dHT indications "local tumor recurrence and compression" and "soft tissue sarcoma" has been temporarily prolonged, again for another 2-year time period. The indications for bladder, pancreatic and rectal cancer lost their reimbursement status (Table 1) [20].

Regarding superficial HT, four indications (specific situations in breast and head and neck cancer, malignant melanoma and palliative indications with local tumor compression), were granted for two years and then without time restrictions [17,19]. However, superficial HT is not within the scope of the present analysis.

To the best of our knowledge, this is the first analysis of an unselected, dHT patient cohort regarding treatment indications, patient and tumor characteristics and treatment schedules. We aimed to perform a pattern of care analysis to shed more light on dHT practice in Switzerland and build a basis for a national strategy to evaluate, consolidate and expand the evidence for dHT.

2. Materials and Methods

All patients presented at the SHN tumor board between January 2017 and June 2021 for the evaluation of radiative dHT+RT based on ESHO guidelines [13,14] were collected in a database. In July 2021, the reimbursed dHT indications changed and, since the end of 2021, a second center in Switzerland has started to apply dHT. This time period included a patient cohort treated by a single dHT center with only one modification of reimbursed dHT indications.

Data from tumor board protocols were independently extracted and crosschecked by two authors regarding reimbursed dHT indications, patient and tumor characteristics and information regarding referring hospitals. These data then were crosschecked and completed with dHT and RT treatment details by three other authors. In case of any discrepancy, a consensus was reached. This project was approved by the local ethics committee (EKNZ2021-01022, 1 July 2021).

Possible candidates for dHT were presented at the weekly national SHN tumor board by their referring physicians. The individual indication for dHT was discussed with at least two radiation oncologists with clinical experience in moderate dHT, including also senior medical oncologists. Indications were approved if the patient exhibited no contraindications for dHT (e.g., metal implant, cardio-pulmonary insufficiency, etc.), if dHT was technically feasible (only treatable lesions in accessible tumor locations) and if there was no other more appropriate treatment option (i.e., RT alone, hormone therapy, chemotherapy or immunotherapy).

2.1. Principles of Application of Deep Hyperthermia

From 2017 to 2021, Kantonsspital Aarau was the only institution providing radiative dHT+RT in accordance with ESHO guidelines [13,14] and therefore received referrals from centers throughout Switzerland. Not only the optimal treatment sequence of HT and RT but also the optimal time interval between RT and HT or vice versa is still a matter of debate. Multiple working mechanisms requiring different optimal temperature ranges contribute to the effectiveness of HT, as comprehensively presented in Oei et al. [40]. In the absence of robust clinical data, the decision on the therapeutic sequence of HT and RT is made individually by the respective center. Preclinical studies indicated that the time interval between RT and HT should be kept as short as possible [41] but clinical studies addressing the time interval are sparse [42–45]. In two retrospective clinical studies investigating the effect of the time interval on treatment outcomes in cervical cancer patients, one revealed a strong correlation of a short time interval between RT and dHT for a better clinical outcome [44], where the other study showed that a time interval up to 4 h has no effect [45]. These contradicting results initiated a comprehensive discussion that depicted the complexity of this topic [46–48]. However, with regard to the dHT standard operating procedure at the Kantonsspital Aarau, dHT is given before RT with a minimal time interval.

dHT was performed with the BSD 2000 3D Hyperthermia Systems© (BSD Medical Corporation/Pyrexar, Salt Lake City, UT, USA) using either the SigmaEye© or Sigma 60© applicator, depending on the diameter of the abdomen or limb. The interval between two dHT treatments was at least 72 h. For pelvic dHT, thermometry probes were inserted in the bladder, the rectum, the vagina, the anal margin and superficially on both groins for continuous thermometry and thermal mapping where possible/necessary. Interstitial thermometry was not performed except for patients receiving interstitial brachytherapy. For all other patients, the hyperthermia treatment planning software Sigma Hyperplan© (M/s Dr. Sennewald Medizintechnik GmbH, Munich, Germany) was used to estimate suitable power and steering parameters to achieve the targeted tumor temperature of 41 °C. A dHT session starts with a warm-up heating phase. The following plateau phase had a duration of 60 min and started when (a) the targeted temperature in the tumor was reached (this option was only possible if the heated tumor was adjacent to an intraluminal thermometry probe), (b) the targeted power and steering parameters were reached or (c) latest after a 30 min warm-up heating phase, respectively. During treatment, vital functions were continuously monitored.

The frequency of dHT was determined individually. Usually, dHT once per week was used for curative indications and dHT twice per week for palliative indications.

As not every patient started RT on a Monday, a reliable subdivision of dHT once versus twice per week was not possible. For the purpose of this study, dHT frequency was therefore categorized as once or once to twice a week. For patients referred from other hospitals, the optimal RT schedule in combination with dHT was discussed at the SHN tumor board; however, the final responsibility for the RT schedule lay with the referring center. Whenever possible, patients were treated within or analogous to an existing treatment protocol.

Some patients treated for bladder, rectal, anal and pancreatic cancer received a trimodal treatment with dHT+RT and concurrent chemotherapy. These patients were treated within [49–51] or analogous to a clinical trial [50–54]. Patients were divided into "in-house" and "referred" patients. Every patient originating from the Kantonsspital Aarau was considered "in-house". Additionally, patients from other hospitals without RT facilities, which referred patients for RT to the Kantonsspital Aarau, were also considered "in-house". Patients from other hospitals with RT facilities who were referred for dHT were classified as "referred patients", independent of where they finally received the RT treatment. To depict the spatial policy of referrals, referring hospitals were further divided into intra-cantonal and extra-cantonal and the distance by road from the referring hospitals to the Kantonsspital Aarau was calculated. There were three options for the organization of the dHT+RT treatment: (1) the patient received both dHT+RT at the Kantonsspital Aarau, (2) the patient received RT at the day of the dHT session at the Kantonsspital Aarau and the remainder of the RT at the referring hospital or (3) the patient received dHT sessions only at Kantonsspital Aarau and all RT sessions at the referring hospital. The latter option was deemed suboptimal based on the standard operating procedure at the Kantonsspital Aarau, wherein dHT should be given before RT with a minimal time interval. If not possible, a latency of 90 min between HT and RT was deemed acceptable. For patients treated with protons at the Paul Scherrer Institute, only option 3 was possible; however, the distance by road was less than 30 km. For referred patients, option 2 was preferred due to the short latency between RT and dHT. During the COVID-19 pandemic, this option was omitted to avoid mixing in-house and external patients to decrease the risk of infection. The time interval between dHT and start of the following RT was measured in patients receiving both dHT and RT at the Kantonsspital Aarau and was defined as the time between switching power off on the dHT device and first beam-on of the RT. Time points were extracted from automatical treatment recordings and stated in minutes.

2.2. Statistics

Descriptive statistics were used to describe patient and tumor characteristics and treatment details, which were presented as mean with standard error, median with (interquartile) range or frequencies with percentages, depending on their distribution.

Data were represented using Statistical Package R (released 2021, 10 August, Version 4.1.1) and the ggplot2 package, version 3.3.5. Due to the combination of the small sample size, many stratification levels and wide heterogeneity of treatment and patient characteristics, statistical inference was not performed beyond the summary tables presented here as it was judged that a qualitative assessment of the data would be more suited to the aims of this study. Continuous values were summarized with mean, standard deviation, median and max/min values. Categorical variables were summarized as frequencies and proportions.

The river plot was generated using the free, internet-based software SankeyMATIC [55].

3. Results

3.1. Patient Flow through the Swiss Hyperthermia Network Tumor Board

Between January 2017 and June 2021, 567 patients were presented for the evaluation of superficial or deep hyperthermia, with 32.3% (183/567) qualifying for dHT. Of these 183 patients, 28.4% (52/183) were deemed unsuitable. The remaining 131 patients were further assessed at a medical consultation and by their ability to tolerate the patient positioning required for dHT. This resulted in the further exclusion of 24.4% of patients (32/131). The reasons are stated in Figure 1a. In total, 54.1% (99/183) of patients initially presented at the SHN tumor board actually received dHT. Four patients had to be excluded due to withdrawal of consent, resulting in a total of 95 patients for analysis. Patients for superficial HT were beyond the scope of this analysis.

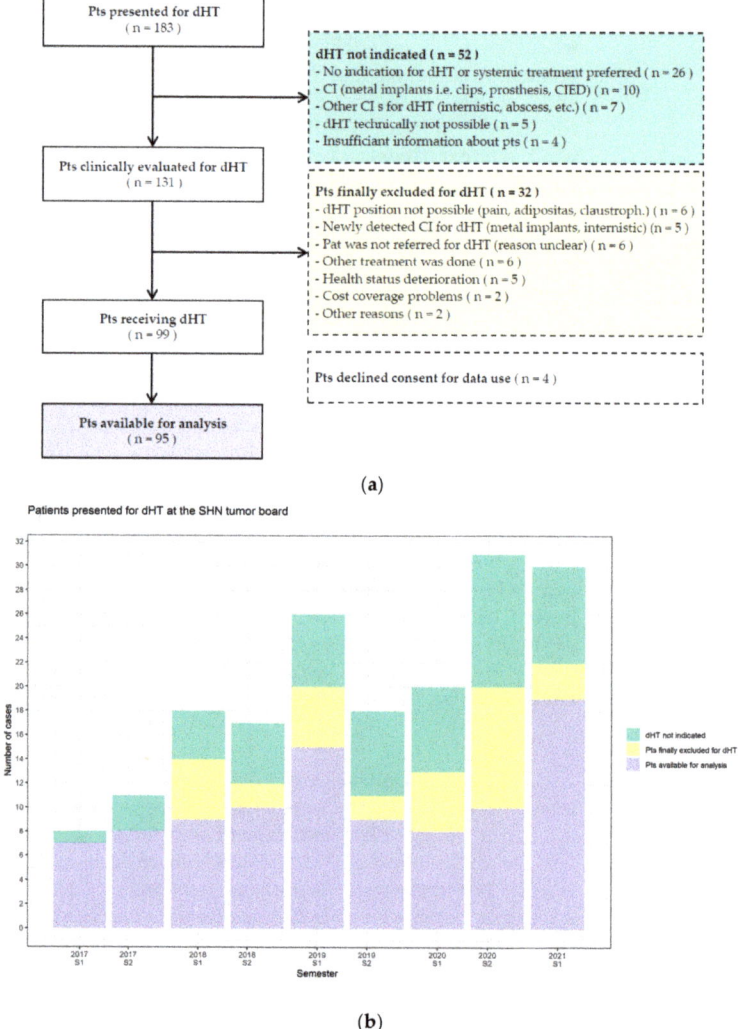

Figure 1. Patient flow through the SHN tumor board. (**a**) Patients presented for dHT were excluded if dHT was not indicated (green) or a physical examination and treatment tolerability check revealed

an exclusion criterion (yellow). Only patients with informed consent were eligible for analysis (violet). Background colors match the corresponding bar chart plot. (**b**) Patients presented at the SHN tumor board from January 2017 to June 2021 were depicted per semester. Events that may have affected the number of patients and indications treated were the two new "reimbursed dHT indications" as of 2019 and the changes in oncological treatment patterns during the COVID-19 pandemic, especially the COVID-19 lockdown in Switzerland (11 March to 26 April 2020; 1st semester 2020). Abbreviations: CI: contraindication, CIED: cardiac implantable electronic device, Claustroph: claustrophobia, dHT: deep hyperthermia, Sem: semester, SHN: Swiss Hyperthermia Network, Pts: patients, S1: 1st semester, S2: 2nd semester.

3.2. Patient Characteristics

The median age of patients receiving dHT was 65 years (range, 18–88). Moreover, 57.9% (55/95) of patients were male and 49.5% (47/95); 41.1% (39/95) and 9.5% (9/95) had an Eastern Cooperative Oncology Group (ECOG) performance score of 0, 1 or 2, respectively. A total of 47.4% (45/95) of patients received dHT with curative intent. Meanwhile, 42.1% (40/95) of patients had been previously irradiated and received dHT combined with re-irradiation (re-RT). In addition, 7.4% (7/95), 23.2% (22/95) and 69.5% (66/95) of patients were treated within a study protocol [49–51], analogous to a protocol [50–54] or as part of routine clinical practice, respectively (Table 2).

Patients were divided into groups based on treatment indication regarding reimbursement status (reimbursed dHT indications vs. indication requiring an individual "request for insurance cover") and based on primary tumor entities, respectively (Table 2, Figure 2, Supplementary Data, Figure S1). This revealed that "local tumor recurrence with compression" was the most common reimbursed dHT indication treated, representing 20.0% (19/95) of patients, followed by "rectal cancer" with 14.7% (14/95) and "bladder cancer" with 13.7% (13/95) of patients. Over the 4.5-year time period, 24.2% of patients (24/95) were treated with an indication not directly covered or not yet covered and therefore required an individual "request for insurance cover" to obtain reimbursement. Details of this patient group are provided in the Supplementary Data in Table S1. 15 of 24 patients who were treated from 2017 to 2018 and therefore before the two new dHT indications ("tumor local recurrence and compression" and "painful bone metastasis") were added, as well as 9/24 patients in the time period from 2019 to the first semester of 2021. Ten of these 15 patients would have fallen within the two new indications, showing that the two new indications covered an existing demand.

Regarding primary cancer entities, the most common was rectal cancer, with 22.1% (21/95), followed by bladder cancer with 15.8% (15/95) and soft tissue sarcoma with 13.7% (13/95) of patients (Table 2). Tumor entities with less than three treated patients are not individually represented but summarized in the group "others", which contributed with 18.9% (18/95). Primary cancer entities, i.e., anal, colon and prostate cancer, presented in a clinical situation belonging to the reimbursed indications "local tumor recurrence and compression", "painful bone metastasis" or to the group "request for insurance cover". The time trend is shown in the Supplementary Data, in Figure S1.

The patient population treated with dHT consisted of 36.8% (35/95) in-house and 63.2% (60/95) of patients referred from external radiation oncology institutions. To depict the spatial policy of referrals, the distance from the referring hospital to the Kantonsspital Aarau was calculated, resulting in a mean of 61.5 km (SD 54.3 km) and a median of 42 km (range 23–238 km) (Table 2).

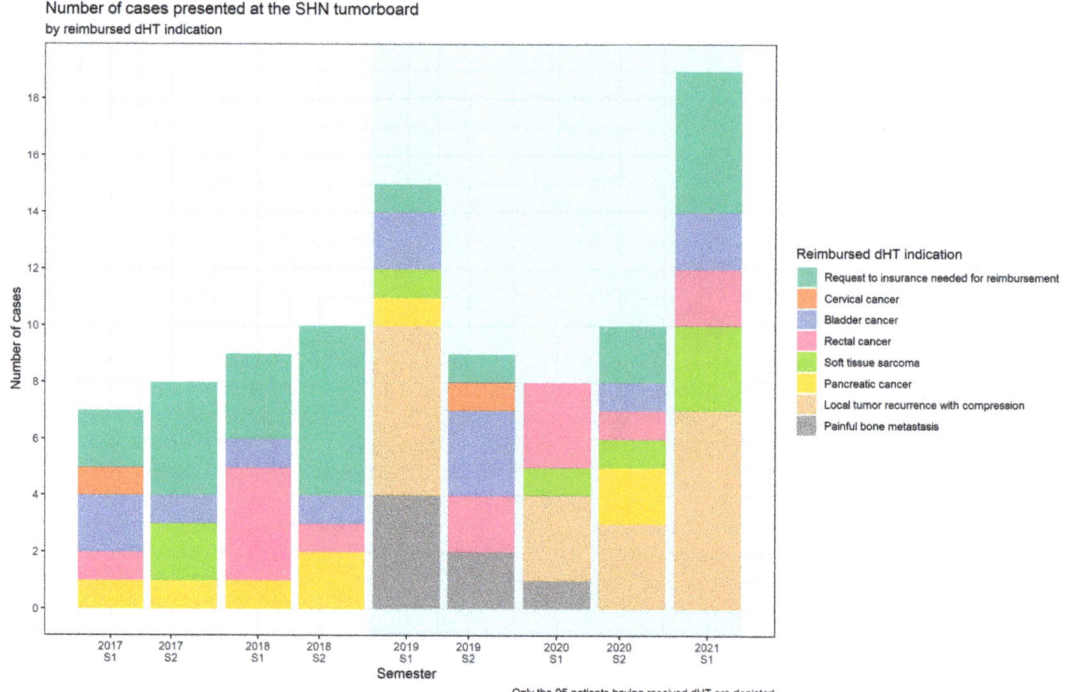

Figure 2. Trend of patients treated with combined deep hyperthermia (dHT) and radiotherapy over time. Bar chart where numbers of patients receiving dHT between January 2017 and June 2021 are depicted per semester (S1 and S2) and divided into "reimbursed dHT indications" with specific subgroups and "request for insurance cover". From 2017 to 2018, a linear increase in patient numbers with approx. 1 patient per semester was showed. Two new reimbursed indications, "local tumor recurrence with compression" and "painful bone metastasis", were granted as from 2019 (blue shaded background). COVID-19 lockdown in Switzerland was during 1st semester 2020 (11 March to 26 April 2020).

All in-house patients received their RT at the Kantonsspital Aarau. Regarding the patients referred from other hospitals, 23.3% (14/60) of them received both, dHT with all irradiations, at the Kantonsspital Aarau. Moreover, 10.0% (6/60) of patients received all irradiations at their referring hospital except at the day of dHT, where RT was applied at the Kantonsspital Aarau to minimize the time delay between HT and RT. In addition, 66.7% (40/60) of patients received only dHT treatment at the Kantonsspital Aarau and were irradiated at their referring hospital (Figure 3).

Patient characteristics are described more in detail in Supplementary Table S2, comparing (1) in-house vs. referred patients, (2) patients receiving dHT in the setting of a re-RT vs. primary RT, (3) patients treated with palliative vs. curative intention or (4) patients treated within a clinical trial, analogous to a trial or in clinical routine practice, respectively (Supplementary Table S3A). Interestingly, (5) a gender difference was noted (Supplementary Table S4).

Table 2. Patient and tumor characteristics with treatment indications, referral status and deep hyperthermia treatment adherence. Specifications of "reimbursed dHT indications" are given in Table 1.

Patient Characteristics	
	Total (*n* = 95)
Sex	
Male	55 (57.9%)
Female	40 (42.1%)
Age	
Mean (SD)	63.1 (14.2)
Median [Min, Max]	65 [18, 88]
ECOG	
0	47 (49.5%)
1	39 (41.1%)
2	9 (9.5%)
Reimbursed dHT indications	
Cervical cancer	2 (2.1%)
Bladder cancer	13 (13.7%)
Rectal cancer	14 (14.7%)
Soft tissue sarcoma	8 (8.4%)
Pancreatic cancer	8 (8.4%)
Local tumor recurrence with compression	19 (20.0%)
Painful bone metastasis	7 (7.4%)
Request for insurance cover	24 (25.3%)
Primary cancer entities	
Cervical cancer	3 (3.2%)
Bladder cancer	15 (15.8%)
Rectal cancer	21 (22.1%)
Soft tissue sarcoma	13 (13.7%)
Pancreatic cancer	8 (8.4%)
Prostate cancer	7 (7.4%)
Anal cancer	4 (4.2%)
Colon cancer	6 (6.3%)
Others	18 (18.9%)
Treatment intention	
Curative	45 (47.4%)
Palliative	50 (52.6%)
Re-irradiation	
No	55 (57.9%)
Yes	40 (42.1%)
Treatment within a study protocol	
No	66 (69.5%)
Yes	7 (7.4%)
Analogous to protocol	22 (23.2%)
Patient origin	
In-house patient	35 (36.8%)
Referred from external hospital	60 (63.2%)
Patient origin (specified)	
Intra-cantonal	26 (43.3%)
Extra-cantonal	34 (56.7%)
Distance to referring hospital (km)	
Median [Min, Max]	42 [23, 238]
Mean (SD)	61.5 (54.3)
Place of treatment	
RT at referring institution, dHT at KSA	40 (42.1%)
dHT+RT at KSA	49 (51.6%)
HT and only RT at the same day at KSA, remaining RT at referring institution	6 (6.3%)
All prescribed dHT sessions received	
No	6 (6.3%)
Yes	89 (93.7%)

Abbreviations: dHT: deep hyperthermia, dHT+RT: combined dHT and RT, ECOG: Eastern Cooperative Oncology Group, intra and extra-cantonal: cantons in Switzerland are equivalent to states, provinces or regions in other countries, KSA: Kantonsspital Aarau (=dHT center), Others: the definition is given in the text, RT: radiotherapy, SD: standard deviation.

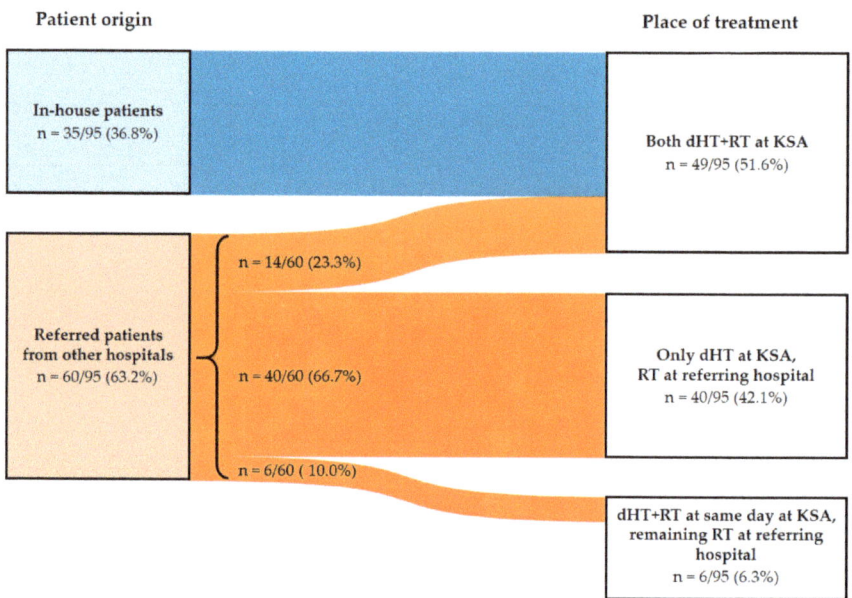

Figure 3. River plot showing the proportions of in-house and referred patients and where the RT and dHT were applied. On the left, patients are grouped according to source of referral. On the right, the three options regarding where and how dHT+RT treatment was applied are stated. The thickness of the connecting flowlines represents the proportion of patients. Abbreviations: dHT: deep hyperthermia, dHT+RT: combined dHT and RT, KSA: Kantonsspital Aarau (dHT center), RT: radiation.

3.3. Treatment Characteristics

One of the 95 treated patients stopped dHT+RT after three RT fractions due to reasons unrelated to treatment. This patient was excluded from treatment schedule analysis. In the whole cohort, a mean of 5.24 (SD ± 1.94) and a median of 5 (range 1–10) dHT sessions were applied, with 52.1% (49/94) of patients receiving it once a week and 47.9% (45/94) once to twice a week. Concurrent dHT was applied with external body RT (EBRT), stereotactic body RT (SBRT), protons and interstitial HDR-brachytherapy in 84% (79/94), 2.1% (2/94), 9.6% (9/94) and 4.3% (4/94) of patients, respectively. The mean total number of fractions was 21.7 (SD ± 8.89), with a median of 25 (range 4–38), a mean dose per fraction of 2.49 Gy (SD ± 1.35) and a median of 2 Gy (range 1.8–9 Gy). The mean total dose was 46.2 Gy (SD ± 12.8), with a median of 50 Gy (range 12.5–76 Gy). Moreover, 20.2% (19/94) of patients received an RT boost. RT was delivered daily in 83% (78/94) of patients (Table 3, Supplementary Table S3B). In total, 55 of 95 patients (57.9%) received dHT followed by RT at the Kantonsspital Aarau. The remaining 40 patients travelled to their referring hospital after the dHT session for the same-day RT (Figure 3). In the first group, the time interval between dHT and RT was available in 98.1% of patients (54/55). The mean and median time between the end of the dHT session and start of the RT was 19 min (SD ± 5.5) and 18 min (range 11–32 min), respectively. Evaluation of the time interval of the 40 patients receiving all RT at their referring institution was not possible due to the retrospective nature of this study and because these patients were irradiated at several RT facilities located all over the country. Treatment characteristics were compared between specific patient subgroups, including in-house vs. referred patients, primary RT vs. re-RT and curative vs. palliative intention (Table 3). The treatment schedules employed are stated per dHT indication and per individual patient in detail in Supplementary Table S5.

Table 3. Treatment characteristics for specific patient subgroups comparing in-house vs. referred patients, primary RT vs. re-RT and curative vs. palliative intention.

	Treatment Characteristics by						
	Referral Status		Re-Irradiation Status		Treatment Intention		
	In-House Patients	Referred from External Hospital	No	Yes	Curative	Palliative	Total
	(n = 35)	(n = 59)	(n = 55)	(n = 39)	(n = 45)	(n = 49)	(n = 94)
HT frequency							
Once per week	14 (40.0%)	35 (59.3%)	36 (65.5%)	13 (33.3%)	32 (71.1%)	17 (34.7%)	49 (52.1%)
Once to twice per week	21 (60.0%)	24 (40.7%)	19 (34.5%)	26 (66.7%)	13 (28.9%)	32 (65.3%)	45 (47.9%)
No. of dHT sessions							
Mean (SD)	5.17 (1.44)	5.29 (2.20)	5.53 (1.91)	4.85 (1.94)	5.60 (1.99)	4.92 (1.86)	5.24 (1.94)
Median [Min, Max]	5 [1, 8]	5 [1, 10]	6 [1, 10]	5 [1, 8]	6 [1, 10]	5 [1, 10]	5 [1, 10]
Total no. of RT fractions							
Mean (SD)	20.1 (8.11)	22.6 (9.27)	24.9 (6.42)	17.1 (9.90)	26.7 (5.98)	17.0 (8.63)	21.7 (8.89)
Median [Min, Max]	23 [4, 35]	25 [4, 38]	27 [10, 35]	15 [4, 38]	28 [4, 38]	15 [4, 35]	25 [4, 38]
Dose/fraction (Gy)							
Mean (SD)	2.46 (1.04)	2.51 (1.51)	2.14 (0.413)	3.00 (1.94)	2.14 (0.950)	2.82 (1.57)	2.49 (1.35)
Median [Min, Max]	2 [1.8, 7.5]	2 [1.8, 9]	2 [1.8, 3]	2.5 [1.8, 9]	2 [1.8, 8]	2.5 [1.8, 9]	2 [1.8, 9]
Boost included							
No	27 (77.1%)	48 (81.4%)	38 (69.1%)	37 (94.9%)	29 (64.4%)	46 (93.9%)	75 (79.8%)
Yes	8 (22.9%)	11 (18.6%)	17 (30.9%)	2 (5.1%)	16 (35.6%)	3 (6.1%)	19 (20.2%)
Total dose (Gy)							
Mean (SD)	43.6 (10.6)	47.6 (13.8)	51.1 (8.85)	39.2 (14.3)	53.3 (8.55)	39.6 (12.7)	46.2 (12.8)
Median [Min, Max]	45 [24, 70]	50 [12.5, 76]	50.4 [30, 71]	32 [12.5, 76]	50.4 [32, 76]	36 [12.5, 71]	50 [12.5, 76]
RT interval							
1×/week	0 (0%)	1 (1.7%)	0 (0%)	1 (2.6%)	0 (0%)	1 (2.0%)	1 (1.1%)
2×/week	2 (5.7%)	4 (6.8%)	0 (0%)	6 (15.4%)	1 (2.2%)	5 (10.2%)	6 (6.4%)
3×/week	0 (0%)	0 (0%)	0 (0%)	0 (0%)	0 (0%)	0 (0%)	0 (0%)
4×/week	4 (11.4%)	5 (8.5%)	7 (12.7%)	2 (5.1%)	4 (8.9%)	5 (10.2%)	9 (9.6%)
5×/week	29 (82.9%)	49 (83.1%)	48 (87.3%)	30 (76.9%)	40 (88.9%)	38 (77.6%)	78 (83.0%)
RT modality							
EBRT	33 (94.3%)	46 (78.0%)	50 (90.9%)	29 (74.4%)	38 (84.4%)	41 (83.7%)	79 (84.0%)
HDR—brachytherapy	0 (0%)	4 (6.8%)	0 (0%)	4 (10.3%)	1 (2.2%)	3 (6.1%)	4 (4.3%)
Protons	0 (0%)	9 (15.3%)	5 (9.1%)	4 (10.3%)	6 (13.3%)	3 (6.1%)	9 (9.6%)
SBRT	2 (5.7%)	0 (0%)	0 (0%)	2 (5.1%)	0 (0%)	2 (4.1%)	2 (2.1%)

One patient stopped treatment very early and was excluded from the treatment characteristics table. Abbreviations: dHT: deep hyperthermia, EBRT: external body radiotherapy, Gy: Gray, HDR: high dose rate, RT: radiotherapy, SBRT: stereotactic body radiotherapy, SD: standard deviation.

The specific treatment schedules were dependent on the treatment indication, aim of treatment, pre-irradiation status, primary tumor entity and tumor stage. Patients treated with curative intent generally received a higher total dose, more RT fractions, usually 2 Gy per fraction and one dHT session per week. Palliative or re-RT treatment schedules mostly consisted of lower total doses, less RT fractions using moderate hypofractionation with 1–2 dHT sessions per week, but nearly the same total number of dHT sessions as in the curative setting. This coincides with the expected current practice in radiation oncology.

3.4. Hyperthermia Treatment Adherence

The adherence to dHT was high, with 94% (89/95) of patients finishing all dHT sessions as initially prescribed. Six patients did not complete the prescribed sessions.

Three of these six patients were treated for bladder cancer, two of them with tetramodal treatment (transurethral resection of bladder tumor (TUR-BT), chemotherapy, dHT+RT) and one with dHT+RT only. The reason for early discontinuation in these three patients was bladder irritation and/or bacterial cystitis, which prevented further catheterization for thermometry. Furthermore, 2/6 patients were treated for rectal cancer with local tumor recurrence with compression with palliative intent and were of ECOG 2. The reason for early discontinuation of dHT was deterioration of health status. The sixth patient was scheduled to receive neoadjuvant dHT+RT for soft tissue sarcoma of the limb. dHT was discontinued after the first HT session due to heat-induced pain in the tumor.

4. Discussion

During the investigated time period, only one RT center in Switzerland provided radiative dHT and seven dHT indications were approved for reimbursement in Switzerland. For other tumor situations that were likely to benefit from combined dHT+RT, an individual request to the patient's insurance company was necessary. A prerequisite for coverage of the costs stipulated by the Swiss Federal Office of Public Health was the presentation and confirmation of the dHT indication at the SHN tumor board.

Our analysis of the patient flow through this tumor board revealed a high number (approximately 50%) of patients who were not approved for dHT. This might be explained not only by the critical evaluation of the dHT indication by an expert panel, thus reflecting the quality of the tumor board decisions, but also by the fact that some referring physicians were not yet familiar with dHT as they presented patients with obvious contraindications, such as metal implants in the tumor region. We noted that only for two patients dHT could not be applied due to lack of cost recovery (Figure 1a), showing that health insurance companies in Switzerland will cover dHT when no other local treatment options than dHT+RT exist and the indication can be justified. The strict supervision of meaningful indications by the SHN tumor board probably contributed to the high acceptance rate of the health insurers. Therefore, we conclude that the SHN tumor board serves not only for the preselection of patients, besides contributing to the transparency and harmonization of treatment schedules, but also plays a role in teaching newcomers to the field.

This analysis presents compelling evidence of an existing clinical demand for dHT for both palliative and curative indications. The majority (74.7%, 71/95) of patients in this analysis were treated based on the seven "reimbursed dHT indications" and only 25.3% (24/95) of patients required an individual "request to the insurance company" to cover the costs of therapy (Table 2). A closer look at the latter group revealed that, in the two years (2017 to 2018) before the introduction of the two new reimbursed dHT indications (local tumor compression and painful bone metastasis), more requests for dHT were submitted to insurance companies (15 vs. 9 patients). From 2017 to 2018, dHT was mainly prescribed for the two indications mentioned above (10 of 15) (Supplementary Table S1). With the approval of these two indications, the number of requests to insurance companies decreased, reflecting that an existing clinical demand had been covered. The linear time trend observed over the first two years, with an increase of one patient per semester, could be interpreted as epidemiological growth or may be due to the fact that hyperthermia achieved more visibility within the Swiss (radiation) oncology society. However, the COVID-19 pandemic has clearly influenced case numbers and indications treated from the first semester of 2020 onwards (Figure 2). Due to this confounding bias, a reliable time trend analysis of patient numbers was not possible; however, it is important to note that an uncontrolled increase in case numbers did not happen despite reimbursement of new treatment indications. Taken together, the dHT indications negotiated jointly by the Swiss Federal Office of Public Health and the SHN appear not to have induced a commercially driven increase in patients treated.

With regard to the referral pattern, our analysis revealed that only 36.8% (35/95) of patients originated in-house and that 63.2% (60/95) patients were referred from external radiation oncology institutions (Figure 3). This shows that a dHT unit in Switzerland, even when integrated into a radiation oncology center, not only treats in-house patients.

Patients have been referred for dHT from university hospitals and as well from the proton therapy center at the Paul Scherer Institute explicitly for the treatment of challenging oncological situations (Supplementary Table S2). This indicates that a dHT unit covers an existing demand for specific oncological situations, such as re-irradiation, organ-preserving treatment combinations (bladder and rectal cancer, soft tissue sarcoma) and other complex situations such as inoperable pancreatic cancer, soft tissue sarcoma or bulky, radioresistant tumors. In Switzerland, HT is frequently and incorrectly regarded as a mainly palliative treatment option. In the present analysis, we refute this by showing that 47.4% (45/95) of patients were treated with a curative treatment approach.

The characteristics of the in-house patients revealed that they generally had a lower performance status and were more likely to be treated with palliative intent. Accordingly, dHT was more often used for the indication "local recurrence and compression". Patients of low performance status are not fit to travel long distances for dHT, even if they would benefit from a radiosensitizer such as dHT, with its good toxicity profile. For palliative indications, the use of dHT could allow for a reduction in RT dose and thereby improve the tolerability and effect of RT, i.e., regarding pain relief, as has been shown by Chi et al. [39] for painful bone metastases. The referred patients in the present cohort travelled a relatively long mean distance of 62.2 km (SD ± 54.6 km), with a maximum of 238 km, to receive dHT (Supplementary Table S2). This effort is unreasonable for palliative and frail patients, which supports the future higher spatial availability of dHT units in Switzerland.

The three most commonly reimbursed dHT indications were "local tumor recurrence with compression" (20%), "rectal cancer" (14.7%) and "bladder cancer" (13.7%) (Table 2). Unfortunately, the approval for reimbursement for the most common curative and organ-preserving indications, "rectal cancer" and "bladder cancer", was withdrawn by July 2021 [20]. Patients treated for the dHT indication "rectal cancer" were mostly referred from external radiotherapy centers (Supplementary Table S2) and predominantly for re-irradiation (71.4%; 10/14 patients, data not shown). More than half (8/14 patients) were treated analogously to the HyRec trial [31] (Supplementary Table S5). The indication "bladder cancer" closes a gap in treatment options for either elderly and frail patients or patients seeking a bladder-sparing treatment approach. Patients were referred from external hospitals for these indications, underlining the demand for this treatment option as well. The SHN board is convinced that there is good evidence for dHT for these two indications [26–29,32], especially in rectal cancer, since two recent studies showed a promising effect of dHT [30,31].

Regarding the other dHT indications, the present analysis revealed that only a few patients are treated for the dHT indication "cervical cancer", although it is associated with the strongest clinical evidence [21–23]. This could be explained by the low incidence of cervical cancer in Switzerland and the fact that this indication only receives direct reimbursement in the case of re-RT and for patients with contraindication to concurrent chemotherapy, which is rarely the case in Switzerland. This is in contrast to, for example, the Netherlands, where dHT is reimbursed in the primary treatment setting in combination with RT and brachytherapy based on evidence from randomized trials [11]. Another observation is the low patient numbers treated for "painful bone metastases", although its superior effect regarding pain control was shown in a phase III randomized trial [39]. At Kantonsspital Aarau, the combination of dHT+RT for the indication of painful bone metastases was intended to be increasingly used in the future, because, with the longer survival of metastatic patients, long-lasting pain control is also becoming more important. However, because, during the COVID-19 pandemic, non-mandatory treatments were minimized and painful bone metastases could be often sufficiently treated with hypofractionated RT schedules alone, dHT was not offered. After returning to normality in the first semester of 2021, dHT patient numbers almost doubled (Figure 2), reaching the limited capacity of treatment slots for dHT. Therefore, patients with curative treatment indications were prioritized and dHT+RT again was not actively offered to patients qualifying for painful bone metastases. With the increasing dHT treatment capacity and controlled establishment of more dHT units in Switzerland, more patients with painful bone metastases could benefit from the increased analgetic effect of dHT+RT.

The present patterns-of-care analysis was conducted as an inventory/survey of current practice and as the basis for a national objective to define standardized treatment schedules in Switzerland. All reimbursed indications, except for the indications "tumor recurrence and compression" and "painful bone metastasis", showed relatively standardized treatment schedules in analogy to clinical trials (Supplementary Table S5). In contrast, the indication group "local tumor recurrence with compression" represents a patient collective with enormous heterogeneity regarding primary cancer entities, re-RT status, RT modalities and treatment schedules. The only common denominator is that they were treated mostly with palliative intent (Supplementary Tables S2 and S5). Importantly, these patients often have no other treatment option apart from dHT+RT and local treatment effect has a high impact on their quality of life. Withholding dHT+RT as a last treatment option from these patients would, in our view, be unethical. Because these patients frequently required individually tailored treatment schedules based on their previous treatment, the standardization of the treatment schedules, especially for clinical trials, would also be difficult. It is therefore clear that an analysis of dHT efficacy in this patient group is a challenge. A good example for the standardization of dHT+RT treatment schedules in patients with tumor recurrences is the subgroup of the HyRec trial from Ott et al. [31,52] and the schedule with 5×4 Gy once weekly combined with weekly wIRA superficial HT in recurrent breast cancer from Notter et al. [56] for superficial HT. Such innovative study designs and further treatment schedules are required to evaluate and consolidate the effect of dHT in these heterogeneous patient groups.

5. Conclusions

To the best of our knowledge, we report the first retrospective analysis of an unselected national patient cohort treated with dHT, evaluating patient numbers over 4.5 years, specific treatment indications, patient characteristics, tumor entities, the referral practice and corresponding treatment schedules in Switzerland.

Nearly 50% of patients were treated with curative intent. Around two thirds of patients were referred from external institutions from all over Switzerland, including from university hospitals and the proton therapy center, for challenging oncologic situations such as re-RT, complex palliative situations, organ-preserving treatment combinations (bladder and rectal cancer, soft tissue sarcoma) and inoperable, bulky or radioresistant tumors. This observation refutes the common prejudice, at least in Switzerland, that HT is only used for palliative situations and clearly underlines the medical need for the combination of dHT+RT.

Patients treated within the reimbursed dHT indications with predominantly curative intent were homogenous subgroups with relatively standardized treatment schedules according to published clinical trials. On the other hand, the present patterns-of-care analysis revealed that patients treated within the two palliative reimbursed indications "tumor local recurrence and compression" and "painful bone metastasis" exhibit immense heterogeneity regarding patient characteristics and treatment schedules, demonstrating the need for standardization as a basis for future clinical studies.

This analysis will provide the basis for standardized national dHT treatment schedules and quality assurance guidelines to consolidate and expand dHT evidence. We think that this insight into dHT practice in Switzerland could be of interest for centers interested in the implementation of a dHT unit and for other HT societies, especially regarding reimbursement policy, and could also foster international study collaborations.

Supplementary Materials: The following are available online at https://www.mdpi.com/article/10.3390/cancers14051175/s1, Figure S1: Number of cases presented at the Swiss Hyperthermia Network tumor board by primary cancer entity. Table S1: Patients and tumor characteristics of patients treated with deep hyperthermia who required an individual request for insurance cover. Table S2: Patient characteristics regarding referral status, re-irradiation status and by treatment indication. Table S3: Patient, tumor and treatment characteristics according to treatment protocol. Table S4: Patient characteristics by gender. Table S5: Deep hyperthermia and combined radiotherapy treatment schedules by specific reimbursed dHT indications.

Author Contributions: Conceptualization, E.S., E.P., S.B. and O.R.; methodology, E.S., A.K., S.B. and O.R.; software, A.K. and E.S.; validation, E.S., E.P., A.A., A.K., R.K., O.T., D.M., M.N., S.B. and O.R.; formal analysis, E.S., A.K. and O.R.; data curation, E.S., A.A., E.P. and R.K.; writing—original draft preparation, E.S.; writing—review and editing, E.S., E.P., A.A., A.K., R.K., O.T., D.M., M.N., S.R., S.B. and O.R.; visualization, E.S. and A.K.; supervision, S.B. and O.R.; funding acquisition, E.S. and O.R. All authors have read and agreed to the published version of the manuscript.

Funding: This research was funded by a Scientific Association of Swiss Radiation Oncology (SASRO) research grant (to E.S.) and by the Swiss Hyperthermia Network (SHN). In addition, this research has received support from the European Union's Horizon 2020 research and innovation programme under the Marie Skłodowska-Curie (MSCA-ITN) grant "Hyperboost" project, no. 955625 (to O.R. and S.B.).

Institutional Review Board Statement: The study was conducted according to the guidelines of the Declaration of Helsinki and approved by the Ethics Committee Nordwest—und Zentralschweiz of Switzerland (protocol code 2021-01022, 1 July 2021).

Informed Consent Statement: Informed consent was obtained from subjects involved in the study. Patients declining use of their data were excluded from analysis, as stated in Figure 1a.

Data Availability Statement: The data presented in this study are available on request from the corresponding author. The data are not publicly available due to privacy and ethical reasons.

Acknowledgments: We thank Sonja Schwenne, for the administrative support.

Conflicts of Interest: The authors declare no conflict of interest.

References

1. van der Zee, J.; Vujaskovic, Z.; Kondo, M.; Sugahara, T. The Kadota Fund International Forum 2004—Clinical group consensus. *Int. J. Hyperth.* **2008**, *24*, 111–122. [CrossRef]
2. Datta, N.R.; Ordóñez, S.G.; Gaipl, U.S.; Paulides, M.M.; Crezee, H.; Gellermann, J.; Marder, D.; Puric, E.; Bodis, S. Local hyperthermia combined with radiotherapy and-/or chemotherapy: Recent advances and promises for the future. *Cancer Treat. Rev.* **2015**, *41*, 742–753. [CrossRef]
3. Peeken, J.C.; Vaupel, P.; Combs, S.E. Integrating Hyperthermia into Modern Radiation Oncology: What Evidence Is Necessary? *Front. Oncol.* **2017**, *7*, 132. [CrossRef]
4. Kok, H.P.; Cressman, E.N.K.; Ceelen, W.; Brace, C.L.; Ivkov, R.; Grüll, H.; Ter Haar, G.; Wust, P.; Crezee, J. Heating technology for malignant tumors: A review. *Int. J. Hyperth.* **2020**, *37*, 711–741. [CrossRef]
5. Lee, S.Y.; Fiorentini, G.; Szasz, A.M.; Szigeti, G.; Szasz, A.; Minnaar, C.A. Quo Vadis Oncological Hyperthermia (2020)? *Front. Oncol.* **2020**, *10*, 1690. [CrossRef]
6. Overgaard, J. The heat is (still) on–the past and future of hyperthermic radiation oncology. *Radiother. Oncol. J. Eur. Soc. Ther. Radiol. Oncol.* **2013**, *109*, 185–187. [CrossRef]
7. Vasanthan, A.; Mitsumori, M.; Park, J.H.; Zhi-Fan, Z.; Yu-Bin, Z.; Oliynychenko, P.; Tatsuzaki, H.; Tanaka, Y.; Hiraoka, M. Regional hyperthermia combined with radiotherapy for uterine cervical cancers: A multi-institutional prospective randomized trial of the international atomic energy agency. *Int. J. Radiat. Oncol. Biol. Phys.* **2005**, *61*, 145–153. [CrossRef]
8. Sauer, R.; Creeze, H.; Hulshof, M.; Issels, R.; Ott, O. Concerning the final report "Hyperthermia: A systematic review" of the Ludwig Boltzmann Institute for Health Technology Assessment, Vienna, March 2010. *Strahlenther. Onkol.* **2012**, *188*, 209–213. [CrossRef]
9. Wild, C. Should hyperthermia be included in the benefit catalogue for oncologic indications? Commercial interests are presumed behind the editorial of R. Sauer et al. *Strahlenther. Onkol.* **2013**, *189*, 81–86. [CrossRef]
10. Myerson, R.J.; Moros, E.G.; Diederich, C.J.; Haemmerich, D.; Hurwitz, M.D.; Hsu, I.C.; McGough, R.J.; Nau, W.H.; Straube, W.L.; Turner, P.F.; et al. Components of a hyperthermia clinic: Recommendations for staffing, equipment, and treatment monitoring. *Int. J. Hyperth.* **2014**, *30*, 1–5. [CrossRef]
11. van der Zee, J.; van Rhoon, G.C. Cervical cancer: Radiotherapy and hyperthermia. *Int. J. Hyperth.* **2006**, *22*, 229–234. [CrossRef] [PubMed]
12. Franckena, M.; Stalpers, L.J.; Koper, P.C.; Wiggenraad, R.G.; Hoogenraad, W.J.; van Dijk, J.D.; Wárlám-Rodenhuis, C.C.; Jobsen, J.J.; van Rhoon, G.C.; van der Zee, J. Long-term improvement in treatment outcome after radiotherapy and hyperthermia in locoregionally advanced cervix cancer: An update of the Dutch Deep Hyperthermia Trial. *Int. J. Radiat. Oncol. Biol. Phys.* **2008**, *70*, 1176–1182. [CrossRef] [PubMed]

13. Bruggmoser, G.; Bauchowitz, S.; Canters, R.; Crezee, H.; Ehmann, M.; Gellermann, J.; Lamprecht, U.; Lomax, N.; Messmer, M.B.; Ott, O.; et al. Quality assurance for clinical studies in regional deep hyperthermia. *Strahlenther. Onkol.* **2011**, *187*, 605–610. [CrossRef] [PubMed]
14. Bruggmoser, G.; Bauchowitz, S.; Canters, R.; Crezee, H.; Ehmann, M.; Gellermann, J.; Lamprecht, U.; Lomax, N.; Messmer, M.B.; Ott, O.; et al. Guideline for the clinical application, documentation and analysis of clinical studies for regional deep hyperthermia: Quality management in regional deep hyperthermia. *Strahlenther. Onkol.* **2012**, *188* (Suppl. S2), 198–211. [CrossRef]
15. Dobšíček Trefná, H.; Crezee, J.; Schmidt, M.; Marder, D.; Lamprecht, U.; Ehmann, M.; Nadobny, J.; Hartmann, J.; Lomax, N.; Abdel-Rahman, S.; et al. Quality assurance guidelines for superficial hyperthermia clinical trials: II. Technical requirements for heating devices. *Strahlenther. Onkol.* **2017**, *193*, 351–366. [CrossRef]
16. Trefná, H.D.; Crezee, H.; Schmidt, M.; Marder, D.; Lamprecht, U.; Ehmann, M.; Hartmann, J.; Nadobny, J.; Gellermann, J.; van Holthe, N.; et al. Quality assurance guidelines for superficial hyperthermia clinical trials: I. Clinical requirements. *Int. J. Hyperth.* **2017**, *33*, 471–482. [CrossRef]
17. Stutz, E.; Datta, N.R.; Puric, E.; Bodis, S. Stellenwert der regionären Hyperthermie in der Krebstherapie. *Swiss Med. Forum [Ger.]* **2017**, *17*, 1074–1076.
18. Verordnung des EDI über Leistungen in der Obligatorischen Krankenpflegeversicherung (Krankenpflege-Leistungsverordnung, KLV) Änderung vom 25. November 2016. Available online: https://www.fedlex.admin.ch/eli/oc/2016/750/de (accessed on 27 January 2022).
19. Verordnung KLV des EDI über Leistungen in der Obligatorischen Krankenpflegeversicherung (Krankenpflege-Leistungsverordnung, KLV) Änderung 30. November 2018. Available online: https://www.fedlex.admin.ch/eli/oc/2018/793/de (accessed on 27 January 2022).
20. Anhang 1 der Krankenpflege-Leistungsverordnung (KLV). Available online: https://www.bag.admin.ch/bag/de/home/versicherungen/krankenversicherung/krankenversicherung-leistungen-tarife/Aerztliche-Leistungen-in-der-Krankenversicherung/anhang1klv.html (accessed on 27 January 2022).
21. Lutgens, L.; van der Zee, J.; Pijls-Johannesma, M.; De Haas-Kock, D.F.; Buijsen, J.; Mastrigt, G.A.; Lammering, G.; De Ruysscher, D.K.; Lambin, P. Combined use of hyperthermia and radiation therapy for treating locally advanced cervix carcinoma. *Cochrane Database Syst. Rev.* **2010**, *2010*, Cd006377. [CrossRef]
22. Datta, N.R.; Rogers, S.; Klingbiel, D.; Gómez, S.; Puric, E.; Bodis, S. Hyperthermia and radiotherapy with or without chemotherapy in locally advanced cervical cancer: A systematic review with conventional and network meta-analyses. *Int. J. Hyperth.* **2016**, *32*, 809–821. [CrossRef]
23. Datta, N.R.; Stutz, E.; Gomez, S.; Bodis, S. Efficacy and Safety Evaluation of the Various Therapeutic Options in Locally Advanced Cervix Cancer: A Systematic Review and Network Meta-Analysis of Randomized Clinical Trials. *Int. J. Radiat. Oncol. Biol. Phys.* **2019**, *103*, 411–437. [CrossRef]
24. Datta, N.R.; Eberle, B.; Puric, E.; Meister, A.; Marder, D.; Tim, O.; Klimov, A.; Bodis, S. Is hyperthermia combined with radiotherapy adequate in elderly patients with muscle-invasive bladder cancers? Thermo-radiobiological implications from an audit of initial results. *Int. J. Hyperth.* **2016**, *32*, 390–397. [CrossRef]
25. Datta, N.R.; Marder, D.; Datta, S.; Meister, A.; Puric, E.; Stutz, E.; Rogers, S.; Eberle, B.; Timm, O.; Staruch, M.; et al. Quantification of thermal dose in moderate clinical hyperthermia with radiotherapy: A relook using temperature-time area under the curve (AUC). *Int. J. Hyperth.* **2021**, *38*, 296–307. [CrossRef]
26. Datta, N.R.; Stutz, E.; Puric, E.; Eberle, B.; Meister, A.; Marder, D.; Timm, O.; Rogers, S.; Wyler, S.; Bodis, S. A Pilot Study of Radiotherapy and Local Hyperthermia in Elderly Patients with Muscle-Invasive Bladder Cancers Unfit for Definitive Surgery or Chemoradiotherapy. *Front. Oncol.* **2019**, *9*, 889. [CrossRef] [PubMed]
27. van der Zee, J.; González González, D.; van Rhoon, G.C.; van Dijk, J.D.; van Putten, W.L.; Hart, A.A. Comparison of radiotherapy alone with radiotherapy plus hyperthermia in locally advanced pelvic tumours: A prospective, randomised, multicentre trial. Dutch Deep Hyperthermia Group. *Lancet (Lond. Engl.)* **2000**, *355*, 1119–1125. [CrossRef]
28. Merten, R.; Ott, O.; Haderlein, M.; Bertz, S.; Hartmann, A.; Wullich, B.; Keck, B.; Kühn, R.; Rödel, C.M.; Weiss, C.; et al. Long-Term Experience of Chemoradiotherapy Combined with Deep Regional Hyperthermia for Organ Preservation in High-Risk Bladder Cancer (Ta, Tis, T1, T2). *Oncologist* **2019**, *24*, e1341–e1350. [CrossRef] [PubMed]
29. Wittlinger, M.; Rödel, C.M.; Weiss, C.; Krause, S.F.; Kühn, R.; Fietkau, R.; Sauer, R.; Ott, O.J. Quadrimodal treatment of high-risk T1 and T2 bladder cancer: Transurethral tumor resection followed by concurrent radiochemotherapy and regional deep hyperthermia. *Radiother. Oncol. J. Eur. Soc. Ther. Radiol. Oncol.* **2009**, *93*, 358–363. [CrossRef]
30. Gani, C.; Lamprecht, U.; Ziegler, A.; Moll, M.; Gellermann, J.; Heinrich, V.; Wenz, S.; Fend, F.; Königsrainer, A.; Bitzer, M.; et al. Deep regional hyperthermia with preoperative radiochemotherapy in locally advanced rectal cancer, a prospective phase II trial. *Radiother. Oncol. J. Eur. Soc. Ther. Radiol. Oncol.* **2021**, *159*, 155–160. [CrossRef]
31. Ott, O.J.; Gani, C.; Lindner, L.H.; Schmidt, M.; Lamprecht, U.; Abdel-Rahman, S.; Hinke, A.; Weissmann, T.; Hartmann, A.; Issels, R.D.; et al. Neoadjuvant Chemoradiation Combined with Regional Hyperthermia in Locally Advanced or Recurrent Rectal Cancer. *Cancers* **2021**, *13*, 1279. [CrossRef]
32. De Haas-Kock, D.F.; Buijsen, J.; Pijls-Johannesma, M.; Lutgens, L.; Lammering, G.; van Mastrigt, G.A.; De Ruysscher, D.K.; Lambin, P.; van der Zee, J. Concomitant hyperthermia and radiation therapy for treating locally advanced rectal cancer. *Cochrane Database Syst. Rev.* **2009**, CD006269. [CrossRef]

33. Prosnitz, L.R.; Maguire, P.; Anderson, J.M.; Scully, S.P.; Harrelson, J.M.; Jones, E.L.; Dewhirst, M.; Samulski, T.V.; Powers, B.E.; Rosner, G.L.; et al. The treatment of high-grade soft tissue sarcomas with preoperative thermoradiotherapy. *Int. J. Radiat. Oncol. Biol. Phys.* **1999**, *45*, 941–949. [CrossRef]
34. Datta, N.R.; Schneider, R.; Puric, E.; Ahlhelm, F.J.; Marder, D.; Bodis, S.; Weber, D.C. Proton Irradiation with Hyperthermia in Unresectable Soft Tissue Sarcoma. *Int. J. Part. Ther.* **2016**, *3*, 327–336. [CrossRef]
35. Issels, R.D.; Lindner, L.H.; Verweij, J.; Wust, P.; Reichardt, P.; Schem, B.C.; Abdel-Rahman, S.; Daugaard, S.; Salat, C.; Wendtner, C.M.; et al. Neo-adjuvant chemotherapy alone or with regional hyperthermia for localised high-risk soft-tissue sarcoma: A randomised phase 3 multicentre study. *Lancet. Oncol.* **2010**, *11*, 561–570. [CrossRef]
36. Rogers, S.J.; Datta, N.R.; Puric, E.; Timm, O.; Marder, D.; Khan, S.; Mamot, C.; Knuchel, J.; Siebenhüner, A.; Pestalozzi, B.; et al. The addition of deep hyperthermia to gemcitabine-based chemoradiation may achieve enhanced survival in unresectable locally advanced adenocarcinoma of the pancreas. *Clin. Transl. Radiat. Oncol.* **2021**, *27*, 109–113. [CrossRef] [PubMed]
37. Datta, N.R.; Pestalozzi, B.; Clavien, P.A.; Siebenhüner, A.; Puric, E.; Khan, S.; Mamot, C.; Riesterer, O.; Knuchel, J.; Reiner, C.S.; et al. "HEATPAC"—A phase II randomized study of concurrent thermochemoradiotherapy versus chemoradiotherapy alone in locally advanced pancreatic cancer. *Radiat. Oncol.* **2017**, *12*, 183. [CrossRef] [PubMed]
38. Maluta, S.; Schaffer, M.; Pioli, F.; Dall'oglio, S.; Pasetto, S.; Schaffer, P.M.; Weber, B.; Giri, M.G. Regional hyperthermia combined with chemoradiotherapy in primary or recurrent locally advanced pancreatic cancer: An open-label comparative cohort trial. *Strahlenther. Onkol.* **2011**, *187*, 619–625. [CrossRef] [PubMed]
39. Chi, M.S.; Yang, K.L.; Chang, Y.C.; Ko, H.L.; Lin, Y.H.; Huang, S.C.; Huang, Y.Y.; Liao, K.W.; Kondo, M.; Chi, K.H. Comparing the Effectiveness of Combined External Beam Radiation and Hyperthermia Versus External Beam Radiation Alone in Treating Patients with Painful Bony Metastases: A Phase 3 Prospective, Randomized, Controlled Trial. *Int. J. Radiat. Oncol. Biol. Phys.* **2018**, *100*, 78–87. [CrossRef]
40. Oei, A.L.; Kok, H.P.; Oei, S.B.; Horsman, M.R.; Stalpers, L.J.A.; Franken, N.A.P.; Crezee, J. Molecular and biological rationale of hyperthermia as radio- and chemosensitizer. *Adv. Drug. Deliv. Rev.* **2020**, *163–164*, 84–97. [CrossRef]
41. Overgaard, J. Simultaneous and sequential hyperthermia and radiation treatment of an experimental tumor and its surrounding normal tissue in vivo. *Int. J. Radiat. Oncol. Biol. Phys.* **1980**, *6*, 1507–1517. [CrossRef]
42. Notter, M.; Piazena, H.; Vaupel, P. Hypofractionated re-irradiation of large-sized recurrent breast cancer with thermography-controlled, contact-free water-filtered infra-red-A hyperthermia: A retrospective study of 73 patients. *Int. J. Hyperth.* **2017**, *33*, 227–236. [CrossRef]
43. Linthorst, M.; van Geel, A.N.; Baaijens, M.; Ameziane, A.; Ghidey, W.; van Rhoon, G.C.; van der Zee, J. Re-irradiation and hyperthermia after surgery for recurrent breast cancer. *Radiother. Oncol.* **2013**, *109*, 188–193. [CrossRef]
44. van Leeuwen, C.M.; Oei, A.L.; Chin, K.; Crezee, J.; Bel, A.; Westermann, A.M.; Buist, M.R.; Franken, N.A.P.; Stalpers, L.J.A.; Kok, H.P. A short time interval between radiotherapy and hyperthermia reduces in-field recurrence and mortality in women with advanced cervical cancer. *Radiat. Oncol.* **2017**, *12*, 75. [CrossRef]
45. Kroesen, M.; Mulder, H.T.; van Holthe, J.M.L.; Aangeenbrug, A.A.; Mens, J.W.M.; van Doorn, H.C.; Paulides, M.M.; Oomen-de Hoop, E.; Vernhout, R.M.; Lutgens, L.C.; et al. The Effect of the Time Interval Between Radiation and Hyperthermia on Clinical Outcome in 400 Locally Advanced Cervical Carcinoma Patients. *Front. Oncol.* **2019**, *9*, 134. [CrossRef] [PubMed]
46. Crezee, H.; Kok, H.P.; Oei, A.L.; Franken, N.A.P.; Stalpers, L.J.A. The Impact of the Time Interval Between Radiation and Hyperthermia on Clinical Outcome in Patients with Locally Advanced Cervical Cancer. *Front. Oncol.* **2019**, *9*, 412. [CrossRef]
47. Kroesen, M.; Mulder, H.T.; van Rhoon, G.C.; Franckena, M. Commentary: The Impact of the Time Interval Between Radiation and Hyperthermia on Clinical Outcome in Patients with Locally Advanced Cervical Cancer. *Front. Oncol.* **2019**, *9*, 1387. [CrossRef] [PubMed]
48. Crezee, J.; Oei, A.L.; Franken, N.A.P.; Stalpers, L.J.A.; Kok, H.P. Response: Commentary: The Impact of the Time Interval Between Radiation and Hyperthermia on Clinical Outcome in Patients with Locally Advanced Cervical Cancer. *Front. Oncol.* **2020**, *10*, 528. [CrossRef] [PubMed]
49. Effects of Deep Regional Hyperthermia in Patients with Anal Carcinoma Treated by Standard Radiochemotherapy (HYCAN) (NCT02369939). Available online: https://clinicaltrials.gov/ct2/show/NCT02369939?term=hyperthermia&cond=anal+cancer&draw=2&rank=1 (accessed on 27 January 2022).
50. Concurrent Hyperthermia and Chemoradiotherapy in LAPC: Phase II Study (HEATPAC) (NCT02439593). Available online: https://clinicaltrials.gov/ct2/show/NCT02439593?cond=NCT02439593&draw=2&rank=1 (accessed on 27 January 2022).
51. A Phase IIB Study of the Tetramodal Therapy of T2-T4 Nx M0 Bladder Cancer with Hyperthermia Combined with Chemoradiotherapy Following TUR-BT. Available online: https://www.ksa.ch/sites/default/files/cms/radio-onkologie/docs/neu-word_vorlage_allgemein_logo_blau.pdf (accessed on 27 January 2022).
52. Neoadjuvant Chemoradiation with 5-FU (or Capecitabine) and Oxaliplatin Combined with Hyperthermia in Rectal Cancer (HyRec) (NCT01716949). Available online: https://clinicaltrials.gov/ct2/show/NCT01716949?term=hyperthermia&cond=rectal+cancer&draw=2&rank=2 (accessed on 27 January 2022).
53. Hyperthermia and Proton Therapy in Unresectable Soft Tissue Sarcoma (HYPROSAR) (NCT01904565). Available online: https://clinicaltrials.gov/ct2/show/NCT01904565?cond=NCT01904565&draw=2&rank=1 (accessed on 27 January 2022).

54. Tran, S.; Puric, E.; Walser, M.; Poel, R.; Datta, N.R.; Heuberger, J.; Pica, A.; Marder, D.; Lomax, N.; Bolsi, A.; et al. Early results and volumetric analysis after spot-scanning proton therapy with concomitant hyperthermia in large inoperable sacral chordomas. *Br. J. Radiol.* **2020**, *93*, 20180883. [CrossRef] [PubMed]
55. SankeyMATIC. Available online: https://sankeymatic.com/build/ (accessed on 15 January 2022).
56. Notter, M.; Thomsen, A.R.; Nitsche, M.; Hermann, R.M.; Wolff, H.A.; Habl, G.; Münch, K.; Grosu, A.L.; Vaupel, P. Combined wIRA-Hyperthermia and Hypofractionated Re-Irradiation in the Treatment of Locally Recurrent Breast Cancer: Evaluation of Therapeutic Outcome Based on a Novel Size Classification. *Cancers* **2020**, *12*, 606. [CrossRef]

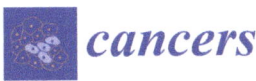

Article

Feasibility, SAR Distribution, and Clinical Outcome upon Reirradiation and Deep Hyperthermia Using the Hypercollar3D in Head and Neck Cancer Patients

Michiel Kroesen [1,2,*], Netteke van Holthe [1], Kemal Sumser [1], Dana Chitu [3], Rene Vernhout [1], Gerda Verduijn [1], Martine Franckena [1], Jose Hardillo [4], Gerard van Rhoon [1] and Margarethus Paulides [1,5]

[1] Department of Radiation Oncology, Erasmus MC Cancer Institute, 3015GD Rotterdam, The Netherlands; tenvijver@xs4all.nl (N.v.H.); k.sumser@erasmusmc.nl (K.S.); r.vernhout@erasmusmc.nl (R.V.); g.verduijn@erasmusmc.nl (G.V.); m.franckena@erasmusmc.nl (M.F.); g.c.vanrhoon@erasmusmc.nl (G.v.R.); m.m.paulides@tue.nl (M.P.)
[2] Holland Proton Therapy Center, 2629JH Delft, The Netherlands
[3] Department of Hematology, HOVON Data Center, Erasmus MC Cancer Institute, 3015GD Rotterdam, The Netherlands; d.chitu@erasmusmc.nl
[4] Department of Otorhinolaryngology—Head and Neck Surgery, Erasmus MC Cancer Institute, 3015GD Rotterdam, The Netherlands; j.hardillo@erasmusmc.nl
[5] Department of Electrical Engineering, Eindhoven University of Technology, 5612AZ Eindhoven, The Netherlands
* Correspondence: m.kroesen@erasmusmc.nl

Citation: Kroesen, M.; van Holthe, N.; Sumser, K.; Chitu, D.; Vernhout, R.; Verduijn, G.; Franckena, M.; Hardillo, J.; van Rhoon, G.; Paulides, M. Feasibility, SAR Distribution, and Clinical Outcome upon Reirradiation and Deep Hyperthermia Using the Hypercollar3D in Head and Neck Cancer Patients. *Cancers* **2021**, *13*, 6149. https://doi.org/10.3390/cancers13236149

Academic Editors: Lorenzo Preda and Primož Strojan

Received: 16 September 2021
Accepted: 5 December 2021
Published: 6 December 2021

Publisher's Note: MDPI stays neutral with regard to jurisdictional claims in published maps and institutional affiliations.

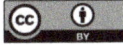

Copyright: © 2021 by the authors. Licensee MDPI, Basel, Switzerland. This article is an open access article distributed under the terms and conditions of the Creative Commons Attribution (CC BY) license (https://creativecommons.org/licenses/by/4.0/).

Simple Summary: Following radiotherapy for head and neck cancer, patients are at risk for developing a recurrent or second tumor. Often reirradiation is required in these patients, which is hampered in dose by the previous irradiation. Besides chemotherapy, hyperthermia can potentially increase the effectivity of the radiotherapy. In this study we have used a new hyperthermia applicator in order to increase the effectivity of the radiotherapy in patients requiring reirradiation. We show that the added hyperthermia treatment is tolerated by patients and that we reach a higher hyperthermia dose to the tumor compared to the previous applicator. In addition, we show that the tumor control and survival as well as toxicity are similar compared to what has been reported in literature using chemotherapy as an additive to reirradiation in head and neck cancer patients.

Abstract: (1) Background: Head and neck cancer (HNC) patients with recurrent or second primary (SP) tumors in previously irradiated areas represent a clinical challenge. Definitive or postoperative reirradiation with or without sensitizing therapy, like chemotherapy, should be considered. As an alternative to chemotherapy, hyperthermia has shown to be a potent sensitizer of radiotherapy in clinical studies in the primary treatment of HNC. At our institution, we developed the Hypercollar3D, as the successor to the Hypercollar, to enable improved application of hyperthermia for deeply located HNC. In this study, we report on the feasibility and clinical outcome of patients treated with the Hypercollar3D as an adjuvant to reirradiation in recurrent or SP HNC patients; (2) Methods: We retrospectively analyzed all patients with a recurrent or SP HNC treated with reirradiation combined with hyperthermia using the Hypercollar3D between 2014 and 2018. Data on patients, tumors, and treatments were collected. Follow-up data on disease specific outcomes as well as acute and late toxicity were collected. Data were analyzed using Kaplan Meier analyses; (3) Results: Twenty-two patients with recurrent or SP HNC were included. The average mean estimated applied cfSAR to the tumor volume for the last 17 patients was 80.5 W/kg. Therefore, the novel Hypercollar3D deposits 55% more energy at the target than our previous Hypercollar applicator. In patients treated with definitive thermoradiotherapy a complete response rate of 81.8% (9/11) was observed at 12 weeks following radiotherapy. Two-year local control (LC) and overall survival (OS) were 36.4% (95% CI 17.4–55.7%) and 54.6% (95% CI 32.1–72.4%), respectively. Patients with an interval longer than 24 months from their previous radiotherapy course had an LC of 66.7% (95% CI 37.5–84.6%), whereas patients with a time interval shorter than 24 months had an LC of 14.3% (95% CI 0.7–46.5%) at 18 months ($p = 0.01$). Cumulative grade 3 or higher toxicity was 39.2% (95% CI 16.0–61.9%);

(4) Conclusions: Reirradiation combined with deep hyperthermia in HNC patients using the novel Hypercollar3D is feasible and deposits an average cfSAR of 80.5 W/kg in the tumor volume. The treatment results in high complete response rates at 12 weeks post-treatment. Local control and local toxicity rates were comparable to those reported for recurrent or SP HNC. To further optimize the hyperthermia treatment in the future, temperature feedback is warranted to apply heat at the maximum tolerable dose without toxicity. These data support further research in hyperthermia as an adjuvant to radiotherapy, both in the recurrent as well as in the primary treatment of HNC patients.

Keywords: head and neck cancer; hyperthermia; reirradiation; treatment outcome

1. Introduction

Recurrent or second primary (SP) head and neck cancer (HNC) after radiotherapy occurs in 30–40% of patients [1–5]. Treatment of previously irradiated patients is a clinical challenge to date, especially when tumors are inoperable, as both the recurrent tumor as well as the renewed radiotherapy course carry substantial risks of morbidity and mortality [5]. Historically, reirradiation with or without sensitizing chemotherapy resulted in poor locoregional control rates [6,7]. In more recent literature, however, treatment with definitive reirradiation with or without chemotherapy showed a local control (LC) rate of 42.7% and an overall survival (OS) of 35.5% at 2 years [5]. Therefore, it seems that in the current era of radiotherapy techniques, reirradiation is becoming a more realistic treatment option for recurrent HNC patients, although careful selection seems warranted [8].

In reirradiation of HNC, chemotherapy is commonly used to sensitize radiotherapy. However, chemotherapy can result in increased side effects from the radiotherapy and carries potential systemic side effects, limiting its use in patients with comorbid disease [7]. Clinical hyperthermia represents an alternative to chemotherapy as a sensitizer of radiotherapy. In primary HNC, elevation of target temperatures to 40–44 °C results in around 20 percent increase in LC [9]. In recurrent HNC, however, the effect of adjuvant hyperthermia to radiotherapy has not been explored thoroughly [2,10,11].

In primary HNC patients, hyperthermia is mostly delivered using capacitive or intraluminal heating devices [12]. These devices can only adequately heat superficial tissues, and treatments in these studies were mostly applied without real-time monitoring. To be able to heat deep-seated tumors and to better steer the energy deposition, we previously developed a medical hyperthermia device incorporating 12 antennas, named the Hypercollar, that can focus microwaves to the target volume [13]. In addition, we developed and validated 3D simulation technology to optimize settings in pretreatment planning and for real-time simulation guided treatment and control [14,15]. We have previously reported on the safety and feasibility of treatment with the Hypercollar [10]. Learning from this experience, we further developed the Hypercollar for improved applicability, patient comfort, and energy steering [12]. This next-generation device, named the Hypercollar3D, has 20 antennas and an improved water bolus fitting for improved heating of the oropharyngeal and nasopharyngeal areas [16]. The better fit also creates a better match between simulation and treatment to improve the simulation-guided treatment.

Since the clinical introduction of the Hypercollar3D in 2014, we have treated 22 patients with recurrent or SP HNC receiving reirradiation with curative intent. The goal of this study was to evaluate the feasibility, acute and late toxicity as well as the clinical outcome in recurrent or SP HNC patients following thermoradiotherapy using the Hypercollar3D.

2. Materials and Methods

2.1. Patient Population

The research protocol for this retrospective study was reviewed by the medical ethics committee of Erasmus MC Cancer Institute, Rotterdam (MEC-2018-1453) and was classified as not falling within the definition and scope of the WMO (Medical Research Involving

Human Subjects Act). Patients included were treated at our institute between 2014 and 2018 for a recurrent or SP HNC with reirradiation combined with deep hyperthermia using the Hypercollar3D with curative intent. Exclusion criteria for deep hyperthermia were systemic temperatures of >39 °C, claustrophobia, tumor caudal to a tracheostomy (this prevents penetration of the microwaves to the tumor), anatomical boundaries of the shoulders prohibiting positioning of the applicator, and the presence of a pacemaker.

2.2. Radiotherapy Treatment

Radiotherapy technique, radiation field, dose, and fractionation were left at the discretion of the treating radiation oncologist and are listed in Table 1. In brief, radiation fields included at least the primary tumor site with or without elective neck irradiation. Radiotherapy techniques used were stereotactic radiotherapy using the Cyberknife (Accuracy Inc., Sunnyvale, CA, USA) in 7 patients and external beam radiotherapy (IMRT or VMAT) in 15 patients. Fractionation schemes are listed in Table 1.

Table 1. General characteristics of patient tumor and treatments.

Characteristic	Categories	Value
Patient/tumor characteristics		
Age (years)	Years (median)	67.0 (IQR 59.5–71.5)
Sex	Male	16 (73.0%)
	Female	6 (27.0%)
Prior surgery (primary tumor)	Yes	13 (59.0%)
	No	9 (41.0%)
Prior systemic therapy (primary tumor)	Yes	7 (32.0%)
	No	15 (68.0%)
Recurrent/SP HNC	Recurrent tumor	14 (64.0%)
	Second primary tumor	8 (36.0%)
Tumor site (recurrent or SP tumor)	Nasopharynx	2 (9.0%)
	Oropharynx	12 (55.0%)
	Oral cavity	2 (9.0%)
	Salivary gland	2 (9.0%)
	Hypopharynx	1 (5.0%)
	Larynx	3 (14.0%)
Histology (recurrent or SP tumor)	Squamous cell carcinoma	19 (86.0%)
	Other	3 (14.0%)
Tumor stage (recurrent or SP tumor)	T0	8 (36.0%)
	T1	1 (5.0%)
	T2	6 (27.0%)
	T3	2 (9.0%)
	T4	4 (18.0%)
	Unknown	1 (5.0%)

Table 1. *Cont.*

Characteristic	Categories	Value
Patient/tumor characteristics		
Nodal stage (recurrent or SP tumor)	N0	9 (41.0%)
	N1	3 (14.0%)
	N2	8 (36.0%)
	N3	1 (5.0%)
	Unknown	1 (5.0%)
Postoperative/ definitivereirradiation + hyperthermia	Postoperative	9 (41.0%)
	Definitive	13 (59.0%)
Fractionation radiotherapy	6 × 5.5 Gy	7 (31.8%)
	10 × 2.0 Gy	1 (4.5%)
	25 × 2.0 Gy	2 (9.0%)
	28 × 1.8 Gy	1 (4.5%)
	30 × 2.0 Gy	9 (40.9%)
	33 × 1.8 Gy	2 (9.0%)
Technique radiotherapy	IMRT	10 (44.5%)
	VMAT	5 (22.7%)
	Cyberknife	7 (31.8%)
Radiation field	Tumor	10 (45.5%)
	Neck	7 (31.8%)
	Both	5 (22,7%)
Time from previous radiotherapy treatment	Months (median)	51.5 (IQR 17.5–122.0)
Number of planned hyperthermia treatments	Number of treatments per patient	Number of patients
	3	7 (31.8%)
	4	1 (4.5%)
	5	2 (9.1%)
	6	11 (50%)
	7	1 (4.5%)
Total number of all treatments	108	22 (100%)
Complete clinical response 12 weeks post-treatment for definitive radiotherapy	Yes	9 (81.8%)
	No	2 (18.2%)

2.3. Hyperthermia Treatment

Hyperthermia (HT) was delivered following the radiotherapy fraction and was delivered weekly. The target volume for hyperthermia was the gross tumor volume (GTV) with a margin to account for planning and positioning inaccuracies. In the postsurgical situation, usually the clinical target volume (CTV) for radiation was the target volume for hyperthermia. If this was too large for adequate heating, a high-risk zone was identified, and the truly elective areas were not primarily heated. For each patient, a 3D patient model was generated by applying automatic segmentation of the planning computed tomography (CT) scan from the radiotherapy treatment [17]. Next, the patient model was imported into SEMCAD-X (Zurich MedTech, Zurich, Switzerland) to calculate the electromagnetic field per antenna. The resultant electric field distributions were imported into in-house developed software VEDO for optimizing the specific absorption rate (SAR) distribution by maximizing the target hotspot quotient (THQ) [15]. THQ is expressed using a total hotspot volume of 1% of the total volume (THQ_1%) [15].

Treatment was started using the preoptimized settings, and total power was gradually increased until the target temperature, a patient indicated hotspot, or a SAR constraint in the masseter region was reached. [10]. As in the earlier protocol, placement of invasive catheters inside the tumor was mandatory in case of a low predicted treatment quality, being 25% iso-SAR coverage (TC25) smaller than 75%, and optional for a TC25 above 75%. In the latter case, placement was often deemed too risky or too troublesome for patients; therefore, no temperatures could be measured. The protocol also included optional measurements of normal tissue temperatures in case distinct hotspots were to be expected based on the predicted SAR distribution.

In all cases, treatment was monitored in real-time using the applied cubic filtered SAR (cf-SAR) estimations [12]. Hereto, the real-time measured power and phase of the signals applied to the antennas were extrapolated into a real-time estimated applied SAR using the pre-calculated electric fields per antenna. Re-optimization of SAR distribution during the treatment was conducted if the patient had discomfort due to hotspots, which was discriminated from other sources of discomfort by briefly turning off total power. The duration of each hyperthermia treatment was 75 min, and heating up to 43 °C in the target or up to the patient's tolerance was applied, aimed at achieving 40–44 °C in the target region for 60 min.

2.4. Collection of Patient and Follow-Up Data

Patient, tumor, and treatment details were extracted from the patients' files. Specific radiotherapy and HT treatment characteristics were extracted from treatment planning and other recording systems. Local recurrence, distant recurrence, survival status, date and cause of death, as well as acute and late toxicity data were extracted and/or retrieved from patient records, referring hospitals, general practitioners, and the civil registry. Toxicity was scored according to CTCAE v4 at baseline, end of radiotherapy treatment, and 3–4 and 12 months post-treatment. Grade 1 toxicities were not included in the analyses because they were considered unreliable due to the retrospective data collection. After evaluation of the first five patients, we decided to introduce measurements of the range of motion (ROM) of the jaw before and after each treatment, as the CTCAE v4 scale is very robust for measuring trismus.

2.5. Hyperthermia Treatment Parameters

Hyperthermia treatment characteristics were collected. The number of hyperthermia treatments, hyperthermia treatment duration, mean applied power, mean estimated applied cf-SAR in tumor, and HTP planning parameters (THQ, TC25, TC50, and TC75) were extracted from the HT treatment files. The hyperthermia treatment session was marked as prematurely aborted if the total duration of the treatment was less than 70 min, since this indicates a problem reported by the patient. The effective treatment time per session was defined as the input power values higher than 1W during the treatment duration. The reported maximum estimated applied cf-SAR in tissues at risk were calculated retrospectively.

2.6. Statistical Analysis

LC and OS were calculated from the start date of radiotherapy until the event. LC was noted as 'failed' when a physician diagnosed a local recurrence either clinically or with imaging (CT/MRI). Patients were censored for LC after the last visit of any physician specifically examining for recurrent disease or death. For OS, patients were censored after the day the civil registry was consulted. LC and OS were analyzed using the Kaplan–Meier method and statistical differences between groups were determined using the log-rank test.

A *p*-value of ≤0.05 was considered statistically significant. All analyses were performed using Stata 15.1 (StataCorp. 2017. Stata Statistical Software: Release 15, StataCorp LLC, College Station, TX, USA).

3. Results

3.1. General Characteristics of Patients, Treatment, and Follow-Up

Patient and radiotherapy characteristics are listed in Table 1. Median follow-up for local recurrence was 17.5 months (IQR 6.0–31.0 months) and for overall survival 24.5 months (IQR 11.0–48.0 months). Thirteen out of twenty-two patients had a local recurrence, fourteen out of twenty-two had any recurrence, and fourteen out of twenty-two died during follow up.

3.2. Hyperthermia Treatment Feasibility

Comparing the clinical performance of the Hypercollar3D with our earlier Hypercollar applicator, we note that the comfort of the treatment as experienced by the patient is comparable, i.e., for the Hypercollar3D applicator in 90% of the treatments the treatment duration was at least 70 min of the intended 75 min, compared to 87% for the earlier Hypercollar design.

Table 2 shows that in total 134.9 W of mean power (range = 49.9–353.0 W) was applied to achieve a mean predicted cfSAR of 104.2 W/kg (range = 36.5–314.8) in the target regions that had a mean volume of 40.8 cc (range = 2.8–233.9 cc). Treatment planning predicted a mean TC25 of 88%, TC50 of 55%, TC75 of 12% and THQ was on average 1.28. In 5/22 patients, temperatures were measured during the first hyperthermia session in the target (4.6%). Measured minimum ("starting") temperatures ranged between 34.3–36.6 °C. This may be an indication that measurements were in general taken very superficially. Measured median temperature (T50) was 39.6 °C (37.2–41.9 °C) but a mean increase of 3.9 °C (1.3–6.2 °C) was achieved.

Because of the incidence of trismus (see toxicity below), after five patients the clinical protocol previously described by Verduijn et al. was adjusted by: (1) decreasing the power increments from 20 W to 10 W per 5 min of treatment time to allow for thermoregulative physiological adjustment, and (2) by applying an absolute SAR threshold of 175 W/kg in the masseter region. Following the adapted instructions, the mean applied power decreased from 278.8 W (first five patients) to 92.5 W (17 patients treated thereafter), and consequently, the mean estimated applied cfSAR in the tumor decreased from 185.0 W/kg to 80.5 W/kg.

In 6/22 patients one or more hyperthermia sessions were prematurely aborted. In four patients this was due to pain from the hyperthermia treatment, and in one of those patients it was due to an increase in pre-existing neuropathic pain. In addition, the last hyperthermia session was not applied in one patient due to tumor progression and for another patient it was due to claustrophobia and fear of technical problems. In 88% of the treatments, the treatment duration was at least 70 min of the intended 75 min. For all patients and treatments, the mean hyperthermia treatment time delivered, reaching 71.5 min or 95.3% of the intended time (75 min).

3.3. Oncological Outcome and Relation with Interval with Previous Radiotherapy

Thirteen patients were treated with definitive thermoradiotherapy, whereas, nine patients were treated with postoperative thermoradiotherapy (Table 1). In patients treated with definitive thermoradiotherapy a complete response rate of 81.8% (9/11; two not recorded) was observed (Table 1). Overall 2-year LC and OS were 36.4% (95% CI 17.4–55.7%) and 54.6% (95% CI 32.1–72.4%), respectively (Figure 1). Comparing postoperative versus definitive thermoradiotherapy, no significant difference was observed in 2-year LC; 33.3% (95% CI 7.8–62.3%) versus 38.5% (95% CI 14.1–62.8%), respectively ($p = 0.97$) (Figure 2).

Table 2. Hyperthermia treatment parameters.

Characteristic	Categories	Value
Hyperthermia treatment characteristics		
HT treatments	n	107
HTV volume	milliliters	40.8 mL (2.8–108.9)
Treatment planning		
TC25	%	90 (44–99)
TC50	%	58 (5–80)
TC75	%	12 (0–48)
THQ_1%	-	1.28 (0.38–3.83)
Mean applied power *	Watts	All 1–22: 134.9 (49.9–353.0)
		Pat 1–5: 278.8 (179.3–353.0)
		Pat 6–22: 92.5 (49.9–123.1)
Mean estimated cf-SAR tumor * (applied power * predicted cf-SAR * efficiency)	W/kg	All 1–22: 104.2 (36.5–314.8)
		Pat 1–5: 185.0 (69.4–314.8)
		Pat 6–22: 80.5 (36.5–145.1)
Target temperature	n (%)	5 (4.6)
Patient reference		A B C D E
Maximum	°C	38.3, 43.9, 40.9, 42.2, 38.0
Median	°C	37.8, 40.8, 40.5, 41.9, 37.2
Minimum	°C	36.5, 36.6, 35.8, 35.7, 34.3
Maximum normal tissue temperature	n (%)	56 (52.3)
Median	°C	40.1 (35.0–42.8)

* After the first five patients, a protocol adaptation lowering the energy in the masseter muscles was introduced.

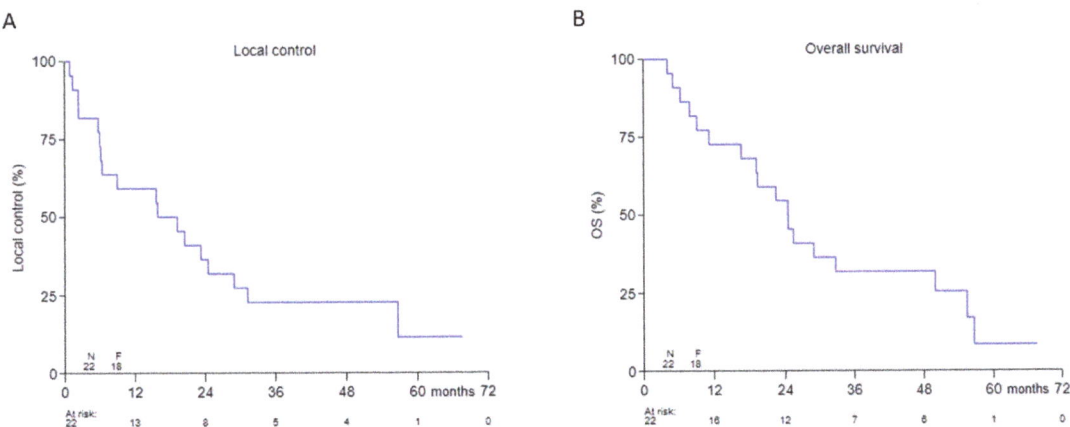

Figure 1. Kaplan-Meier analysis for LC (**A**) and OS (**B**) in 22 patients with a recurrent or second primary head and neck cancer.

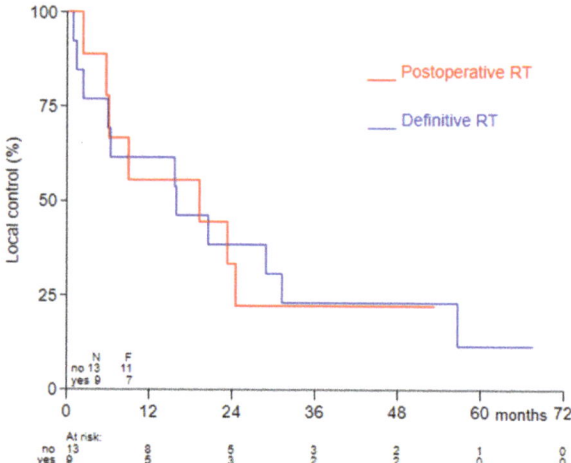

Figure 2. Kaplan-Meier curves for LC were compared for definitive versus postoperative treatment using the log-rank test.

The time interval between the first and the subsequent radiotherapy courses was previously reported to predict clinical outcome [5]. The median time from previous radiotherapy in our cohort was 51.5 months (IQR 17.5–122.0 months). Similar to observation by others, an interval of >24 months was significantly associated with higher LC; 18-month LC was 14.3% (95% CI 0.7–46.5%) for an interval of <24 months versus 66.7% (95% CI 37.5–84.6%) for an interval of >24 months ($p = 0.01$) (Figure 3).

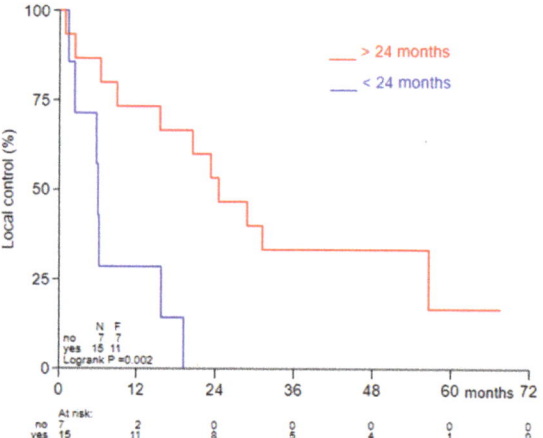

Figure 3. Kaplan-Meier curves for LC were compared for long (>24 months) and short (<24 months) time intervals between radiotherapy courses using the log-rank test.

3.4. Toxicity

The overall incidence of late grade 3 or higher toxicity at 2-years using Kaplan-Meier analysis was 39.2% (95% CI 16.0–61.9%), and the combined incidence of late grade 3 or higher toxicity or local recurrence at 2-years was 81.0% (95% CI 69.2–92.8%) (Figure 4). A detailed overview of type and grade of the toxicity at baseline, shortly after the radiotherapy course, 3–4 and 12 months is provided in Table 3. Of note, no grade IV or V toxicities were observed.

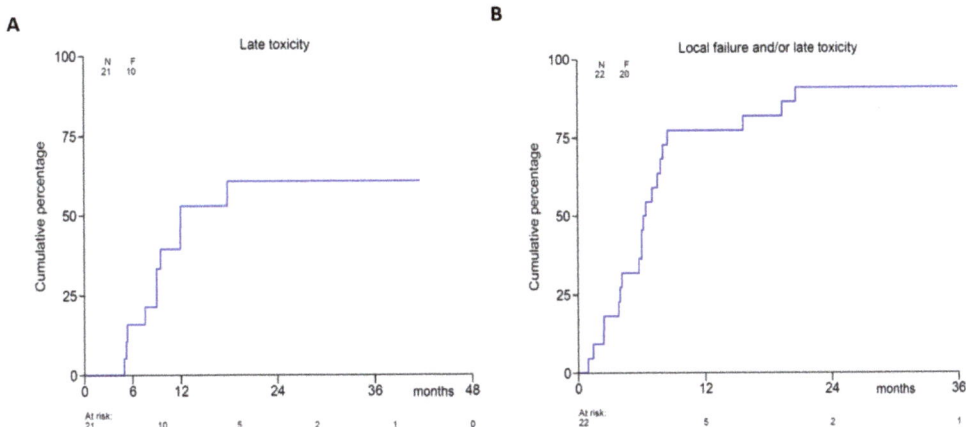

Figure 4. Kaplan-Meier analysis of late (>4 months) grade 3 or higher toxicity (**A**) and grade 3 or higher toxicity and/or local recurrence (**B**).

Table 3. Description of toxicity at baseline, end of radiotherapy treatment, 3–4 months and 12 months post-treatment.

Toxicity	Grade	Baseline $N = 22$ Number (%)	End RT $N = 18$ Number (%)	3–4 Months Post-Treatment $N = 18$ Number (%)	12 Months Sost-Treatment $N = 10$ Number (%)
Xerostomia	2	0	1 (6%)	1 (6%)	0
	3	0	1 (6%)	1 (6%)	1 (10%)
Altered taste	2	0	2 (11%)	1 (6%)	0
	3	0	0	0	0
Dysphagia	2	6 (27%)	6 (33%)	5 (28%)	5 (50%)
	3	3 (14%)	5 (28%)	3 (17%)	2 (20%)
Edema face	2	0	2 (11%)	0	1 (10%)
	3	0	0	0	0
Erythema skin	2	0	0	0	0
	3	0	0	0	0
Ulcus skin	2	0	1 (6%)	2 (11%)	2 (20%)
	3	0	0	0	1 (10%)
Trimus	2	2 (9%)	5 (28%)	4 (22%)	3 (30%)
	3			1 (6%)	1 (10%)
Osteoradionecrosis	Yes	0	0	3 (17%)	1 (10%)
	No	22 (100%)	18 (100%)	15 (83%)	9 (90%)
Burn wound	Yes	0	0	0	0
	No	22 (100%)	18 (100%)	18 (100%)	10 (100%)
Vertigo	Yes	0	0	0	0
	No	22 (100%)	18 (100%)	18 (100%)	10 (100%)
Tube feeding	Yes	2 (9%)	6 (33%)	3 (17%)	2 (20%)
	No	20 (91%)	12 (67%)	15 (83%)	8 (80%)

Table 3. Cont.

Toxicity	Grade	Baseline N = 22 Number (%)	End RT N = 18 Number (%)	3–4 Months Post-Treatment N = 18 Number (%)	12 Months Sost-Treatment N = 10 Number (%)
Opioid use	Yes	4 (18%)	9 (50%)	6 (33%)	1 (10%)
	No	18 (82%)	9 (50%)	12 (66%)	9 (90%)
Other grade 3 or higher toxicity	Yes	1 (5%)	1 (6%)	1 (6%)	1 (10%)
	No	21 (95%)	17 (94%)	17 (94%)	9 (90%)
Tracheostoma	Yes	4 (18%)	4 (22%)	1 (6%)	1 (10%)
	No	18 (82%)	13 (72%)	17 (94%)	9 (90%)

Notably, after evaluation of the first five patients treated with the HyperCollar3D, we saw that three patients had developed clinically relevant trismus; one patient developed grade I and two patients developed grade II trismus relatively early on in the course of treatment as an unexpected side effect. One of them also experienced grade III vertigo after the first treatment and a grade II vertigo after consecutive treatments. Two patients also developed a grade II edema of the neck. We adjusted the clinical protocol after our first evaluation (see feasibility) as explained earlier. After the introduction of the adapted treatment protocol, the occurrence of treatment-induced trismus at the end of the treatment decreased from 3/5 to 5/17. In the group of patients treated following the adapted protocol, the incidence of newly induced trismus at 3–4 months decreased further to 1/17 patients. For the other four patients with trismus at 3–4 months post treatment, two were in the first five patients having a high SAR value at the masseter and two already had trismus at start of the treatment and were not altered in grade by the treatment (Table 3).

4. Discussion

In this retrospective cohort study, we found that application of deep hyperthermia using the Hypercollar3D is feasible, and the oncological outcome is similar to other patient series of reirradiation with or without chemotherapy in HNC patients [5]. This study warrants further clinical studies using thermoradiotherapy in recurrent as well as in primary HNC patients.

In a meta-analysis in 2016 from Datta et al., five randomized trials and one nonrandomized trial, comparing radiotherapy versus radiotherapy plus hyperthermia in non-surgical patients, were analyzed [9]. This meta-analysis showed an overall improvement of the complete remission rate going from 39.6% (range 31.3–46.9%) with radiotherapy alone to 62.5% (range 33.9–83.3%) with radiotherapy plus hyperthermia [9]. Notably, the radiotherapy and hyperthermia treatments used in these studies were mostly performed using less advanced techniques compared to the current hyperthermia technique and/or applicator [18,19]. The CR rate of 81.8% for reirradiation plus hyperthermia observed in nine patients with definitive thermoradiotherapy is in the same range of the literature values, although patient selection and radiotherapy dosage may differ. This indicates the potency of hyperthermia to sensitize radiotherapy, also in the setting of reirradiation. This potency is well-studied in breast cancer, showing again higher complete response rates when hyperthermia is added to radiotherapy [20]. There are few studies reporting on the addition of hyperthermia to radiotherapy in recurrent or SP HNC [11,21]. Recently, we have published the clinical outcome using our previous head and neck applicator, the Hypercollar, in 27 HNC patients, including 18 recurrent or SP HNC patients [10]. In these latter patients, we observed a 2-year LC and OS of 36% and 33%, retrospectively. In our current cohort, we found similar 2-year LC and OS rates of 37% and 53%, respectively.

Comparing the outcome of our current cohort to recurrent HNC patients treated with chemoradiotherapy, several reported studies should be considered. In a randomized trial, albeit in the postoperative setting, full dose reirradiation with chemotherapy resulted in a

2-year LC of 60% [22]. In a recent cohort using IMRT, 2-year LC following reirradiation was reported as high as 64% [8]. More recently, a large, 'real-world practice' study by Ward et al. analyzed 412 recurrent or SP HNC patients [5]. Local regional control rate at 2 years was 42.7% for definitive reirradiation with or without chemotherapy [5]. We observed a local control rate of 37.5% at 2 years. In agreement with the data of Ward et al., we also observed a significantly worse local control when reirradiation was applied within 24 months from the previous radiotherapy course. Our data and the data from Ward et al. collectively support the careful selection of patients on the basis of the time interval with the previous radiotherapy course in order to prevent treatment related toxicity in patients having a dismal prognosis.

Cumulative Grade 3 or higher late toxicity was 33.5% in the study by Ward et al. and 39.2% in our cohort. Most of the important late toxicities were local, including xerostomia, dysphagia, osteoradionecrosis and trismus (Table 3). There were no grade IV or V toxicities and, although not measured, no systemic toxicities are to be expected from the hyperthermia treatment. Thus, the local toxicity following reirradiation is substantial but does not seem to be higher compared to reirradiation with or without chemotherapy [5]. In addition, hyperthermia is not expected to induce the potential systemic side effects of chemotherapy, like gastrointestinal, renal, neurological, and hematological side effects [23,24].

The average mean estimated applied cfSAR to the tumor volume for the Hypercollar3D was 80.5 W/kg for the last 17 patients treated with the adapted protocol, which is 55% higher than the 52 W/kg achieved with our earlier Hypercollar applicator. The gain in the improved cfSAR value achieved at the tumor volume can be explained by the fact that for the Hypercollar3D treatment, the VEDO software selects 12 antennas that make the largest contributions to the cfSAR at the tumor volume from the 20 available antennas. Further, the improved design of the water bolus, i.e., improved shape retention, results in a more efficient transfer of the EM energy.

With respect to hyperthermia related toxicity, the incidence of acute trismus grade II in three of the first five patients treated with the Hypercollar3D prompted us to an early evaluation of our treatment protocol. The adapted treatment protocol effectively reduced incidence of grade II trismus, but also resulted in a lower energy deposition in the target region from 185 W/kg to 81 W/kg. As invasive thermometry was not mandatory in our protocol, the effect of our protective measure for the normal tissues on the thermal dose to target could not be determined. We were also not able to unequivocally determine the safety of the applied reduction in energy deposition. Nevertheless, the fact that the late toxicity and oncological outcomes in our cohort were comparable with those reported in literature was reassuring. Further research is needed to confirm the safety and validity of the SAR thresholds used. For example, by introducing more extensive online temperature modeling whereby during treatment, temperatures are measured at several noninvasive reference locations. These measurements could be considered as a reference to calibrate predicted tissue temperatures for tumors and organs at risk. This could result in further treatment optimization and potentially prevent under treatment of the target area.

The feasibility to apply deep hyperthermia in HNC patients, as shown by our study, has potential implications for future clinical research. Besides recurrent or SP HNC patients, there are two important HNC patient groups that may especially benefit from thermoradiotherapy as opposed to chemoradiotherapy or radiotherapy alone [22]. The first group is HNC patients over 70 years old, in whom the additive effect of chemotherapy has not been demonstrated [23–26]. The second group is patients with a human papilloma virus (HPV) associated HNC, having a more favorable prognosis compared to HPV negative HNC patients [27,28]. Efforts are ongoing to de-escalate current treatment with radiotherapy by decreasing the dose. For example, in a phase 2 trial, HPV positive HNC patients were treated with induction chemotherapy. Complete or partial responders received only 54 Gy, resulting in a favorable progression free survival of 92% at 2 years [29]. The induction chemotherapy, however, induced grade III leucopenia and neutropenia in 39% and 11% of patients, retrospectively. Also in this report, the toxicity of deep hyperthermia of the head and neck is reported to be generally mild, and the radiotherapy toxicity was not enhanced in randomized trials [9,30]. One can hypothesize that adding hyperthermia to a reduced radiotherapy dose can result in a similar long term clinical outcome as the high dose radiotherapy but with less late toxicity from the radiotherapy.

Drawbacks of the current study are the retrospective nature with the potential for confounding data misinterpretation and missing data. In addition, the relatively small sample size, inhomogeneous patient group, and variability in radiotherapy and hyperthermia treatment and doses. Toxicity was not recorded in a standardized manner at our institute during follow-up. In our data collection process, however, toxicity was scored retrospectively by an independent data management team according to the CTCAE criteria and, when in doubt, the treating physician and an experienced head and neck surgeon were consulted (JAUH) to provide a final grading score. The optimal sequence and timing of the hyperthermia is still under debate. Similar to cervix carcinoma patients, we applied the hyperthermia after the radiotherapy fraction within four hours. In cervix carcinoma patients, this results in a clear thermal dose effect of the hyperthermia while the timing does not affect outcome, as long as the treatment is applied within four hours after radiotherapy [31,32]. Whether this is the optimal timing and whether these results can be extrapolated to HNC patients, is still a subject for future studies.

5. Conclusions

Deep hyperthermia using the Hypercollar3D in combination with reirradiation of recurrent and SP HNC is feasible in terms of patient tolerance and SAR deposition in the target area. The introduction of the Hypercollar3D resulted in an improved focused delivery with an increase in the SAR delivered to the tumor by 52 W/kg compared to the previous system. Good thermometry at target and normal tissues is needed to exploit this feature in future trials. The oncologic outcome as well as toxicity in our cohort were comparable to (chemo) radiotherapy in similar clinical settings. The data from our study are encouraging, although the relationship among SAR, tumor response, and toxicity requires further clinical validation. Our data warrant further prospective studies of deep hyperthermia using the Hypercollar3D. In the case of reirradiation, we are planning for a prospective registration study including, not only hyperthermia as an adjuvant, but also chemotherapy or reirradiation alone. In primary HNC we are aiming for a feasibility trial in patients who are not eligible for adjuvant chemotherapy. In this patient group we also aim to be able to have more invasive thermometry due to less pre-existent morbidity. When hyperthermia proves to be feasible in these patients and we have gained better understanding of the relation between SAR, temperature, and toxicity, a larger phase II clinical trial in primary HNC patients can be envisioned.

Author Contributions: Data curation, D.C. and R.V.; Formal analysis, K.S. and D.C.; Supervision, G.v.R. and M.P.; Writing—original draft, M.K.; Writing—review & editing, N.v.H., G.V., M.F. and J.H. All authors have read and agreed to the published version of the manuscript.

Funding: This research was supported in part by KWF Kankerbestrijding (Dutch Cancer Society), grant number 11368 and Sensius BV.

Institutional Review Board Statement: The study was conducted according to the guidelines of the Declaration of Helsinki, and approved by the Ethics Committee of Erasmus MC Cancer Institute, Rotterdam (MEC-2018-1453).

Informed Consent Statement: Patient consent was waived due to the retrospective nature of the study without the use of identifying information. Also, most patients had deceased and/or were lost to follow-up. We estimated that gaining informed consent of the remaining patients would be too much of a burden for these patients after such long time following their initial treatment.

Data Availability Statement: The data presented in this study are available on request from the corresponding author. The data will be kept for at least 15 years after this publication at a secure location at Erasmus University Hospital in Rotterdam.

Acknowledgments: The authors wish to acknowledge I.A.M.F. Derks and E.A.J. Berenschot-Huijbregts for their contribution in the database building and data collection.

Conflicts of Interest: G.v.R and M.P. have financial interest in Sensius BV, a manufacturer of thermotherapy solutions. All other authors declare no conflict of interest.

References

1. Ang, K.K.; Zhang, Q.; Rosenthal, D.I.; Nguyen-Tan, P.F.; Sherman, E.J.; Weber, R.S.; Galvin, J.M.; Bonner, J.A.; Harris, J.; El-Naggar, A.K. Randomized phase III trial of concurrent accelerated radiation plus cisplatin with or without cetuximab for stage III to IV head and neck carcinoma: RTOG 0522. *J. Clin. Oncol.* **2014**, *32*, 2940–2950. [CrossRef]
2. Adelstein, D.J.; Li, Y.; Adams, G.L.; Wagner, H., Jr.; Kish, J.A.; Ensley, J.F.; Schuller, D.E.; Forastiere, A.A. An intergroup phase III comparison of standard radiation therapy and two schedules of concurrent chemoradiotherapy in patients with unresectable squamous cell head and neck cancer. *J. Clin. Oncol.* **2003**, *21*, 92–98. [CrossRef]
3. Forastiere, A.A.; Zhang, Q.; Weber, R.S.; Maor, M.H.; Goepfert, H.; Pajak, T.F.; Morrison, W.; Glisson, B.; Trotti, A.; Ridge, J.A.; et al. Long-term results of RTOG 91-11: A comparison of three nonsurgical treatment strategies to preserve the larynx in patients with locally advanced larynx cancer. *J. Clin. Oncol.* **2013**, *31*, 845–852. [CrossRef]
4. Vargo, J.A.; Ward, M.C.; Caudell, J.J.; Riaz, N.; Dunlap, N.E.; Isrow, D.; Zakem, S.J.; Dault, J.; Awan, M.J.; Higgins, K.A.; et al. A Multi-institutional Comparison of SBRT and IMRT for Definitive Reirradiation of Recurrent or Second Primary Head and Neck Cancer. *Int. J. Radiat. Oncol. Biol. Phys.* **2018**, *100*, 595–605. [CrossRef] [PubMed]
5. Ward, M.C.; Riaz, N.; Caudell, J.J.; Dunlap, N.E.; Isrow, D.; Zakem, S.J.; Dault, J.; Awan, M.J.; Vargo, J.A.; Heron, D.E.; et al. Refining Patient Selection for Reirradiation of Head and Neck Squamous Carcinoma in the IMRT Era: A Multi-institution Cohort Study by the MIRI Collaborative. *Int. J. Radiat. Oncol. Biol. Phys.* **2018**, *100*, 586–594. [CrossRef]
6. De Crevoisier, R.; Bourhis, J.; Domenge, C.; Wibault, P.; Koscielny, S.; Lusinchi, A.; Mamelle, G.; Janot, F.; Julieron, M.; Leridant, A.M.; et al. Full-dose reirradiation for unresectable head and neck carcinoma: Experience at the Gustave-Roussy Institute in a series of 169 patients. *J. Clin. Oncol.* **1998**, *16*, 3556–3562. [CrossRef]
7. Spencer, S.A.; Harris, J.; Wheeler, R.H.; Machtay, M.; Schultz, C.; Spanos, W.; Rotman, M.; Meredith, R.; Ang, K.K. Final report of RTOG 9610, a multi-institutional trial of reirradiation and chemotherapy for unresectable recurrent squamous cell carcinoma of the head and neck. *Head Neck* **2008**, *30*, 281–288. [CrossRef]
8. Sulman, E.P.; Schwartz, D.L.; Le, T.T.; Ang, K.K.; Morrison, W.H.; Rosenthal, D.I.; Ahamad, A.; Kies, M.; Glisson, B.; Weber, R.; et al. IMRT reirradiation of head and neck cancer-disease control and morbidity outcomes. *Int. J. Radiat. Oncol. Biol. Phys.* **2009**, *73*, 399–409. [CrossRef]
9. Datta, N.R.; Rogers, S.; Ordonez, S.G.; Puric, E.; Bodis, S. Hyperthermia and radiotherapy in the management of head and neck cancers: A systematic review and meta-analysis. *Int. J. Hyperth.* **2016**, *32*, 31–40. [CrossRef]
10. Verduijn, G.M.; de Wee, E.M.; Rijnen, Z.; Togni, P.; Hardillo, J.A.U.; Ten Hove, I.; Franckena, M.; van Rhoon, G.C.; Paulides, M.M. Deep hyperthermia with the HYPERcollar system combined with irradiation for advanced head and neck carcinoma—A feasibility study. *Int. J. Hyperth.* **2018**, *34*, 994–1001. [CrossRef]
11. Zschaeck, S.; Weingartner, J.; Ghadjar, P.; Wust, P.; Mehrhof, F.; Kalinauskaite, G.; Ehrhardt, V.H.; Hartmann, V.; Tinhofer, I.; Heiland, M.; et al. Fever range whole body hyperthermia for re-irradiation of head and neck squamous cell carcinomas: Final results of a prospective study. *Oral Oncol.* **2021**, *116*, 105240. [CrossRef]
12. Paulides, M.M.; Verduijn, G.M.; Van Holthe, N. Status quo and directions in deep head and neck hyperthermia. *Radiat. Oncol.* **2016**, *11*, 21. [CrossRef]
13. Paulides, M.M.; Bakker, J.F.; Neufeld, E.; van der Zee, J.; Jansen, P.P.; Levendag, P.C.; van Rhoon, G.C. Winner of the "New Investigator Award" at the European Society of Hyperthermia Oncology Meeting 2007. The HYPERcollar: A novel applicator for hyperthermia in the head and neck. *Int. J. Hyperth.* **2007**, *23*, 567–576. [CrossRef]
14. Verhaart, R.F.; Verduijn, G.M.; Fortunati, V.; Rijnen, Z.; van Walsum, T.; Veenland, J.F.; Paulides, M.M. Accurate 3D temperature dosimetry during hyperthermia therapy by combining invasive measurements and patient-specific simulations. *Int. J. Hyperth.* **2015**, *31*, 686–692. [CrossRef] [PubMed]
15. Rijnen, Z.; Bakker, J.F.; Canters, R.A.; Togni, P.; Verduijn, G.M.; Levendag, P.C.; Van Rhoon, G.C.; Paulides, M.M. Clinical integration of software tool VEDO for adaptive and quantitative application of phased array hyperthermia in the head and neck. *Int. J. Hyperth.* **2013**, *29*, 181–193. [CrossRef]
16. Cappiello, G.; Drizdal, T.; Mc Ginley, B.; O'Halloran, M.; Glavin, M.; van Rhoon, G.C.; Jones, E.; Paulides, M.M. The potential of time-multiplexed steering in phased array microwave hyperthermia for head and neck cancer treatment. *Phys. Med. Biol.* **2018**, *63*, 135023. [CrossRef]
17. Verhaart, R.F.; Fortunati, V.; Verduijn, G.M.; van Walsum, T.; Veenland, J.F.; Paulides, M.M. CT-based patient modeling for head and neck hyperthermia treatment planning: Manual versus automatic normal-tissue-segmentation. *Radiother. Oncol.* **2014**, *111*, 158–163. [CrossRef]
18. Perez, C.A.; Pajak, T.; Emami, B.; Hornback, N.B.; Tupchong, L.; Rubin, P. Randomized phase III study comparing irradiation and hyperthermia with irradiation alone in superficial measurable tumors. Final report by the Radiation Therapy Oncology Group. *Am. J. Clin. Oncol.* **1991**, *14*, 133–141. [CrossRef]

19. Datta, N.R.; Bose, A.K.; Kapoor, H.K.; Gupta, S. Head and neck cancers: Results of thermoradiotherapy versus radiotherapy. *Int. J. Hyperth.* **1990**, *6*, 479–486. [CrossRef] [PubMed]
20. Linthorst, M.; Baaijens, M.; Wiggenraad, R.; Creutzberg, C.; Ghidey, W.; van Rhoon, G.C.; van der Zee, J. Local control rate after the combination of re-irradiation and hyperthermia for irresectable recurrent breast cancer: Results in 248 patients. *Radiother. Oncol. J. Eur. Soc. Ther. Radiol. Oncol.* **2015**, *117*, 217–222. [CrossRef]
21. Gabriele, P.; Ferrara, T.; Baiotto, B.; Garibaldi, E.; Marini, P.G.; Penduzzu, G.; Giovannini, V.; Bardati, F.; Guiot, C. Radio hyperthermia for re-treatment of superficial tumours. *Int. J. Hyperth.* **2009**, *25*, 189–198. [CrossRef]
22. Janot, F.; de Raucourt, D.; Benhamou, E.; Ferron, C.; Dolivet, G.; Bensadoun, R.J.; Hamoir, M.; Gery, B.; Julieron, M.; Castaing, M.; et al. Randomized trial of postoperative reirradiation combined with chemotherapy after salvage surgery compared with salvage surgery alone in head and neck carcinoma. *J. Clin. Oncol. Off. J. Am. Soc. Clin. Oncol.* **2008**, *26*, 5518–5523. [CrossRef]
23. Hurria, A.; Togawa, K.; Mohile, S.G.; Owusu, C.; Klepin, H.D.; Gross, C.P.; Lichtman, S.M.; Gajra, A.; Bhatia, S.; Katheria, V.; et al. Predicting chemotherapy toxicity in older adults with cancer: A prospective multicenter study. *J. Clin. Oncol.* **2011**, *29*, 3457–3465. [CrossRef] [PubMed]
24. Pignon, J.P.; le Maitre, A.; Maillard, E.; Bourhis, J.; Mach-Nc Collaborative Group. Meta-analysis of chemotherapy in head and neck cancer (MACH-NC): An update on 93 randomised trials and 17,346 patients. *Radiother. Oncol.* **2009**, *92*, 4–14. [CrossRef]
25. Szturz, P.; Vermorken, J.B. Treatment of Elderly Patients with Squamous Cell Carcinoma of the Head and Neck. *Front. Oncol.* **2016**, *6*, 199. [CrossRef]
26. Machtay, M.; Moughan, J.; Trotti, A.; Garden, A.S.; Weber, R.S.; Cooper, J.S.; Forastiere, A.; Ang, K.K. Factors associated with severe late toxicity after concurrent chemoradiation for locally advanced head and neck cancer: An RTOG analysis. *J. Clin. Oncol.* **2008**, *26*, 3582–3589. [CrossRef]
27. Lassen, P.; Eriksen, J.G.; Hamilton-Dutoit, S.; Tramm, T.; Alsner, J.; Overgaard, J. Effect of HPV-associated p16INK4A expression on response to radiotherapy and survival in squamous cell carcinoma of the head and neck. *J. Clin. Oncol.* **2009**, *27*, 1992–1998. [CrossRef]
28. Kobayashi, K.; Hisamatsu, K.; Suzui, N.; Hara, A.; Tomita, H.; Miyazaki, T. A Review of HPV-Related Head and Neck Cancer. *J. Clin. Med.* **2018**, *7*, 241. [CrossRef]
29. Chen, A.M.; Felix, C.; Wang, P.C.; Hsu, S.; Basehart, V.; Garst, J.; Beron, P.; Wong, D.; Rosove, M.H.; Rao, S.; et al. Reduced-dose radiotherapy for human papillomavirus-associated squamous-cell carcinoma of the oropharynx: A single-arm, phase 2 study. *Lancet Oncol.* **2017**, *18*, 803–811. [CrossRef]
30. Huilgol, N.G.; Gupta, S.; Sridhar, C.R. Hyperthermia with radiation in the treatment of locally advanced head and neck cancer: A report of randomized trial. *J. Cancer Res. Ther* **2010**, *6*, 492–496. [CrossRef]
31. Kroesen, M.; Mulder, H.T.; van Holthe, J.M.L.; Aangeenbrug, A.A.; Mens, J.W.M.; van Doorn, H.C.; Paulides, M.M.; Oomen-de Hoop, E.; Vernhout, R.M.; Lutgens, L.C.; et al. The Effect of the Time Interval Between Radiation and Hyperthermia on Clinical Outcome in 400 Locally Advanced Cervical Carcinoma Patients. *Front. Oncol.* **2019**, *9*, 134. [CrossRef] [PubMed]
32. Kroesen, M.; Mulder, H.T.; van Holthe, J.M.L.; Aangeenbrug, A.A.; Mens, J.W.M.; van Doorn, H.C.; Paulides, M.M.; Oomen-de Hoop, E.; Vernhout, R.M.; Lutgens, L.C.; et al. Confirmation of thermal dose as a predictor of local control in cervical carcinoma patients treated with state-of-the-art radiation therapy and hyperthermia. *Radiother. Oncol.* **2019**, *140*, 150–158. [CrossRef]

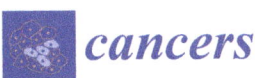

Article

Feasibility of Temperature Control by Electrical Impedance Tomography in Hyperthermia

Redi Poni [1,2], Esra Neufeld [1,2,*], Myles Capstick [2], Stephan Bodis [2,3], Theodoros Samaras [4] and Niels Kuster [1,2]

1. Department of Information Technology and Electrical Engineering, Swiss Federal Institute of Technology (ETH), 8092 Zurich, Switzerland; rponi@ethz.ch (R.P.); kuster@itis.swiss (N.K.)
2. Foundation for Research on Information Technologies in Society (IT'IS), 8004 Zurich, Switzerland; capstick@itis.swiss (M.C.); stephan.bodis@ksa.ch (S.B.)
3. Center of Radiation Oncology KSA-KSB, Kantonsspital Aarau, 5001 Aarau, Switzerland
4. Department of Physics, Aristotle University of Thessaloniki, 54124 Thessaloniki, Greece; theosama@auth.gr
* Correspondence: neufeld@itis.swiss

Simple Summary: Online treatment monitoring is an important tool to ensure the safety and effectiveness of hyperthermia cancer therapy. However, current solutions provide only sparse/inaccurate data, demand extensive access to complex and expensive infrastructure, or are associated with increased toxicity. In this study, we present a simulation-based evaluation of the feasibility of electrical impedance tomography (EIT) for hyperthermia treatment monitoring. EIT is a low cost, information-rich, non-invasive technique that could potentially be adapted and employed to reconstruct conductivity changes and translate them to temperature- and perfusion-change maps. Using an innovative reconstruction methodology that leverages (ideally personalized) treatment simulations, physics-motivated constraints, multiple frequencies, measurement-derived compensation, and novel numerical approaches, we investigated the impact of factors such as noise and reference model accuracy on the temperature- and perfusion-reconstruction accuracy. Results suggest that EIT can provide valuable real-time monitoring capabilities. As a next step, experimental confirmation under real-world conditions is needed to validate our results.

Abstract: We present a simulation study investigating the feasibility of electrical impedance tomography (EIT) as a low cost, noninvasive technique for hyperthermia (HT) treatment monitoring and adaptation. Temperature rise in tissues leads to perfusion and tissue conductivity changes that can be reconstructed in 3D by EIT to noninvasively map temperature and perfusion. In this study, we developed reconstruction methods and investigated the achievable accuracy of EIT by simulating HT treatmentlike scenarios, using detailed anatomical models with heterogeneous conductivity distributions. The impact of the size and location of the heated region, the voltage measurement signal-to-noise ratio, and the reference model personalization and accuracy were studied. Results showed that by introducing an iterative reconstruction approach, combined with adaptive prior regions and tissue-dependent penalties, planning-based reference models, measurement-based reweighting, and physics-based constraints, it is possible to map conductivity-changes throughout the heated domain, with an accuracy of around 5% and cm-scale spatial resolution. An initial exploration of the use of multifrequency EIT to separate temperature and perfusion effects yielded promising results, indicating that temperature reconstruction accuracy can be in the order of 1 °C. Our results suggest that EIT can provide valuable real-time HT monitoring capabilities. Experimental confirmation in real-world conditions is the next step.

Keywords: perfusion estimation; temperature monitoring; conductivity reconstruction

Citation: Poni, R.; Neufeld, E.; Capstick, M.; Bodis, S.; Samaras, T.; Kuster, N. Feasibility of Temperature Control by Electrical Impedance Tomography in Hyperthermia. *Cancers* **2021**, *13*, 3297. https://doi.org/10.3390/cancers13133297

Academic Editor: Thoralf Niendorf

Received: 11 May 2021
Accepted: 25 June 2021
Published: 30 June 2021

Publisher's Note: MDPI stays neutral with regard to jurisdictional claims in published maps and institutional affiliations.

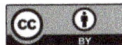

Copyright: © 2021 by the authors. Licensee MDPI, Basel, Switzerland. This article is an open access article distributed under the terms and conditions of the Creative Commons Attribution (CC BY) license (https://creativecommons.org/licenses/by/4.0/).

1. Introduction

Noninvasive imaging techniques such as electrical impedance tomography (EIT) are valuable tools for medical applications. EIT is used to image the electrical conductivity of tissues in the human body. EIT usage was first suggested in the 1970s [1]. Despite its relatively low cost, safety, and high temporal resolution, EIT has not been as widely adopted as other medical imaging methods, such as magnetic resonance imaging (MRI) and computed tomography (CT) [2,3].

The applications of functional EIT include pulmonary investigations [4], cardiac and gastrointestinal tract monitoring, breast cancer screening, and functional brain imaging [5]. Multiple devices have been introduced for clinical research [6], mainly in applications with functional imaging, such as bedside lung monitoring. Other applications, such as temperature estimation where accurate quantitative conductivity (or change in conductivity) reconstruction is needed, are more challenging compared with those in which only the volume with high dielectric change must be reconstructed.

One of the main challenges in EIT is that image reconstruction from measured voltages is an ill-posed problem [7]. Changes in the whole domain correspond to an infinite number of degrees of freedom (DOF) that must be reconstructed from a limited number of electrode measurements. Nevertheless, knowledge about distribution smoothness adds constraints, and regularization methods can be employed to facilitate reconstruction. Another issue with EIT is that impedances are affected by the entire volume rather than a single slice. Therefore, 2D reconstructions are merely an approximation of the real 3D problem [8]. While linearization methods combined with prior knowledge about the conductivity distribution and difference imaging have been used to further improve image reconstruction, the problem is nonlinear. Nonlinear reconstruction methods are more sensitive to inaccuracies in electrode models and positions. The literature on reconstruction algorithms for EIT [9] suggests that linear reconstruction methods should be combined with nonlinear iterative approaches to improve overall accuracy. From an instrumentation perspective, measurement noise, electrode positioning accuracy, signal generation, and sensing techniques impact overall EIT quality [10]. Further advances in EIT require improvements in both instrumentation and image reconstruction. Improvements are especially needed for applications that require the quantitative imaging of conductivity.

A potential application of EIT is in hyperthermic oncology. Hyperthermia (HT) therapy aims to selectively heat tumor tissue to temperatures ranging from 40 °C to 45 °C for a duration of about one hour. It is typically used as an adjuvant to radio- and/or chemotherapy in cancer treatment. In the case of deep-seated tumors, selective heating is usually achieved through coherent interference of electromagnetic (EM) energy from multiple radiating elements [11]. A significant challenge is noninvasive temperature monitoring in deep-seated tissue. The achieved temperature is difficult to predict, but it is important for tracking the achieved thermal dose in the tumor and avoiding potential treatment-limiting hotspots in healthy tissue. Treatment planning [12,13], which involves patient-specific EM simulation, optimization of energy deposition, and thermal prediction of the treatment, has been introduced as a tool for improving the prediction of thermal distribution. However, high uncertainty about the actual temperatures (e.g., due to perfusion changes during treatment) remains [14–16]. Research progress has been made in noninvasive monitoring using magnetic resonance thermometry (MRT) [17], but the accuracy of measurement is susceptible to patient movements, magnetic field drift over time, and limited sensitivity in fatty tissues, among others. In addition, the cost associated with MRT and the integration complexity with HT are high [18]. Alternatively, EIT can offer a low-cost, low-complexity solution for estimating temperature increases and perfusion changes during HT treatment.

Temperature elevation impacts tissue conductivity in two different ways. First, temperature changes the conductivity of intra- and extracellular fluids, which can be modeled by a linear relationship and described by a temperature coefficient (T_c)—the ratio of relative conductivity increases per degree centigrade. Second, in tissues in which thermoregulation-induced perfusion changes (e.g., vasodilatory response) are high, fluid flow in the extracellular environment increases, resulting in additional tissue conductivity change. At lower frequencies, current flows mainly in the extracellular region, whereas at higher frequencies, current flow is more uniform across all tissue compartments. Multifrequency EIT is considered as a method to distinguish changes in conductivity directly related to temperature (i.e., T_c-related part) from changes in conductivity due to perfusion increase [19]. Earlier studies have achieved temperature estimation accuracies ranging from 1.5 °C to 5 °C [20]. The results of these and other studies [21–25] suggest that to enable clinical EIT for HT and ablation treatment monitoring, improvements in conductivity reconstruction and temperature estimation are essential and consequently require accurate models of temperature-induced conductivity changes and the ability to distinguish temperature-related changes from tissue changes or damage-related changes, both permanent and temporary.

Recently, there has been increased interest and progress in applying EIT as a monitoring tool for thermal ablation, both in experimental and simulation studies [26–29], which motivates revisiting EIT for HT monitoring. New tools for EIT simulations have been introduced [30,31], and the computational power has increased considerably. Additionally, developments in tissue segmentation [32], combined with knowledge about tissue properties [33], enable the simulation of patient-specific treatment scenarios. Similarly, more realistic anatomical models can be used to perform sensitivity analyzes to improve the design of instruments. Most experimental studies in EIT are performed in tanks with simple geometrical shapes and few objects with different conductivities; hence, results cannot directly be translated to real human application. Since human anatomy is highly heterogeneous and geometrically complex, accurate representation in a model requires high resolution and many discretization elements. Notably, higher resolution negatively impacts reconstruction accuracy since total error minimization involves residuum minimization for more degrees of freedom, while the number of voltage electrode measurements remains the same [34].

Accurate temperature and/or perfusion estimation requires accurate knowledge about the relationship between temperature and conductivity, in addition to accurate conductivity imaging. In this paper, we focus on the achievable EIT reconstruction accuracy by using existing tools, such as electrical impedance tomography and diffuse optical tomography reconstruction (EIDORS) [31]), in conjunction with high-resolution anatomical models [35]. We aim to exploit HT treatment planning-based prior information and investigate the reconstruction of conductivity changes in the range expected for the given application. We also identify potential practical issues specific to hyperthermic oncology and their impact on the accuracy of conductivity change reconstruction to further improve temperature estimation.

2. Materials and Methods

To investigate the potential application of EIT in HT treatment planning and treatment monitoring, we performed simulations using the Virtual Population (ViP) Duke (age: 34, height: 1.77 m, BMI: 22.4 kg/m^2) and Glenn (age: 84, height: 1.73 m, BMI: 20.4 kg/m^2) anatomical models [35]. Two anatomical models were used to assess the impact of intersubject variability, as well as the importance of using personalized reference models. The models were discretized using a tetrahedral mesh in EIDORS v3.9. We first describe single iteration reconstruction using EIDORS. In Section 2.2, we present novel reconstruction approaches capable of overcoming the limitations of existing methods in our application of interest, their implementation, and the investigation scenarios. While considering the high heterogeneity of the human body, we then determined if the reconstruction accuracy improved when using a tissue-dependent penalty (TiD) parameter. A sensitivity analysis regarding the location and size of the simulated region was also performed.

In difference imaging, a reference model with an initial conductivity assignment is required. The measured changes in the electrode voltages are used to reconstruct the changes in conductivity from the reference model. As reference patient models may display anatomical segmentation inaccuracies, we investigated their impact on the reconstruction accuracy by considering a scenario where a volume outside the prior region, i.e., the volume, where an increased sensitivity is achieved by applying a penalty value [36], exhibited a large deviation ($\Delta\sigma$) from the reference model conductivity (σ_{ref}).

Noise in the measurement acquisition chain is also present in practical implementations. We assessed the impact of different electrode voltage noise levels (signal-to-noise ratio, SNR) on reconstruction accuracy using different reconstruction parameter values.

Finally, a realistic bladder tumor HT treatment scenario was considered as an EIT application case, using the two anatomical models (different body shapes and heating patterns). The clinical value of treatment planning-based EIT and the importance of personalizing the reference model were also assessed.

2.1. Single Iteration Reconstruction

EIDORS includes multiple algorithms for two- and three-dimensional (2D/3D) image reconstruction. In this study, we used difference imaging reconstruction on a 3D body. Single iteration reconstruction assumes small variations in conductivity, for which the relationship between voltage and conductivity can be approximated linearly as follows:

$$y = Jx + n, \quad (1)$$

where $J_{ij} = \frac{\partial y_i}{\partial x_j}$ is the Jacobian, $x = \sigma - \sigma_{ref}$ is the difference of the actual conductivity distribution and the reference value, $y = v - v_{ref}$ is a vector with electrode voltage differences of the actual measurement to the reference measurement, and n is the measurement noise. Regularization techniques are used to solve this problem [36–38]. We used the one-step linear Gauss–Newton method to estimate $\hat{x}$ by minimizing the sum of quadratic norms for:

$$||y - J\hat{x}||^2 + \lambda^2 ||x||^2. \quad (2)$$

The solution of the above formulation is:

$$\hat{x} = \left(J^T W J + \lambda^2 R \right)^{-1} J^T W y = By. \quad (3)$$

To reduce computational time by decreasing the size of the matrix to be inverted, B can be rewritten as follows:

$$B = P J^T \left(J P J^T + \lambda^2 V \right)^{-1}, \quad (4)$$

where $P = R^{-1}$ and $[R]_{ii} = [J^T J]_{ii}^{0.5}$. Effectively, R is a diagonal regularization matrix scaled with the sensitivity of each element and λ is a regularization parameter. $V = W^{-1} = I$ represents difference imaging EIT with identical channels. Two important and frequently used parameters in the reconstruction are the hyperparameter (λ) and the penalty parameter. When known changes are likely to occur in a smaller subdomain, a penalty parameter is used to implement an increased sensitivity in this region: $[R]_{ii} = [J^T J]_{ii}^{0.5} [Penalty]_{ii}$, for i in the subdomain. More details about derivations can be found in existing publications [36,37,39].

2.2. Pipeline and Simulation Setup

The ViP Duke model comprised of tissue properties from the IT'IS tissue database [33] was imported into EIDORS. Only a 20 cm portion of the torso (620 k elements) was used for further analysis.

Using difference imaging, we exploited prior information about the geometry and the conductivity distribution. Hence, we focused on reconstructing the conductivity change ($\Delta\sigma_{rec}$):

$$\Delta\sigma_{rec} = INV\left(v_{ref}, v, \sigma_{ref} \right), \quad (5)$$

where reference conductivity (baseline for EIT difference reconstruction) is σ_{ref}. INV is the function to solve the inverse problem using v and v_{ref} from the electrode voltages calculated from solving the forward problem or from current injection measurements for σ, respectively σ_{ref}. The actual conductivity change ($\Delta\sigma = \sigma - \sigma_{ref}$) is referred to as "modified conductivity", since a range of conductivity change configurations will be created by modifying the reference conductivity to investigate difference image reconstruction scenarios.

HT treatment planning workflows already include a tissue segmentation step. The segmented anatomical model can be assigned tissue properties, while considering the EIT frequency, to establish the reference model.

Difference imaging reconstruction is less sensitive to the modeling of the electrodes and contact impedance, as we assume the same conditions are present in both reference and additional measurements of the model to be reconstructed [9,40]. Therefore, we did not investigate the impact of the electrode parameters in this study; however, changes in the contact quality in experimental measurements will affect the reconstruction accuracy.

The reconstruction pipeline used in this study is shown in Figure 1. The reference model includes the tissue conductivity assignments. In nonablative HT treatment, the target region can reach temperatures of up to 45 °C. In addition to the direct temperature-related conductivity change contribution modeled with temperature coefficients (~2%/°C), σ can also change due to perfusion changes, thus altering the tissue extracellular fluid distribution. From the reference model, modified models were created by changing the tissue conductivity by up to 40%, a level similar to the experimental measurement study by Gersing [25]. The reference conductivity was multiplied by a 3D Gaussian shape mimicking heating during an HT treatment, as shown in Figure 2. At the end of the simulation pipeline, we compared the reconstructed model conductivity with the modified model conductivity.

For current injection and measurement, we positioned electrodes in single nodes, distributed as two rows of eight electrodes to form an interleaved arrangement. Current injection was applied transversely through single pairs (1–8, 2–9, etc.) and the voltage difference was calculated in all adjacent pairs (v_{34}, v_{45}, etc.) except for the electrodes used for current injection. Injecting currents through transversal, nonadjacent electrodes increases the current density, and hence, the sensitivity of EIT to changes in deeper tissues. Theoretically, a larger number of electrodes should improve the reconstruction accuracy. However, for the same injected current, which is limited by safety considerations, the voltage difference of more densely placed electrodes will be lower and, in practice, we will obtain more voltage measurements with lower SNR. An additional drawback of using numerous electrodes is the increased computational reconstruction effort. The torso model and electrode placements used in this study are shown in Figure 2.

In HT applications, the prior region can be determined either from the volume with highest HT power deposition or from a preliminary thermal simulation, which does not have to exactly reproduce the real patient tissue parameters. Although prior regions improve reconstruction by focusing on changes in a smaller volume, changes outside the prior region may be attributed to changes inside the region.

Simulations were interpolated to a structured rectilinear grid. A spatial averaging filter (cubic volume of 1.2 cm edge length) was applied to $\Delta\sigma$ (%), mimicking the expected smoothness of the heat distribution in tissue. Finally, the reconstruction accuracy across different tissues was analyzed.

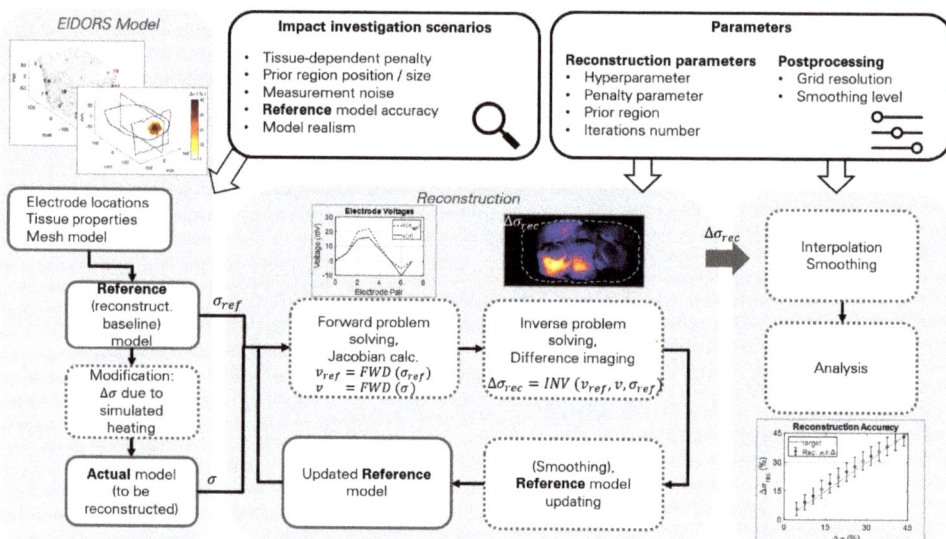

Figure 1. Illustration of the implemented reconstruction pipeline and the scenarios investigated in this study. Boxes with continuous outlines represent data, while the dotted ones represent processes. First, the actual and the reference model are generated, based on a discretized dielectric model of the patient and electrodes. Reconstruction proceeds through multiple iterations of forward (FWD) and inverse (INV) problem solving. The reconstruction results have been analyzed to study the impact of reconstruction approaches, noise, as well as reference model realism and accuracy.

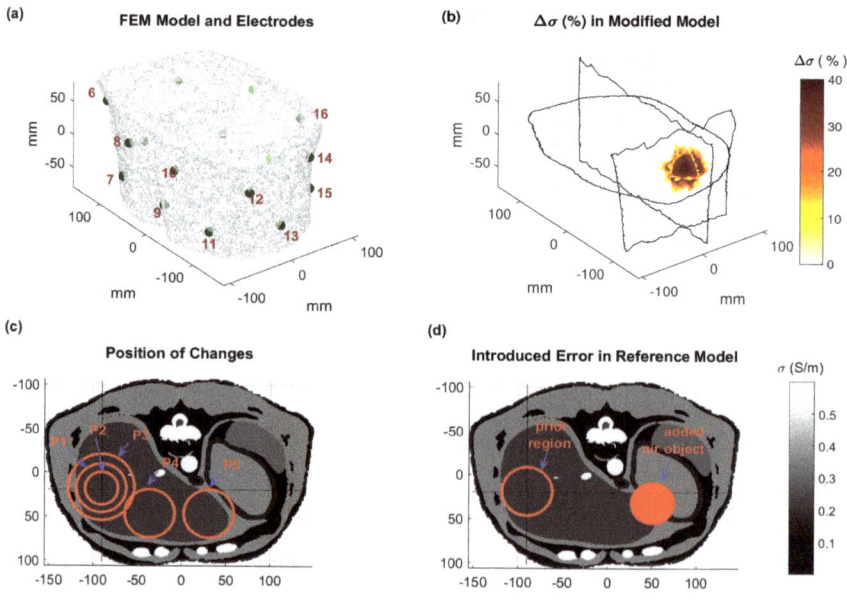

Figure 2. (**a**) FEM model of the Duke anatomical model torso with electrode locations indicated in green; (**b**) slices of the modified model $\Delta\sigma(\%)$ for a heated region in the liver; (**c**) locations and sizes of the different heated region scenarios; (**d**) setup featuring changes outside the prior region.

2.3. Investigation Scenarios

2.3.1. Tissue-Dependent Penalty

As the human body is highly heterogeneous, a wide range of low frequency σ values can be found, from close to $0\,\text{S/m}$ (internal air) to over $0.36\,\text{S/m}$ (muscle) and $3\,\text{S/m}$ (urine). The prior region can encompass a multitude of tissues covering a broad σ range, which makes adequate change detection throughout the entire range without overestimation or underestimation challenging. Information from the reference model σ_{ref} allows for the use of tissue-dependent penalty values, as constant penalty changes in low σ tissues are overestimated and changes in tissues with high σ, such as muscle, are underestimated, since the reconstruction algorithm minimizes the overall electrode voltage differences. In this study, we compared the reconstruction accuracy in different tissues when using a constant penalty value versus a tissue-dependent penalty in a single iteration reconstruction without applying any averaging or smoothing filter.

2.3.2. Region Location and Size

It is necessary to compare the reconstruction accuracy for different heating locations and sizes. The size of the region where the conductivity was changed should correspond to the typical extent of focused heating in HT treatment. For the first investigated location, spherical heating regions of different diameters were considered. A simulated heating was applied to a spherical region, as illustrated in Figure 2, by multiplying the conductivity inside the sphere with $1 + 0.4 \cdot e^{-\frac{r^2}{2R^2}}$ (r: radial distance, $R = 3$ cm, peak σ-increase of 40%). Depending on the location, the region can contain more than one tissue type. The modified regions are shown in Table 1 and illustrated in Figure 2. In these scenarios, we assumed that the prior region is perfectly known, and corresponds to the heated region.

Table 1. Size and position of simulated heated region and the added air object for the case of changes outside the focus region. See Figure 2 for the location of the origin (0, 0, 0).

Simulation	P1	P2	P3	P4	P5	Air Object
Center (x, y, z) [mm]	(−90, 20, 15)	(−90, 20, 15)	(−90, 20, 15)	(−40, 50, 15)	(30, 50, 15)	(50, 30, 15)
Diameter [mm]	60	40	80	60	60	50

2.3.3. Impact of Inaccurate Reference Model

The reconstruction is sensitive to the accuracy of the reference model. Even if the reference model is accurate at the beginning of the treatment, organ shifts and air movement in the bowels can occur during the treatment, since the HT treatment duration is relatively long. We simulated such a scenario, where in addition to the changes due to the simulated heating, the modified model included a spherical region with a 50 mm diameter and $\sigma = 0\,\text{S/m}$ (same as air), as illustrated in Figure 2. The setup corresponds to P1 (Table 1), such that results can be compared with the ideal case of an accurate reference model (see Sections 2.4 and 3.3.1 regarding the impact of not using a personalized reference anatomy).

In addition to the iterative approach with a fixed prior region, we also introduced an adaptive prior region approach. An initial mask was obtained by reconstructing the conductivity change without prior region and thresholding locations, where a high change was obtained. Subsequently, the mask was used as a prior region and a relatively relaxed penalty value of 0.1 was assigned before obtaining an adapted or more focal mask. On the basis of the obtained reconstruction, three additional reconstruction iterations with a stricter penalty value were performed in the usual manner. This adaptive approach increased the reconstruction sensitivity to changes outside of the classic prior region. Both the change in the simulated heated region and the unexpected change outside the prior region were simultaneously reconstructed. To achieve this, five (1 + 1 + 3) iterations instead of three were required.

2.3.4. Voltage Measurement Noise

The reconstruction problem is ill-conditioned. Minor voltage differences in the electrode measurements can lead to large changes in estimated conductivity. As a result, electrode voltage measurement noise is expected to significantly corrupt the reconstruction quality. Here, we investigated its impact on the conductivity reconstruction in the Duke anatomical model with a large number of mesh elements. Specifically, we assessed the impact of the noise level by adding noise with different SNR levels in setup P1. A noisy voltage vector (v_n) was generated by adding noise to the electrode voltages (v) from the forward problem solution of the modified model (σ).

$$v_n = v + n, \qquad (6)$$

where n is zero mean white Gaussian noise with standard deviation σ_n. The SNR is calculated as follows:

$$SNR = 20 \log\left(\frac{\Delta v_{rms}}{\sigma_n}\right), \qquad (7)$$

where $\Delta v = v - v_{ref}$.

2.4. Simulated HT Treatment Reconstruction

In this part of the study, we used a setup that mimicked the targeting of a bladder tumor using locoregional HT, where heat was delivered to a larger region encompassing the tumor (see Figure 3). This scenario provides increased realism and avoids the simplifying symmetries of the previous sections.

The procedure for the simulation was as follows:

1. We performed two thermal simulations of a one-hour treatment (T_{Opt} and T_{Pess}) using the same specific absorption rate (SAR) distribution. The Pennes bioheat equation (PBE) [41] with temperature-dependent perfusion models was used for the thermal simulations (see Equation (8)). The applied power level was the same in both cases, but the temperature-dependent perfusion models for muscle, fat, and tumor tissues were different (see Figure 4), to illustrate the impact of perfusion uncertainty;
2. We translated the temperature increase to a modified conductivity map, which included a component directly related to temperature ($\Delta\sigma_{temp}$) and a perfusion-related indirect component ($\Delta\sigma_{perf}$);
3. We reconstructed and analyzed the changes in conductivity based on the "ground truth" temperature simulation (T_{Pess}), using the conductivity at 37 °C as the reference model (Scenario 1) or the conductivity for the "planned" T_{Opt} (Scenario 2). The reconstructed conductivity was then converted into a reconstructed temperature estimation map.

The procedure is illustrated in Figure 5.

The PBE couples thermal diffusion with a heat-sink term that is proportional to the local perfusion and to the difference between the local tissue temperature ($T(t)$) at time t and the arterial blood temperature (T_a):

$$\rho c \frac{\partial T}{\partial t} = \nabla k \nabla T + w_b \rho_b c_b (T_a - T) + q_m + q_{ext}, \qquad (8)$$

where ρ represents density (kg/m^3), c is the specific heat capacity (J/kg°C), k is the thermal conductivity (J/(s·m·°C)), w_b is the perfusion rate (kg/(s·m^3)), ρ_b is the density of blood, c_b is the specific heat capacity of blood, q_m is the metabolic heat generation rate (J/(s·m^3)), and q_{ext} is the electromagnetic power deposition. w_b can be temperature dependent to account for vasodilation.

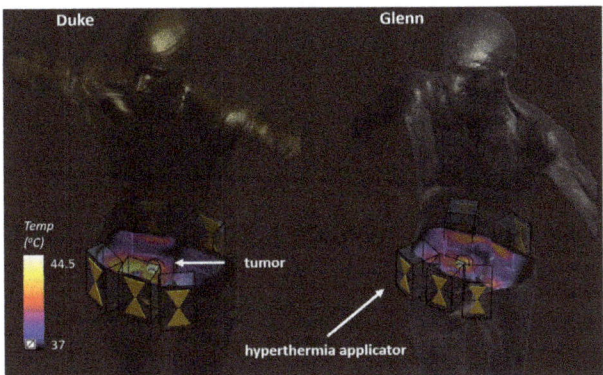

Figure 3. Simulated HT treatment in the Duke and Glenn anatomical models. Five modular applicator elements were placed circumferentially around the tumor, and their phases and amplitudes were optimized to preferentially heat the tumor. Two different anatomical models were used to investigate the impact of anatomical variability, as well as the impact of using a nonpersonalized reference model for reconstruction.

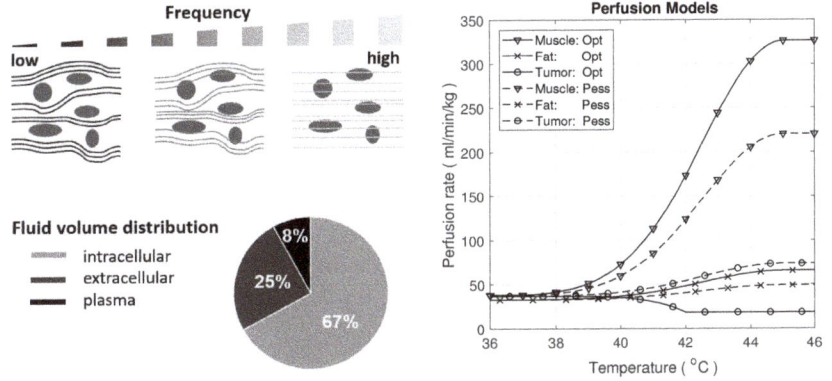

Figure 4. Current flow at different frequencies and fluid distribution in the human body [42] (**left**); optimistic and pessimistic perfusion models for muscle, fat, and tumor tissue [14,43] (**right**).

2.4.1. Change in Conductivity Due to Temperature Increase

The change in conductivity during a HT treatment can be modeled with two components:

$$\Delta\sigma(T) = \Delta\sigma_{temp}(T) + \Delta\sigma_{perf}(T), \tag{9}$$

where the change in conductivity directly due to the increase in temperature ($\Delta T = T - T_{ref}$) is $\Delta\sigma_{temp}(T) = T_c \cdot \Delta T$, with the temperature coefficient T_c (we assume $T_c = 2\%/°C$ in all tissues).

The conductivity change due to perfusion depends on the tissue as well as the frequency. At lower frequencies (kHz, LF), current flows mainly in the extracellular compartment, whereas at higher frequencies (MHz, HF), current flow tends to be more uniform across all tissue (see Figure 4).

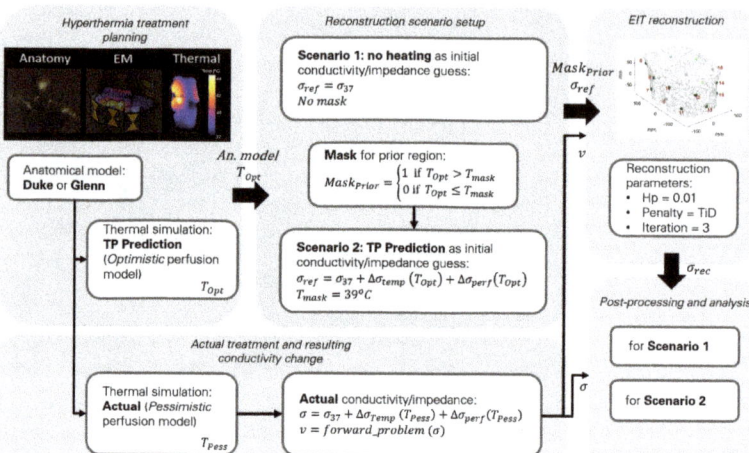

Figure 5. Conductivity changes reconstruction pipeline for two investigated EIT scenarios: EIT attempts to reproduce the voltage measurement signal of the "actual" model by reconstructing temperature and perfusion changes with regard to the reconstruction reference. (Scenario 1) uses the conductivity at 37 °C as reconstruction reference, while (Scenario 2) uses the modified conductivity as predicted by computational modeling of induced heating, perfusion response, and resulting conductivity change (but wrongly assuming an "Optimistic" perfusion, while the "actual" conductivity change is based on the "Pessimistic" perfusion model). Scenario 2 also employs masking based on the predicted temperature increase (prior region) to improve reconstruction.

For the purpose of this study, a simple model representing the difference between high and low frequency EIT and perfusion effects was constructed. Large uncertainties were associated with the temperature dependence of the perfusion $\Delta \sigma_{perf}$. However, as long as the model reproduced the general magnitude and behavior in terms of perfusion impact on conductivity and heating, it did not affect the generality of the study conclusions. To model the different frequencies, we neglected other dispersive effects and assumed that:

$$G_{HF} = G_{icHF} + G_{ecHF} + G_{pHF}, \tag{10}$$

and

$$G_{LF} = G_{ecLF} + G_{pLF}, \tag{11}$$

where G_{LF} and G_{HF} are the LF and HF conductance, respectively. G_{ic}, G_{ec}, G_p, correspond to intracellular, extracellular (without the blood plasma), and plasma conductance. We used the average human body volume ratio of these compartments from [42], as illustrated in Figure 4, as the conductance ratio between compartments to model the perfusion impact on conductance. Actual values are tissue-dependent.

The change in perfusion affects the total conductance by changing the relative contributions of the three compartments; therefore, the plasma volume increases as the perfusion increases. Assuming that the relative tissue volume change related to a perfusion increase is small and the plasma conductivity is the principal contributor to the overall conductivity, we obtain:

$$\Delta \sigma_{perf}(T) = \frac{\Delta V_p(T)}{V_{total}} (1 + T_c \cdot \Delta T), \tag{12}$$

where $\Delta V_p(T) = V_{p,0} \cdot \left(\sqrt{\omega(T)} - 1 \right)$ is the plasma volume change due to perfusion, and $\omega(T)$ is the relative perfusion change. $\alpha = \frac{V_{p,0}}{V_{total}}$ is the relative amount of plasma prior to heating, which is taken uniformly as 8% (see Figure 4), while in reality it varies across tissues and individuals. The -1 accounts for the plasma volume prior to heating, which is already included in the $\Delta\sigma_{temp}$ term. The square root approximates the relationship between blood vessel cross-sectional area and perfusion increase and is obtained under the assumption of a constant pressure drive and laminar flow [44].

Perfusion-related changes were considered for muscle, fat, and tumor tissues, particularly for prominent tissues with strong temperature dependence of perfusion and an important impact on the predicted temperature, using the two perfusion models shown in Figure 4, according to [14]. Tumor perfusion has a high associated uncertainty [14] due to irregular vascularization.

Disentangling Temperature and Perfusion

Distinguishing $\Delta\sigma_{temp}$ from $\Delta\sigma_{perf}$ to identify temperature and perfusion changes is not the subject of this paper. However, a possible approach is provided here:
$\Delta\sigma = \Delta\sigma_{temp} + \Delta\sigma_{perf}$, where $\Delta\sigma_{temp} = T_c \cdot \Delta T$ and $\Delta\sigma_{perf} = \alpha \cdot (\sqrt{\omega} - 1) \cdot (1 + T_c \cdot \Delta T)$. If α is known at two frequencies for a tissue of interest (in this study, we assumed $\alpha_{LF} = 24\%$ and $\alpha_{HF} = 8\%$ for all tissues), we obtain

$$\Delta\sigma_{LF} - \frac{\alpha_{LF}}{\alpha_{HF}} \cdot \Delta\sigma_{HF} = \left(1 - \frac{\alpha_{LF}}{\alpha_{HF}}\right) \cdot T_c \cdot \Delta T \tag{13}$$

and

$$\Delta\sigma_{LF} - \Delta\sigma_{HF} = (\alpha_{LF} - \alpha_{HF}) \cdot (\sqrt{\omega} - 1) \cdot (1 + T_c \cdot \Delta T). \tag{14}$$

The former can be used to estimate ΔT, while the latter can be used to obtain ω (either using the ΔT estimated using Equation (13), or ΔT from the simulation, or neglecting the term $T_c \cdot \Delta T$ in Equation (14)). In practice, α_{LF} and α_{HF} might not be known, as the exact form of the temperature and perfusion dependences likely deviates from Equation (12), and the reconstructed $\Delta\sigma_{LF}$ and $\Delta\sigma_{HF}$ contain reconstruction errors. For a brief analysis of the latter, see Section 3.3.2.

2.4.2. Reconstruction Scenarios

Temperature predictions have uncertainties; hence, the need for online monitoring of temperature during treatment. Here, we assumed that a temperature distribution (T_{Pess}) corresponds to the actual thermal treatment administered to a patient with a bladder tumor. Using the equations and assumptions above, we calculated the actual conductivity change corresponding to T_{Pess} and the corresponding EIT voltages were used for reconstruction. Two scenarios were considered: one without previous knowledge and one with an imperfect thermal simulation-based treatment plan. In Scenario 1 (see Figure 5), we reconstructed conductivity changes using the values at 37 °C (no heating applied) as the reference conductivity. In Scenario 2, temperature distributions from simulations using T_{Opt} were used to define the prior region for reconstruction; the incorrect perfusion information was used to introduce uncertainty similar to expected outcomes in a real treatment. Despite not using accurate perfusion values, Scenario 2 provided a better starting point than Scenario 1 for the reconstruction, as the conductivity difference to be reconstructed is smaller.

In both scenarios, we determined the prior region by thresholding T_{Opt} at a temperature above a temperature threshold (T_{Mask}). For Scenario 2, a T_{Mask} of 39 °C was used, whereas for Scenario 1, no mask is applied. In Scenario 1, we expected changes in the whole volume, whereas in Scenario 2, the prior region was smaller, as differences were more localized. Suitable temperature thresholds were identified by studying the resulting reconstruction accuracy in a range of setups. Higher thresholds prevent the reconstruction outside the masked volume, resulting in an overall increased error, while lower thresholds lead to underestimation of tumor heating, as the impedance changes are attributed to a larger region.

To investigate the importance of using personalized reference models, reconstruction was performed again using the Duke reference model, but with a simulated HT treatment measurement of Glenn (similar element placement, same steering parameters).

As reconstruction with 16 elements was unsuccessful (see Section 3.3.1), eight-element reconstruction was investigated further. Subsequently, changes in anatomy (Glenn has a smaller cross-section area than Duke) were compensated by rescaling the voltages with the ratio of the voltages prior to heating. The additional constraint of demanding a positive temperature increase was imposed by zeroing all negative conductivity changes prior to each reconstruction iteration (note: negative conductivity changes cannot be excluded completely, e.g., due to geometry changes during treatment or perfusion redistribution; performing the reconstruction step after zeroing does allow to account for some of that). Finally, the expected temperature distribution smoothness was mimicked by convolution with a Gaussian filter (radius: 1 cm; chosen based on the characteristic lengths of the PBE Green's function in muscle, bone, fat, and tumor at the initial temperature).

For the analysis of the reconstruction accuracy, the conductivity change in the heated reference model was compared with the conductivity change in the reconstruction.

Both the LF and the HF EIT cases were simulated. In the LF case, the contribution of perfusion to the conductivity change is higher. Thus, the same temperature distribution resulted in a higher total change in conductivity. Ultimately, EIT at multiple frequencies was used to distinguish conductivity changes related to T_c from indirect conductivity changes related to perfusion changes and to monitor both the temperature and the perfusion distribution. In this study, we focused on the feasibility of conductivity reconstruction, and only briefly considered multifrequency EIT-enabled contribution separation.

3. Results

3.1. Reconstruction Time

A typical reconstruction for a setup with ~6E5 tetrahedral elements, 16 electrodes, and 182 voltage measurements requires less than 5 min on a personal computer with an Intel i7-4770 processor (3.4 GHz, 4 cores). If less than three iterations are used, the reconstruction speed can be further accelerated. In view of the characteristic heating time in hyperthermic oncology, this provides sufficient temporal resolution.

3.2. Investigation Scenarios

3.2.1. Tissue-Dependent Penalty

Second order polynomials were fitted to the scatter plots of actual conductivity change ($\Delta\sigma = \sigma - \sigma_{ref}$; in %, relative to nonheated baseline conductivity) vs. reconstructed conductivity ($\Delta\sigma_{rec} = \sigma_{rec} - \sigma_{ref}$). Figure 6 shows the results from a single iteration without any averaging filter after the reconstruction. The fits were performed separately for all tissues present in the heated regions. Results showed that a constant penalty value applied to all the tissues leads to an overestimation for low σ tissues and an underestimation in the reconstruction of the high σ tissues. Tissue-dependent penalty values improve the reconstruction across all tissues.

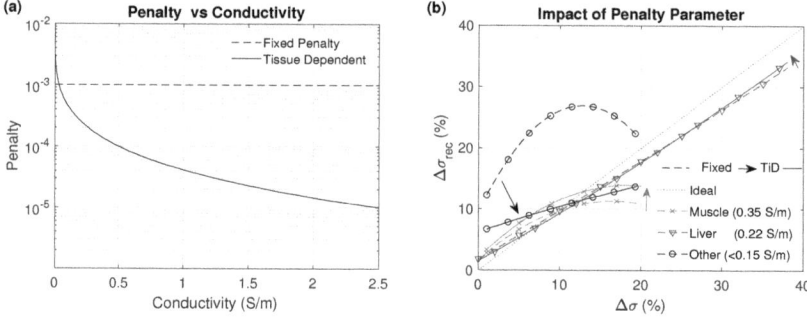

Figure 6. (a) "Tissue-dependent Penalty" and "Fixed Penalty" values. (b) Plot by tissue of the fitted relationship between reconstructed ($\Delta\sigma_{rec}$) versus reference ($\Delta\sigma$) changes in conductivity using "Fixed Penalty" (dashed line) and "Tissue-dependent Penalty" (solid line).

3.2.2. Multiple Regions

For scenario P1 from Table 1, Figure 7 shows the $\Delta\sigma_{rec}$ (%) versus $\Delta\sigma$ (%), mean, and $\pm$ standard deviation after computing a sliding histogram every 1% of $\Delta\sigma$. The results for all other cases are shown as the error in conductivity reconstruction ($\Delta\sigma_{err} = \Delta\sigma_{rec} - \Delta\sigma$ in %) from the modified $\Delta\sigma$ (%). The magnitude of the deviations of the reconstructed conductivity changes from the actual changes, as well as their variability, are similar and moderate (well below 10%) in all cases. The largest deviation from the target is observed in the case of smaller region (P2), which corresponds to the situation with the highest dielectric contrast at the heating region surface.

3.2.3. Impact of Inaccurate Reference Model

When investigating the impact of changes outside the prior region, which is also equivalent to an inaccurate reference model conductivity, both the penalty parameter and the hyperparameter values are important. The hyperparameter shows the reliance of the reconstructed model on the reference model σ. The penalty, however, impacts how much the reconstruction focuses on changes within the prior region and how much it relies on the absence of no changes outside of the prior region. Since both of these parameters are related to the accuracy of the reference model, results for different values of these parameters are presented in Figure 8.

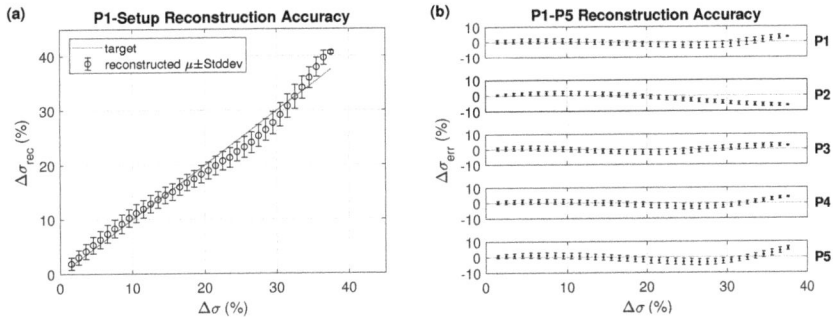

Figure 7. (a) Reconstructed conductivity $\Delta\sigma_{rec}$ (%) for the P1 setup from Figure 2 and (b) its deviation from the actual conductivity change ($\Delta\sigma_{err} = \Delta\sigma_{rec} - \Delta\sigma$) for all the setups P1–P5, as shown in Table 1 and illustrated in Figure 2, (right), using three iterations, tissue-dependent (TiD) penalty, and Hp = 0.01.

Initially, we observed that the reconstruction error resulting from the important conductivity changes outside the prior region can be large when using the same penalty and hyperparameter values, such as for the ideal case. Relaxing those parameters reduced the standard deviation of the error, but the reconstructed conductivity still did not follow the expected change across the whole range. After introducing adaptive prior regions, an improvement of the results was obtained, as shown for TiD penalties in Figure 8. Refer to Section 3.3.1 regarding reconstruction using a nonpersonalized reference anatomical model.

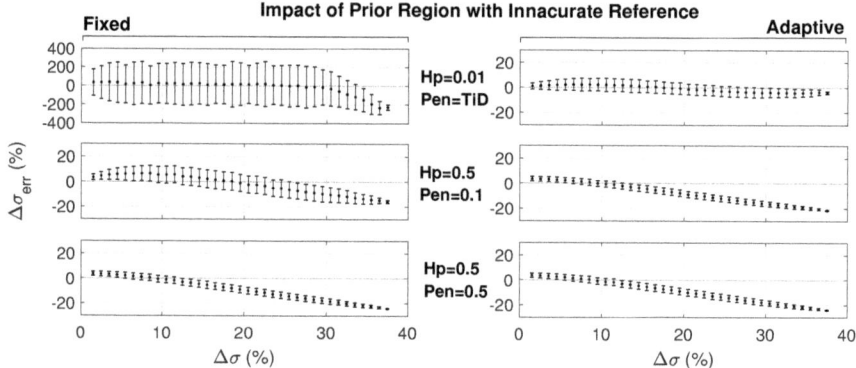

Figure 8. Reconstructed deviation in an inaccurate reference model (large inserted air sphere) for a fixed prior region using three iterations (**left**) and an adaptive prior region using 1 + 1 + 3 iterations (**right**)—note the different scale in the upper left graph.

3.2.4. Voltage Measurement Noise

Figure 9 shows the results for heating scenario P1, when voltage measurements with different levels of SNR are mimicked. Since we wanted to focus on the impact of noise, the prior region was fixed and there were no changes outside the prior region in the reference model. The SNR was calculated with respect to the voltage difference, not the absolute voltages. As expected, noise strongly deteriorated the reconstruction accuracy, especially with low hyperparameter values. In the reconstruction algorithm, this gives more weight to the voltage measurements, which have poor SNR in this case, and less to the reference conductivity in the regularization part.

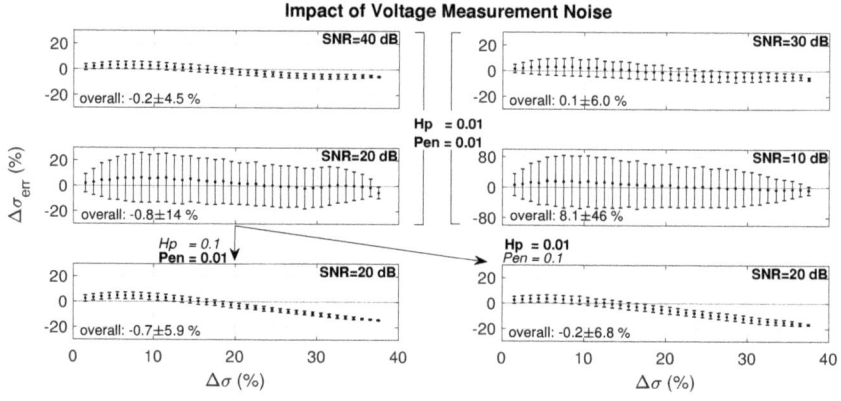

Figure 9. Impact of electrode voltage SNR (see Section 2.3.4 for the SNR calculation) on the reconstruction accuracy using three iterations for four levels of SNR (10, 20, 30, 40 dB), and in the 20 dB SNR case for varying combinations of reconstruction parameters (hyperparameter and penalty)—note the different scale in the 10 dB SNR case.

3.3. Simulated HT Treatment Reconstruction

Slice views of simulated HT treatment temperatures, conductivity maps, and reconstructions are shown for Scenario 1 and 2 (Duke model, LF EIT) in Figure 10. Simulations were performed using the Duke and Glenn anatomical models for LF and HF EIT, using reconstruction Scenarios 1 and 2, resulting in a total of eight cases. For all these cases, we also calculated the estimated temperature change error ($T_{err} = T_{rec} - T_{actual}$) for fat, muscle, tumor, and all tissues combined by using the reconstructed conductivity (see Figure 11).

T_{rec} was calculated using the inverse of the function $\Delta\sigma(T)$ that was used to translate the temperature distribution to a modified conductivity map (see Section 2.3). This only served to provide an interpretable error metric for analysis purposes. In practical applications, the uncertainties associated with the temperature dependence of conductivity prevented reliable inversion and multifrequency EIT measurements instead permitted direct temperature reconstruction by separating direct temperature-related from perfusion-related conductivity changes (see Section 3.3.2).

In Scenario 1, there was higher error across the whole range of change, as a result of the much larger conductivity changes (up to 55%) and the large required prior region. In Scenario 2, we observed an improved reconstruction accuracy, except for the tumor. Even though there were relatively high changes in tumor conductivity (up to 20%), tumor volume was relatively small and the reconstruction attributed the associated impedance changes to small conductivity changes in a larger volume. As a result, changes in tumor conductivity were only partially reconstructed for Scenario 2.

HF reconstruction resulted in lower temperature prediction errors compared to the LF case. This was mainly due to the smaller range of the conductivity change that required reconstruction.

Similar observations were made for the Duke and Glenn anatomical models, with slightly better results for Glenn, perhaps due to his smaller body size. The heating pattern in Glenn was more focused compared to Duke, resulting in a smaller region of significant conductivity changes and thus a smaller prior region, facilitating reconstruction.

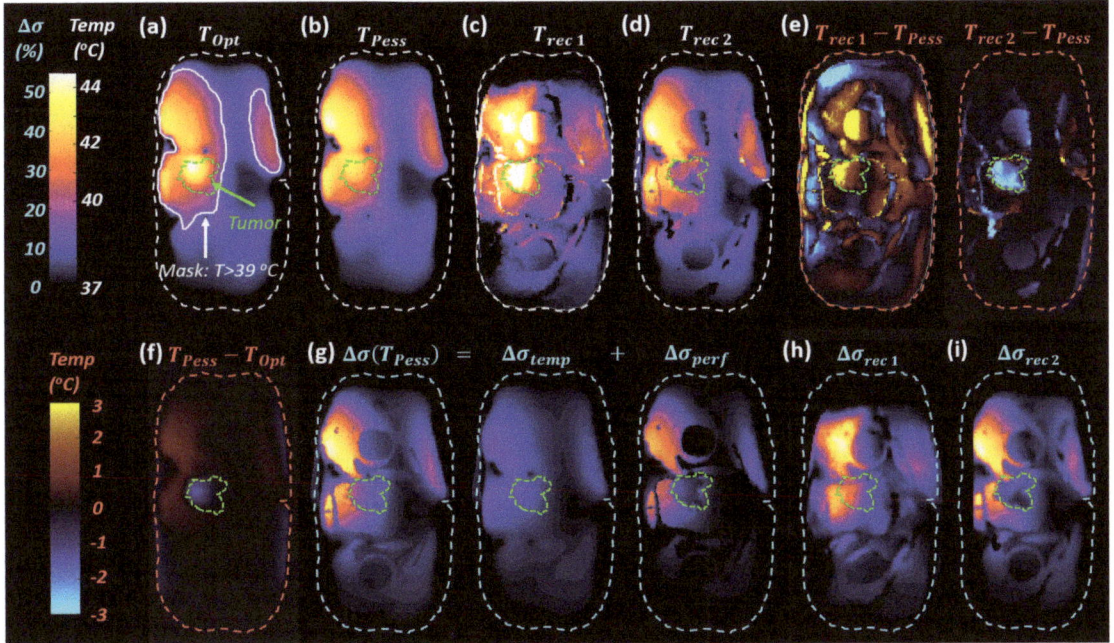

Figure 10. Reconstruction results from realistic HT treatment modeling (LF, Duke anatomical model): (**a**) axial slice from the thermal simulation with the optimistic perfusion model (T_{Opt}), (**b**) axial slice from thermal simulation with the pessimistic perfusion model (T_{Pess}) and (**f**) difference between T_{Pess} and T_{Opt}; (**c**,**d**) reconstructed temperature results from Scenario 1 (T_{rec1}, using the reference conductivity at 37 °C) and Scenario 2 (T_{rec2}, using the reference conductivity $\Delta\sigma(T_{Opt})$), as calculated from the reconstructed $\Delta\sigma_{rec}$ in (**h**,**i**), respectively; (**e**) temperature estimation error for both scenarios; (**g**) $\Delta\sigma(T_{Pess})$ with its direct temperature-related ($\Delta\sigma_{temp}$) and the perfusion-related $\Delta\sigma_{perf}$ contributions.

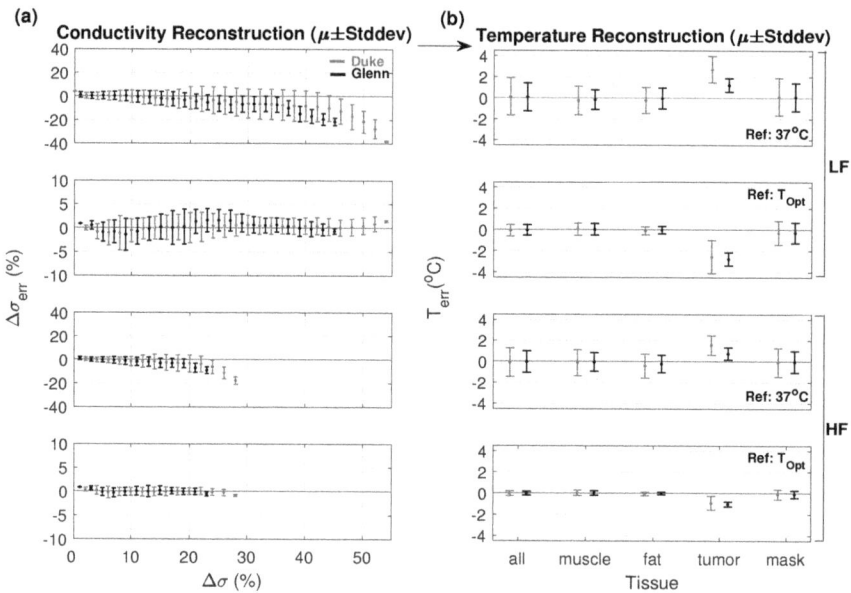

Figure 11. (a) Reconstructed mean and standard deviation of conductivity ($\Delta\sigma_{err}$) and (b) estimated temperature error (T_{err}). Reconstructions were performed for the Duke and Glenn anatomical models, for low frequency (LF) and high frequency (HF) current injection, using the conductivity map at 37 °C as the reference (baseline for EIT difference reconstruction) or the one predicted by thermal simulations with the (inaccurate) optimistic perfusion model (T_{Opt}). Mean and standard deviation of temperature error for muscle, fat, tumor, the prior region mask, and all tissues combined are shown. TiD penalty and Hp = 0.01 were used.

For the simulated HT treatment on the Duke model, Table 2 shows the electrode voltage levels obtained by solving the forward problem when injecting a 1 mA current at the stimulating electrodes. The injection current was limited by safety constraints. For frequencies above 100 kHz, the stimulating current should not exceed 10 mA regardless of the pulse shape. In a practical implementation, depending on the SNR and the acquisition system capabilities, the conductivity-change-induced reconstruction-relevant voltage differences can be of a similar magnitude as the noise.

Table 2. Mean and standard deviation of the electrode voltages (v_{ref}) and voltage differences at each iteration of reconstruction for two cases (reconstruction using reference conductivity, σ_{ref}, at 37 °C and T_{Opt}).

	Electrode Voltages Levels at 1 mA Injection Current			
Simulation	v_{ref}	|Δv| at Iteration		
		1	2	3
Reference 37 °C	5.1 ± 4.8 mV	390 ± 370 µV	42 ± 45 µV	1.7 ± 1.7 µV
Reference T_{Opt}	4.7 ± 4.5 mV	30 ± 26 µV	0.9 ± 0.8 µV	0.9 ± 0.8 µV

The results presented in Table 2 also show that in Scenario 2 the remaining difference between the reference and reconstruction-based voltage in the second and third iteration was much smaller than for Scenario 1. This was a consequence of using T_{Opt} as a starting guess, which was closer than Scenario 1 to the target distribution. In fact, in Scenario 2, the first iteration would be sufficient. Nevertheless, three iterations were maintained, in case of important conductivity changes within or outside the prior region, which cannot be excluded in advance. The expected electrode voltages and voltage changes are important for defining the hardware requirements.

3.3.1. Personalized Reference Model

When the voltages from a simulated Glenn HT treatment were reconstructed using a Duke reference model, no meaningful results were obtained (Figure 12). Matching the impedances from 16 contacts and 192 voltage measurements resulted in overfitting or extreme conductivity variations that rely on compensation to achieve accurate impedance matches. Thus, reconstruction from eight electrodes was performed. While this produced inferior results when using a subject-specific reference model (lower reconstruction resolution and accuracy), it considerably improved reconstruction using a nonpersonalized reference (Figure 12). Further improvements were obtained when (i) rescaling voltages based on the measurable preheating voltages to compensate for anatomical differences (see Figure 13), (ii) constraining conductivity changes to be positive, and (iii) smoothing the temperature distribution based on the characteristic thermal length (~1 cm). The latter two improvements are not specific to using personalized reference models.

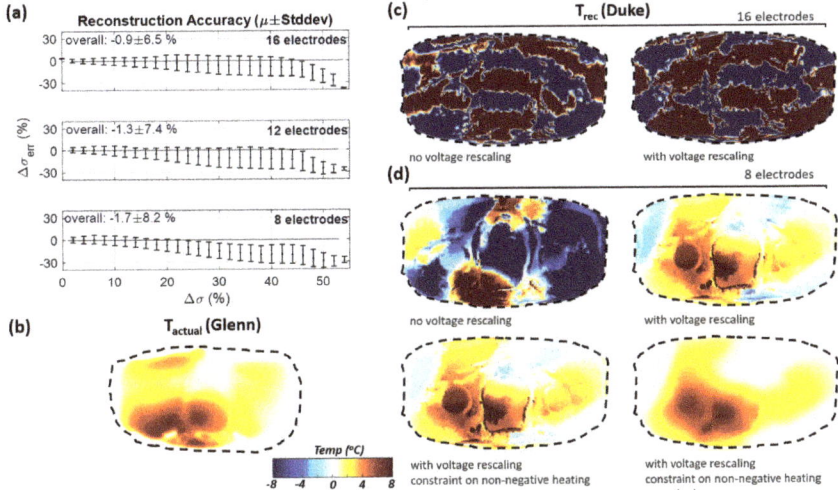

Figure 12. (a) Conductivity reconstruction error ($\Delta\sigma_{err} = \Delta\sigma_{rec} - \Delta\sigma$ in %) using 16, 12, or 8 electrodes, when the actual treatment (along with the extraction of the measurement voltages) is applied to the Duke model, (b) actual heating on Glenn, (c,d) reconstruction is performed using the Duke model as reconstruction reference, to study nonpersonalized reconstruction of heating on Glenn. While avoiding the generation of patient-specific models for reconstruction considerably reduces the involved effort, an important factor in a clinical environments, it also results in reduced reconstruction accuracy. As hyperthermia QA guidelines recommend personalized treatment planning for deep-seated tumors, personalized models are frequently available already. The important reconstruction errors in (a) reflect the use of the Duke conductivity distribution at 37 °C as reconstruction reference, while the reconstruction approaches in (c,d) employ nonpersonalized, Duke-based treatment planning (incl. thermal modeling) instead. (c) displays reconstruction results obtained using 16 electrodes with or without voltage-rescaling to compensate for the absence of a personalized reference model. (d) displays reconstruction results obtained when reducing the number of electrodes to 8, using voltage-rescaling, introducing constraints (non-negative temperature changes), and applying Green's-function-based smoothing. These measures result in increasingly accurate temperature increase estimations.

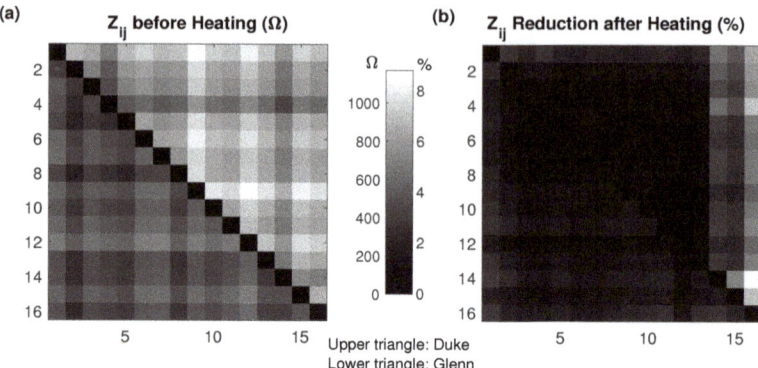

Figure 13. (a) Preheating impedance Z_{ij} per electrode pair (in Ω) and (b) impedance reduction due to heating (in %). Upper and lower triangle values correspond to the Duke and Glenn anatomical models, respectively. The numbering follows Figure 2.

3.3.2. Temperature and Perfusion Mapping

Figure 14 illustrates the perfusion and temperature increase maps obtained using the multifrequency approach from Section 2.4.1 (shown for the Duke case, using the optimistic perfusion model as the reconstruction reference; see Section 2.4). The two-frequency reconstruction resulted in a superior reconstruction of the temperature maps (error < 2 °C), when compared to the single frequency one. The perfusion reconstruction showed important deviations in the tumor. The superiority of the temperature mapping over the perfusion mapping could be related to the differing conductivity reconstruction error magnitudes at the two frequencies. Equation (13) adds different weights to the reconstructions at the two frequencies, such that the two errors are compensated when computing the temperature map, while Equation (14) subtracts the two without weighting, such that part of the conductivity reconstruction error remains and affects the perfusion mapping.

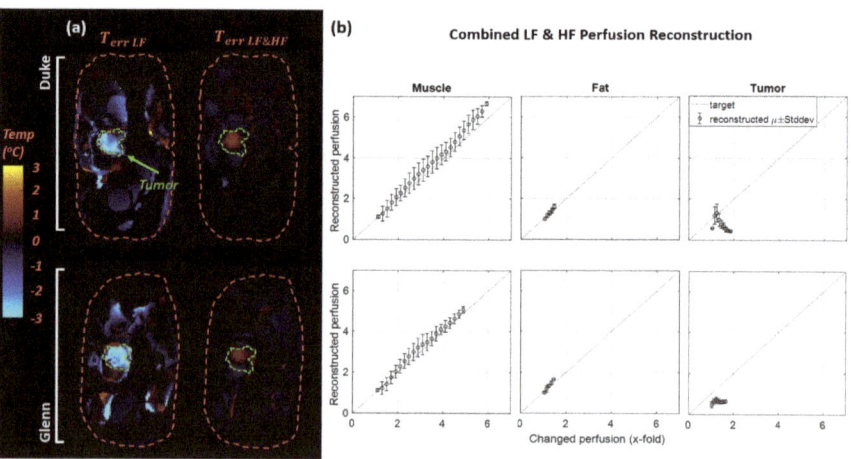

Figure 14. Reconstruction results from multifrequency EIT on Duke and Glenn: (a) cross-sectional view of the temperature error distribution; (b) reconstructed perfusion versus underlying perfusion plotted separately for muscle, fat, and tumor tissues.

3.3.3. Summary of Temperature Reconstruction Accuracy

Table 3 summarizes the impact of the reconstruction approach and scenario on reconstruction accuracy. It illustrates the improvements relative to the prior state-of-the-art (baseline) afforded by the newly introduced iterative approach, adaptive prior regions, and tissue-dependent penalties. The mean and standard deviation of the reconstruction error in the masked prior region are reported (note that the prior region changes when adaptive prior regions are used). The crucial improvements afforded by the use of planning-based reference models, measurement-based reweighting, and physics-based constraints are not reflected in the table, as the chosen metrics to not allow for a direct comparison across changing anatomies—the relevant information can instead be found in Figure 12. For the generic scenarios, in which the conductivity was changed in a given spherical region, the conductivity reconstruction accuracy was converted to an equivalent temperature accuracy by dividing by $T_c = 2\%/°C$. The limitations of the reconstruction accuracy estimations are discussed in Table 4.

Table 3. Summary of the impact of the reconstruction approach (parameters, iterations, adaptive penalties and prior regions, reference model) and scenario (generic local σ change, detailed treatment scenario, perfusion changes, EIT frequency/frequencies) on the reconstruction accuracy (mean and standard deviation in the prior region). For the realistic HT therapy heating pattern scenarios, the worst case from the investigated Glenn and Duke scenarios is reported. Accuracy of nonpersonalized reconstruction scenarios is not reported here, since the chosen metrics are not applicable.

Condition	Accuracy (Mean/Stddev °C)
Temperature Estimation Accuracy	
Ideal: generic local (spherical) σ change	
1-iter., No Penalty, Hp = 0.01	−3.9/4.9 °C
1-iter., Penalty = 0.001, Hp = 0.01 (*baseline*)	−0.6/1.7 °C
1-iter., Penalty = TiD, Hp = 0.01	−0.6/1.4 °C
3-iter., Penalty = TiD, Hp = 0.01	−0.1/1.1 °C
Nonideal: noise/σ change outside prior region	
3-iter., Penalty = TiD, Hp = 0.01, σ *change outside prior region*	Unusable with Fixed prior region; 0/2.4 °C with Adaptive prior region
3-iter., Penalty = 0.01, Hp = 0.1, SNR = 20 dB	−0.4/3 °C
Hyperthermia treatment scenarios, temperature increase and perfusion changes	
3-iter., Penalty = TiD, HP = 0.01, Ref 37 °C	0.2/1.8 °C (LF) −0.1/1.4 °C (HF)
3-iter., Penalty = TiD, HP = 0.01, *personalized Ref T_{Opt}*	−0.3/1.1 °C (LF) −0.1/0.5 °C (HF)
3-iter., Penalty = TiD, HP = 0.01, *Multifrequency*	−0.1/0.3 °C

Figure 10 suggests that under ideal conditions and when using personalized reference models, a spatial reconstruction accuracy in the centimeter-range is achievable, which is similar to the inherent thermal length-scale (diffusion related characteristic length of the PBE Green's function [45]). However, Figure 12 suggests that imperfections, such as the use of nonpersonalized models, reduce the achievable spatial accuracy to multiple centimeters. The ability of detecting highly localized temperature features, e.g., near important cooling arteries, has not been assessed.

4. Discussion

In this study, we investigated the potential application of EIT as a low-cost, noninvasive technique for HT treatment monitoring.

For estimation accuracy, if only changes in conductivity associated with T_c are considered, a 2% deviation from the actual conductivity leads to 1 °C error in temperature. Due to the presence of perfusion-related conductivity changes, the total conductivity sensitivity to temperature is higher, which can facilitate temperature mapping, if accurate information about the temperature dependence of perfusion is provided. However, the relation between the conductivity error and the temperature or perfusion estimation error becomes more complex. In the absence of well-known temperature–perfusion relationships, distinguishing between perfusion and temperature changes using multifrequency EIT is crucial. To simultaneously map perfusion and temperature changes, the use of more than two measurement frequencies and postprocessing techniques should be further investigated, considering the limited accuracy of conductivity map reconstruction and the limited knowledge about α.

Using a tissue-dependent penalty along with adaptive prior regions are key to achieving conductivity mapping in highly heterogeneous anatomical models. Information from thermal simulations can be used to further improve the accuracy, as shown in the simulated HT treatment scenario. Under ideal conditions, reconstruction in a simulated HT treatment achieves a mean deviation in the order of 1 °C (see Figure 11) in the heated domain. Having a good reference model is important, and a priori personalized models should be used. When using a nonspecific anatomical reference, fewer measurement electrodes should be used and voltages should be rescaled based on preheating measurements. An extreme scenario was investigated to assess local reference model inaccuracies (e.g., passing air bubble). Regarding local reference model inaccuracies (e.g., passing air bubble), an extreme scenario was investigated. We found that using adaptive prior regions in combination with a tissue-dependent penalty successfully enabled reconstruction. Nonablative HT is a relatively long treatment ($\sim$40–60 min) and the heating time constant is in the order of minutes. Therefore, changes during treatment, except for body movements, occur slowly compared with the potential voltage acquisition speed. Continuous monitoring can be combined with continuous prior region adaptation to handle slow tissue environment changes and to adapt the reference model.

Measurement noise is problematic as the number of cells in the model to be reconstructed is large compared to the number of voltage measurements. Figure 9 illustrates the quantifiable impact of SNR on the reconstruction error from 40 dB to 10 dB SNR, while keeping the same reconstruction parameters results in an increase of the reconstruction error by an order of magnitude. The SNR can be improved by averaging multiple acquisitions, and voltage measurements with poor SNR should be detected.

The combination of HT treatment planning with EIT has multiple advantages: Treatment planning typically includes imaging and segmentation for personalized treatment optimization, and a personalized reference model is important for the reconstruction. Electromagnetic and thermal simulations from HT planning can be used in EIT to determine the region where changes in conductivity are expected and which can serve as a prior region. A good reference model for the heated state also facilitates reconstruction (smaller $\Delta\sigma$). In turn, EIT-reconstructed changes in conductivity converted to perfusion/temperature changes can be used for an online adaptation of the treatment plan and of the applied parameters.

For the simulated HT scenarios with the Duke and Glenn ViP models, additional investigations were performed that are not presented in this paper due to space constraints. The following parameters were varied: masking threshold level (37–40 °C), hyperparameter value (0.0001–1), and the number of electrodes (8–32) and electrode rows (2–4). The masking threshold affects the reconstruction of regions with relatively high changes that are left outside the mask, if too high, or the accuracy of high temperature region reconstruction, if too low. The impact of the hyperparameter is dependent on the masking threshold and the mask and penalty values; however, in most of the cases, 0.01 was considered a good choice. Increasing both the number of rows and electrodes did not yield significant improvements compared to two rows with 16 electrodes and resulted in smaller voltage differences between nearby electrodes, making the system more susceptible to noise and measurement uncertainty in practical implementations.

Table 4 lists study limitations that should be considered.

Table 4. List of limitations in this study and their implications.

Limitation	Discussion
Generality	The present study focused on two anatomies, one realistic tumor location in addition to a few spherical heating cases, a fixed exposure element type and placement, and stable EIT electrode placement. While the reconstruction parameters were not particularly tweaked to obtain the presented results, it is important to investigate whether these parameters are indeed generalizable.
Anatomical model accuracy	Personalized anatomical model generation—or intersubject variability, if presegmented models are used—affect the simulation fidelity and are likely to be one of the main sources of reconstruction errors.
Constant T_c	A constant $T_c = 2\%/°C$ was used in this study. However, reported values in tissue vary between 0.6–2.1%/°C; refs. [14,46] with a typical value around 2.0%/°C. Although it is unclear how much is measurement-accuracy-related, large intertissue or intersubject variability affects the reconstruction.
Frequency and temperature dependence of conductivity	There is a high degree of uncertainty associated with the temperature dependence of perfusion and electric conductivity. However, since this study focused on conductivity change reconstruction, this uncertainty does not affect our conclusions. If multifrequency EIT can separate direct temperature effects from perfusion-related ones, the uncertainty is reduced to that of T_c.
Inaccurate conductivity values	The reference model and the model to be reconstructed use tissue properties from a tissue properties database; however, uncertainty and variability associated with these properties affect the achievable reconstruction accuracy. EIT prior to therapy application can help obtain more accurate property maps.
Nonlocal changes of perfusion and local vascular cooling	Although we assumed that increased blood flow circulation occurred in the heated region, nonlocal effects, such as whole-body thermoregulation, convective transport by medium-sized blood vessels, and the stealing effects or blood-flow reduction in a tissue resulting from an increase in neighboring tissue were not considered. Additionally, the localized cooling by sufficiently large blood vessels is not considered by the employed PBE, which assumes distributed perfusion.
Fixed body core temperature	In our simulations, we assumed that body-core temperature was constant. However, the high energy delivery during HT therapy can result in a body-core temperature increase which affects overall tissue temperature.
Electrode modeling and positioning	We modeled point electrodes with precisely known locations. The impact of inaccurate electrode positioning and compensation methods have already been studied [47–49]. We assume that accurate placement of electrodes can be assured during treatment. Replacing the point electrodes with extended electrodes will affect the current density in the vicinity of the electrode, and thus the reconstruction sensitivity in that region; this is easily handled and not the subject of this study, which focused on EIT for deep heating monitoring.
Fixed patient geometry	We assumed that the patient geometry did not change between the treatment model creation and the treatment administration. Precise and reproducible patient positioning is required in the clinic, and it is already a requirement for high-quality HT treatment administration. Changes in the internal organ geometry have been investigated in this study, and are handled using adaptive prior regions. Nevertheless, large changes were shown to deteriorate the reconstruction accuracy.
Reconstruction parameter choice	Further investigations are necessary to determine if the reconstruction parameters identified in this study also provide the best reconstruction results across other scenarios.

5. Conclusions

In this study, we investigated the feasibility of EIT difference imaging for detecting conductivity changes during HT therapy. Realistic scenarios were considered for the practical implementation of EIT in HT monitoring. We implemented an iterative reconstruction in which the reference model was updated for each iteration. The results suggest that a single iteration may be sufficient if there are only small changes.

By using highly heterogeneous anatomical models, we showed that a tissue-dependent penalty parameter improves reconstruction accuracy throughout the modeled volume. We also showed that reconstruction performance has no apparent dependence on the location and extent of the heated region when placing heated spheres with sizes typical of HT heating volumes in relevant torso treatment locations.

Simulated HT treatment with realistic heating patterns revealed large errors in the reconstruction, mainly due to conductivity changes within most of the volume. Using simulated treatment plans as references yields better reconstructions, despite modeling-inherent inaccuracies (e.g., of the tissue parameters). A personalized reference model is thus required; however, a nonspecific reference model can be used if the number of electrodes is reduced and a rescaling of voltages based on preheating measurements is performed.

In view of real-world limitations, we considered the impact of voltage measurement noise and strong localized inaccuracies in the reference model (large air bubble). Both can lead to significant errors, if reconstruction parameters for ideal conditions (no noise, accurate reference model) are used. However, important improvements can be achieved by relaxing reconstruction parameters and introducing prior region adaptation in the reconstruction.

For the successful application of EIT to monitor temperature and perfusion during HT therapy, all factors contributing to the deterioration of the accuracy must be addressed and mitigated. Essentially, accurate reference models (geometry and conductivity) and accurate impedance measurements are required. The results indicate that a temperature estimation accuracy in the order of 1 °C is achievable under the considered conditions and assumptions based on the novel methodologies in this study (iterative reconstruction with adaptive prior regions, planning-based references, measurement-based reweighting, tissue-dependent penalties, and positive heating constraints). The achievable mapping accuracy will depend on how well multifrequency EIT measurements can be leveraged to distinguish direct temperature-related impedance changes from changes caused by perfusion adaptation.

As a next step, experimental realization and validation of the presented approach is required. Initial work could focus on the reconstruction of heating distributions when applying HT ex vivo, where perfusion changes are irrelevant and measurement access is better. Subsequent work would then shift to in vivo situations and rely on strategically placed thermometry catheters, or information from MR thermometry and MR perfusion mapping. Compatibility issues associated with the presence of EIT electrodes during HT application must be considered.

Author Contributions: Conceptualization and methodology, N.K., T.S., R.P., E.N. and M.C.; implementation and simulations, R.P.; data analysis, R.P. and E.N.; writing—original draft preparation, R.P. and E.N.; writing—review and editing, M.C., E.N. and T.S.; clinical perspective, S.B.; supervision and funding, N.K. and S.B. All authors have read and agreed to the published version of the manuscript.

Funding: This project was cofunded by the University of Zurich.

Institutional Review Board Statement: Not applicable.

Informed Consent Statement: Not applicable.

Data Availability Statement: No measurement datasets were generated or used in this study. The generated simulations are available on request from the corresponding author. The data cannot be shared publicly due to the licensed anatomical models involved.

Acknowledgments: We are grateful to Simone Callegari and Bryn Lloyd for their support with the anatomical models, to Eduardo Carrasco for his guidance on EIT, Sabine Regel (sr-scientific.com) for her inputs and thorough review of the manuscript, and Taylor Newton for reviewing the figures.

Conflicts of Interest: The authors declare no conflict of interest.

References

1. Henderson, R.P.; Webster, J.G. An impedance camera for spatially specific measurements of the thorax. *IEEE Trans. Biomed. Eng.* **1978**, *3*, 250–254. [CrossRef] [PubMed]
2. Brown, B.H. Electrical impedance tomography (EIT): A review. *J. Med. Eng. Technol.* **2003**, *27*, 97–108. [CrossRef] [PubMed]
3. Holder, D. *Electrical Impedance Tomography: Methods, History and Applications*; CRC Press: Boca Raton, FL, USA, 2004.
4. Frerichs, I. Electrical impedance tomography (EIT) in applications related to lung and ventilation: A review of experimental and clinical activities. *Physiol. Meas.* **2000**, *21*, R1. [CrossRef]
5. Bayford, R.; Tizzard, A. Bioimpedance imaging: An overview of potential clinical applications. *Analyst* **2012**, *137*, 4635–4643. [CrossRef]
6. Lobo, B.; Hermosa, C.; Abella, A.; Gordo, F. Electrical impedance tomography. *Ann. Transl. Med.* **2018**, *6*, 2. [CrossRef]

7. Adler, A.; Grychtol, B.; Bayford, R. Why is EIT so hard, and what are we doing about it. *Physiol. Meas.* **2015**, *36*, 1067–1073. [CrossRef]
8. Lionheart, W.R. Uniqueness, shape, and dimension in EIT. *Ann. N. Y. Acad. Sci.* **1999**, *873*, 466–471. [CrossRef]
9. Lionheart, W.R. EIT reconstruction algorithms: Pitfalls, challenges and recent developments. *Physiol. Meas.* **2004**, *25*, 125. [CrossRef] [PubMed]
10. McEwan, A.; Cusick, G.; Holder, D. A review of errors in multi-frequency EIT instrumentation. *Physiol. Meas.* **2007**, *28*, S197. [CrossRef] [PubMed]
11. Chicheł, A.; Skowronek, J.; Kubaszewska, M.; Kanikowski, M. Hyperthermia–description of a method and a review of clinical applications. *Rep. Pract. Oncol. Radiother.* **2007**, *12*, 267–275. [CrossRef]
12. Lagendijk, J. Hyperthermia treatment planning. *Phys. Med. Biol.* **2000**, *45*, R61. [CrossRef]
13. Paulides, M.M.; Stauffer, P.R.; Neufeld, E.; Maccarini, P.F.; Kyriakou, A.; Canters, R.A.; Diederich, C.J.; Bakker, J.F.; Van Rhoon, G.C. Simulation techniques in hyperthermia treatment planning. *Int. J. Hyperth.* **2013**, *29*, 346–357. [CrossRef]
14. Rossmann, C.; Haemmerich, D. Review of temperature dependence of thermal properties, dielectric properties, and perfusion of biological tissues at hyperthermic and ablation temperatures. *Crit. Rev. Biomed. Eng.* **2014**, *42*, 467–492. [CrossRef] [PubMed]
15. Song, C.W. Effect of local hyperthermia on blood flow and microenvironment: A review. *Cancer Res.* **1984**, *44*, 4721s–4730s.
16. De Greef, M.; Kok, H.; Correia, D.; Bel, A.; Crezee, J. Optimization in hyperthermia treatment planning: The impact of tissue perfusion uncertainty. *Med. Phys.* **2010**, *37*, 4540–4550. [CrossRef]
17. Numan, W.C.; Hofstetter, L.W.; Kotek, G.; Bakker, J.F.; Fiveland, E.W.; Houston, G.C.; Kudielka, G.; Yeo, D.T.; Paulides, M.M. Exploration of MR-guided head and neck hyperthermia by phantom testing of a modified prototype applicator for use with proton resonance frequency shift thermometry. *Int. J. Hyperth.* **2014**, *30*, 184–191. [CrossRef] [PubMed]
18. Winter, L.; Oberacker, E.; Paul, K.; Ji, Y.; Oezerdem, C.; Ghadjar, P.; Thieme, A.; Budach, V.; Wust, P.; Niendorf, T. Magnetic resonance thermometry: Methodology, pitfalls and practical solutions. *Int. J. Hyperth.* **2016**, *32*, 63–75. [CrossRef]
19. Esrick, M.; McRae, D. The effect of hyperthermia-induced tissue conductivity changes on electrical impedance temperature mapping. *Phys. Med. Biol.* **1994**, *39*, 133. [CrossRef] [PubMed]
20. Paulsen, K.; Moskowitz, M.; Ryan, T.; Mitchell, S.; Hoopes, P. Initial in vivo experience with EIT as a thermal estimator during hyperthermia. *Int. J. Hyperth.* **1996**, *12*, 573–591. [CrossRef]
21. Conway, J.; Hawley, M.; Seagar, A.; Brown, B.; Barber, D. Applied potential tomography (APT) for noninvasive thermal imaging during hyperthermia treatment. *Electron. Lett.* **1985**, *21*, 836–838. [CrossRef]
22. Conway, J.; Hawley, M.; Mangnall, Y.; Amasha, H.; Van Rhoon, G. Experimental assessment of electrical impedance imaging for hyperthermia monitoring. *Clin. Phys. Physiol. Meas.* **1992**, *13*, 185. [CrossRef] [PubMed]
23. Gersing, E.; Kruger, W.; Osypka, M.; Vaupel, P. Problems involved in temperature measurements using EIT. *Physiol. Meas.* **1995**, *16*, A153. [CrossRef]
24. Moskowitz, M.; Ryan, T.; Paulsen, K.; Mitchell, S. Clinical implementation of electrical impedance tomography with hyperthermia. *Int. J. Hyperth.* **1995**, *11*, 141–149. [CrossRef] [PubMed]
25. Gersing, E. Monitoring Temperature-Induced Changes in Tissue during Hyperthermia by Impedance Methods a. *Ann. N. Y. Acad. Sci.* **1999**, *873*, 13–20. [CrossRef]
26. Katrioplas, K.; Samaras, T. Monitoring of microwave ablation treatment with electrical impedance tomography. In Proceedings of the 2018 EMF-Med 1st World Conference on Biomedical Applications of Electromagnetic Fields (EMF-Med), Split, Croatia, 10–13 September 2018; pp. 1–2.
27. Nguyen, D.M.; Qian, P.; Barry, T.; McEwan, A. The region-of-interest based measurement selection process for electrical impedance tomography in radiofrequency cardiac ablation with known anatomical information. *Biomed. Signal Process. Control* **2020**, *56*, 101706. [CrossRef]
28. Nguyen, D.M.; Andersen, T.; Qian, P.; Barry, T.; McEwan, A. Electrical Impedance Tomography for monitoring cardiac radiofrequency ablation: A scoping review of an emerging technology. *Med. Eng. Phys.* **2020**, *84*, 36–50. [CrossRef]
29. Bottiglieri, A.; Dunne, J.; McDermott, B.; Cavagnaro, M.; Porter, E.; Farina, L. Monitoring Microwave Thermal Ablation using Electrical Impedance Tomography: An experimental feasibility study. In Proceedings of the 2020 14th European Conference on Antennas and Propagation (EuCAP), Copenhagen, Denmark, 15–20 March 2020; pp. 1–5.
30. Vauhkonen, M.; Lionheart, W.R.; Heikkinen, L.M.; Vauhkonen, P.J.; Kaipio, J.P. A MATLAB package for the EIDORS project to reconstruct two-dimensional EIT images. *Physiol. Meas.* **2001**, *22*, 107. [CrossRef]
31. Adler, A.; Boyle, A.; Crabb, M.; Grychtol, B.; Lionheart, W.; Tregidgo, H.; Yerworth, R. EIDORS Version 3.9. In Proceedings of the 18th International Conference on Biomedical Applications of Electrical Impedance Tomography (EIT2017), Thayer School of Engineering at Dartmouth, Hanover, NH, USA, 21–24 June 2017.
32. Withey, D.J.; Koles, Z.J. A review of medical image segmentation: Methods and available software. *Int. J. Bioelectromagn.* **2008**, *10*, 125–148.
33. Hasgall, P.; Di Gennaro, F.; Baumgartner, C.; Neufeld, E.; Lloyd, B.; Gosselin, M.; Payne, D.; Klingenböck, A.; Kuster, N. IT'IS Database for Thermal and Electromagnetic Parameters of Biological Tissues. Technical Report VIP21000-04-0, Version 4.0. 15 May 2018. Available online: www.itis.swiss/database (accessed on 11 May 2021).
34. Adler, A.; Arnold, J.H.; Bayford, R.; Borsic, A.; Brown, B.; Dixon, P.; Faes, T.J.; Frerichs, I.; Gagnon, H.; Gärber, Y.; et al. GREIT: A unified approach to 2D linear EIT reconstruction of lung images. *Physiol. Meas.* **2009**, *30*, S35. [CrossRef]

35. Gosselin, M.C.; Neufeld, E.; Moser, H.; Huber, E.; Farcito, S.; Gerber, L.; Jedensjö, M.; Hilber, I.; Di Gennaro, F.; Lloyd, B.; et al. Development of a new generation of high-resolution anatomical models for medical device evaluation: The Virtual Population 3.0. *Phys. Med. Biol.* **2014**, *59*, 5287. [CrossRef] [PubMed]
36. Adler, A.; Lionheart, W.R. Uses and abuses of EIDORS: An extensible software base for EIT. *Physiol. Meas.* **2006**, *27*, S25. [CrossRef]
37. Cheney, M.; Isaacson, D.; Newell, J.C.; Simske, S.; Goble, J. NOSER: An algorithm for solving the inverse conductivity problem. *Int. J. Imaging Syst. Technol.* **1990**, *2*, 66–75. [CrossRef]
38. Adler, A.; Guardo, R. Electrical impedance tomography: Regularized imaging and contrast detection. *IEEE Trans. Med. Imaging* **1996**, *15*, 170–179. [CrossRef]
39. Adler, A.; Dai, T.; Lionheart, W.R. Temporal image reconstruction in electrical impedance tomography. *Physiol. Meas.* **2007**, *28*, S1. [CrossRef] [PubMed]
40. Barber, D.; Brown, B. Errors in reconstruction of resistivity images using a linear reconstruction technique. *Clin. Phys. Physiol. Meas.* **1988**, *9*, 101. [CrossRef] [PubMed]
41. Pennes, H.H. Analysis of tissue and arterial blood temperatures in the resting human forearm. *J. Appl. Physiol.* **1948**, *1*, 93–122. [CrossRef]
42. Tobias, A.; Mohiuddin, S.S. Physiology, Water Balance. In *StatPearls [Internet]*; StatPearls Publishing: Treasure Island, FL, USA, 2019.
43. Lang, J.; Erdmann, B.; Seebass, M. Impact of nonlinear heat transfer on temperature control in regional hyperthermia. *IEEE Trans. Biomed. Eng.* **1999**, *46*, 1129–1138. [CrossRef] [PubMed]
44. Pontiga, F.; Gaytán, S.P. An experimental approach to the fundamental principles of hemodynamics. *Adv. Physiol. Educ.* **2005**, *29*, 165–171. [CrossRef] [PubMed]
45. Yeung, C.J.; Atalar, E. A Green's function approach to local rf heating in interventional MRI. *Med. Phys.* **2001**, *28*, 826–832. [CrossRef] [PubMed]
46. Duck, F. *Physical Properties of Tissue: A Comprehensive Reference Book*; Academic Press: London, UK, 1990.
47. Kiber, M.; Barber, D.; Brown, B. Estimation of object boundary shape from the voltage gradient measurements. In Proceedings of the A Meeting on Electrical Impedance Tomography, Copenhagen, Denmark, 14–16 July 1990; pp. 52–59.
48. Kolehmainen, V.; Lassas, M.; Ola, P. The inverse conductivity problem with an imperfectly known boundary. *SIAM J. Appl. Math.* **2005**, *66*, 365–383. [CrossRef]
49. Soleimani, M.; Gómez-Laberge, C.; Adler, A. Imaging of conductivity changes and electrode movement in EIT. *Physiol. Meas.* **2006**, *27*, S103. [CrossRef] [PubMed]

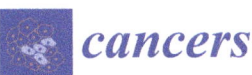

Article

A Novel Framework for the Optimization of Simultaneous ThermoBrachyTherapy

Ioannis Androulakis [1,*], Rob M. C. Mestrom [2], Miranda E. M. C. Christianen [1], Inger-Karine K. Kolkman-Deurloo [1] and Gerard C. van Rhoon [1,3,*]

1. Department of Radiotherapy, Erasmus MC Cancer Institute, University Medical Center Rotterdam, 3015 Rotterdam, The Netherlands; m.christianen@erasmusmc.nl (M.E.M.C.C.); i.kolkman-deurloo@erasmusmc.nl (I.-K.K.K.-D.)
2. Department of Electrical Engineering, Eindhoven University of Technology, 5600 Eindhoven, The Netherlands; r.m.c.mestrom@tue.nl
3. Department of Radiation Science and Technology, Delft University of Technology, 2629 Delft, The Netherlands
* Correspondence: i.androulakis@erasmusmc.nl (I.A.); g.c.vanrhoon@erasmusmc.nl (G.C.v.R.)

Simple Summary: ThermoBrachyTherapy, a combination therapy where radiation and heat are simultaneously applied using needle-shaped applicators from within the target, is a potentially very effective treatment for prostate cancer. When radiation and thermal therapies are applied, the dose coverage of each treatment is preplanned without considering the combined effect of the two dose distributions. In this study, we propose a method to automatically plan the thermal dose in such a treatment, based on the combined effect with the radiation. Furthermore, we apply the method on 10 patients and compare the treatment to a brachytherapy-only treatment plan. In this way, we show that, with properly optimized ThermoBrachyTherapy, we can provide equivalent combined dose coverages to the prostate, while reducing the dose delivered to critical organs surrounding the prostate, which might translate to reduced toxicity of the treatment.

Abstract: In high-dose-rate brachytherapy (HDR-BT) for prostate cancer treatment, interstitial hyperthermia (IHT) is applied to sensitize the tumor to the radiation (RT) dose, aiming at a more efficient treatment. Simultaneous application of HDR-BT and IHT is anticipated to provide maximum radiosensitization of the tumor. With this rationale, the ThermoBrachyTherapy applicators have been designed and developed, enabling simultaneous irradiation and heating. In this research, we present a method to optimize the three-dimensional temperature distribution for simultaneous HDR-BT and IHT based on the resulting equivalent physical dose (EQD_{phys}) of the combined treatment. First, the temperature resulting from each electrode is precomputed. Then, for a given set of electrode settings and a precomputed radiation dose, the EQD_{phys} is calculated based on the temperature-dependent linear-quadratic model. Finally, the optimum set of electrode settings is found through an optimization algorithm. The method is applied on implant geometries and anatomical data of 10 previously irradiated patients, using reported thermoradiobiological parameters and physical doses. We found that an equal equivalent dose coverage of the target can be achieved with a physical RT dose reduction of 20% together with a significantly lower EQD_{phys} to the organs at risk (p-value < 0.001), even in the least favorable scenarios. As a result, simultaneous ThermoBrachyTherapy could lead to a relevant therapeutic benefit for patients with prostate cancer.

Keywords: hyperthermia; induced; brachytherapy; prostatic neoplasms; interstitial hyperthermia; treatment plan optimization; prostate; thermoradiotherapy; linear quadratic model; biological modeling

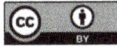

1. Introduction

High-dose-rate brachytherapy (HDR-BT) is a well-established treatment option in localized prostate cancer treatment [1]. Radiobiological clinical data have shown that prostate cancer, in contrast to most tumor sites, has a very low α/β ratio (α/β = 0.9–2.2 Gy) [2]. This is a value very close to or lower than the α/β of nearby organs at risk (OAR), with the urethra estimated at an α/β = 0.5–1 Gy [3] and the rectum estimated at an α/β = 1.6–3.1 Gy [4], depending on the considered toxicity endpoint. This very low α/β ratio is the reason that radiotherapy for prostate cancer is aimed towards hypofractionation, with extensive use of HDR-BT as a boost to external beam radiation therapy (EBRT) or even as a standalone therapy (monotherapy) [5,6].

In HDR-BT monotherapy for prostate cancer, several clinical trials have shown that even ultrahypofractionated treatments of 2–4 fractions lead to excellent overall disease-free survival in low-risk and favorable intermediate-risk cancer patients [6–8]. On the other hand, the treatments are still linked with genitourinary and gastrointestinal toxicities [9]. Moreover, further reduction to a single fraction treatment has shown very poor results in multiple studies, with the reasons for those poor results not yet clear. Furthermore, ultrahypofractionated HDR-BT monotherapy is currently not recommended in higher-risk patients [10,11].

The abovementioned drawbacks could be overcome if the treatment could further escalate the radiation dose in the prostate without affecting the OAR, or if the same dose could be reached in the prostate with a reduced dose in the OAR. A way to achieve this could be by selective target radiosensitization. One of the most potent sensitizers to radiation is hyperthermia [12,13]. It has also been shown in clinical data that hyperthermia reduces the α/β of tumors [14] and, hence, makes the tumors more favorable to hypofractionation. This is also evident in multiple in vitro experiments on specific prostate cancer cell lines [15–17]. Other than that, the ability of hyperthermia to increase perfusion, increase reoxygenation, and overcome radiation-resistant hypoxia [18] could enable a reinvestigation of single fraction treatments, since the lack of reoxygenation and hypoxic cells are presumed to be a possible cause of failure, according to Morton and Hoskin [19].

Together with HDR-BT, interstitial hyperthermia (IHT) can be used to sensitize the target [20]. This is especially convenient if the same catheters used for the HDR-BT treatment can also be used for the IHT application. IHT has been applied in various early clinical trials [21,22] and, lately, in a phase II clinical trial ongoing for salvage prostate cancer treatment [23], where three fractions of IHT (1 h at 40–43 °C) followed by 10 Gy HDR-BT were applied over three weeks.

Historical biological research has clearly shown that thermal radiosensitization depends on the time interval between radiation and hyperthermia, with the highest radiosensitization reached at simultaneous (i.e., radiation during hyperthermia) application of the two modalities [13,24]. Based on this rationale, we have developed novel Thermo-Brachytherapy (TBT) applicators that enable the simultaneous application of HDR-BT and capacitive coupled radiofrequency (CC-RF) interstitial heating [25]. The improved temperature-related technical characteristics of these applicators are described in our earlier publication [25].

The challenge in simultaneous thermal radiosensitization is that, according to Overgaard [26], normal tissue might be sensitized as much as the target tissue. Hence, in order to reach a therapeutic benefit with simultaneous application of the two modalities, both treatment modalities need to be confined to the target as much as possible [27]. In prostate cancer treatment, this is a challenging task, with OAR very close to (rectum, bladder) or in direct contact with (urethra) the target volume. Therefore, very precise treatment plan optimization is needed to reach a therapeutic benefit, taking into account the combined effect of both hyperthermia and radiation.

In recent years, substantial progress has been made in theoretical modeling to calculate and quantify the combined effect of radiation and hyperthermia [28–31]. Most notably, this has resulted in the temperature-dependent linear-quadratic (TDLQ) model [29] and its extended version, including direct temperature-induced cytotoxicity [30]. While these models have been used to evaluate existing treatment plans retrospectively, there has been no attempt for pretreatment plan optimization based on the combined effect of radiation and hyperthermia.

In general, research on IHT treatment plan (IHT-TP) optimization is limited and rarely applied in clinical practice [20]. In [32], Chen et al. proposed an automated optimization algorithm for ultrasound-based IHT-TP. In [33], Salgaonkar et al. validated temperature superpositioning for faster optimization of ultrasound-based IHT-TP. In [34], Kok et al. proposed a framework for fast automated temperature optimization using basic temperature-based objective functions that can also be applied on CC-RF IHT. In [35], we validated a highly accurate fast calculation method for the power deposition of the TBT applicators. The next step in producing fast IHT-TP is to automate the treatment planning process.

This study presents the framework to optimize the IHT-TP parameters based on the equivalent RT dose resulting from the TDLQ model. This optimization framework is applied on real anatomical and implant data from 10 patients. The results demonstrate that, under clinically realistic circumstances, HDR-BT combined with simultaneous IHT using the TBT applicators has the potential to lead to a relevant therapeutic benefit in terms of OAR sparing or escalation of the equivalent physical dose.

2. Materials and Methods

2.1. Overview of Optimization Framework

In the following paragraphs, we detail all steps that constitute the optimization framework (Figure 1). To reach the optimal thermoradiobiological TBT plan, first, the planning CT images (Figure 1 Item 1) are used to create the patient tissue model (Figure 1 Item 2). The position of the TBT applicators is reconstructed, and the electromagnetic (EM) fields and temperature distributions are precomputed per electrode (Figure 1 Items 3 and 4). The dwell times and dwell positions, defining the physical radiation dose, are optimized autonomously using the standard clinical HDR-BT protocol and workflow (Figure 1 Item 5). The IHT-TP parameters are then optimized based on the combined effect of the temperature distribution and the radiation distribution (Figure 1 Item 8). To evaluate the combined effect in terms of equivalent physical dose (EQD_{phys}), the TDLQ model is applied (Figure 1 Item 6) with thermoradiobiological parameters from the literature. The optimization uses the standard clinical objectives and constraints as applied in the HDR-BT-only plans (Figure 1 Item 7).

2.2. Patient Anatomy Modeling

The patient tissues are modeled (Figure 1 Item 2) using information derived from computed tomography (CT) images taken as for HDR-BT planning (Figure 1 Item 1), with the dual function TBT applicators implanted into the patient. Prostate, urethra, rectum, bladder, bone, fat, muscle, and air volumes are distinguished. Prostate, urethra, rectum, and bladder volumes are defined by manual segmentation by an expert radiotherapy technologist using Oncentra® Brachy (Elekta Brachytherapy Solutions, Veenendaal, The Netherlands), and approved by a radiation oncologist. For the other tissues, an automated workflow, based on thresholding, developed for clinical deep hyperthermia treatment planning is used (MIM Software, Cleveland, OH, USA). An example CT image with implanted afterloading catheters instead of TBT applicators can be seen in Figure 2a. The corresponding tissue model on the same slice can be seen in Figure 2b. The TBT applicator visualization and positioning are expected to be identical to the afterloading catheters used in standard HDR-BT treatment.

2.3. TBT Applicator Modeling, Positioning, and E-Field Calculation

Each TBT applicator consists of two 20-mm-long cylindrical electrodes with a 5-mm separation deposited on a needle-shaped flexible polyoxymethylene afterloading catheter and coated with a thin Parylene C coating. The two electrodes are connected to a power source through two feeding lines running parallel to the catheter up to the proximal end of the applicator. A detailed description of the applicator can be found in [25]. In the patient model, the TBT applicators are located and reconstructed as shown in the planning CT images (Figure 2c).

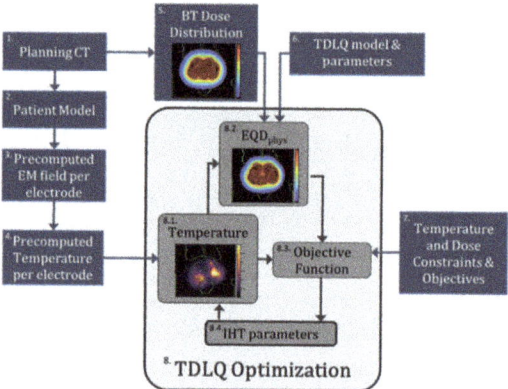

Figure 1. Graphical summary of the proposed optimization framework. 1. The planning CT is the initial input of the process. 2. The patient model is generated. 3. The EM field per electrode is precalculated. 4. The temperature distribution per electrode is precalculated. 5. The BT dose distribution is imported from the BT treatment planning software. 6. The TDLQ model is used for the calculation of the combined effect. 7. Both temperature and dose constraints and objectives are used for the optimization process. 8. The TDLQ optimization process optimizes the IHT parameters (8.4) that generate a temperature distribution (8.1) from which an EQD$_{phys}$ distribution is generated (8.2). This EQD$_{phys}$ distribution is used to compute the objective function, which needs to be minimized (8.3).

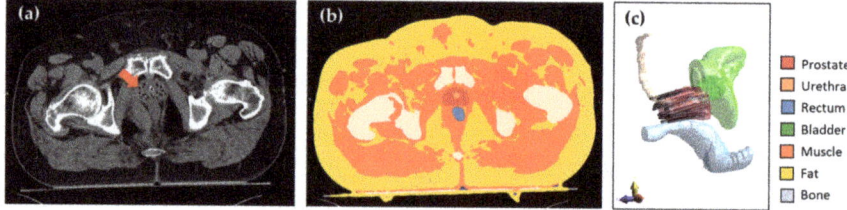

Figure 2. (a) Axial CT slice showing the anatomy of a patient with afterloading catheters (visible as black dots indicated by the arrow) inserted in the prostate. (b) Same axial slice of the resulting patient model after segmentation of all tissues. (c) Lateral 3D view of the prostate, OAR, and simulated TBT applicators in the same patient.

The electric field (E-field) is calculated for each electrode i as described in [35], using a finite element method solver for the electroquasistatic approximation [36]:

$$\nabla \cdot (\sigma + j2\pi f \varepsilon)\nabla V_i = 0, \quad (1a)$$

$$E_i = -\nabla V_i \quad (1b)$$

where σ is the electrical conductivity, f is the frequency of the alternating E-field, ε is the dielectric permittivity, and V_i is the scalar potential of electrode i. The E-field E_i is calculated for each electrode from Equation (1b).

For a set of n different electrodes i, with amplitude settings v_i, all E_i can be superposed to obtain the total E-field E_{tot} as:

$$E_{tot} = \sum_{i=1}^{n} E\, v_i = \mathbf{Ev}. \tag{2}$$

The power loss density (P) produced by the total field can then be derived from:

$$P = \sigma \frac{|E_{tot}|^2}{2} = \frac{\sigma}{2}\mathbf{v}^H \mathbf{E}^H \mathbf{E v} = \mathbf{v}^H \mathbf{P v}, \tag{3}$$

where $\mathbf{P}$ is an $n \times n$ matrix, and $\mathbf{E}^H$ and $\mathbf{v}^H$ are the Hermitian transpose of $\mathbf{E}$ and $\mathbf{v}$, respectively.

For the E-field calculation (Figure 1 Item 3), the electric tissue properties are assigned according to the IT'IS database [37]. The electric properties of all used tissues, as well as those of the TBT applicator materials, are summarized in Table 1. All E-field and power calculations are performed in Sim4Life v6.2 (ZMT, Zurich, Switzerland).

Table 1. Electric and thermal properties of the applicator materials and the tissues used in the simulations.

Tissue	ρ (kg/m³)	σ @27 MHz (S/m)	ε_r @27 MHz	c (J/kg/K)	k (W/m/K)	ω (ml/kg/min)
Applicator Dielectric [38,39]	1289	1×10^{-5}	2.4	712	0.084	-
Air [37]	1.164	0	1.0	1004	0.0273	-
Muscle [37]	1090.4	0.654	95.8	3421	0.495	40
Fat [37]	911	0.061	17.9	2348	0.211	33
Bone [37]	1908	0.052	21.8	1313	0.320	10
Prostate [37]	1045	0.838	120.1	3760	0.512	394
Rectum [37]	1045	0.654	95.8	3801	0.557	0
Urethra [37]	1102	0.375	88.8	3306	0.462	394
Bladder [37]	1086	0.276	31.5	3581	0.522	78

2.4. Temperature Calculation and Superpositioning

The temperature distribution (T) resulting from all electrodes can be calculated by solving the Pennes' bioheat equation [40,41]:

$$\rho c \frac{\partial T}{\partial t} = \nabla \cdot (k \nabla T) + \rho Q + P - \rho_b c_b \rho \omega (T - T_b) \tag{4}$$

where k is the thermal conductivity, c is the specific heat capacity, Q denotes the specific metabolic heat generation rate, and ω is the perfusion rate. ρ is the mass density of the medium. T_b, ρ_b, and c_b are the temperature, mass density, and specific heat capacity of blood, respectively. According to Das et al. [42], the temperature solution can be rewritten as:

$$T = \mathbf{v}^H \mathbf{T v} + T \tag{5}$$

where $\mathbf{T}$, similar to $\mathbf{P}$ in (3), is an $n \times n$ matrix, and T_b is equal to the baseline temperature in the case of Dirichlet boundary conditions.

A fast optimization process is essential when applying simultaneous HDR-BT and IHT. To achieve faster temperature optimization, we use temperature superpositioning per electrode (Figure 1 Item 4), as proposed by Salgaonkar et al. for ultrasound-based IHT-TP [33]. In this method, all off-diagonal terms of $\mathbf{T}$ are neglected, reducing the complexity of the problem. With ΔT_i, the temperature increase resulting from the power loss density P_i, Equation (5) is simplified to:

$$T = \sum_{i=1}^{n} v_i^2 \Delta T + T_b \tag{6}$$

Under the above assumption (temperature superpositioning per electrode), the temperature T_i generated by each electrode i can be computed by solving the Pennes' bioheat Equation as in (4). The precomputed temperature distributions per electrode were calculated using a finite element method (FEM) solver in Sim4Life v6.2 (ZMT, Zurich, Switzerland).

2.5. HDR-BT Treatment Plan and Dose Calculation

The HDR-BT treatment planning protocol is defined using dose–volume metrics. The prescribed radiation dose (D_p) needs to be reached in at least 95% of the total target volume ($V_{100\%} \geq 95\%$). For the OAR, the dose in a particular volume x (D_x) is constrained to an organ-specific limit. The detailed HDR-BT treatment planning protocol is summarized in Table 2 and is based on [8].

Table 2. Fraction dose objectives and constraints of the clinical HDR-BT protocol.

Tissue	Criterion	Aim	Type
Prostate	$V_{100\%}$	$\geq 95\%$	Objective
	$V_{150\%}$	$<30\%$	Soft Constraint
	$V_{200\%}$	$<8\%$	Soft Constraint
Urethra	$D_{0.1cc}$	$<115\%$	Hard Constraint
Rectum	D_{1cc}	$<75\%$	Hard Constraint
Bladder	D_{1cc}	$<75\%$	Soft Constraint

The HDR-BT treatment plan (Figure 1 Item 5) is generated by expert radiotherapy technologists, based on inverse planning by simulated annealing [43] and manual finetuning, using the Oncentra® Brachy treatment planning software, and reviewed by a radiation oncologist. The HDR-BT treatment plan is based solely on the radiation dose generated by an HDR ^{192}Ir Flexisource, without considering the effect of the IHT. For the radiation dose calculation, a dose kernel based on the TG-43 standard is used [44].

2.6. Thermoradiobiological Modeling

To calculate the combined effect of the radiation and hyperthermia dose, thermoradiobiological modeling was performed (Figure 1 Item 6). The TDLQ model was applied [29]:

$$S(D,T) = \exp\left[-\alpha(T) \cdot D - \beta(T) \cdot D^2\right], \quad (7)$$

where $S(D,T)$ is the surviving fraction of tissue when simultaneously exposed to a radiation dose D and a temperature T for 1 h, assuming that the parameters $\alpha(T)$ and $\beta(T)$ are exponentially dependent on the temperature according to:

$$\alpha(T) = \alpha(37) \cdot \exp\left[\frac{T-37}{T_{ref}-37} \cdot \ln\left[\frac{\alpha(T_{ref})}{\alpha(37)}\right]\right], \quad (8a)$$

$$\beta(T) = \beta(37) \cdot \exp\left[\frac{T-37}{T_{ref}-37} \cdot \ln\left[\frac{\beta(T_{ref})}{\beta(37)}\right]\right], \quad (8b)$$

where T_{ref} is a reference temperature at which the $\alpha(T_{ref})$ and $\beta(T_{ref})$ have known values.

With this model, the equivalent dose received by a tissue, taking the thermal radiosensitization into account, is:

$$EQD_{ref} = \frac{\alpha(T) \cdot D + G \cdot \beta(T) \cdot D^2}{\alpha(37) + \beta(37) \cdot d_{ref}}, \quad (9)$$

where d_{ref} is the fraction dose to which the dose is normalized, and G is the Lea-Catcheside dose protraction factor, which is equal to 1 for a high dose rate source.

In our implementation, the equivalent dose is calculated normalized to the physical dose D. From Equations (8) and (9), this is calculated as:

$$EQD_{phys} = \frac{\frac{\alpha(37)}{\beta(37)} exp\left[\frac{T-37}{T_{ref}-37} \cdot ln\left[\frac{\alpha(T_{ref})}{\alpha(37)}\right]\right] \cdot D + exp\left[\frac{T-37}{T_{ref}-37} \cdot ln\left[\frac{\beta(T_{ref})}{\beta(37)}\right]\right] \cdot D^2}{\frac{\alpha(37)}{\beta(37)} + D} \quad (10)$$

where the values of the radiobiological parameter $\alpha/\beta = \alpha(37)/\beta(37)$, and the thermoradiobiological parameters $\alpha(T_{ref})/\alpha(37)$ and $\beta(T_{ref})/\beta(37)$ for a given temperature T_{ref} are needed for each tissue. The thermoradiobiological parameters for prostate tissue are assigned according to the in vitro data on the PC-3 and DU-145 prostate cancer cell lines in Pajonk et al. [16]. For normal tissues, there are no thermoradiobiological data available. Based on Overgaard [26], we can assume α and β parameters of normal tissue to have a similar thermal radiosensitization pattern as tumor tissue for the setting of simultaneous irradiation and hyperthermia; hence, we assigned the same $\alpha(T_{ref})/\alpha(37)$ and $\beta(T_{ref})/\beta(37)$ values to normal tissue. The radiobiological parameter α/β is conservatively set equal to 3 for all tissues at a normal temperature of 37 °C [45]. The values of all parameters are summarized in Table 3. Note that, in all following dose volume and dose coverage criteria in this article, dose is quantified in terms of EQD_{phys}, which is temperature-dependent in the case of TBT and equal to the physical dose, D, in the case of BT only.

Table 3. Thermoradiobiological parameters applied in this study, with T_{ref} = 43 °C.

Tissue	$\alpha(37)/\beta(37)$	$\alpha(43)/\alpha(37)$	$\beta(43)/\beta(37)$
Prostate	3		
PC-3 [16]		2.4	6.8
DU-145 [16]		0.8	1.8
Normal Tissue	3		

2.7. Thermoradiobiological Objective Function and Optimization Algorithm

For the optimization of the electrode amplitudes v_i in the TBT treatment, an equivalent physical dose (EQD_{phys}) based optimization algorithm is used (Figure 1 Item 8). The objectives are based on the criteria as reported in Table 2, combined with an overall upper temperature limit of T_{max} = 47.5 °C [20]. This is formulated in a minimization problem containing penalty functions PF_i for every violated constraint i, and objective scoring functions SF_j that return lower values for better performance for an objective j:

$$\Omega = W \sum_i PF_i + \sum_j SF_j. \quad (11)$$

The penalty functions PF_i are in the form of:

$$PF_i = \max[0, p_i(C - L_i)], \quad (12a)$$

where the values for C_i and L_i are according to Table 4 and the polarity factor p_i is +1 for low pass constraints and −1 for high pass constraints. The scoring functions SF_j are in the form of:

$$SF_i = -w_j|O_j - G_j|, \quad (12b)$$

where the values for O_j, G_j, and w_j are according to Table 4 (Figure 1 Item 7). The penalty weight factor W is set to a constant $W = 10^3$ for all constraints in order to ensure a high penalty for every constraint violation. The objective function Ω is minimized using a particle swarm optimization algorithm in MATLAB (MathWorks Inc., Natick, MA, USA).

2.8. Temperature Superpositioning Validation

While the temperature superpositioning method for fast temperature calculations has been validated for interstitial ultrasound power sources [33], we also perform a validation in our approach. To validate the accuracy of the temperature superpositioning method, we calculated a temperature distribution using the superpositioning method and we recalculated the temperature distribution resulting from the same power amplitudes using the FEM solver. In this way, we investigated the assumption of Equation (4) that the off-diagonal terms in **T** not contributing significantly to the total temperature distribution is correct. The agreement between the two calculation methods was scored using three-dimensional γ-index analysis [46,47].

Table 4. Constraints and objectives applied in the objective function.

Constraints	Tissue	Criterion (C_i)	Limit (L_i)	Type
	Prostate	$V_{100\%}$	Value of BT-only	High pass
	Urethra	$D_{0.1cc}$	Value of BT-only	Low pass
	Rectum	D_{1cc}	Value of BT-only	Low pass
	Bladder	D_{1cc}	Value of BT-only	Low pass
	All	T_{max}	47.5 °C	Low pass
Objectives	**Tissue**	**Criterion (O_j)**	**Goal (G_j)**	**Weight (w_i)**
	Urethra	$D_{0.1cc}$	0	1
	Rectum	D_{1cc}	0	1
	Prostate	$V_{150\%}$	30% of volume	0.01

2.9. Implementation on Patient Data

To evaluate the proposed TBT treatment plan, we used data of 10 prostate cancer patients treated at our institution with HDR-BT monotherapy in two fractions of D_p = 13.5 Gy in a single day with a single implantation. For the first fraction, the patients were treated with a US-based HDR-BT treatment and, for the second fraction, they were treated with a CT-based HDR-BT treatment [35]. To validate the implementation of our treatment plan, we simulated a replacement for the second fraction by a TBT treatment and compared the resulting EQD_{phys} distribution to the original HDR-BT-only physical dose distribution by assuming that the TBT applicators are placed at the same position as the flexible 6F ProGuide afterloading needles (Elekta Brachytherapy Solutions, Veenendaal, The Netherlands).

The TBT treatment plan used a uniformly scaled-down version of the original HDR-BT dose distribution that had been clinically generated [35]. Different plans were generated using various combinations for the thermoradiobiological parameters $\alpha(43)/\alpha(37)$ and $\beta(43)/\beta(37)$, according to Table 3. The BT dose distributions were scaled from 70% to 95% of the original clinical dose. This process is illustrated in Figure 3.

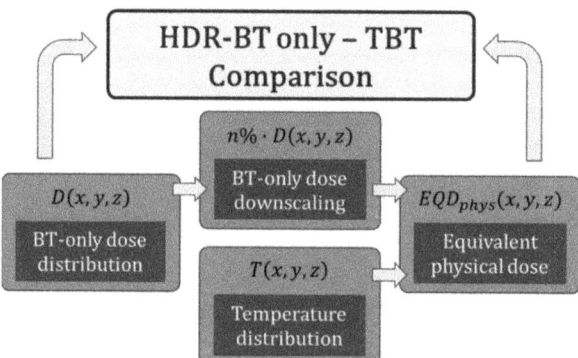

Figure 3. Flowchart illustrating how the TBT EQD_{phys} distribution is generated from and compared with the original BT-only dose distribution.

3. Results

3.1. Temperature Superpositioning Validation

The temperature distribution in a simulated patient with 18 applicators with given electrode amplitudes was calculated using both the superpositioning method (Figure 4a) and an FEM recalculation (Figure 4b). With the FEM-recalculated temperature as a reference, a γ-index analysis was performed. Applying 5%/0.5 mm dose difference and distance to agreement criteria, a passing rate >95% was observed, suggesting a good match to the reference (Figure 4c). As can be seen in Figure 4c, the highest gamma index values were positioned in the far-field of the temperature increase, where temperature values were low.

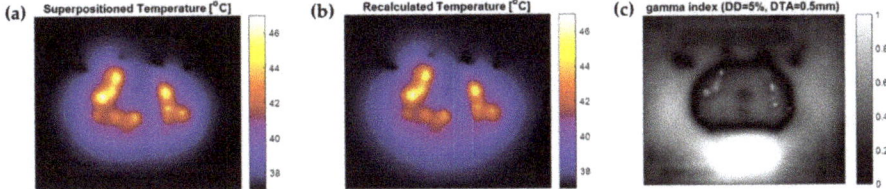

Figure 4. Comparison between superpositioned temperature calculation and FEM recalculation on the central axial slice in the prostate. (**a**) Temperature map using superpositioning of separate FEM calculations for each electrode. (**b**) Temperature map using a single FEM calculation for the same, combined, electrode settings. (**c**) γ-index map of the comparison.

3.2. Thermal Radiosensitization

To illustrate the thermal radiosensitization that is expected in prostate cancer cells, we applied the values of Table 3 to Equation (10) and visualized the results for different radiation doses and temperatures. How those values affect the EQD_{phys} dose resulting from a TBT treatment can be seen in Figure 5. As can be seen, there is a considerable difference in thermal radiosensitization between the PC-3 and DU-145 cell lines. Indicatively, the thermal enhancement caused by a 43 °C temperature in PC-3 is approximately threefold that of DU-145.

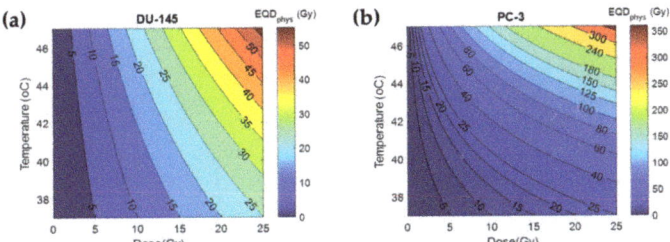

Figure 5. Isodose curves for the EQD_{phys} resulting from different combinations of physical dose and temperature for 1 h: (**a**) EQD_{phys} assuming DU-145 data; (**b**) EQD_{phys} assuming PC-3 data.

3.3. Treatment Planning Results

We optimized the temperature distribution for the 10 simulated patient plans for different scalings of the HDR-BT dose. Figure 6 shows the results for a single patient with an HDR-BT dose scaling of 80%. The $\alpha(43)/\alpha(37)$ and $\beta(43)/\beta(37)$ values are assumed equal to the average between DU-145 and PC-3 data, which gives $\alpha(43)/\alpha(37) = 1.6$ and $\beta(43)/\beta(37) = 4.3$. The EQD_{phys} volume histogram shows that the same target coverage is reached (96.6%), while $D_{0.1cc}$ for the urethra, and D_{1cc} for the rectum and bladder are reduced by 6.1%, 4.9%, and 8.2% of the prescribed dose, respectively. On the other hand, the $V_{150\%}$ and $V_{200\%}$ are higher by 12.1% and 12.4% of prostate volume, respectively.

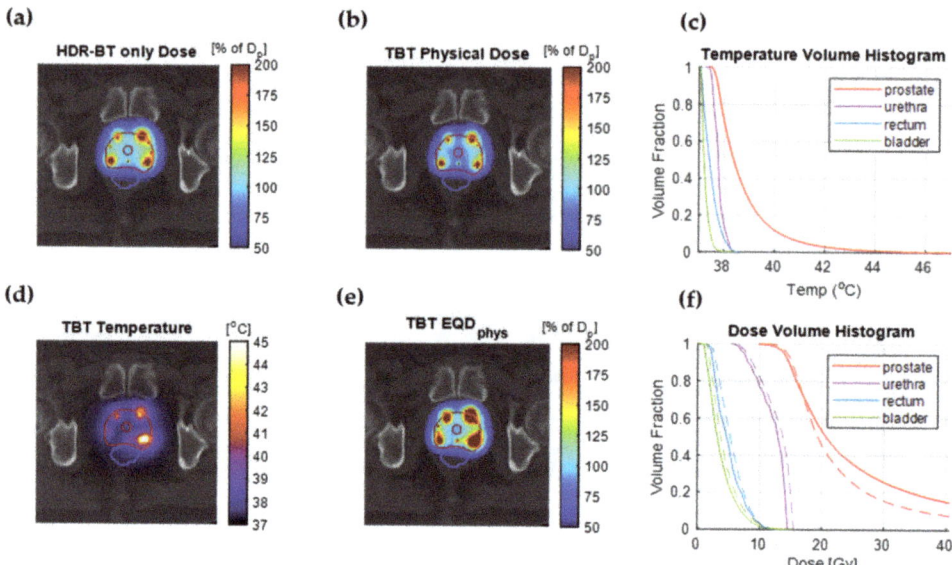

Figure 6. TBT TP results assuming thermoradiobiological parameters equal to the average between DU-145 and PC-3 data. (**a**) The original clinically applied HDR-BT dose fraction. (**b**) The applied TBT physical dose (80% of original). (**c**) Temperature volume histogram showing the temperature coverage in the prostate and OARs. (**d**) The temperature distribution calculated for the optimal TBT plan. (**e**) The TBT EQD_{phys} resulting from the combined treatment. (**f**) Dose volume histogram of the prostate and OARs for the HDR-BT-only dose (dashed line) and the TBT EQD_{phys} dose (solid line).

Figure 7 summarizes the results over all simulated patients (showing average values and standard deviations) for the prostate. From this figure, it can be seen that the required target coverage can be reached when using at least 80% of the original physical dose of the HDR-BT-only treatment (Figure 7a) for the less thermosensitive DU-145 cells. This result is valid for all three evaluated values of $\alpha(43)/\alpha(37)$ and $\beta(43)/\beta(37)$: PC-3, DU-145, and average. For radiosensitization according to the more thermosensitive PC-3 cells, this is as low as 70% of the original physical dose. It is evident that the addition of IHT contributes to considerably higher values for $V_{150\%}$ and $V_{200\%}$. This should be expected, since the IHT sources and HDR-BT sources irradiate from the same positions: the TBT applicator.

Figure 8 shows the T_{10}, T_{50}, and T_{90} values (temperature reached in at least 10%, 50%, and 90% of the total volume, respectively) over all simulated patients. It is evident that higher T_{10}, T_{50}, and T_{90} values are required for lower physical doses and for lower thermal sensitivity of the tumor. Furthermore, T_{50} and T_{90} values are mainly under the 39 °C value. This means that hyperthermia values are not needed in the whole prostate to reach the optimal EQD_{phys} distribution. On the other hand, the temperature is, as is the radiation dose, per definition, heterogeneous in the prostate.

For the OAR there are no data available on their sensitivity. Therefore, we evaluated the dose metrics for two extreme cases: assuming sensitization as high as in tumor tissue [26] and assuming no sensitization. The actual sensitization is expected to be somewhere in between the two extreme values. The OAR dose metrics reached with the different TBT plans are visualized in Figure 9. For all evaluated cases, the $D_{0.1cc}$ of the urethra, the D_{1cc} of the rectum, and the D_{1cc} of the bladder are lower with the TBT plan than with the HDR-BT-only plan (p-value < 0.001, paired two-sided Wilcoxon signed rank test).

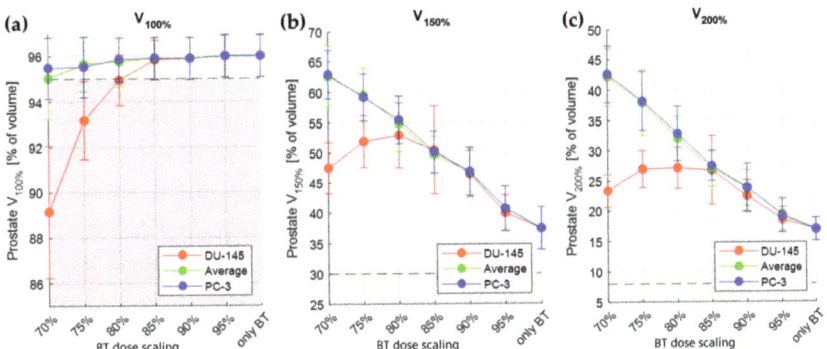

Figure 7. Average values (±standard deviation) over 10 simulated patients of TBT prostate $V_{100\%}$ (**a**), $V_{150\%}$ (**b**), and $V_{200\%}$ (**c**) for different scalings of the original HDR-BT dose. The different colors correspond to the plans generated based on different thermoradiotherapeutic values (red for DU-145, blue for PC-3, and green for the average between DU-145 and PC-3). It is evident that the original prostate coverage is met when the physical dose is scaled over 80% of the original value. The vertical bars correspond to standard deviation. The horizontal dashed lines correspond to the objective ($V_{100\%}$) and soft constraint ($V_{150\%}$ and $V_{200\%}$) limits. The green and red areas correspond to targeted and constrained values, respectively.

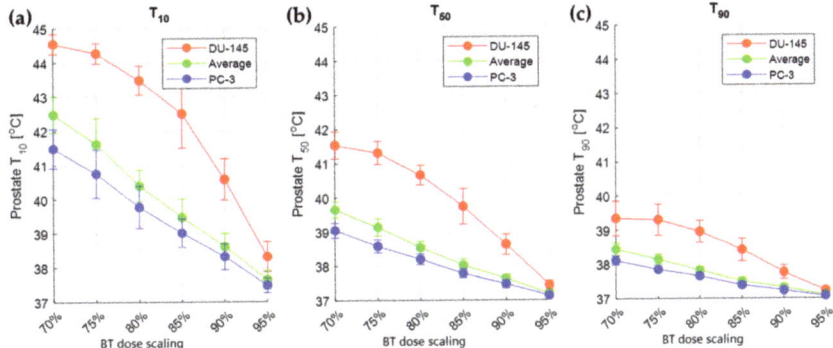

Figure 8. Average values (±standard deviation) over 10 simulated patients of the optimal TBT prostate T_{10} (**a**), T_{50} (**b**), and T_{90} (**c**) for different scalings of the original HDR-BT dose. The different colors correspond to the plans generated based on different thermoradiotherapeutic values (red for DU-145, blue for PC-3, and green for the average between DU-145 and PC-3). The vertical bars correspond to standard deviation.

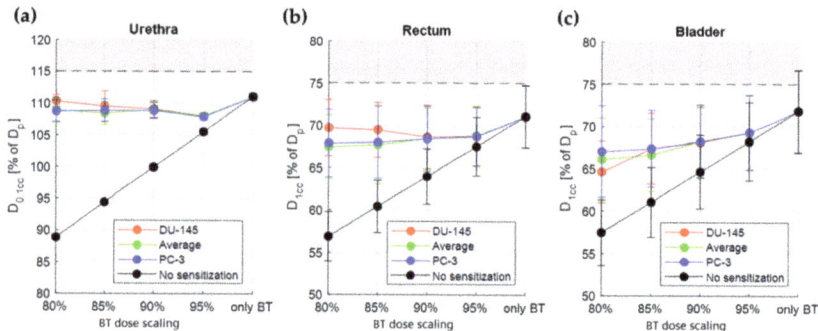

Figure 9. Average values (±standard deviation) over 10 simulated patients of the TBT TP parameters for different scaling of the original dose: urethra $D_{0.1cc}$ (**a**), rectum D_{1cc} (**b**), and bladder D_{1cc} (**c**). The different colors correspond to the plans generated based on different thermoradiotherapeutic values (red for DU-145, blue for PC-3, and green for the average between DU-145 and PC-3). The black line shows the lowest possible value, assuming no radiosensitization of the normal tissue. The horizontal dashed lines correspond to the constraint limit for each criterion. The red areas correspond to constrained values for each criterion.

4. Discussion

Extensive biological studies have indicated that hyperthermia is a potent sensitizer to radiotherapy, especially when applied simultaneously with the radiation dose [12,13]. To benefit from the high radiosensitization achieved in such a setting, both the thermal and radiation dose have to be focused sufficiently well to the target. In the TBT setting, both doses are administered from within the target region, which makes it the ideal method for simultaneous application. The highly localized deposition of both doses requires, however, good planning of the electrode amplitudes, dwell times, and dwell positions for good thermal and radiation coverage of the target and OAR sparing.

From a thermoradiobiological point of view, three-dimensional evaluation of combined radiotherapy and hyperthermia treatments is possible using the TDLQ model [29]. It is challenging to meet the set dose targets and constraints with the resulting EQD_{phys} without optimizing the temperature distribution according to those criteria. Given the high number of variables that need to be tuned, an automated method to optimize the temperature distribution is necessary for an optimal TBT treatment. Therefore, with the proposed optimization method, we can optimize the temperature on radiotherapeutic dose criteria.

To produce fast calculations of the temperature distribution, temperature superpositioning was used. We showed in our evaluation that this is a reasonable estimation of the temperature distribution, with a passing rate >95% for 5%/0.5 mm dose difference and distance to agreement criteria. It is important to note that the temperature calculation method showed the best results where high temperature elevations and consequently high radiosensitization were present (Figure 4), with the lower temperature regions mainly in the rectum showing less agreement with the single FEM temperature calculation. Therefore, with the current temperature calculation method, simulated rectum temperatures might not be reliable enough. For a more accurate estimation of the final temperature distribution, one could consider recalculating the final temperature distribution based on the optimal IHT-TP settings for evaluation purposes. Another option is to apply the method of Das et al. [42] (Equation (4)), although it would lead to slower optimizations due to the high number of electrodes producing an E-field.

We showed in our results (Figure 7) that the calculated TBT EQD_{phys} distribution can meet the prostate coverage $V_{100\%} \geq 95\%$ for different values of $\alpha(43)/\alpha(37)$ and $\beta(43)/\beta(37)$ with up to 20% decrease in physical dose (80% of original HDR-BT dose). For the required temperature elevations (Figure 8), it is evident that temperature homogeneity in the target

(Figure 6d) is not necessary to meet the prescribed target coverage. In the clinical feasibility study of the MECS applicator by van Vulpen et al. [48], it was noted that the observed high temperature gradients (T_{10} = 45.7 °C, T_{90} = 39.4 °C) were an undesired effect. By looking at the temperature distribution as a radiation dose sensitizer, we see that we can still reach significant improvements to the treatment, since only underdosed regions of the target are in need of a temperature increase.

Since there is no information available about the radiosensitization of normal tissues, we assumed in our optimization process a worst-case scenario of equal radiosensitization for normal and tumor tissue. With this assumption, we saw EQD_{phys} sparing for all three OAR (2.2 ± 1.7%, 2.6 ± 2.1%, and 4.2 ± 2.2% decrease for urethra $D_{0.1cc}$, rectum D_{1cc}, and bladder D_{1cc}, respectively). In practice, we can expect a lower normal tissue radiosensitization than tumor tissue radiosensitization, especially since human prostate cancer cells are remarkably thermosensitive [15]. Therefore, we also evaluated the maximum potential decrease in the OAR by assuming no thermal radiosensitization in normal tissue (Figure 9). It is evident that OAR sparing can be significant in such a scenario (i.e., urethra $D_{0.1cc}$ as low as 90% of D_p). To draw definitive conclusions on the level of OAR sparing, the availability of thermoradiobiological data for normal tissues is an absolute requirement. Should the OAR sparing be insufficient, one can also investigate OAR cooling. Another option would be to investigate whether sequential TBT is beneficial. However, in sequential TBT the level of tumor radiosensitization is lower and the sequential procedure could prolong overall treatment time.

While OAR sparing can be expected, it is also evident from Figure 7 that the high target doses ($V_{150\%}$ and $V_{200\%}$) become even higher in the TBT setting. Namely, scaling down the physical dose increases the $V_{150\%}$ and $V_{200\%}$ to a saturation point where the $V_{100\%}$ target can be reached (for DU-145, this is visible at 80% target coverage in Figure 7). This effect is expected, given the fact that both modalities are delivered to the target from within the same applicator. Whether this is a negative effect or not can be debated. On the one hand, clinical treatment protocols strive to decrease extreme heterogeneity in the tumor by applying soft constraints on the high prostate doses, as is also carried out in the current study [6,49]. On the other hand, guidelines on prostate HDR-BT do not restrict high doses [10,11]. This can be explained by the fact that a saturation dose beyond which no further injury can occur likely exists in prostate brachytherapy [50,51].

In this study, we only optimize the temperature distribution based on the combined treatment. We expect that also optimizing the radiation dose distribution based on the combined effect has the potential to lead to more enhancement, i.e., better results, given the higher number of degrees of freedom. This additional optimization opportunity should, therefore, be considered in future research.

The TDLQ model is not complete in describing the combined effect of radiation and temperature elevation. The extended TDLQ model incorporating direct temperature-induced cytotoxicity has also been proposed and evaluated for cervical cancer cell lines [30]. There are currently not enough data to apply the same model for prostate cancer. However, in our application, where very high radiation fraction doses are applied, it can be presumed that most of the cell death is caused by radiation rather than temperature increase. In any case, should there be enough radiobiological data available, a more elaborate model could easily be applied to this algorithm as well.

In Figure 8, we showed that the calculated T_{10}, T_{50}, and T_{90} values needed for sufficient target coverage are, in some cases, lower than what is commonly regarded as adequate temperature elevation in hyperthermia treatments. These values are, however, set for an IHT treatment duration of 1 h. It is debatable whether temperatures under 39 °C can cause tumor radiosensitization at all [52]. One can, therefore, choose to normalize the length of the treatment to achieve the same thermal dose in, i.e., $CEM43$ [12] or AUC [52]. This is also convenient in a simultaneous TBT treatment, since an HDR-BT treatment has a delivery time of approximately 10–20 min.

We have presented a method for automated IHT-TP optimization based on thermoradiotherapeutic criteria when IHT is used simultaneously with HDR-BT. We also showed that the results of the optimization are very dependent on the thermosensitivity of the tumor and normal tissue. With information on thermosensitivity of the involved tissues not yet available, the full potential use of this algorithm still needs to be determined. However, it can already serve as a promising tool for further development of IHT in combination with HDR-BT.

5. Conclusions

In this study, we presented a framework to optimize the temperature for simultaneous HDR-BT and IHT, based on the resulting EQD_{phys} of the combined treatment. This gives the opportunity of treatment planning on the same radiotherapeutic dose constraints and objectives as for HDR-BT only. We established that the fast calculation of the temperature distribution is accurate. Furthermore, on a sample of 10 patients, the calculated equivalent dose distribution predicts a favorable reduction in the dose in OARs. At the same time, the target dose coverage remains at the same level as prescribed in the standard protocol, while the high-dose regions ($V_{150\%}$ and $V_{200\%}$) get considerably higher values. While this framework offers a valuable tool for simultaneous thermobrachytherapy treatment plan optimization, further research on the biological effects of both heat and radiation is needed to confirm the clinical relevance of a simultaneous thermobrachytherapy treatment.

Author Contributions: Conceptualization, I.A., G.C.v.R., I.-K.K.K.-D., R.M.C.M. and M.E.M.C.C.; methodology, I.A.; software, I.A.; validation, I.A., R.M.C.M. and I.-K.K.K.-D.; formal analysis, I.A.; investigation, I.A.; resources, G.C.v.R., I.-K.K.K.-D. and M.E.M.C.C.; writing—original draft preparation, I.A.; writing—review and editing, G.C.v.R., R.M.C.M., M.E.M.C.C. and I.-K.K.K.-D.; visualization, I.A.; supervision, G.C.v.R., M.E.M.C.C., R.M.C.M. and I.-K.K.K.-D.; project administration, G.C.v.R.; funding acquisition, G.C.v.R. All authors have read and agreed to the published version of the manuscript.

Funding: This research was funded by Elekta, grant number 106932, task 4.

Institutional Review Board Statement: The study was conducted according to the guidelines of the Declaration of Helsinki, and approved by the Institutional Review Board (or Ethics Committee) of Erasmus Medical Center Rotterdam (METC 2018-1711, date of approval 14-01-2019).

Informed Consent Statement: Informed consent was obtained from all subjects involved in the study.

Data Availability Statement: The data presented in this study can be made available upon request to the corresponding author.

Conflicts of Interest: The authors declare no conflict of interest. The funders had no role in the design of the study; in the collection, analyses, or interpretation of data; in the writing of the manuscript, or in the decision to publish the results.

References

1. Litwin, M.S.; Tan, H.-J. The Diagnosis and Treatment of Prostate Cancer: A Review. *JAMA* **2017**, *317*, 2532–2542. [CrossRef] [PubMed]
2. Miralbell, R.; Roberts, S.A.; Zubizarreta, E.; Hendry, J.H. Dose-Fractionation Sensitivity of Prostate Cancer Deduced from Radiotherapy Outcomes of 5,969 Patients in Seven International Institutional Datasets: α/β = 1.4 (0.9–2.2) Gy. *Int. J. Radiat. Oncol. Biol. Phys.* **2012**, *82*, e17–e24. [CrossRef] [PubMed]
3. Gocho, T.; Hori, M.; Fukushima, Y.; Someya, M.; Kitagawa, M.; Hasegawa, T.; Tsuchiya, T.; Hareyama, M.; Takagi, M.; Hashimoto, K. Evaluation of the Urethral α/β Ratio and Tissue Repair Half-Time for Iodine-125 Prostate Brachytherapy with or without Supplemental External Beam Radiotherapy. *Brachytherapy* **2020**, *19*, 290–297. [CrossRef] [PubMed]
4. Brand, D.H.; Brüningk, S.C.; Wilkins, A.; Fernandez, K.; Naismith, O.; Gao, A.; Syndikus, I.; Dearnaley, D.P.; Tree, A.C.; van As, N. Estimates of Alpha/Beta (α/β) Ratios for Individual Late Rectal Toxicity Endpoints: An Analysis of the CHHiP Trial. *Int. J. Radiat. Oncol. Biol. Phys.* **2021**, *110*, 596–608. [CrossRef] [PubMed]
5. Morton, G.C. High-Dose-Rate Brachytherapy Boost for Prostate Cancer: Rationale and Technique. *J. Contemp. Brachyther.* **2014**, *6*, 323. [CrossRef] [PubMed]

6. Tselis, N.; Hoskin, P.; Baltas, D.; Strnad, V.; Zamboglou, N.; Rödel, C.; Chatzikonstantinou, G. High Dose Rate Brachytherapy as Monotherapy for Localised Prostate Cancer: Review of the Current Status. *Clin. Oncol. R. Coll. Radiol.* **2017**, *29*, 401–411. [CrossRef] [PubMed]
7. Hoskin, P.; Rojas, A.; Lowe, G.; Bryant, L.; Ostler, P.; Hughes, R.; Milner, J.; Cladd, H. High-Dose-Rate Brachytherapy Alone for Localized Prostate Cancer in Patients at Moderate or High Risk of Biochemical Recurrence. *Int. J. Radiat. Oncol.* **2012**, *82*, 1376–1384. [CrossRef]
8. Nagore, G.; Guerra, J.L.L.; Krumina, E.; Lagos, M.; Ovalles, B.; Miró, A.; Beltran, L.; Gómez, E.; Praena-Fernandez, J.M.; del Campo, E.R.; et al. High Dose Rate Brachytherapy for Prostate Cancer: A Prospective Toxicity Evaluation of a One Day Schedule Including Two 13.5 Gy Fractions. *Radiother. Oncol.* **2018**, *127*, 219–224. [CrossRef]
9. Aluwini, S.; Busser, W.M.; Alemayehu, W.G.; Boormans, J.L.; Kirkels, W.J.; Jansen, P.P.; Praag, J.O.; Bangma, C.H.; Kolkman-Deurloo, I.-K.K. Toxicity and Quality of Life after High-Dose-Rate Brachytherapy as Monotherapy for Low- and Intermediate-Risk Prostate Cancer. *Radiother. Oncol.* **2015**, *117*, 252–257. [CrossRef]
10. Hoskin, P.; Colombo, A.; Henry, A.; Niehoff, P.; Hellebust, T.P.; Siebert, F.-A.; Kovacs, G. GEC/ESTRO Recommendations on High Dose Rate Afterloading Brachytherapy for Localised Prostate Cancer: An Update. *Radiother. Oncol.* **2013**, *107*, 325–332. [CrossRef]
11. Yamada, Y.; Rogers, L.; Demanes, D.J.; Morton, G.; Prestidge, B.R.; Pouliot, J.; Cohen, G.; Zaider, M.; Ghilezan, M.; Hsu, I.-C. American Brachytherapy Society consensus guidelines for high-dose-rate prostate brachytherapy. *Brachytherapy* **2012**, *11*, 20–32. [CrossRef]
12. Van Rhoon, G.C. Is CEM43 Still a Relevant Thermal Dose Parameter for Hyperthermia Treatment Monitoring? *Int. J. Hyperth.* **2016**, *32*, 50–62. [CrossRef]
13. Horsman, M.R.; Overgaard, J. Hyperthermia: A Potent Enhancer of Radiotherapy. *Clin. Oncol.* **2007**, *19*, 418–426. [CrossRef]
14. Datta, N.R.; Bodis, S. Hyperthermia with Radiotherapy Reduces Tumour Alpha/Beta: Insights from Trials of Thermoradiotherapy vs. Radiotherapy Alone. *Radiother. Oncol.* **2019**, *138*, 1–8. [CrossRef]
15. Ryu, S.; Brown, S.L.; Kim, S.-H.; Khil, M.S.; Kim, J.H. Preferential Radiosensitization of Human Prostatic Carcinoma Cells by Mild Hyperthermia. *Int. J. Radiat. Oncol.* **1996**, *34*, 133–138. [CrossRef]
16. Pajonk, F.; Van Ophoven, A.; McBride, W.H. Hyperthermia-Induced Proteasome Inhibition and Loss of Androgen Receptor Expression in Human Prostate Cancer Cells. *Cancer Res.* **2005**, *65*, 4836–4843. [CrossRef]
17. Rajaee, Z.; Khoei, S.; Mahdavi, S.R.; Ebrahimi, M.; Shirvalilou, S.; Mahdavian, A. Evaluation of the Effect of Hyperthermia and Electron Radiation on Prostate Cancer Stem Cells. *Radiat. Environ. Biophys.* **2018**, *57*, 133–142. [CrossRef]
18. Elming, P.B.; Sørensen, B.S.; Oei, A.L.; Franken, N.A.P.; Crezee, J.; Overgaard, J.; Horsman, M.R. Hyperthermia: The Optimal Treatment to Overcome Radiation Resistant Hypoxia. *Cancers* **2019**, *11*, 60. [CrossRef]
19. Morton, G.C.; Hoskin, P.J. Single Fraction High-Dose-Rate Brachytherapy: Too good to Be True? *Int. J. Radiat. Oncol. Biol. Phys.* **2019**, *104*, 1054–1056. [CrossRef]
20. Dobšíček Trefná, H.; Schmidt, M.; van Rhoon, G.C.; Kok, H.P.; Gordeyev, S.S.; Lamprecht, U.; Marder, D.; Nadobny, J.; Ghadjar, P.; Abdel-Rahman, S.; et al. Quality Assurance Guidelines for Interstitial Hyperthermia. *Int. J. Hyperth.* **2019**, *36*, 276–293. [CrossRef]
21. Prionas, S.D.; Kapp, D.S.; Goffinet, D.R.; Ben-Yosef, R.; Fessenden, P.; Bagshaw, M.A. Thermometry of Interstitial Hyperthermia Given as an Adjuvant to Brachytherapy for the Treatment of Carcinoma of the Prostate. *Int. J. Radiat. Oncol.* **1994**, *28*, 151–162. [CrossRef]
22. Williams, V.L.; Puthawala, A.; Phan, T.P.; Sharma, A.; Syed, A.N. Interstitial Hyperthermia during HDR Brachytherapy Monotherapy for Treatment of Early Stage Prostate Cancer with Benign Prostate Hyperplasia (BPH). *Brachytherapy* **2007**, *6*, 86. [CrossRef]
23. Kukiełka, A.; Hetnał, M.; Dąbrowski, T.; Walasek, T.; Brandys, P.; Nahajowski, D.; Kudzia, R.; Dybek, D.; Reinfuss, M. Salvage Prostate HDR Brachytherapy Combined with Interstitial Hyperthermia for Local Recurrence after Radiation Therapy Failure. *Strahlenther. Onkol.* **2013**, *190*, 165–170. [CrossRef]
24. Mei, X.; Ten Cate, R.; Van Leeuwen, C.M.; Rodermond, H.M.; De Leeuw, L.; Dimitrakopoulou, D.; Stalpers, L.J.A.; Crezee, J.; Kok, H.P.; Franken, N.A.P.; et al. Radiosensitization by Hyperthermia: The Effects of Temperature, Sequence, and Time Interval in Cervical Cell Lines. *Cancers* **2020**, *12*, 582. [CrossRef]
25. Androulakis, I.; Mestrom, R.M.C.; Christianen, M.E.M.C.; Kolkman-Deurloo, I.-K.K.; van Rhoon, G.C. Design of the Novel ThermoBrachy Applicators Enabling Simultaneous Interstitial Hyperthermia and High Dose Rate Brachytherapy. *Int. J. Hyperth.* **2021**, *38*, 1660–1671. [CrossRef]
26. Overgaard, J. Simultaneous and Sequential Hyperthermia and Radiation Treatment of an Experimental Tumor and Its Surrounding Normal Tissue in Vivo. *Int. J. Radiat. Oncol.* **1980**, *6*, 1507–1517. [CrossRef]
27. Overgaard, J. The Heat Is (still) on—The Past and Future of Hyperthermic Radiation Oncology. *Radiother. Oncol.* **2013**, *109*, 185–187. [CrossRef]
28. Kok, H.P.; Crezee, J.; Franken, N.; Stalpers, L.J.; Barendsen, G.W.; Bel, A. Quantifying the Combined Effect of Radiation Therapy and Hyperthermia in Terms of Equivalent Dose Distributions. *Int. J. Radiat. Oncol.* **2014**, *88*, 739–745. [CrossRef]
29. Van Leeuwen, C.M.; Crezee, J.; Oei, A.L.; Franken, N.A.P.; Stalpers, L.J.A.; Bel, A.; Kok, H.P. 3D Radiobiological Evaluation of Combined Radiotherapy and Hyperthermia Treatments. *Int. J. Hyperth.* **2016**, *33*, 160–169. [CrossRef]
30. Van Leeuwen, C.M.; Oei, A.L.; Cate, R.T.; Franken, N.A.P.; Bel, A.; Stalpers, L.J.A.; Crezee, J.; Kok, H.P. Measurement and Analysis of the Impact of Time-Interval, Temperature and Radiation Dose on Tumour Cell Survival and Its Application in Thermoradiotherapy Plan Evaluation. *Int. J. Hyperth.* **2017**, *34*, 30–38. [CrossRef]

31. De Mendoza, A.M.; Michlíková, S.; Berger, J.; Karschau, J.; Kunz-Schughart, L.A.; McLeod, D.D. Mathematical Model for the Thermal Enhancement of Radiation Response: Thermodynamic Approach. *Sci. Rep.* **2021**, *11*, 5503. [CrossRef] [PubMed]
32. Chen, X.; Diederich, C.; Wootton, J.H.; Pouliot, J.; Hsu, I.-C. Optimisation-Based Thermal Treatment Planning for Catheter-Based Ultrasound Hyperthermia. *Int. J. Hyperth.* **2010**, *26*, 39–55. [CrossRef] [PubMed]
33. Salgaonkar, V.A.; Prakash, P.; Diederich, C.J. Temperature Superposition for Fast Computation of 3D Temperature Distributions during Optimization and Planning of Interstitial Ultrasound Hyperthermia Treatments. *Int. J. Hyperth.* **2012**, *28*, 235–249. [CrossRef] [PubMed]
34. Kok, H.P.; Kotte, A.N.T.J.; Crezee, J. Planning, Optimisation and Evaluation of Hyperthermia Treatments. *Int. J. Hyperth.* **2017**, *33*, 593–607. [CrossRef]
35. Androulakis, I.; Mestrom, R.M.C.; Christianen, M.E.M.C.; Kolkman-Deurloo, I.-K.K.; van Rhoon, G.C. Simultaneous Thermo-Brachytherapy: Electromagnetic Simulation Methods for Fast and Accurate Adaptive Treatment Planning. *Sensors* **2022**, *22*, 1328. [CrossRef]
36. Haus, H.A.; Melcher, J.R. *Electromagnetic Fields and Energy*; Prentice Hall Englewood Cliffs: Hoboken, NJ, USA, 1989; Volume 107.
37. Hasgall, P.A.; Di Gennaro, F.; Baumgartner, C.; Neufeld, E.; Lloyd, B.; Gosselin, M.C.; Payne, D.; Klingenböck, A.; Kuster, N. *IT'IS Database for Thermal and Electromagnetic Parameters of Biological Tissues*; Version 4.0; IT'IS Foundation: Zürich, Switzerland, 2018.
38. Khawaji, I.H.; Chindam, C.; Awadelkarim, O.O.; Lakhtakia, A. Dielectric Properties of and Charge Transport in Columnar Microfibrous Thin Films of Parylene C. *IEEE Trans. Electron. Devices* **2017**, *64*, 3360–3367. [CrossRef]
39. Kahouli, A.; Sylvestre, A.; Jomni, F.; Yangui, B.; Legrand, J. Experimental and Theoretical Study of AC Electrical Conduction Mechanisms of Semicrystalline Parylene C Thin Films. *J. Phys. Chem. A* **2012**, *116*, 1051–1058. [CrossRef]
40. Pennes, H.H. Analysis of Tissue and Arterial Blood Temperatures in the Resting Human Forearm. *J. Appl. Physiol.* **1948**, *1*, 93–122. [CrossRef]
41. Wissler, E.H. Pennes' 1948 Paper Revisited. *J. Appl. Physiol.* **1998**, *85*, 35–41. [CrossRef]
42. Das, S.K.; Clegg, S.T.; Samulski, T.V. Computational Techniques for Fast Hyperthermia Temperature Optimization. *Med. Phys.* **1999**, *26*, 319–328. [CrossRef]
43. Lessard, E.; Pouliot, J. Inverse Planning Anatomy-Based Dose Optimization for HDR-Brachytherapy of the Prostate Using Fast Simulated Annealing Algorithm and Dedicated Objective Function. *Med. Phys.* **2001**, *28*, 773–779. [CrossRef]
44. Perez-Calatayud, J.; Ballester, F.; Das, R.K.; DeWerd, L.A.; Ibbott, G.S.; Meigooni, A.S.; Ouhib, Z.; Rivard, M.J.; Sloboda, R.S.; Williamson, J.F. Dose Calculation for Photon-Emitting Brachytherapy Sources with Average Energy Higher than 50 keV: Report of the AAPM and ESTRO. *Med. Phys.* **2012**, *39*, 2904–2929. [CrossRef]
45. Roos, M.; Kolkman-Deurloo, I.-K.; De Pan, C.; Aluwini, S. Single Fraction HDR Brachytherapy as Monotherapy in Patients with Prostate Cancer: What Is the Optimal Dose Level? *Brachytherapy* **2016**, *15*, S167–S168. [CrossRef]
46. Low, D.A.; Harms, W.B.; Mutic, S.; Purdy, J.A. A Technique for the Quantitative Evaluation of Dose Distributions. *Med. Phys.* **1998**, *25*, 656–661. [CrossRef]
47. De Bruijne, M.; Samaras, T.; Chavannes, N.; van Rhoon, G.C. Quantitative Validation of the 3D SAR Profile of Hyperthermia Applicators Using the Gamma Method. *Phys. Med. Biol.* **2007**, *52*, 3075. [CrossRef]
48. Van Vulpen, M.; Raaymakers, B.W.; Lagendijk, J.J.W.; Crezee, J.; Leeuw, A.A.C.D.; Van Moorselaar, J.R.A.; Ligtvoet, C.M.; Battermann, J.J. Three-Dimensional Controlled Interstitial Hyperthermia Combined with Radiotherapy for Locally Advanced Prostate Carcinoma—A Feasibility Study. *Int. J. Radiat. Oncol.* **2002**, *53*, 116–126. [CrossRef]
49. Christianen, M.; De Vries, K.; Jansen, P.; Luthart, L.; Kolkman-Deurloo, I.; Nout, R. PO-0244 HDR Brachytherapy Monotherapy with 2 × 13.5 Gy for Localized Prostate Cancer: Short Term Follow Up. *Radiother. Oncol.* **2021**, *158*, S203–S204. [CrossRef]
50. Ling, C.; Roy, J.; Sahoo, N.; Wallner, K.; Anderson, L. Quantifying the Effect of Dose Inhomogeneity in Brachytherapy: Application to Permanent Prostatic Implant with 125I Seeds. *Int. J. Radiat. Oncol.* **1994**, *28*, 971–977. [CrossRef]
51. Fatyga, M.; Williamson, J.F.; Dogan, N.; Todor, D.; Siebers, J.V.; George, R.; Barani, I.; Hagan, M. A Comparison of HDR BrachyTherapy and IMRT Techniques for Dose Escalation in Prostate Cancer: A Radiobiological Modeling Study. *Med. Phys.* **2009**, *36*, 3995–4006. [CrossRef]
52. Datta, N.R.; Marder, D.; Datta, S.; Meister, A.; Puric, E.; Stutz, E.; Rogers, S.; Eberle, B.; Timm, O.; Staruch, M.; et al. Quantification of Thermal Dose in Moderate Clinical Hyperthermia with Radiotherapy: A Relook Using Temperature—Time Area under the Curve (AUC). *Int. J. Hyperth.* **2021**, *38*, 296–307. [CrossRef]

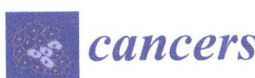

Article

Theoretical Evaluation of the Impact of Hyperthermia in Combination with Radiation Therapy in an Artificial Immune—Tumor-Ecosystem

Stephan Scheidegger [1,*], Sergio Mingo Barba [1,2] and Udo S. Gaipl [3]

1 ZHAW School of Engineering, Zurich University of Applied Sciences, 8401 Winterthur, Switzerland; ming@zhaw.ch
2 Faculty of Science and Medicine, University of Fribourg, 1700 Fribourg, Switzerland
3 Translational Radiobiology, Department of Radiation Oncology, Universitätsklinikum Erlangen, 91054 Erlangen, Germany; Udo.Gaipl@uk-erlangen.de
* Correspondence: scst@zhaw.ch

Simple Summary: Radio-sensitizing effects of moderate or mild hyperthermia (heating up tumor cells up to 41–43 °C) in combination with radiotherapy (thermoradiotherapy) have been evaluated for decades. However, how this combination might modulate an anti-tumor immune response is not well known. To investigate the dynamic behavior of immune–tumor ecosystems in different scenarios, a model representing an artificial adaptive immune system in silico is used. Such a model may be far removed from the real situation in the patient, but it could serve as a laboratory to investigate fundamental principles of dynamics in such systems under well-controlled conditions and it could be used to generate and refine hypothesis supporting the design of clinical trials. Regarding the results of the presented computer simulations, the main effect is governed by the cellular radio-sensitization. In addition, the application of hyperthermia during the first radiotherapy fractions seems to be more effective.

Abstract: There is some evidence that radiotherapy (RT) can trigger anti-tumor immune responses. In addition, hyperthermia (HT) is known to be a tumor cell radio-sensitizer. How HT could enhance the anti-tumor immune response produced by RT is still an open question. The aim of this study is the evaluation of potential dynamic effects regarding the adaptive immune response induced by different combinations of RT fractions with HT. The adaptive immune system is considered as a trainable unit (perceptron) which compares danger signals released by necrotic or apoptotic cell death with the presence of tumor- and host tissue cell population-specific molecular patterns (antigens). To mimic the changes produced by HT such as cell radio-sensitization or increase of the blood perfusion after hyperthermia, simplistic biophysical models were included. To study the effectiveness of the different RT+HT treatments, the Tumor Control Probability (TCP) was calculated. In the considered scenarios, the major effect of HT is related to the enhancement of the cell radio-sensitivity while perfusion or heat-based effects on the immune system seem to contribute less. Moreover, no tumor vaccination effect has been observed. In the presented scenarios, HT boosts the RT cell killing but it does not fundamentally change the anti-tumor immune response.

Keywords: systems medicine; immune system in silico; perceptron; antigen pattern; danger signal; fractionation; immune response

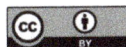

1. Introduction

Preclinical and, to some extent, clinical research demonstrated that radiotherapy (RT) is able to modulate anti-tumor immune responses [1–4]. The idea of activating the immune system by radiation leads to the question of how hyperthermia (HT) in combination with RT could help to trigger or amplify such an anti-tumor response.

Radio-sensitizing effects of HT in combination with RT (thermoradiotherapy, HT-RT) have been evaluated for decades. Effects have been investigated on molecular [5–7], cellular [8,9], and tissue scale [10–12]. Regarding the tissue level, increased perfusion leading to a removal of acidic metabolites [13–15] and re-oxygenation [16–18] have been discussed by several authors. Re-oxygenation is known as a radio-sensitizing factor [19,20], but the effect of, e.g., combining 3–6 of total 32 fractions of RT with HT may be very limited [21], especially when considering time gaps between application of HT and RT of 30–120 or more minutes in clinical routine treatments. However, the wash-out of acidic metabolites by increased perfusion below 42–43 °C could improve the immune system response [22–25]. In addition, increased perfusion may improve the accessibility for immune cells, leading to a better detection of antigenic patterns and enhanced tumor–immune cell interaction via related to danger signals such as Heat Shock Proteins (HSP) [26–28]. There seem to be many contributing factors and it is difficult to identify the key processes leading to the clinically observed improved therapy outcome of HT-RT. Whereas on the cellular level, more or less controlled experiments in vitro may help to understand molecular or cellular aspects of the additive or synergistic heat- and radiation-induced responses, the dynamic interaction of the immune system with the tumor tissue is patient-specific and would require a time-resolved monitoring of immune cell activity in the body or at least, in the tumor environment. This information is hard to access during clinical trials since, for example, repeated (frequent) biopsy material has to be sampled from the patients and analyzed.

However, treatment optimization would require a profound understanding of the dynamic response of tumor and host tissue as well as the immune system. Whereas clinical trials may generate knowledge about the effectiveness of specific aspects such as fractionation schemes and can be seen as acid tests for novel approaches for anti-cancer treatments, the investigation of the dynamic behavior should include the analysis of time-resolved data representing the complex interaction in the tumor-host-immune system. Such a tumor-host-immune system may be considered as an ecosystem [29–31]. This may include the interaction between sub-populations of tumor cells, tumor-associated cells (e.g., fibroblasts), host tissue, endothelial cells, and immune cells. Understanding the dynamics in such a complex ecosystem may be pivotal as soon as the therapy outcome is governed by the dynamic interactions between the different actors in the system. Regarding the immune system as a part of the whole, the complexity is enormous since not only the immune cells (e.g., T-cells or macrophages) in the tumor compartment but the systemic response has to be considered as well [32].

At a first glance, there seems to be no way to get a profound insight into the complex dynamic interactions in such an immune–tumor ecosystem. Regarding the effects of HT, the processes taking place on different scale levels may influence the system in an obscure manner, but the identification of key processes would support the optimization of hyperthermia in combination with RT (e.g., timing of HT sessions and RT fractions). The different therapy regimens may be tested in clinical trials. Mathematical models and computer simulations could be used to guide the search for optimal conditions for HT-RT. The complexity will probably hamper the development of predictive models covering all the aspects relevant for therapy response in vivo or in patient. The situation may be different as soon as not prediction is sought. Artificial immune–tumor ecosystems may be far removed from the real situation in the living organism, but they could serve as a laboratory to investigate fundamental principles of dynamics in such systems under well-controlled conditions. As a complementary approach to biological experiments in vitro, ex vivo, in vivo, or clinical trials, such sandbox games could be used to generate and refine hypothesis supporting the design of clinical trials. Scheidegger et al. [33] proposed an artificial immune–tumor model system covering two essential aspects: ecosystem dynamics between host tissue and different tumor sub-clones and antigen pattern recognition by a learning (adaptive) immune system. The proposed model exhibited some interesting aspects: as a response to radiation treatments, host tissue becomes immune-suppressive whereas the tumor-related response is improved by the re-growing tumor cell populations and subsequent necrosis. This behavior is dependent on the interaction strength (competition) between the host tissue and the different tumor sub-populations. Regarding these results, an interesting question is whether there are parameters influencing the specific anti-tumor immune response in this model which are related to effects of HT. Therefore, the purpose of this study is to identify such model parameters and to investigate the potential effect of combining HT sessions with different RT fractionation schemes in the framework of the proposed artificial system. In contrast to other mathematical models for immune–tumor systems [1,34], we consider the adaptive immune system as a trainable (programmable) unit and anti-cancer treatments as means to train the immune system to battle against cancer.

2. Materials and Methods

The artificial immune–tumor ecosystem proposed by Scheidegger et al. [33] consists of two major components: a tumor ecosystem, including host tissue and immune cells in the tumor compartment, and a perceptron [35] for antigen pattern recognition (Figure 1). The idea of using a perceptron to mimic the immune system's ability of pattern recognition is based on the danger model proposed by P. Matzinger [36]. Following this concept, the immune system is only activated when a danger signal and antigens are coincidently present (adjuvanticity plus antigenicity). The proposed model uses a very simplistic approach for danger signal generation, which is assumed to be proportional to the amount of necrotic or immune system-activating apoptotic cells [37–39]. In the following, the model equations are presented (a detailed explanation of the model is given by Scheidegger et al. [33]). The dynamic interaction between the different tumor sub-clones T_{ik} and the host tissue H is given by the following system of ordinary differential equations:

$$\frac{dT_{11}}{dt} = (k_{T11} - k_{mut} - k_{eT} - r_{11}k_{IT} - k_{HT}H - k_{TT}T - (\alpha_T + 2\beta_T\Gamma) \cdot R) \cdot T_{11}$$

$$\frac{dT_{ik}}{dt} = (k_{Tik} - k_{eT} - r_{ik}k_{IT} - k_{HT}H - k_{TT}T - (\alpha_T + 2\beta_T\Gamma) \cdot R) \cdot T_{ik} + k_{mut} \cdot q_{il}T_{lk} \quad (1)$$

$$\frac{dH}{dt} = (k_{aH} - k_{eH} - r_{H}k_{IH} - k_{bH}H - k_{TH}T - (\alpha_H + 2\beta_H\Gamma) \cdot R) \cdot H$$

where $k_{Tik} \cdot T_{ik}$ is the reproduction rate of the tumor sub-population T_{ik} (the tumor sub-clones are assumed to form a mutation tree with branches k; $k_{T11} \cdot T_{11}$ denotes the reproduction rate of the population $i = 1$ and $k = 1$, for the host tissue, the corresponding rate is $k_{aH} \cdot H$); $k_{eT} \cdot T_{ik}$ (and $k_{eH} \cdot H$ for host tissue) represents the rate of cell elimination (death rate) independent from radiation-induced cell killing and immune system-mediated cell elimination; the immune system-related elimination rate is calculated by $r_{ik}k_{IT} \cdot T_{ik}$ with an interaction coefficient k_{IT} (assumed to be the same for all tumor sub-clones, r_{ik} defines the match with antigen-receptor binding sites and will be explained later; for host tissue, a different coefficient k_{IH} is used); $k_{mut} \cdot q_{il}T_{lk}$ gives the rate of mutation (q_{il} is a matrix representing the topology of the population network, see [33]). Competition between the different tumor sub-populations is included by $k_{TT}T \cdot T_{ik}$ (with the total amount of tumor cells T) and for host tissue by $k_{TH}T \cdot H$; $k_{bH} \cdot H^2$ represents the self-inhibition of host tissue growth. For radiation-induced cell killing, a dynamic linear-quadratic law with a transient biological dose equivalent Γ [40] is used. The radiation-induced death rate is dependent on the radiation dose rate R, the radio-sensitivity coefficients α_H and β_H for host and α_T and β_T for tumor cells (in this study assumed to be the same for all tumor sub-clones). The transient biological dose equivalent Γ is rising with the dose rate R and decaying with a repair constant γ:

$$\frac{d\Gamma_{T,H,I}}{dt} = R - \gamma_{T,H,I}\Gamma_{T,H,I} \quad (2)$$

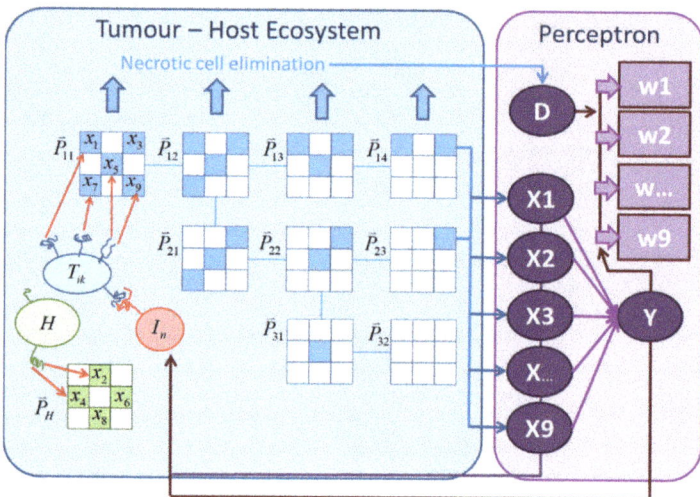

Figure 1. Structure of the tumor–immune system model and mutation tree/tumor sub-clones with associated antigen pattern vectors $\vec{P}_{ik}$. Vector components may represent epitopes on a specific complex protein or may be distributed over different proteins. According to the presence antigen vector components, an antigen signal X_n together with the danger signal D generate a perceptron response Y which induces the growth and immigration of effector cells (I_n).

The indices are indicating that—depending on the cellular repair capability–different repair rate constants γ have to be applied for tumor cells, host tissue, and immune cells (effector cells, the exchange of these cells in the tumor compartment leads to a certain "repair" effect which depends on the immigration speed of these cells).

The different cell death processes will lead to apoptotic and necrotic cells. Apoptotic cell death seems not to be equally considered as a danger signal compared to necrotic cell death [41], where the release of intracellular Heat Shock Proteins (HSP's) may be involved [28]. Apoptosis may generate danger signals [42–44] but this usually happens in particular situations and they can be pro- or anti-inflammatory [45,46]. In the presented model, we distinguish only between immune-stimulating and non-stimulating cell elimination processes. As immune-stimulating cell death processes, inflammatory processes, necrotic cells, non-cleared apoptotic cells which undergo secondary necrosis, or immunogenic apoptosis can be seen as immune-stimulating processes [47] and will contribute to the danger signal. The calculation of this signal is based on the amount of these cells which are "transformed" damaged pre-immune-stimulatory tumor cells $N_{p,ik}$ and damaged pre-immune-stimulatory host tissue cells $N_{p,H}$. Only host tissue cells are considered to be able to undergo a non-immune-stimulatory elimination pathway (e.g., apoptotic cell death processes that are characterized by dying cells with still intact membrane integrity and that do not generate any danger signal) by the rate $k_{ap}N_{p,H}$:

$$\frac{dN_{p,11}}{dt} = (k_{eT} + r_{11}k_{IT} + (\alpha_T + 2\beta_T \Gamma) \cdot R) \cdot T_{11} - k_{pn}N_{p,11}$$

$$\frac{dN_{p,ik}}{dt} = (k_{eT} + r_{ik}k_{IT} + (\alpha_T + 2\beta_T \Gamma) \cdot R) \cdot T_{ik} - k_{pn}N_{p,ik} \quad (3)$$

$$\frac{dN_{p,H}}{dt} = (k_{eH} + r_H k_{IH} + (\alpha_H + 2\beta_H \Gamma) \cdot R) \cdot H - (k_{pn} + k_{ap}) \cdot N_{p,H}$$

According Equations (1) and (3), only the elimination processes related to radiation, immune system-mediated response, and other cell death described by the death rate parameters k_{eT} and k_{eH} are considered to produce dying cells, which subsequently are transformed to immune-stimulatory necrotic or apoptotic cells at the rate $k_{pn}N_{n,ik}$ and $k_{pn}N_{n,H}$. These cells are calculated by:

$$\frac{dN_{11}}{dt} = k_{pn}N_{p,11} - k_n N_{11}$$

$$\frac{dN_{ik}}{dt} = k_{pn}N_{p,ik} - k_n N_{ik} \quad (4)$$

$$\frac{dN_H}{dt} = k_{pn}N_{p,H} - k_n N_H$$

In summary—and in contrast to the model presented by Scheidegger et al. [33]—the danger signal generation includes a two-step process with lethally damaged cells which subsequently transforms to "immune-system-activating" cells as described above. For calculating the danger signal, a sigmoidal relationship between the signal strength and the amount of dying cells is assumed:

$$D = \frac{\left[\sum_{i,k} N_{ik} + N_H\right]^2}{L_{act}^2 + \left[\sum_{i,k} N_{ik} + N_H\right]^2} \quad (5)$$

L_{act} governs the steepness of this sigmoidal relation between the amount of immune-stimulatory necrotic or apoptotic cells and the D (activation response).

The task of the adaptive immune system in principle is the detection of antigen patterns and a response generation based on the presence of the danger signal D. To mimic this process, Scheidegger et al. [33] proposed a perceptron as a structure which enables the immune system's adaptability and ability to learn, along with molecular danger signals and antigen-antibody (or antigen-receptor) interactions. For this, an antigen pattern vector $\vec{X} = X_i$ can be defined. Every cell of a specific population (tumor sub-clones and host tissue) bears a corresponding pattern, which is defined by the elements of the antigen pattern vector. The presence of a component of the pattern vector (molecular signal) is considered to be dependent on the number of cells bearing this specific component. According to the pattern used in this study (Figure 1), the antigen signal strength of the first component for example is given by:

$$X_1 = \frac{\left(\tilde{T}_{11} + \tilde{T}_{12} + \tilde{T}_{13} + \tilde{T}_{14}\right)^2}{(X_{act})^2 + \left(\tilde{T}_{11} + \tilde{T}_{12} + \tilde{T}_{13} + \tilde{T}_{14}\right)^2} \quad (6)$$

with $\tilde{T}_{ik} = T_{ik} + \eta N_{p,ik} + \chi N_{ik}$: pre-immune-stimulatory and immune-stimulatory necrotic or apoptotic cells are considered to contribute to the presence of antigens, but with the weighting factors η and χ. Similar to the sigmoidal relation in Equation (5), X_{act} influences the activation response. Depending on the presence of a specific antigen signal, the perceptron is used to adapt corresponding antigen weights w_i for generating the perceptron response by comparing the actual danger signal strength D with the perceptron response Y:

$$\frac{dw_i}{dt} = a \cdot (D - Y) \cdot X_i \quad (7)$$

with the perceptron response $Y = \Sigma^{\xi}/(Y_{act}^{\xi} + \Sigma^{\xi})$ and $\Sigma = \sum_{i=1}^{9} w_i X_i$. Even here, the perceptron response is modelled by a sigmoidal function, whose shape can be adapted by the powers ξ and the activation response parameter Y_{act}.

The perceptron response Y directly governs the production effector cells by the production rate $k_I Y X_n$. The presented model does not distinguish between the different immune-response pathways and is based on a simplistic elimination process, where the receptor binding of an effector cell of the population I_n with a tumor cell bearing the corresponding antigen will contribute to the tumor cell elimination. The match of antigen pattern with the effector cell population vector $I_n = \vec{I}$ is evaluated by the dot product between $\vec{I}$ and an antigen pattern vector $\vec{P}$ with components = 1 for bearing a specific antigen corresponding to the antigen pattern vector component X_n and 0 otherwise: $r_{ik} = \vec{I} \bullet \vec{P}_{ik}$. Finally, the elimination of effector cells is considered by the elimination rate constant k_{eI} and the radiation-induced elimination by a TBDE-based LQ model with the radio-sensitivity coefficients α_I and β_I. At this point, it is important to keep in mind that only the immune cells in the tumor compartment are irradiated and that compared to the stem cells in the red bone marrow, the radio-sensitivity of these effector cells may be lower. The very simplistic concept used here may be more suitable for describing the T-cell–mediated response. Summing up these rates, the temporal change of the antigen or immune cell population can be calculated by:

$$\frac{dI_n}{dt} = k_I Y X_n - (k_{eI} + (\alpha_I + 2\beta_I \Gamma_I) \cdot R) \cdot I_n - k_{IT} \cdot \left(\sum_{i,k} r_{ik} T_{ik} \right)_n \quad (8)$$

The selection of parameter values (Tables 1–3) used in this study is representing a scenario where the radiation sensitivity of irradiated immune cells or antibodies in the tumor compartment are assumed to be less than the sensitivity of tumor cells but more than the host tissue. The repair parameter γ_I in the kinetic model for Γ_I (TBDE for effector cells, Equation (2)) is not only determined by the intrinsic repair of cells (if there is repair) but by the replacement of effector cells in the irradiated compartment. Therefore, the value for γ_I should be above the one of k_{eI}. For the radio-sensitivity of tumor cells, a value close to colon cancer lines is used [48,49]. It is important to note here that the alpha and beta values cannot be directly compared with the standard LQ model since the kinetic model for the TBDE will reduce cell killing by repair. The effective alpha and beta values are therefore lower in this model (with $\gamma_T = 3\,d^{-1}$: $\alpha_{T,eff} = 0.128\,\text{Gy}^{-1}$ and $\beta_{T,eff} = 0.020\,\text{Gy}^{-1}$), representing more radio-resistant tumor cells such as, e.g., cervix carcinoma cells.

Table 1. Model parameters for ecosystem interactions: parameters used for the investigated scenario; parameters considered as susceptible for hyperthermia are indicated by an asterisk. Parameters are normalized to 10^9 cells.

Parameter/Unit	Description	Default Value
$k_{T11} = k_{Tik}/d^{-1}$	tumor growth rate constant	$3 \times 46 \times 10^{-2}$
k_{mut}/d^{-1}	mutation rate constant	10^{-3}
k_{eT}/d^{-1}	tumor cell elimination rate constant	4×10^{-3}
k_{TT}/d^{-1}	tumor cell growth inhibition	10^{-4}
k_{IT}/d^{-1}	immunogenic tumor cell elimination	1
k_{HT}/d^{-1}	host-tumor cells interaction	10^{-5}
k_{TH}/d^{-1}	tumor-host cells interaction	$2 \times 2 \times 10^{-4}$
k_{aH}/d^{-1}	host cell growth	3×10^{-2}
k_{bH}/d^{-1}	host cell growth inhibition	$1 \times 2 \times 10^{-4}$
k_{eH}/d^{-1}	host cell elimination	10^{-5}
k_{pn}/d^{-1}	necrotic transformation rate constant	0×5
k_n/d^{-1}	necrotic cell elimination	5
k_{ap}/d^{-1}	apoptosis rate constant	2
k_{IH}/d^{-1}	immunogenic host cell elimination	1
k_I/d^{-1}	immune cell production and migration *	10
k_{eI}/d^{-1}	immune cell elimination	1

Table 2. Model parameters for pattern-recognition: parameters used for the investigated scenario; parameters considered as susceptible for hyperthermia are indicated by an asterisk.

Parameter/Unit	Description	Default Value
Y_{act}	danger signal activation level	3
ξ	power of perceptron response function	9
X_{act}	pattern recognition level *	2
η	pattern presence weight for pre-necrotic cells	0.5
χ	pattern presence weight for necrotic cells	0.2
L_{act}	danger signal param. (Equation (7)) *	3
$a/1 \times d^{-1}$	perceptron learning rate	5

Table 3. Model parameters for radiobiological model: parameters used for the investigated scenario; parameters considered as susceptible for hyperthermia are indicated by an asterisk.

Parameter/Unit	Description	Default Value
α_T/Gy^{-1}	radiation sensitivity coefficient tumor cells *	0.28
β_T/Gy^{-2}	radiation sensitivity coefficient tumor cells *	0.05
α_H/Gy^{-1}	radiation sensitivity coefficient host tissue	0.05
β_H/Gy^{-2}	radiation sensitivity coefficient host tissue	0.01
α_I/Gy^{-1}	radiation sensitivity coefficient immune cells (effector cells)	0.1
β_I/Gy^{-2}	radiation sensitivity coefficient immune cells (effector cells)	0.01
γ_T/d^{-1}	radiobiol. repair constant for tumor cells	3
γ_H/d^{-1}	radiobiol. repair constant for host tissue	10
γ_I/d^{-1}	radiobiol. repair constant for immune cells	2
$R/\text{Gy/min}$	radiation dose rate	0.14

The tumor and host tissue growth parameters have been selected based on the following criteria: the tumor is considered as a fast-growing tumor (doubling time of 20 days for all tumor sub-populations; $k_{Tik} = 3.46 \cdot 10^{-2} d^{-1}$), whereas the host tissue is assumed to repopulate slightly slower. The equilibrium level H_{eq} for host tissue (homeostasis) is determined by the values of k_{aH} and k_{eH} to 250 (2.50×10^{11} cells). Assuming an average volume of $2 \cdot 10^3$ µm³ per cell, the initial compartmental volume is 500 cm³. The equilibrium levels for host (H_{eq}) and tumor (T_{eq}) cell population can be calculated by the equilibrium conditions from Equation (1):

$$T_{eq} = \frac{k_{Tik} - k_{eT}}{k_{TT}} \text{ and } H_{eq} = \frac{k_{aH} - k_{eH}}{k_{bH}} \qquad (9)$$

The equilibrium level for the tumor cell population without immunogenic elimination is set to 306 (3.06×10^{11} cells). This corresponds to a scenario where the tumor has less growth limitation than the host tissue.

As stated in the introduction, many processes may contribute to the effect of HT. Biophysical models may be used for the description of temperature-dependent effects such as inhibition of repair proteins or perfusion changes. Even non-thermal effects could be considered. It is important to clarify here that this study does not focus on the detailed mode of action of HT. The proposed model describes the tumor–host tissue evolution over about 5 years and focusses on large time scales. Therefore, a multi-scale approach including HT-effects in an implicit manner is used. The parameters in the following Sections 2.1 and 2.2 are considered to be susceptible for hyperthermia.

2.1. Cellular Radiobiological Parameters

Assuming that tumor cells are radio-sensitized by heat-induced impair of the repair system [50–52], the radio-sensitivity parameters α_T and β_T are modified according to the biophysical model proposed by van Leeuwen et al. [53]. The temperature during HT treatment (duration 60 min per session) was fixed to 42 °C and the time gap was assumed to be the same for all HT-RT treatments (30 min). Calculating the enhancement factor for the radio-sensitivity parameters for SiHa and HeLa cells using this model gives for both cell lines a similar value: $\alpha_T(42°C) \approx 1.96 \cdot \alpha_T(37°C)$ and $\beta_T(42°C) \approx 0.34 \cdot \beta_T(37°C)$. These are the values used in this study to mimic the effect of HT in combination with RT. In the dynamic LQ-model, an additional parameter for repair kinetics, γ_T may be influenced by HT. In contrast to the well-established LQ formula, repair kinetics is separated from α_T and β_T; these coefficients can be considered to describe a baseline radio-sensitivity. Since the important aspect in the immune–tumor ecosystem model is the amount of radiation-induced necrotic cells, there is no principal difference in the effect when modifying only radio-sensitivity by α_T and β_T instead of γ_T. Tumor tissue is assumed to have slow repair; therefore, this value was set to 3 d^{-1} for RT only (incomplete repair between the RT fraction; 10 d^{-1} corresponds to more or less complete repair between the RT fractions). Hyperthermia was assumed to reduce repair speed (repair protein inhibition) specifically for tumor cells. Therefore, we tested the sensitivity of the model to changes of γ_T. The effect of these variations is small and does not change the dynamics in the system. To keep the model simple, the full effect of HT was only considered by the given factors for α_T and β_T.

2.2. Parameters Influencing the Tumour–Immune System Interaction

Besides the radio-sensitivity parameters describing the cellular response to HT-RT (indirect immune activation via production of necrotic or immune-stimulatory apoptotic cells), thermal-induced modifications of immune system response are related to processes on cellular as well as tissue or systemic level. Thermally induced changes in perfusion and vascular permeability may enhance the accessibility of immune cells (not only effector cells) to the tumor compartment. To model the perfusion enhancement, the data from Song et al. [11,54] are used for a simple model: the perfusion enhancement factor PEF is calculated by a first order kinetic model: $d\theta/dt = k_{perf1} - k_{perf2} \cdot \theta$ with the condition $k_{perf1}/k_{perf2} = 1$ and $PEF = 1 + \theta$. This leads to a perfusion enhancement of a factor 2 which is reported by Song [11] for tumor tissue heated up to 42 °C. To achieve the temporal course of perfusion changes observed by Song et al. [54], the values for k_{perf1} and k_{perf2} are set to 200 d^{-1}. According to the data from Song [54], modification of perfusion can be considered as a fast process, where during heating, perfusion increases to a factor 2 within 30–40 min and decreases within 30 min after heating to the baseline level.

In contrast to this fast process, a second slower process was included in the model to describe some "long-term" effects of HT. This model has the same structure but the rate parameters are set to lower values: $d\phi/dt = k_{ims1} - k_{ims2} \cdot \phi$. The values for these immune stimulating parameters ($k_{ims1} = 7d^{-1}$ and $k_{ims2} = 7d^{-1}$) are selected to mimic the experimental data for MHC class I antigen presentation after hyperthermia from Ito et al. [27], where rat T-9 glioma cells were heated up to 43 °C for one hour. According the data from Ito et al. [27], the enhancement of antigen expression starts 24 h after heating, reaches a maximum (two-fold increase) at 48 h after heating, and then decays to the baseline expression level cells at 72 h. To simulate this scenario, one day after a hyperthermia treatment the parameter k_{ims1} was "switched on" for 24 h. The immune stimulation factor is defined by: $ISF = 1 + \phi$.

Regarding the effect of perfusion, effector cells are considered to have a better accessibility to the tumor compartment. Since k_I does not only describe the production rate of effector cells but includes migration speed to the irradiated compartment as well, this parameter is modified for HT by the perfusion enhancement factor: $k_{I,HT} = PEF \cdot k_I$.

The antigen pattern detectability (parameter X_{act}) may be influenced by HT via in increased antigen presentation which is related to an enhanced recognition by the immune cells (macrophages, APCs). By decreasing the value for X_{act}, the signal "antigen present" will increase stronger (steeper slope) at small numbers of tumor cells bearing the corresponding antigen. In this model, the shift of X_{act} is considered to be related with the slow process: $X_{act,HT} = X_{act}/ISF$.

The danger signal parameter L_{act} can be used to describe HT-induced modifications of the danger signal generation. Regarding Equation (5), the danger signal in the proposed model is assumed to be dependent on the amount of immune-stimulatory necrotic or apoptotic cells. The amplification of this danger signal for example by excess HSP release is considered by varying parameter values of L_{act}. In analogy to X_{act}, this HT-related modification is assumed to be related to the slow process (more HSP production, lowering of L_{act} shifts the response curve to the left: $L_{act,HT} = L_{act}/ISF$). For comparison, scenarios for both parameters have been studied for the fast (directly perfusion-related) process ($X_{act,HT} = X_{act}/PEF$; $L_{act,HT} = L_{act}/PEF$) as well.

2.3. Investigated Scenarios and Fractionation Schemes

In this study, nine antigen pattern components and nine tumor sub-clones according to Scheidegger et al. [33] were used. The structure of mutation tree is displayed in Figure 1.

Different fractionation schemes and combinations with HT have been evaluated (Figure 2). The tumor control probability TCP was calculated by the total amount of tumor cells T: $TCP = e^{-T}$. The TCP was evaluated at the time point with the lowest value of T during or after RT or HT-RT application. In the computer simulations, the artificial immune–tumor ecosystem evolved 560–570 days before irradiation. The total simulation time was set to 1800 days. For numerical integration, a Runge-Kutta algorithm with a time increment of $dt = 10^{-3}$ d was selected.

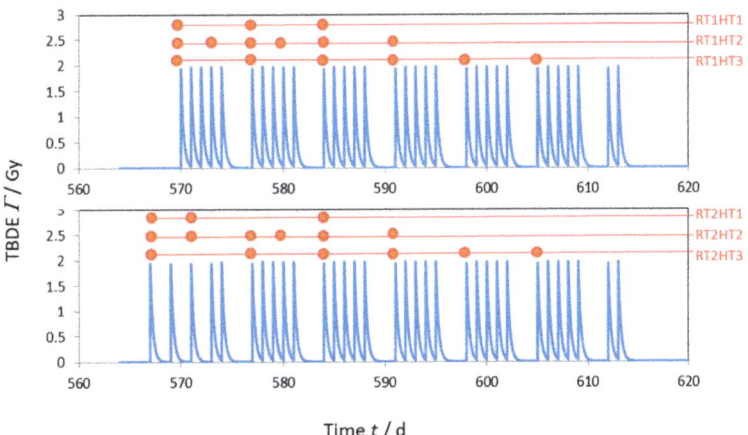

Figure 2. Different scenarios for fractionation and HT sessions: RT is applied in 32 fractions with 2 Gy per fraction, The HT scheme in RTxHT2 corresponds to the HYCAN trial [55], RTxHT3 to the KSA bladder trial [56].

3. Results

For the different treatment schemes displayed in Figure 2, the TCP has been calculated. The parameter values for the selected scenarios are adapted to achieve a baseline TCP of 0.8 without HT. In Table 4, the resulting TCP for the evaluated parameters are summarized. The highest TCP was achieved by RT1HT2 protocol (0.990) and a scenario where all HT-susceptible parameters where modified.

Table 4. TCP values after RT and HT-RT for the different combination of varying parameter values: k_I is assumed to be perfusion-limited only (fast process only); the column "all parameters" shows the combined effect of all parameter values modified by HT. Protocols according to Figure 2.

Protocol	α_T, β_T	α_T, β_T, k_I	$\alpha_T, \beta_T, X_{act}$	$\alpha_T, \beta_T, L_{act}$	All
RT1HT0	0.798 [2]	no HT	no HT	no HT	no HT
RT1HT1	0.933	0.934	0.935 (0.933) [1]	0.952 (0.935) [1]	0.960
RT1HT2	0.979	0.980	0.980 (0.979) [1]	0.988 (0.980) [1]	0.990
RT1HT3	0.980	0.980	0.981 (0.981) [1]	0.986 (0.980) [1]	0.988
RT2HT0	0.801 [2]	no HT	no HT	no HT	no HT
RT2HT1	0.931	0.932	0.931 (0.931) [1]	0.951 (0.931) [1]	0.951
RT2HT2	0.979	0.979	0.980 (0.979) [1]	0.983 (0.979) [1]	0.984
RT2HT3	0.979	0.979	0.980 (0.980) [1]	0.981 (0.979) [1]	0.982

[1] Fast process (perfusion-limited modifications) for X_{act} and L_{act}; [2] No HT applied.

The range of TCP values for treatments with HT was 0.931–0.990. In general, the differences between the corresponding HT protocols for the two RT fractionation schemes (RT1 and RT2) are less than $\Delta TCP = 0.01$ and clearly smaller than the impact of HT (TCP-rise of 0.130–0.192). Regarding the slow and fast process according to the HT models for X_{act} and L_{act} in Section 2.2, the perfusion-like process almost does not affect the TCP value while the slower process slightly improves it when it is applied to the L_{act} parameter. However, the main improvement of the treatment outcome produced by hyperthermia is the cell radio-sensitization effect, i.e., the change in the α_T and β_T parameters. For this reason, the HT1-Protocols have the lowest impact due to the smaller number of HT sessions.

In Figure 3, the resulting course of the host and tumor populations are shown. All the studied scenarios followed the same behavior with two tumor growth phases: the first one before RT and the second one after RT (tumor recurrence). Hyperthermia does not change qualitatively this course; however, it delays the second tumor regrowth by enhancing the radiation-induced cytotoxicity and the immune system response.

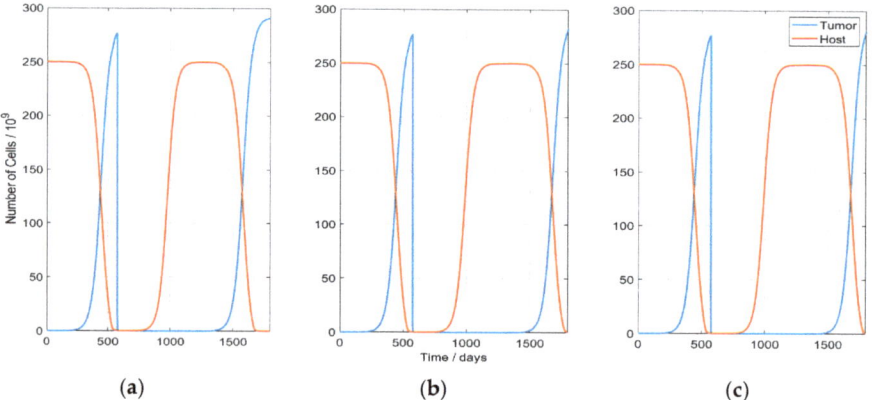

Figure 3. Development of the host—and tumor—cell populations: The sudden drop in the tumor population indicates the time point of RT start (day 570). After RT, the tumor starts to regrowth and approaches in every scenario the equilibrium level of 306×10^6 cells. The scenarios presented here correspond to: (**a**) Case with no HT (RT1HT0); (**b**) Case RT1HT3; (**c**) Case RT1HT2.

In Figure 4, the evolution of the effector cell populations is presented. Hyperthermia clearly increases the immune cells production during the first phase of treatment. However, no antitumor-vaccination effect is observed in any of the cases: This is clearly visible in the lower diagrams of Figure 4, where the immune cell numbers are plotted with a linear scale. In the upper part of Figure 4 (logarithmic plots), the weak responses during host and tumor regrowth become visible. A fundamental behavior of the system is visible during host tissue repopulation after treatment: In a first phase (around day 800), the host-related immune cell population (I2) rises, based on the previously evolved perceptron weights and the increasing presence of host tissue cells. Due to the lack of a danger signal during host tissue regrowth, the effector cell production and immigration drop after an initial rise. This is related to an evolution of perceptron weights (Equation (7)) to negative values. Comparing the three displayed scenarios, no substantial changes are observed between the different hyperthermia schemes, so the immune response is similar in all the cases.

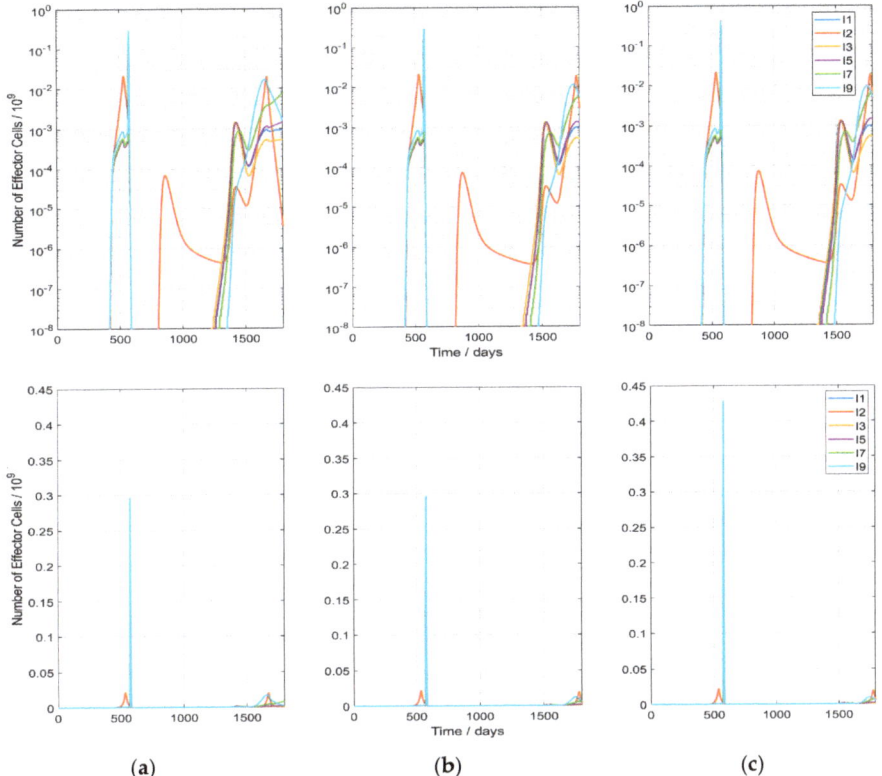

Figure 4. Development of effector immune cells in case of HT-induced modification of all parameters (last column in Table 4): For the host-related effector cells, only the population I2 (red line) is displayed; the other host-associated populations behave identically. The scenarios presented here correspond to (**a**) Case with no HT (RT1HT0); (**b**) Case RT1HT3; (**c**) Case RT1HT2; upper figures with logarithmic axis.

The immune response after RT is only produced during the first 10 days of treatment (Figure 5). This explains why the hyperthermia treatment HT2, which is the one with more hyperthermia sessions during those days, results in the highest TCP value. Additionally, spikes are visible at the position of each RT fraction because of the radiation-mediated effector cell elimination. On the other hand, rises in the effector cell production are visible after each hyperthermia session (Figure 5b,c): one just after HT produced by the perfusion like effects and another one 1–2 days after because of slow processes. In this figure, it is also observed that the anti-host immune response after RT is augmented by HT.

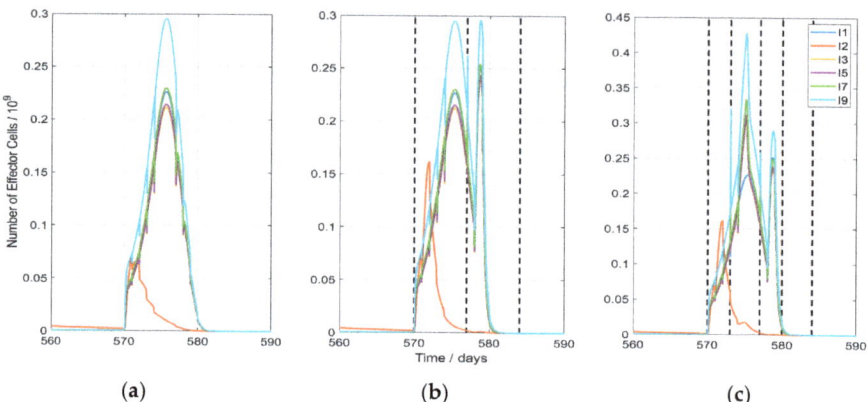

Figure 5. Development of effector immune cells during RT and HT-RT (in case of HT-induced modification of all parameters, according last column in Table 4). The impact of every RT fraction (5 fractions in the first week starting at day 570 and 4 of 5 fractions of the 2nd week starting at day 577) on the effector cells is visible as a spike-shaped drop of the cell number. The scenarios presented here correspond to (**a**) Case with no HT (RT1HT0); (**b**) Case RT1HT3; (**c**) Case RT1HT2. A dashed line is plotted each time a HT session is performed.

4. Discussion

As stated in the introduction, the results of this study cannot be applied directly to clinical treatments since they represent the behavior of an artificial system. Besides the uncertainty of many of the used parameters, a very simplistic description of the immune system is used. One of the main shortcomings is the lack of an immunological memory. In addition, only the local response in the tumor compartment is regarded. The anti-host immune reaction observed in our simulations may be interpreted as a local inflammatory process after radiation. In the case of additional compartments containing only non-irradiated neighboring host tissue, the training of the perceptron may result in different weights for host tissue and a subsequent modification of the anti-host response. Regarding this aspect, a multi-compartmental model would be closer to the real patient.

In addition, the inclusion of HT in the model follows simplistic concepts leading to the question of whether they are appropriate. In particular, thermo-tolerance is not considered. Therefore, the conclusions may not be appropriate for shorter intervals of HT sessions at higher temperatures (above 41–42 °C). Interestingly, the influence of variations in the HT sub-models does not lead to large differences in the outcome. This can be seen as an indication that—at least for larger time scales—the dynamic interplay between the adaptive immune system (perceptron training) and tumor-host ecosystem may be more important, independently of the details of the different sub-models.

The analysis of infiltrating immune cells in biopsy material can be compared to the time course of the effector cell populations in the model. The problems of comparing the model with such real-world data derived by biopsy material of cancer patients are manifold. The analysis of tumor samples by Holl et al. [57] revealed a percentage of overall lymphocytes of 2–39% of totally living cells. Not all of these cells can be considered as effector cells in the sense of our model. Therefore, it can be expected that the number of effector cells acting against the tumor should be clearly below (in the presented simulations, a percentage of 0.1–0.5% can be observed). Real world data give an indication for an upper limit (the simulation results are clearly below this limit) but also exhibit a large variation of patient—and tumor—specific responses.

Besides the percentage of effector cells in the peak of the immune response, a comparison of the production/invasion and elimination speed with real-world data would be interesting. According the work of Krosl et al. [58], the immigration (infiltration) of cells of the innate immune system seems to be very fast: neutrophils peak around 5 min and mast cells exhibit a pronounced rise during the first 25 min after Photodynamic Therapy (PDT) in CH3/HeN mice with implanted squamous cell carcinoma. No lymphocytes have been observed during the first 8 h after PDT. In our simulations, the effector cell number rise after the first RT fractions with a delay of 1 h at a high rate during 2–3 h followed by a slower increase over days. Regarding the point that these effector cells are part of the adaptive immune system, a slower process compared to the innate immune response can be expected, although the artificial immune system in our simulations was pre-exposed to the tumor antigens prior to the first RT fraction by necrotic tumor cells.

A stringent comparison with clinical trials is at the moment not possible and would require a sufficient number of patients in the different HT-RT treatment schemes (HTxRTy). A coarse indication may be obtained by a comparison with a clinical trial including patients with UICC stage I-IV anal cancer who received chemo-radiotherapy [55]: 50 out of the 112 patients received additional hyperthermia treatments. After 5 years follow-up, the overall response was significantly increased in the hyperthermia group (95.8 vs. 74.5%). The local recurrence-free after 5 years follow-up was 97.7% (HT) vs. 78.7% (no HT). These values are in agreement with the presented results. It is important to note here that only the case without HT (RT only) was adjusted to a TCP of 0.8. The fact that a comparable impact of HT, as observed by Ott et al. [55], was reached is based on the HT models used in the simulations.

During this study, a large number of simulations with varying conditions and parameter values have been executed (not shown). Over a large range of different parameter values, similar behavior of the system was observed. In this light, the semantic approach used for modelling in this study leads to the observation of some fundamental dynamic patterns which may allow general conclusions concerning the basic dynamics in such systems. However, the following conclusions are more or less restricted to the investigated scenarios and the proposed artificial immune–tumor ecosystem.

5. Conclusions

For the first time, a simulation for investigating the effect of a full HT-RT treatment on an artificial adaptive immune–tumor ecosystem is presented. In the investigated scenarios, RT leads to an anti-tumor as well as an anti-host response during RT. This effect is—especially for tumor cells—increased by the application of HT prior to selected RT fractions. The main effect of HT (ΔTCP = 0.13–0.18) is based on the adaption of the radio-sensitivity coefficients indicating a pivotal role of heat-induced, intra-cellular modifications. Perfusion or heat-based effects on the immune system seem to contribute less ($\Delta TCP = 0.003 - 0.019$) in the investigated system. In addition, the influence onto the TCP between the two RT fractionation schemes is very small ($\Delta TCP = 0.001 - 0.011$) and the RT2-fractionation turned out to be slightly less effective, in contrast to the findings by Scheidegger and Fellermann [59]. Even for the different HT protocols, the main rise of TCP is achieved by the early HT sessions. This is the reason why the HT2-protocol (as used for the HYCAN trial) exhibits a slightly better response. This is based on the fact that at the beginning of the therapy, more tumor cells are present and the effect of radiation-induced cell killing and immune activation is therefore stronger. As a possible consequence for clinical treatments, more HT sessions at the beginning of a HT-RT treatment seems to be favorable, as long as no thermo-tolerance will be induced.

During RT and HT-RT, a pronounced immune response contributes to tumor cell elimination by activation of the immune system via the perceptron response (rise of perceptron weights). As the tumor regrows after treatment, the secondary (late) immune response remains weak in all simulations and no radiation—or heat—induced anti-tumor vaccination effect was observed. The perceptron weights for host tissue evolve during the regrowth phase into negative values. This leads together with the decreased weights for the different tumor sub-clones to an immune-suppressive effect. This effect is based on the dynamic interplay between population (re-) growth and the perceptron training. If the immune system in patient would behave similar, this effect would be added to other effects based on the immune-suppressive strategies of tumor cells such as the release of immune-regulatory cytokines or changes in the microenvironment [60]. In general, the therapy outcome is strongly influenced by the combination of ecosystem dynamics and perceptron training. By implementing an immunological memory in the model, it would be interesting to search for scenarios where HT enhance or induce a memory-based anti-tumor response (HT-induced anti-tumor vaccination).

As a more general conclusion, a stringent and systematic comparison between the presented simulation and clinical trials requires trials with sufficient patients receiving treatments using similar fractionation schemes and with a careful documentation/reporting of achieved temperature courses during treatments (and time gaps between HT and RT).

Author Contributions: Conceptualization, S.S. and U.S.G.; methodology, S.S.; software, S.S. and S.M.B.; validation, S.M.B., S.S. and U.S.G.; formal analysis, S.S. and S.M.B.; investigation, S.S. and S.M.B.; writing—original draft preparation, S.S.; writing—review and editing, U.S.G. and S.M.B.; visualization, S.S. and S.M.B.; supervision, S.S.; project administration, S.S.; funding acquisition, S.S. All authors have read and agreed to the published version of the manuscript.

Funding: This project (Hyperboost; www.Hyperboost-h2020.eu (accessed on 10 November 2021)) has received funding from the European Union's Horizon 2020 research and innovation programme under the Marie Skłodowska-Curie grant agreement No 955625.

Institutional Review Board Statement: Not applicable.

Informed Consent Statement: Not applicable.

Data Availability Statement: Program code is available on request to scst@zhaw.ch.

Conflicts of Interest: The authors declare no conflict of interest.

References

1. Alfonso, J.C.L.; Papaxenopoulou, L.A.; Mascheroni, P.; Meyer-Hermann, P.; Hatzikirou, H. On the Immunological Consequences of Conventionally Fractionated Radiotherapy. *iScience* **2020**, *23*, 100897. [CrossRef] [PubMed]
2. Di Maggio, F.; Di Maggio, M.; Minafra, L.; Forte, G.I.; Cammarata, F.P.; Lio, D.; Messa, C.; Gilardi, M.C.; Bravatà, V. Portrait of inflammatory response to ionizing radiation treatment. *J. Inflamm.* **2015**, *12*, 14. [CrossRef] [PubMed]
3. Frey, B.; Rückert, M.; Deloch, L.; Rühle, P.F.; Derer, A.; Fietkau, R.; Gaipl, U.S. Immuno-modulation by ionizing radiation-impact for design of radio-immunotherapies and for treatment of inflammatory diseases. *Immunol. Rev.* **2017**, *280*, 231–248. [CrossRef] [PubMed]
4. Rosado, M.M.; Pioli, C. Cancer-host battles: Measures and countermeasures in radiation-induced caspase activation and tumor immunogenicity. *Cell. Mol. Immunol.* **2020**, *17*, 1022–1023. [CrossRef]
5. Bergs, J.W.J.; Krawczyk, P.M.; Borovski, T.; Cate, R.T.; Rodermond, H.M.; Stap, J.; Medema, J.P.; Haveman, J.; Essers, J.; van Bree, C.; et al. Inhibition of homologous recombination by hyperthermia shunts early double strand break repair to non-homologous end-joining. *DNA Repair* **2013**, *12*, 38–45. [CrossRef]
6. Iliakis, G.; Wu, W.; Wang, M. DNA double strand break repair inhibition as a cause of heat radiosensitization: Re-evaluation considering backup pathways of NHEJ. *Int. J. Hyperth.* **2008**, *24*, 17–29. [CrossRef] [PubMed]
7. Hildebrandt, B.; Wust, P.; Ahlers, O.; Dieing, A.; Sreenivasa, G.; Kerner, T.; Felix, R.; Riess, H. The cellular and molecular basis of hyperthermia. *Crit. Rev. Oncol. Hematol.* **2002**, *43*, 33–56. [CrossRef]
8. Dewey, W.C.; Hopwood, L.E.; Sapareto, S.A.; Gerweck, L.E. Cellular responses to combinations of hyperthermia and radiation. *Radiology* **1977**, *123*, 463–474. [CrossRef] [PubMed]
9. Hall, E.J.; Roizin-Towle, L. Biological Effects of Heat. *Cancer Res.* **1984**, *44*, 4708s–4713s.
10. Reinhold, H.S.; Endrich, B. Tumour microcirculation as a target for hyperthermia. *Int. J. Hyperth.* **1986**, *2*, 111–137. [CrossRef]
11. Song, C.W. Effect of Local Hyperthermia on Blood Flow and Microenvironment: A Review. *Cancer Res.* **1984**, *44*, 4721s–4730s.
12. Winslow, T.B.; Eranki, A.; Ullas, S.; Singh, A.K.; Repasky, E.A.; Sen, A. A pilot study of the effects of mild systemic heating on human head and neck tumour xenografts: Analysis of tumour perfusion, interstitial fluid pressure, hypoxia and efficacy of radiation therapy. *Int. J. Hyperth.* **2015**, *31*, 693–701. [CrossRef]
13. Wike-Hooley, J.L.; van der Zee, J.; van Rhoon, G.C.; van den Berg, A.P.; Reinhold, H.S. Human tumour pH changes following hyperthermia and radiation therapy. *Eur. J. Cancer Clin. Oncol.* **1984**, *20*, 619–623. [CrossRef]
14. Ohishi, T.; Nukuzuma, C.; Seki, A.; Watanabe, M.; Tomiyama-Miyaji, C.; Kainuma, E.; Inoue, M.; Kuwano, Y.; Abo, T. Alkalization of blood pH is responsible for survival of cancer patients by mild hyperthermia. *Biomed. Res.* **2009**, *30*, 95–100. [CrossRef]
15. Thistlethwaite, A.J.; Leeper, D.B.; Moylan, D.J.; Nerlinger, R.E. pH distribution in human tumors. *Int. J. Radiat. Oncol. Biol. Phys.* **1985**, *11*, 1647–1652. [CrossRef]

16. Brizel, D.M.; Scully, S.P.; Harrelson, J.M.; Layfield, L.J.; Dodge, R.K.; Charles, H.C.; Samulski, T.V.; Prosnitz, L.R.; Dewhirst, M.W. Radiation Therapy and Hyperthermia Improve the Oxygenation of Human Soft Tissue Sarcomas. *Cancer Res.* **1996**, *56*, 5347–5350. [PubMed]
17. Sun, X.; Xing, L.; Ling, C.C.; Li, G.C. The effect of mild temperature hyperthermia on tumour hypoxia and blood perfusion: Relevance for radiotherapy, vascular targeting and imaging. *Int. J. Hyperth.* **2010**, *26*, 224–231. [CrossRef]
18. Song, C.W.; Shakil, A.; Osborn, J.L.; Iwata, K. Tumour oxygenation is increased by hyperthermia at mild temperatures. *Int. J. Hyperth.* **1996**, *12*, 367–373. [CrossRef]
19. Harrison, L.B.; Chadha, M.; Hill, R.J.; Hu, K.; Shasha, D. Impact of Tumor Hypoxia and Anemia on Radiation Therapy Outcomes. *Oncologist* **2002**, *7*, 492–508. [CrossRef] [PubMed]
20. Moulder, J.E.; Rockwell, S. Hypoxic fractions of solid tumors: Experimental techniques, methods of analysis, and a survey of existing data. *Int. J. Radiat. Oncol. Biol. Phys.* **1984**, *10*, 695–712. [CrossRef]
21. Scheidegger, S.; Bonmarin, M.; Timm, O.; Rhodes, S.; Datta, N.R. Estimating radio-sensitisation based on re-oxygenation after hyperthermia by using dynamic models. *Panminerva Med.* **2014**, *56* (Suppl. 1), 24.
22. Husain, Z.; Huang, Y.; Seth, P.; Sukhatme, V.P. Tumor-Derived Lactate Modifies Antitumor Immune Response: Effect on Myeloid-Derived Suppressor Cells and NK Cells. *J. Immunol.* **2013**, *191*, 1486–1495. [CrossRef] [PubMed]
23. Calcinotto, A.; Filipazzi, P.; Grioni, M.; Iero, M.; De Milito, A.; Ricupito, A.; Cova, A.; Canese, R.; Jachetti, E.; Rossetti, M.; et al. Modulation of microenvironment acidity reverses anergy in human and murine tumor-infiltrating T lymphocytes. *Cancer Res.* **2012**, *72*, 2746–2756. [CrossRef]
24. Bosticardo, M.; Ariotti, S.; Losana, G.; Bernabei, P.; Forni, G.; Novelli, F. Biased activation of human T lymphocytes due to low extracellular pH is antagonized by B7/CD28 costimulation. *Eur. J. Immunol.* **2001**, *31*, 2829–2838. [CrossRef]
25. Erra Díaz, F.; Dantas, E.; Geffner, J. Unravelling the interplay between extracellular acidosis and immune cells. *Mediat. Inflamm.* **2018**, *2018*, 1218297. [CrossRef] [PubMed]
26. Milani, V.; Noessner, E.; Ghose, S.; Kuppner, M.; Ahrens, B.; Scharner, A.; Gastpar, R.; Issels, R.D. Heat shock protein 70: Role in antigen presentation and immune stimulation. *Int. J. Hyperth.* **2002**, *18*, 563–575. [CrossRef]
27. Ito, A.; Shinkai, M.; Honda, H.; Wakabayashi, T.; Yoshida, J.; Kobayashi, T. Augmentation of MHC class I antigen presentation via heat shock protein expression by hyperthermia. *Cancer Immunol. Immunother.* **2001**, *50*, 515–522. [CrossRef]
28. Srivastava, P. Roles of heat-shock proteins in innate and adaptive immunity. *Nat. Rev. Immunol.* **2002**, *2*, 185–194. [CrossRef]
29. Pienta, K.J.; McGregor, N.; Axelrod, R.; Axelrod, D.E. Ecological therapy for cancer: Defining tumors using an ecosystem paradigm suggests new opportunities for novel cancer treatments. *Transl. Oncol.* **2008**, *1*, 158–164. [CrossRef] [PubMed]
30. Basanta, D.; Anderson, A.R.A. Exploiting ecological principles to better understand cancer progression and treatment. *Interface Focus* **2013**, *3*, 20130020. [CrossRef]
31. Merlo, L.M.F.; Pepper, J.W.; Reid, B.J.; Maley, C.C. Cancer as an evolutionary and ecological process. *Nat. Rev. Cancer* **2006**, *6*, 924–935. [CrossRef] [PubMed]
32. Frey, B.; Rückert, M.; Weber, J.; Mayr, X.; Derer, A.; Lotter, M.; Bert, C.; Rödel, F.; Fietkau, R.; Gaipl, U.S. Hypofractionated Irradiation Has Immune Stimulatory Potential and Induces a Timely Restricted Infiltration of Immune Cells in Colon Cancer Tumors. *Front. Immunol.* **2017**, *8*, 231. [CrossRef]
33. Scheidegger, S.; Mikos, J.; Fellermann, H. Modelling Artificial Immune—Tumor Ecosystem Interaction During Radiation Therapy Using a Perceptron—Based Antigen Pattern Recognition. In Proceedings of the 2020 Conference on Artificial Life, Online, Montréal, QC, Canada, 13–18 July 2020; MIT Press: Cambridge, MA, USA, 2020; pp. 541–548.
34. Eftimie, R.; Bramson, J.L.; Earn, D.J.D. Interactions between the immune system and cancer: A brief review of non-spatial mathematical models. *Bull. Math. Biol.* **2011**, *73*, 2–32. [CrossRef]
35. Rosenblatt, F. The perceptron: A probabilistic model for information storage and organization in the brain. *Psychol. Rev.* **1958**, *65*, 386–408. [CrossRef]
36. Matzinger, P. The danger model: A renewed sense of self. *Science* **2002**, *296*, 301–305. [CrossRef] [PubMed]
37. Golden, E.B.; Frances, D.; Pellicciotta, I.; Demaria, S.; Barcellos-Hoff, M.H.; Formetti, S.C. Radiation fosters dose-dependent and chemotherapy-induced immunogenic cell death. *Oncoimmunology* **2014**, *3*, e28518. [CrossRef]
38. Abhishek, D.; Agostinis, P. Cell death and immunity in cancer: From danger signals to mimicry of pathogen defense responses. *Immunol. Rev.* **2017**, *280*, 126–148.
39. Rodriguez-Ruiz, M.E.; Vitale, I.; Harrington, K.J.; Melero, I.; Galluzzi, L. Immunological impact of cell death signaling driven by radiation on the tumor microenvironment. *Nat. Immunol.* **2020**, *21*, 120–134. [CrossRef]
40. Scheidegger, S.; Lutters, G.; Bodis, S. A LQ-based kinetic model formulation for exploring dynamics of treatment response of tumours in patients. *Z. Med. Phys.* **2011**, *21*, 164–173. [CrossRef]
41. Grimsley, C.; Ravichandran, K.S. Cues for apoptotic cell engulfment: Eat-me, don't eat-me and come-get-me signals. *Trends Cell Biol.* **2003**, *13*, 648–656. [CrossRef] [PubMed]
42. Zhou, J.; Wang, G.; Chen, Y.; Wang, H.; Hua, Y.; Cai, Z. Immunogenic cell death in cancer therapy: Present and emerging inducers. *J. Cell. Mol. Med.* **2019**, *23*, 4854–4865. [CrossRef]
43. Park, S.J.; Kim, J.M.; Kim, J.; Hur, J.; Park, S.; Kim, K.; Shin, H.J.; Chwae, Y.J. Molecular mechanisms of biogenesis of apoptotic exosome-like vesicles and their roles as damage-associated molecular patterns. *Proc. Natl. Acad. Sci. USA* **2018**, *115*, E11721–E11730. [CrossRef]

44. Nagata, S.; Tanaka, M. Programmed cell death and the immune system. *Nat. Rev. Immunol.* **2017**, *17*, 333–340. [CrossRef]
45. Faouzi, S.; Burckhardt, B.E.; Hanson, J.C.; Campe, C.B.; Schrum, L.W.; Rippe, R.A.; Maher, J.J. Anti-Fas Induces Hepatic Chemokines and Promotes Inflammation by an NF-κB-independent, Caspase-3-dependent Pathway. *J. Biol. Chem.* **2001**, *276*, 49077–49082. [CrossRef]
46. Willems, J.J.L.P.; Arnold, B.P.; Gregory, C.D. Sinister Self-Sacrifice: The Contribution of Apoptosis to Malignancy. *Front. Immunol.* **2014**, *5*, 299. [CrossRef] [PubMed]
47. Monico, B.; Nigro, A.; Casolaro, V.; Col, J.D. Immunogenic Apoptosis as a Novel Tool for Anticancer Vaccine Development. *Int. J. Mol. Sci.* **2018**, *19*, 594. [CrossRef] [PubMed]
48. Leith, J.T.; Padfield, G.; Faulkner, L.E.; Quinn, P.; Michelson, S. Effects of feeder cells on the X-ray sensitivity of human colon cancer cells. *Radiother. Oncol.* **1991**, *21*, 53–59. [CrossRef]
49. van Leeuwen, C.M.; Oei, A.L.; Crezee, J.; Bel, A.; Franken, N.A.P.; Stalpers, L.J.A.; Kok, H.P. The alfa and beta of tumours: A review of parameters of the linear-quadratic model, derived from clinical radiotherapy studies. *Radiat. Oncol.* **2018**, *13*, 96. [CrossRef]
50. Wang, Z.; Armour, E.P.; Corry, P.M.; Martinez, A. Elimination of dose-rate effects by mild hyperthermia. *Int. J. Radiat. Oncol. Biol. Phys.* **1992**, *24*, 965–973. [CrossRef]
51. Armour, E.P.; Wang, Z.; Corry, P.M.; Martinez, A. Sensitization of Rat 9L Gliosarcoma Cells to Low Dose Rate Irradiation by Long Duration 41 °C Hyperthermia. *Cancer Res.* **1991**, *51*, 3088–3095. [PubMed]
52. Hunt, C.R.; Pandita, R.K.; Laszlo, A.; Higashikubo, R.; Agarwal, M.; Kitamura, T.; Gupta, A.; Rief, N.; Horikoshi, N.; Baskaran, R.; et al. Hyperthermia activates a subset of ataxia-telangiectasia mutated effectors independent of DNA strand breaks and heat shock protein 70 status. *Cancer Res.* **2007**, *67*, 3010–3017. [CrossRef] [PubMed]
53. van Leeuwen, C.M.; Oei, A.L.; Cate, R.T.; Franken, N.A.P.; Bel, A.; Stalpers, L.J.A.; Crezee, J.; Kok, H.P. Measurement and analysis of the impact of time-interval, temperature and radiation dose on tumour cell survival and its application in thermoradiotherapy plan evaluation. *Int. J. Hyperth.* **2018**, *34*, 30–38. [CrossRef] [PubMed]
54. Song, C.W.; Choi, I.B.; Nah, B.S.; Sahu, S.K.; Osborn, J.L. Microvasculature and Perfusion in Normal Tissues and Tumors. In *Thermoradiotherapy and Thermochemotherapy*; Seegenschmiedt, M.H., Fessenden, P., Vernon, C.C., Eds.; Springer: Berlin/Heidelberg, Germany; New York, NY, USA, 1995; pp. 139–156.
55. Ott, O.J.; Schmidt, M.; Semrau, S.; Strnad, V.; Matzel, K.E.; Schneider, I.; Raptis, D.; Uter, W.; Grützmann, R.; Fietkau, R. Chemoradiotherapy with and without deep regional hyperthermia for squamous cell carcinoma of the anus. *Strahlenther. Onkol.* **2019**, *195*, 607–614. [CrossRef]
56. Datta, N.R.; Stutz, E.; Puric, E.; Eberle, B.; Meister, A.; Marder, D.; Timm, O.; Rogers, S.; Wyler, S.; Bodis, S. A Pilot Study of Radiotherapy and Local Hyperthermia in Elderly Patients with Muscle-Invasive Bladder Cancers Unfit for Definitive Surgery or Chemoradiotherapy. *Front. Oncol.* **2019**, *9*, 889. [CrossRef] [PubMed]
57. Holl, E.K.; Frazier, V.N.; Landa, K.; Beasley, G.M.; Hwang, E.S.; Nair, S.K. Examining peripheral and tumor cellular in patients with cancer. *Front. Immunol.* **2019**, *10*, 1767. [CrossRef]
58. Krosl, G.; Korbelik, M.; Dougherty, G.J. Induction of immune cell infiltration into murine SCCVII tumour by Photofrin-based photodynamic therapy. *Br. J. Cancer* **1995**, *71*, 549–555. [CrossRef] [PubMed]
59. Scheidegger, S.; Fellermann, H. Optimizing Radiation Therapy Treatments by Exploring Tumour Ecosystem Dynamics in-silico. In Proceedings of the 2019 Conference on Artificial Life, Online, Newcastle, UK, 29 July–2 August 2019; MIT Press: Cambridge, MA, USA, 2019; pp. 236–242.
60. Rabinovich, G.A.; Gabrilovich, D.; Sotomayor, E.M. Immunosuppressive strategies that are mediated by tumor cells. *Annu. Rev. Immunol.* **2007**, *25*, 267–296. [CrossRef]

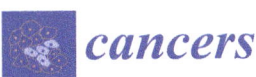

Article

Fast Adaptive Temperature-Based Re-Optimization Strategies for On-Line Hot Spot Suppression during Locoregional Hyperthermia

H. Petra Kok * and Johannes Crezee

Department of Radiation Oncology, Amsterdam UMC, University of Amsterdam, Cancer Center Amsterdam, 1105 AZ Amsterdam, The Netherlands; h.crezee@amsterdamumc.nl
* Correspondence: h.p.kok@amsterdamumc.nl

Simple Summary: When treatment limiting hot spots occur during locoregional hyperthermia (i.e., heating tumors to 40–44 °C for ~1 h), system settings are adjusted based on experience. In this study, we developed and evaluated treatment planning with temperature-based re-optimization and compared the predicted effectiveness to clinically applied protocol/experience-based steering. Re-optimization times were typically ~10 s; sufficiently fast for on-line use. Effective hot spot suppression was predicted, while maintaining adequate tumor heating. Inducing new hot spots was avoided. Temperature-based re-optimization to suppress treatment limiting hot spots seemed feasible to match the effectiveness of long-term clinical experience and will be further evaluated in a clinical setting. When numerical algorithms are proven to match long-term experience, the overall treatment quality within hyperthermia centers can significantly improve. Implementing these strategies would then imply that treatments become less dependent on the experience of the center/operator.

Abstract: Background: Experience-based adjustments in phase-amplitude settings are applied to suppress treatment limiting hot spots that occur during locoregional hyperthermia for pelvic tumors. Treatment planning could help to further optimize treatments. The aim of this research was to develop temperature-based re-optimization strategies and compare the predicted effectiveness with clinically applied protocol/experience-based steering. Methods: This study evaluated 22 hot spot suppressions in 16 cervical cancer patients (mean age 67 ± 13 year). As a first step, all potential hot spot locations were represented by a spherical region, with a user-specified diameter. For fast and robust calculations, the hot spot temperature was represented by a user-specified percentage of the voxels with the largest heating potential (HPP). Re-optimization maximized tumor T90, with constraints to suppress the hot spot and avoid any significant increase in other regions. Potential hot spot region diameter and HPP were varied and objective functions with and without penalty terms to prevent and minimize temperature increase at other potential hot spot locations were evaluated. Predicted effectiveness was compared with clinically applied steering results. Results: All strategies showed effective hot spot suppression, without affecting tumor temperatures, similar to clinical steering. To avoid the risk of inducing new hot spots, HPP should not exceed 10%. Adding a penalty term to the objective function to minimize the temperature increase at other potential hot spot locations was most effective. Re-optimization times were typically ~10 s. Conclusion: Fast on-line re-optimization to suppress treatment limiting hot spots seems feasible to match effectiveness of ~30 years clinical experience and will be further evaluated in a clinical setting.

Keywords: hyperthermia; hyperthermia treatment planning; adaptive planning; temperature optimization

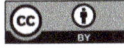

1. Introduction

Mild hyperthermia treatments, i.e., heating tumors to 40–44 °C, enhance the effect of radiotherapy and chemotherapy [1–7]. Treatment outcome depends on both the achieved temperature and treatment duration [8–12]. Therefore, the thermal dose is often expressed as the number of equivalent minutes at 43 °C [13]. The standard treatment duration is typically ~1 h to ensure both a good therapeutic effect and patient tolerance. The risk of thermal toxicity to normal tissue also depends on the local temperature and exposure time [14]. In clinical practice, hyperthermia-associated toxicity is rarely observed when temperatures remain below the pain sensation level (~45 °C [15]). The maximum achievable tumor temperature is usually limited when such treatment limiting hot spots occur.

Tumor temperatures should be monitored to ensure adequate heating. Standard clinical thermometry feedback uses (minimally invasive) thermometry probes. For some specific tumor sites (e.g., soft tissue sarcoma or tumors in extremities), non-invasive MR-thermometry can be utilized [16,17], however for patients with thoracic, abdominal or pelvic tumors, the reliability is limited due to organ movement and blood flow [18]. Therefore, quality assurance guidelines [19] prescribe treatment guidance based on thermometry probe information and patient feedback about the incidence of hot spots.

Locoregional hyperthermia is usually applied for heating pelvic tumors, administered by means of phased-array systems, consisting of four or more antennas organized in one or more rings around the patient [20]. Commercially available systems are the BSD-2000 systems and the ALBA-4D system, operating between 60 and 120 MHz [21–24]. The phases and amplitudes of the antennas can be adjusted such that interference yields a heating focus at the tumor location. However, due to inhomogeneities in dielectric and thermal tissue properties, treatment limiting hot spots can occur at tissue interfaces [25]. The operator should determine phase-amplitude settings to maximize tumor heating, while avoiding treatment limiting normal tissue hot spots. Phase-amplitude steering is presently usually based on experience of the operator and empirical steering protocols.

Hyperthermia treatment planning can improve treatment quality [26,27]. Ideally, inverse treatment planning, i.e., 'inverting' the optimal specific absorption rate (SAR)/temperature distribution to obtain phase-amplitude settings that generate that optimal distribution, as also used for radiotherapy, would be applied. A numerical optimization routine would then be used to prescribe optimal phases and amplitudes. Many research groups have worked on such methods, either based on SAR [28–33] or temperature [25,31,34,35]. However, due to the uncertainties in predicted SAR and temperature levels, caused by the lack of information about patient-specific tissue properties and local blood perfusion, treatment limiting hot spots can still occur when applying such optimized phase-amplitude settings and on-line adjustments during treatment remain necessary [36,37].

Thus, inverse pre-treatment optimization methods cannot provide a quantitatively reliable and robust treatment plan. However, previous studies have shown qualitative reliability, i.e., when adjusting phase-amplitude settings, the resulting simulated and measured changes in heating patterns do correlate [38,39]. The deviation between measured and predicted changes in temperature after phase-amplitude steering was accurate within ± 0.1 °C for most events [39]. This makes adaptive planning during treatment possible. Hyperthermia treatment planning can be very useful in assisting phase-amplitude steering in response to hot spots and to optimize tumor heating [39–41]. Visualizing the predicted effect of different steering strategies can help the operator to find more effective phase-amplitude steering strategies [40,41]. In analogy with radiotherapy, this can be considered as 'forward adaptive planning'.

Inverse adaptive planning strategies based on SAR have been proposed by Canters et al. [42]. In case of a hot spot, the power density in the hot spot region was reduced by adding a penalty term to the objective function. Target temperatures in the therapeutic range were achieved in patients using this complaint-adaptive steering strategy [42]. A cross-over trial with 36 patients further confirmed feasibility of SAR-based complaint-adaptive steering, yet also revealed some challenges in hot spot suppression [43].

Although SAR and temperature are correlated [39], temperature-based treatment planning might be more effective for complaint-adaptive steering strategies. SAR-based treatment planning does not account for the influence of relevant thermal processes as conduction, blood perfusion and water bolus cooling, which makes that SAR hot spots will not always coincide with temperature hot spots. Furthermore, SAR-based treatment planning strategies, as described above, account for hot spots using a penalty term, but do not use normal tissue constraints to suppress and/or avoid hot spots. Temperature-based optimization maximizes the target temperature with constraints to normal tissue temperatures [25]. This makes temperature-based optimization more intuitive to use and potentially more effective to suppress hot spots. However, on-line re-optimization needs to be fast, preferably a few seconds, and at least less than 1 min. A drawback of temperature-based optimization is that it is computationally more expensive than SAR-based optimization, despite efficient computation strategies that have been developed [34,44].

In this study we developed fast temperature-based re-optimization strategies for on-line use, and we evaluated the possible effectiveness of these strategies for 22 hot spots in 16 cervical cancer patients using simulations. Results for re-optimized phase-amplitude settings were compared to measured/predicted results of experience/protocol-based clinically applied steering in terms of hot spot reduction and target temperatures.

2. Materials and Methods
2.1. Treatment Planning Workflow

Hyperthermia treatment planning is part of the standard clinical workflow at the Amsterdam UMC. First a 60 cm long CT scan is made in the treatment position, i.e., on a water bolus and mattresses, with the thermometry catheters in situ. The radiation oncologist delineates the target region and this standard DICOM structure set and the CT data set are imported by Plan2Heat, a versatile in-house developed finite difference-based software package for hyperthermia treatment planning [45]. Hyperthermia treatment planning is performed by a physicist. Further tissue segmentation is based on Hounsfield Units, distinguishing muscle, fat, bone and lung/air. This process also segments the plastic thermometry catheters as bone, which is corrected manually, along with other segmentation artefacts, if present.

This segmented anatomy is downscaled to $2.5 \times 2.5 \times 2.5$ mm^3 and combined with a hyperthermia applicator model; in our case the 70 MHz ALBA-4D system with 4 waveguides (top, bottom, left, right). The literature-based dielectric and thermal tissue properties are assigned, with (tissue-dependent) enhanced perfusion values accounting for a physiological response to a temperature rise in the hyperthermic range [46–50]. All voxels labelled in the same tissue category are assigned homogeneous properties. Table 1 summarizes these properties. Using this patient-applicator model, electromagnetic field, SAR and temperature simulations are performed.

Table 1. Values of the dielectric and thermal tissue properties at 70 MHz used in the simulations.

Tissue	σ (S m^{-1})	ε_r (-)	ρ (kg m^{-3})	c (J kg^{-1} °C^{-1})	k (W m^{-1} °C^{-1})	W_b (kg m^{-3} s^{-1})
Air	0	1	1.29	1000	0.024	0
Bone	0.05	10	1595	1420	0.65	0.12
Fat	0.06	10	888	2387	0.22	1.1
Muscle	0.75	75	1050	3639	0.56	3.6
Tumor	0.74	65	1050	3639	0.56	1.8

electrical conductivity (σ [S m^{-1}]); relative permittivity (ε_r [-]); density (ρ [kg m^{-3}]); specific heat capacity (c [J kg^{-1} °C^{-1}]); thermal conductivity (k [W m^{-1} °C^{-1}]) and perfusion (W_b [kg m^{-3} s^{-1}]). NB: perfusion values are enhanced to account for a physiological response to a temperature rise in the hyperthermic range [48,51].

2.2. Potential Hot Spots

At Amsterdam UMC hot spot complaints occurring during clinical hyperthermia treatments are registered in the treatment report. To facilitate this process each potential hot spot location is identified by a unique number (1–39), projected onto an anatomical picture (Figure 1A). This helps communication between the patient and the operator and to assess the hot spot location corresponding to the present pain complaint.

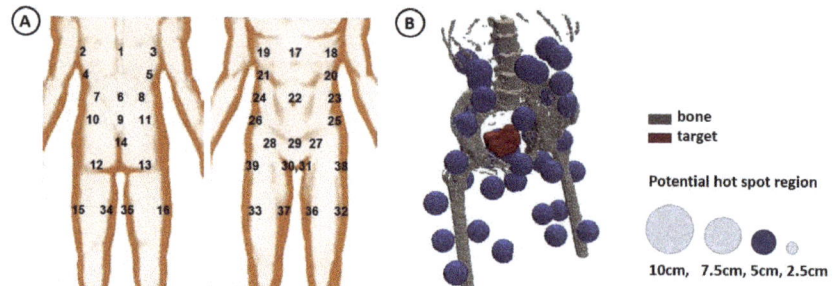

Figure 1. (**A**) Anatomical picture with all potential hot spot locations identified by a unique number, as used during clinical hyperthermia treatments. (**B**) 3D illustration of the spherical regions representing the potential hot spot locations, together with the bony anatomy for a cervical cancer patient. In this study, the potential hot spot diameter was varied between 2.5 and 10 cm. In this visualization a potential hot spot diameter of 5 cm is shown.

In the treatment planning process, these potential hot spot locations were represented by spherical regions, with a user-specified diameter. For a semi-automatic generation of potential hot spot regions, a dedicated module was added to Plan2Heat, in which the user should specify the desired diameter and eight world coordinates. The first six coordinates represent the center of the spherical region for the potential hot spot locations at the pubic bone (29), tail bone (9), left and right hip (25 + 26), left and right belly (23 + 24). The other two coordinates represent the center of the upper legs at the end of the water bolus, which are used in combination with the six hot spots to approximate the other 33 potential hot spot regions by interpolation. At these coordinates, spherical potential hot spot regions are created. If desired, the user can manually correct specific hot spot locations. A 3D example of reconstructed potential hot spot locations is shown in Figure 1B.

2.3. Temperature-Based Re-Optimization

Thermal predictions were based on the commonly applied Pennes' bioheat equation, where perfusion is modelled as a heat sink [52]. The steady-state temperature T (°C) was defined as the steady state solution to:

$$c\rho \frac{\partial T}{\partial t} = \nabla \cdot (k \nabla T) - c_b W_b (T - T_{art}) + \rho \cdot \text{SAR} \qquad (1)$$

with c_b (J kg^{-1} °C^{-1}) the specific heat capacity of blood (~3600 J kg^{-1} °C^{-1}) and T_{art} the local arterial or body core temperature (assumed to be 37 °C). For efficient calculations during temperature-based optimization, the temperature at voxel (x,y,z) was calculated using superposition by:

$$T(x, y, z) = v^H \underline{T} v + T_{00} \qquad (2)$$

where v is the feed vector containing the amplitudes and phases, $\underline{T}$ is a complex $N \times N$ Hermitian matrix (N: number of antennas) and T_{00} is a constant representing the thermal boundary conditions. For more details on derivation of these matrix elements, the reader is referred to previously published articles on this topic [25,34]. Quadratic programming was used to optimize a specified objective function, subject to normal tissue and antenna constraints. This was conducted five times with different random initial phase-amplitude settings, after which the best overall result was selected. Objectives and constraints are defined in the subsections below.

2.3.1. Constraints

Normal tissue temperature evaluation is one of the most time consuming operations during constrained temperature-based optimization due to the very large number of normal tissue voxels. Therefore, normal tissue evaluation is reduced to the 39 potential hot spot regions, which are represented by 39 normal tissue constraints. Averaging the hot spot temperature in these regions allows extremely fast calculation, since an average temperature matrix can be used. However, this would largely smooth peak temperatures and thus not be effective in hot spot suppression. Continuously searching for the maximum temperature per hot spot region during optimization is again time consuming and, thus, also not suitable for on-line applications.

To realize effective and fast hot spot temperature calculations, the potential hot spot temperatures were determined by the average temperature of the hot spot voxels with the largest heating potential. The heating potential of a voxel is represented by the maximum eigenvalue of its temperature matrix [34]. The 1 cm outer rim of the patient was excluded in this process, since although these voxels have a large heating potential, no temperature hot spots will occur in the most superficial layers due to strong bolus cooling. The percentage of voxels with the largest heating potential can be selected by the user. In the present study, percentages of 1, 10, 50 and 100% were evaluated.

In case of a treatment limiting hot spot, the re-optimization of phase-amplitude settings was performed with a hard constraint to suppress the indicated hot spot. The real hot spot temperature was assumed to be 45 °C, since that is the level at which a pain sensation is experienced, and which can lead to irreversible tissue damage after too long exposure [15]. In a previous clinical pilot study, on-line adaptive treatment planning was applied to suppress hot spots, and in those patient cases the mean and median hot spot temperature reduction was ~1 °C [40]; also assuming the real hot spot temperature to be 45 °C. Therefore, in this study, a constraint was set to the treatment limiting hot spot location to realize a temperature reduction of 1 °C, after re-scaling the hot spot temperature to 45 °C. To avoid introducing new hot spots, hard constraints were set to all other potential hot spot locations, such that the current temperature level will increase at most 0.5 °C. Furthermore, power constraints were applied to the waveguides to avoid clinically unrealistic amplitude settings. A waveguide should at least deliver 10% of the total power, although not more than 40%. The total applied power should remain constant.

2.3.2. Objective Functions

The aim in clinical hyperthermia is always to maximize the tumor temperature, and T90, i.e., the temperature at least achieved in 90% of the tumor volume is an important clinical parameter. Therefore, the objective functions used maximized T90. Hard constraints were applied to avoid a large temperature increase at other potential hot spot locations; to further minimize this temperature increase, also the use of additional penalty terms was evaluated. Penalty terms were defined for either the maximum increase in all potential hot spot temperatures, or the sum of the increase in potential hot spot temperatures. This yields the following three optimization goals:

$$\max \left(T_{90} - \max_{\substack{\text{potential} \\ \text{hot spots}}} \max(0, (T_{new} - T_{old})) \right) \quad (3)$$

$$\max \left(T_{90} - \sum_{\substack{\text{potential} \\ \text{hot spots}}} \max(0, (T_{new} - T_{old})) \right) \quad (4)$$

$$\max(T_{90}) \quad (5)$$

all subject to hard normal tissue and antenna constraints, as described in Section 2.3.1. T_{old} and T_{new} represent the hot spot temperature before and after the re-optimization, respectively.

2.4. Patient and Event Selection

For evaluation of the re-optimization algorithms, we used the patient group from Kok et al. (2018) [39], where SAR/temperature changes after phase-amplitude steering were evaluated for patients with pelvic tumors to determine the correlation between measurements and simulations. All these patients received the hyperthermia treatment according to our standard clinical protocol, with protocol/experience-based steering. We selected steering events that were registered as action to suppress treatment limiting hot spots. Bladder cancer patients were excluded for this study, since the correlation between measured and simulated SAR/temperature changes in the bladder was rather weak (due to convection in the bladder fluid, not accounted for in standard treatment planning), and the target temperature is an optimization/evaluation parameter. This selection resulted in 22 phase-amplitude steering events in 16 locally advanced cervical cancer patients (mean age 67 ± 13 y). The average tumor size was 111 ± 69 cc. The average fat percentage in the patient models was 51.4 ± 9.4%; for muscle and bone these percentages were 42.2 ± 8.8% and 4.7 ± 0.7%, respectively. The registered hot spot locations per event and patients are listed in Table 2; in some cases two hot spots occurred simultaneously.

Table 2. Registered treatment limiting hot spot locations for the patients and events included in this study. Anatomical location of hot spot location identifiers is shown in Figure 1A.

Event	Patient	Hot Spot Identifier
1	1	14
2	2	29
3	2	8
4	3	7
5	3	27 + 28
6	4	5
7	4	11
8	5	29
9	6	9
10	7	10
11	7	25 + 26
12	8	14
13	8	6
14	9	25
15	10	6
16	10	6
17	11	14
18	12	22
19	13	25 + 26
20	14	29
21	15	6
22	16	6 + 17

2.5. Evaluation

For each hot spot event in Table 2, re-optimization of phase-amplitude settings was performed to suppress the hot spot (or hot spots). To assess clinical feasibility for on-line use the re-optimization time was evaluated for each of the different strategies (i.e., objective Equations (3)–(5) and maximum eigenvalue percentages of 1, 10, 50 and 100%). To evaluate effectiveness in hot spot suppression, all voxels in the treatment limiting hot spot region were evaluated and the predicted maximum temperature reduction was determined. To evaluate the risk of newly induced hot spots, the overall maximum increase in the other potential hot spot regions and the change in predicted overall maximum in the whole patient volume were determined. For each re-optimization strategy, these predictions were compared with predictions for the clinically applied protocol/experience-based phase-amplitude adjustments.

Regarding the target temperatures, the predicted T90 and the temperature changes along the thermometry probes were evaluated. To reconstruct the simulated temperature along the thermometry probe trajectories in the cervix, track paths were delineated from the CT scan using the Plan2Heat module jTracktool [45]. Using these track paths the temperature was extracted from the simulated distributions with a 5 mm interval (i.e., the sensor spacing of the thermocouple probes) along the track. Spatial average values were calculated and simulated average temperatures were scaled per location with a factor such that the simulated value before changing the antenna settings corresponds to the measurement value. Next, the change in temperature due to adapting the antenna settings was determined. For each re-optimization strategy, we compared these predicted temperature changes along the probe with predictions for the clinically applied phase-amplitude adjustments, as well as with the real measurements.

All evaluations were first performed for a potential hot spot region diameter of 5 cm. For the most effective strategy, the influence of the hot spot diameter was also evaluated, comparing diameters of 2.5, 5, 7.5 and 10 cm.

3. Results

The effect of different re-optimization strategies on treatment limiting hot spot suppression as well as the maximum temperature increase at other potential hot spot locations and the overall normal tissue temperature maximum, are shown in Figure 2. The hot spot diameter was 5 cm. The effect of the clinically applied steering strategy by experienced treatment operators, is also shown. We observed that effective treatment limiting hot spot suppression was predicted for all strategies, which is, with exception of a few outliers, equally effective as the clinical strategy (Figure 2A). The difference in predicted mean hot spot temperature change compared to the clinical strategy was less than 0.2 °C for all strategies, and the standard deviation differed less than 0.1 °C. Considering the individual difference in predicted hot spot reductions between planning-based and clinical strategies for all 22 hot spots and steering actions, we see that the overall mean difference is -0.1 -- -0.2 °C (± 0.3–0.4 °C). This indicates a mild trend that planning-based steering yields a slightly larger reduction in hot spot temperature. However, since real and predicted temperature changes might deviate ± 0.1 °C [39] and small differences might not be perceptible by the patient, this difference is not considered clinically relevant and planning-based and clinical strategies are considered equally effective. Although hard constraints were applied to other potential hot spot locations to avoid inducing new hot spots, adding a penalty term was an effective strategy to further avoid a large temperature increase at other locations (Figure 2B,C). Both penalties in goal function (3) and (4) were effective. As expected, the risk of insufficiently suppressing the treatment limiting hot spot and/or inducing new hot spots increased when a larger number of voxels was included to determine the average hot spot temperature. In case voxels with the 50% or 100% largest heating potential were used (50% max EV and 100% max EV), this averaging often underestimates the hot spot temperature and a higher temperature increase at other potential hot spot locations was observed and the risk of outliers increased (Figure 2A,B). These outliers represent the limited number of cases where the average temperature estimating the hot spot temperature in the model, deviated largely from the real maximum temperature in the hot spot region. The fact that there are few outliers with a large temperature increase indicates that this averaging strategy to realize fast calculations works well, especially when only those voxels with the largest heating potential are included (i.e., 1% and 10% max EV). In those cases, and when including penalty terms, the average difference in predicted maximum potential hot spot increase and overall maximum temperature change compared to the clinical strategy was less than 0.15 °C (and with a comparable spread), which is not a clinically relevant difference and thus the strategies can be considered equally effective.

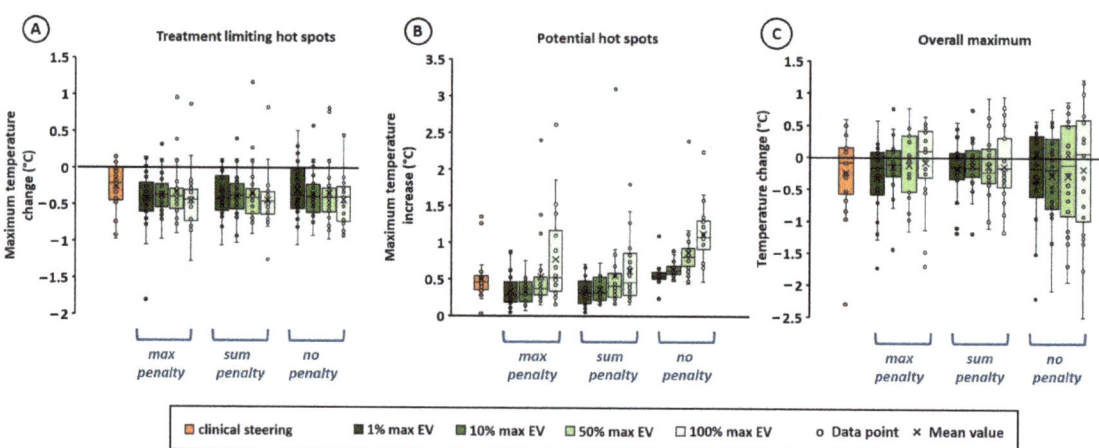

Figure 2. Effect of different re-optimization strategies on the predicted temperature at treatment limiting hot spot locations (**A**), other potential hot spot locations (**B**) and the overall maximum temperature (**C**). Results are compared to simulations for the clinically applied protocol/experience-based steering strategy during treatment. Max penalty, sum penalty and no penalty refer to the re-optimization goal functions in Equations (3), (4) and (5), respectively. To efficiently calculate a hot spot temperature during optimization, the average temperature of the voxels with the x% largest heating potential was calculated, which are the voxels with the largest maximum eigenvalues (EV) of their temperature matrix ($\underline{T}$ in Equation (2)). Values of x of 1, 10, 50 and 100% were evaluated. The hot spot diameter was 5 cm.

Figure 3A shows that for all re-optimization strategies, the simulated target T90 after re-optimization was quite comparable to the initial value before re-optimization, and also quite similar to the simulated T90 for the clinically applied steering strategy based on experience. Both mean and standard deviation were equal within 0.1 °C, which is not a clinically relevant difference. Considering the individual absolute difference in predicted T90 between planning-based and clinical strategies for all 22 hot spots and steering actions, we see that the mean absolute difference is also very low, i.e., 0.1 ± 0.1 °C when applying a penalty term and 1% or 10% max EV. When evaluating the change in temperature along the thermometry probes (Figure 3B), it was observed that this was approximately 0 °C for the clinically applied strategy, both simulated and measured during treatment. For both optimization goal functions using a penalty term, the predicted temperature change along the probes was comparable to the clinical strategy. When only re-optimizing T90, without a penalty term, a slight increase of typically 0.1–0.2 °C is observed. However, this is not considered clinically relevant and as indicated in Figure 2B,C, this also yields a risk of inducing new hot spots at other locations. The re-optimization time was quite similar for all re-optimization strategies (Figure 3C). Re-optimization of the phase-amplitude settings took typically ~10 s (mean ± std = 12 ± 9 s) on an Intel Xeon® E5-1650 v3 3.5 GHz running CentOS 6.8, and always less than 1 min, which is sufficiently fast for on-line application. In about 3% of the cases (i.e., 9 out of the overall total of 22 × 4 × 3 = 264 re-optimizations), no feasible solution satisfying all constraints was found. As a back-up solution for these situations, a form of standard steering was implemented. The power of the waveguide closest to the selected treatment limiting hot spot location was then reduced by 15%, which was redistributed over the other waveguides to maintain a fixed power level; e.g., in case of hot spot 29, pubic bone, the power supplied by the top waveguide is reduced by 15%. This is quite similar to commonly applied clinical steering strategies.

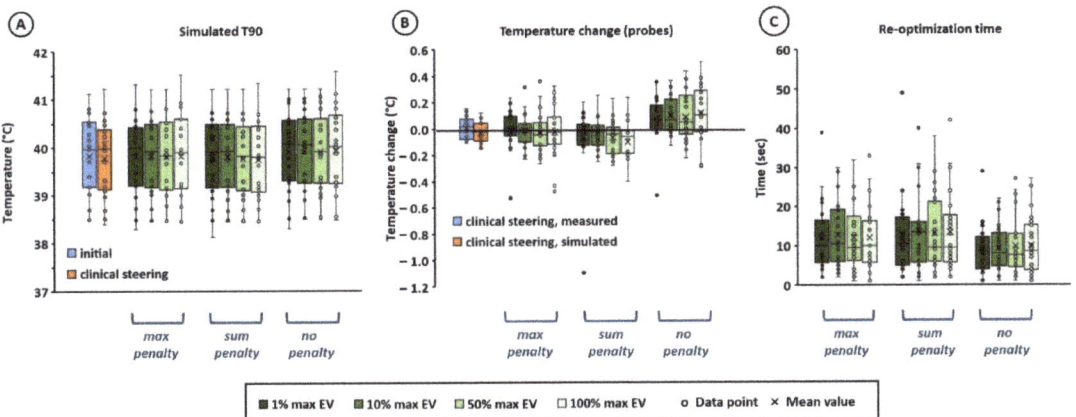

Figure 3. Effect of different re-optimization strategies on the simulated T90 (**A**) and the temperature change along the thermometry probes (**B**). The re-optimization calculation time per strategy is indicated in (**C**) for an Intel Xeon® E5-1650 v3 3.5 GHz running CentOS 6.8. Results are compared to simulations for the clinically applied protocol/experience-based steering strategy during treatment (**A**,**B**), as well as to probe measurements (**B**). Max penalty, sum penalty and no penalty refer to the re-optimization goal functions in Equations (3), (4) and (5), respectively. To efficiently calculate a hot spot temperature during optimization, the average temperature of the voxels with the x% largest heating potential was calculated, which are the voxels with the largest maximum eigenvalues (EV) of their temperature matrix ($\underline{T}$ in Equation (2). Values of x of 1, 10, 50 and 100% were evaluated. The hot spot diameter was 5 cm.

Thus, based on the results summarized in Figures 2 and 3, an objective function including a penalty term would be most effective. Next, the influence of the hot spot diameter was evaluated for the most effective strategy. Both a penalty term for the maximum temperature increase in all potential hot spots (Equation (3)), and the sum of the increase in potential hot spot temperatures (Equation (4)) were effective, with no clearly pronounced difference. However, Equation (3) was selected for further evaluation, since Figure 3B shows a weak trend that using Equation (4), temperatures along the thermometry probe decrease slightly, and since the risk of not finding a solution was slightly lower in case of Equation (3). The potential hot spot diameter was varied between 2.5, 5, 7.5, and 10 cm and Figure 4 shows the effect of different re-optimization strategies on treatment limiting hot spot suppression as well as the maximum temperature increase at other potential hot spot locations and the overall normal tissue temperature maximum. Again, it was observed that the risk of insufficiently suppressing the treatment limiting hot spot and/or inducing new hot spots increased when a larger number of voxels was included to determine the average hot spot temperature (50% max EV and 100% max EV). No pronounced effect of the diameter was observed. When using 1% max EV or 10% max EV, the average predicted decrease in treatment limiting hot spot temperature deviated less than 0.2 °C from the clinical steering strategy, and the standard deviation differed less than 0.1 °C, for all hot spot diameters. Similarly, the average maximum increase in other potential hot spot locations deviated less than 0.2 °C from the clinical steering strategy, and the standard deviation differed less than 0.15 °C. The overall mean maximum temperature change deviated less than 0.1 °C from the clinical steering strategy, and the standard deviation differed less than 0.25 °C. As observed also in Figure 2, there is a mild trend that planning-based steering yields a slightly larger reduction in hot spot temperature. However, since real and predicted temperature reductions might deviate ±0.1 °C [39] and small differences might not be perceptible by the patient, these small differences are not considered clinically relevant and thus the strategies can be considered equally effective.

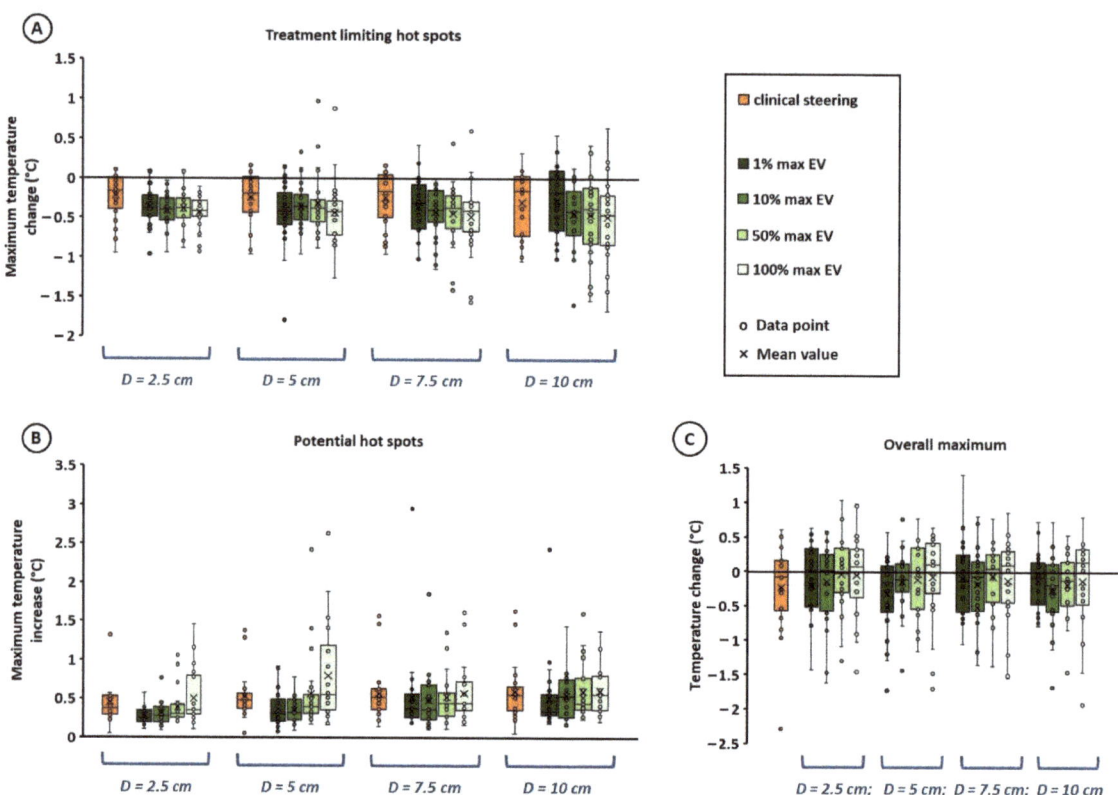

Figure 4. Effect of potential hot spot diameter (D = 2.5, 5, 7.5 or 10 cm) on the predicted temperature at treatment limiting hot spot locations (**A**), other potential hot spot locations (**B**) and the overall maximum temperature (**C**), when using a re-optimization goal function with a penalty term for the maximum increase of all potential hot spot temperatures (Equation (3)). Results are compared to simulations for the clinically applied protocol/experience-based steering strategy during treatment. To efficiently calculate a hot spot temperature during optimization, the average temperature of the voxels with the x% largest heating potential was calculated, which are the voxels with the largest maximum eigenvalues (EV) of their temperature matrix ($\underline{T}$ in Equation (2)). Values of x of 1, 10, 50 and 100% were evaluated.

Figure 5 shows the effect of the potential hot spot diameter on the simulated T90 and the temperature change along the thermometry probes. For all diameters, the simulated target T90 after re-optimization was quite comparable to the initial value before re-optimization, and also quite similar to the simulated T90 for the clinically applied steering strategy based on experience (Figure 5A). Both mean and standard deviation were equal within 0.1 °C, which is not a clinically relevant difference. Considering the individual absolute difference in predicted T90 between planning-based and clinical strategies for all 22 hot spots and steering actions, we see that the mean absolute difference is again also very low, i.e., typically 0.1 ± 0.2 °C. When evaluating the temperature along the thermometry probes (Figure 5B), it was observed that this temperature remains quite constant for any diameter, and similar to the clinically applied strategy. The mean temperature change was less than 0.1 °C. No pronounced influence of the diameter was observed, although the risk of outliers slightly increased for a larger potential hot spot region diameter, since a larger number of voxels is included in the averaging to estimate the hot spot temperature. As expected, the hot spot diameter also had no influence on re-optimization calculation times (Figure 5C).

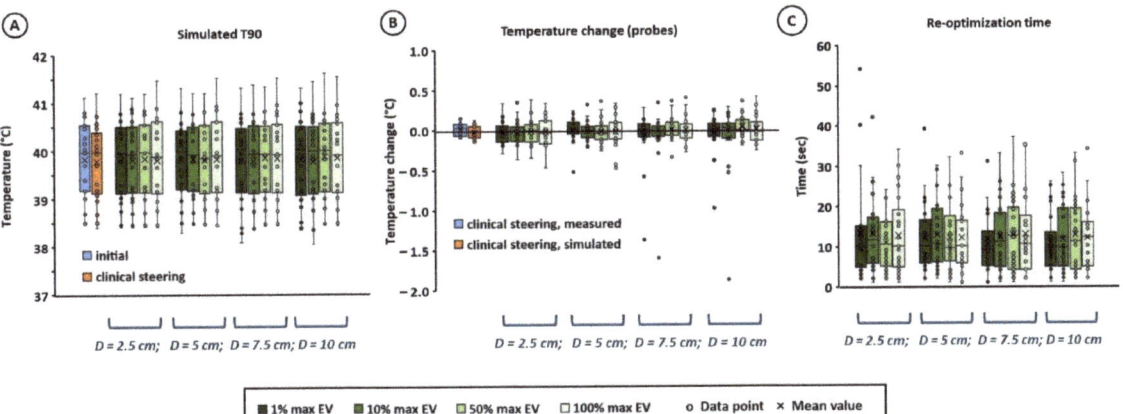

Figure 5. Effect of potential hot spot diameter (D = 2.5, 5, 7.5 or 10 cm) on the simulated T90 (**A**) and on the temperature change along the thermometry probes (**B**), when using a re-optimization goal function with a penalty term for the maximum increase in all potential hot spot temperatures (Equation (3)). The re-optimization calculation time is indicated in (**C**) for an Intel Xeon® E5-1650 v3 3.5 GHz running CentOS 6.8. Results are compared to simulations for the clinically applied protocol/experience-based steering strategy during treatment (**A**,**B**), as well as to probe measurements (**B**). To efficiently calculate a hot spot temperature during optimization, the average temperature of the voxels with the x% largest heating potential was calculated, which are the voxels with the largest maximum eigenvalues (EV) of their temperature matrix ($\underline{T}$ in Equation (2)). Values of x of 1, 10, 50 and 100% were evaluated.

Similarities were observed in the steering strategies, when comparing clinically applied phase-amplitude settings with numerically re-optimized settings. Clinical steering for hot spot suppression predominantly uses amplitude steering while keeping phases quite constant to maintain a focus at the target location. Numerically achieved re-optimized settings generally also prescribed amplitude steering. For amplitude steering, a similarity in steering direction was also observed in many cases, i.e., when an amplitude was increased or decreased in clinical steering, numerical optimization also resulted in increase/decrease, albeit with different amplitudes. Figure 6 shows clinically applied phase-amplitude adjustments and numerically re-optimized settings for a potential hot spot diameter of 5 cm, using a re-optimization goal function with a penalty term for the maximum increase in all potential hot spot temperatures (Equation (3)) and using voxels with the 10% maximum heating potential to calculate the hot spot temperature (10% max EV).

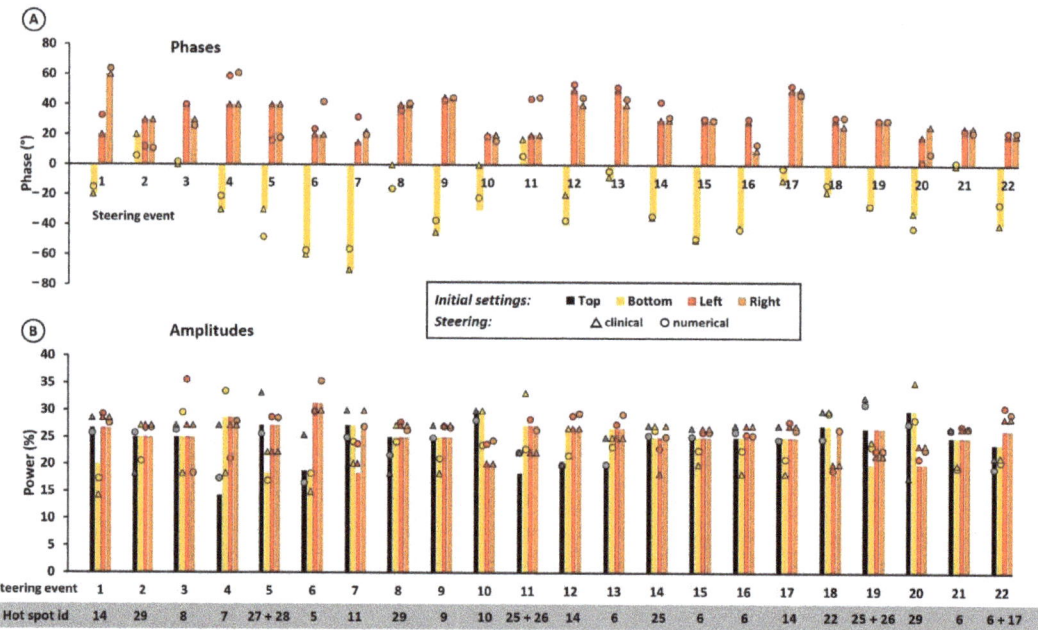

Figure 6. Clinically applied protocol/experience-based phase (**A**) and amplitude (**B**) adjustments and numerically re-optimized settings for a potential hot spot diameter of 5 cm, using a re-optimization goal function with a penalty term for the maximum increase in all potential hot spot temperatures (Equation (3)) and using voxels with the 10% maximum heating potential to calculate the hot spot temperature (10% max EV). The top antenna was always used as a reference, i.e., phase 0°. Hot spot id refers to the anatomical locations in Figure 1A.

4. Discussion

In this paper, we presented fast and advanced temperature-based strategies for adaptive on-line re-optimization of phase-amplitude settings, to overcome treatment limiting hot spots during locoregional hyperthermia treatments. Considering target and hot spot temperatures, results were compared to predictions and tumor temperature measurements for clinically applied protocol/experience-based steering strategies. A similar effectiveness to clinical experience was predicted. This is a very promising result in view of there being about 30 years of experience with locoregional hyperthermia and experience-based steering at our department. When numerical algorithms can match such long-term experience, the overall treatment quality in hyperthermia centers can significantly improve. The results also imply that treatments become less dependent on the experience of the center/operator by implementing these planning-based strategies.

Although temperature-based optimization is computationally more expensive than the commonly applied SAR-based optimization, we managed to achieve average re-optimization times of about 10 s. This was realized by efficient superposition to calculate steady-state temperatures (Equation (2)) and limiting the number of normal tissue constraints to only the potential hot spot regions, with their temperature represented by the average temperature of the voxels with the largest heating potential. Superposition was possible due to the use of constant enhanced perfusion levels. In reality, perfusion is temperature-dependent and thermal models including temperature-dependent perfusion have been proposed [51,53]. Ignoring the temperature-dependency of perfusion can result in under/overestimation of absolute temperatures levels [36,37]. However, the use of temperature-dependent perfusion values will not necessarily improve the quality of adaptive treatment planning as proposed in this study, since changes in simulated temperatures are used as a predictor, rather than the absolute values. Furthermore, including temperature-dependent perfusion values does not allow fast superposition to calculate temperatures, which makes calculations much more computationally expensive and not feasible for on-line re-optimization.

Our clinical steering strategy mainly applies amplitude adjustments (Figure 6). Amplitude adjustments are a preferred and effective strategy adopted in empirical steering guidelines by our and other experienced centers [54]. This makes sense as phase settings mainly determine the location of the heating focus, so avoiding significant phase changes and applying amplitude steering ensures maintaining the focus at the target location, as optimized at the start of treatment. Furthermore, the location of treatment limiting hot spots is usually relatively superficial, and amplitude adjustments directly affect the local temperature close to the antenna. We observed that numerical re-optimization also identified this principle as an optimal solution to suppress hot spots while maintaining optimal target heating; numerical re-optimization also predominantly prescribed amplitude steering.

Based on the positive results of this simulation study, a next step would be clinical evaluation of temperature-based adaptive re-optimization and comparing this with clinical experience. A cross-over trial by Franckena et al. comparing SAR-based treatment planning-guided steering with experience-based steering demonstrated the feasibility of treatment planning-based steering [43]. In the first half of a patient's treatment series, similar target temperatures were achieved with both planning-guided and empirical steering. However, in the second half of the treatment series, planning-guided steering resulted in significantly lower (~0.5 °C) target temperatures, indicating the necessity to further improve treatment planning-based steering. Several (technical and patient) factors could explain this decreasing reliability and require further research, such as planning strategy, decreasing patient tolerance and a changing anatomy over the treatment course, while the planning is based on anatomical information of the initial planning CT scan.

The planning strategy applied in the trial of Franckena et al. was a SAR-based re-optimization, developed as an add-on to Sigma HyperPlan, and using adjusted weight factors to reduce the SAR in treatment limiting hot spot regions [42,43]. Although there is some correlation between SAR and temperature, the local temperature determines whether a hot spot becomes treatment limiting or not. The temperature at a potential hot spot location depends on SAR. However, it also depends on thermal processes, such as thermal conduction, blood perfusion and bolus cooling, which are not accounted for in SAR-based (re-)optimization. Furthermore, SAR-based optimization is less intuitive for the operator and it is difficult to determine how much SAR reduction is required to resolve a hot spot complaint. This might partly explain the challenges Franckena et al. encountered in solving hot spot-related complaints. Our temperature-based approach accounts for relevant thermal processes and is more practical and intuitive for clinical use. Moreover, a unique approach is that our strategy not only aims to reduce the temperature at treatment limiting hot spot locations, but also to prevent inadvertently inducing new hot spots at other potential hot spot locations while adjusting the phase-amplitude settings to suppress the original hot spot. This feature would make it more robust for clinical applications compared to existing SAR-based strategies.

Another important aspect of re-optimization algorithms is robustness in terms of specification of potential hot spot locations. Since the operating frequency of the ALBA-4D system is 70 MHz, the wavelength in muscle tissue is approximately 50 cm. This means that true small scale steering is not possible and the re-optimization results will not be very sensitive to the exact specified position of the potential hot spots [55]. This is confirmed by the observation that the potential hot spot region diameter did not significantly affect re-optimization results (Figures 4 and 5). The fact that the diameter is not an important factor implies that results are also not strongly dependent on the exact potential hot spot location indicated by the user. Since all locoregional heating systems operate in the frequency range between 60 and 120 MHz [20], this will probably also hold when combining this temperature-based optimization strategy with other locoregional devices. Results of the present study can certainly be extrapolated to the widely used BSD Sigma-60 system, with four antenna pairs and similar heating characteristics as the ALBA-4D system [56]. With an increased number of antennas and thus an increased number of degrees of freedom, e.g., for the BSD Sigma-Eye system, the exact hot spot location could be slightly more important, requiring further investigation. However, re-optimization is still expected to be quite robust to potential hot spot location because of the large wavelengths used in locoregional heating systems.

The relatively large wavelength of locoregional heating systems can also explain why no improvement in tumor temperature was predicted compared to experience-based steering. This is in line with simulation study results of Canters et al., who evaluated the possible gain in tumor temperatures by optimization for the BSD Sigma-60 system [55]. They showed that the potential of treatment planning to optimize the SAR distribution is limited [55]. The maximum improvement was in the order of 5%, which would lead to a temperature increase of about 0.2 °C [43,55]. Although the performance of planning-based re-optimization is expected to improve using temperature-based strategies, the number of degrees of freedom is relatively small with four antennas or antenna pairs and a wavelength in the order of 50 cm, so the steering possibilities remain a limitation. Using heating systems with higher frequencies and/or more antennas, such as the AMC-8 system and the BSD Sigma-Eye system, more flexible steering and thus a tumor temperature increase is expected to be possible [57,58]. However, clinical use of these systems showed that realizing improved tumor heating by exploiting the increased steering possibilities remains challenging [59]. Thus, investigation of advanced (adaptive) treatment planning tools to fully exploit the benefits of such systems enabling 3D steering is worthwhile [59,60].

Evaluation of the benefit of using temperature-based planning during hyperthermia treatment is a subject of ongoing research within our department. After positive results in pilot studies with treatment planning and planning-assisted manual re-optimization [40,41], we will continue to investigate the benefit of automatic re-optimization as proposed in this paper. To ensure optimal patient safety, operators will always have to check the re-optimized phase-amplitude settings and manually apply them to the heating system. Furthermore, continuous monitoring of the thermometry probe registrations and patient feedback, as part of our standard treatment protocol, remains important. When successful, treatment planning-based steering would match empirical steering by very experienced operators, realizing a constant operator-independent heating quality. Subsequently, effective treatment limiting hot spot suppression and absence of new hot spots could allow a total power increase to realize a better heating quality.

5. Conclusions

Fast and advanced temperature-based strategies for adaptive on-line re-optimization of phase-amplitude settings were presented to suppress treatment limiting hot spots which may occur during locoregional hyperthermia treatments. An effectiveness similar to re-optimization based on long-term clinical experience was predicted. A major advantage is that treatments would become less dependent on the experience of the hyperthermia center/operator, thereby improving the overall treatment quality in hyperthermia centers. Further clinical evaluation is a subject of ongoing research.

Author Contributions: Conceptualization, H.P.K. and J.C.; methodology, H.P.K. and J.C.; software, H.P.K.; validation, H.P.K.; formal analysis, H.P.K.; investigation, H.P.K.; resources, H.P.K.; writing—original draft preparation, H.P.K.; writing—review and editing, H.P.K. and J.C.; visualization, H.P.K.; project administration, H.P.K.; funding acquisition, H.P.K. and J.C. All authors have read and agreed to the published version of the manuscript.

Funding: This work was financially supported by the Dutch Cancer Society (Grant number 10873).

Institutional Review Board Statement: The study was approved by the Medical Ethics Committee of the Amsterdam UMC (W21_422) approval date 11 October 2021.

Informed Consent Statement: The Medical Ethics Review Committee of the Academic Medical Center confirmed that the Medical Research Involving Human Subjects Act (WMO) did not apply.

Data Availability Statement: The data presented in this study are available on reasonable request. The data are not publicly available due to privacy.

Conflicts of Interest: The authors declare no conflict of interest.

References

1. Issels, R.D.; Lindner, L.H.; Verweij, J.; Wessalowski, R.; Reichardt, P.; Wust, P.; Ghadjar, P.; Hohenberger, P.; Angele, M.; Salat, C.; et al. Effect of Neoadjuvant Chemotherapy Plus Regional Hyperthermia on Long-term Outcomes Among Patients With Localized High-Risk Soft Tissue Sarcoma: The EORTC 62961-ESHO 95 Randomized Clinical Trial. *JAMA Oncol.* **2018**, *4*, 483–492. [CrossRef]
2. Van der Zee, J.; González González, D.; Van Rhoon, G.C.; van Dijk, J.D.P.; van Putten, W.L.J.; Hart, A.A. Comparison of radiotherapy alone with radiotherapy plus hyperthermia in locally advanced pelvic tumours: A prospective, randomised, multicentre trial. Dutch Deep Hyperthermia Group. *Lancet* **2000**, *355*, 1119–1125. [CrossRef]
3. Overgaard, J.; González González, D.; Hulshof, M.C.C.M.; Arcangeli, G.; Dahl, O.; Mella, O.; Bentzen, S.M. Randomised trial of hyperthermia as adjuvant to radiotherapy for recurrent or metastatic malignant melanoma. European Society for Hyperthermic Oncology. *Lancet* **1995**, *345*, 540–543. [CrossRef]
4. Wust, P.; Hildebrandt, B.; Sreenivasa, G.; Rau, B.; Gellermann, J.; Riess, H.; Felix, R.; Schlag, P.M. Hyperthermia in combined treatment of cancer. *Lancet Oncol.* **2002**, *3*, 487–497. [CrossRef]
5. Vernon, C.C.; Hand, J.W.; Field, S.B.; Machin, D.; Whaley, J.B.; Van der Zee, J.; van Putten, W.L.J.; Van Rhoon, G.C.; van Dijk, J.D.P.; González González, D.; et al. Radiotherapy with or without hyperthermia in the treatment of superficial localized breast cancer: Results from five randomized controlled trials. International Collaborative Hyperthermia Group. *Int. J. Radiat. Oncol. Biol. Phys.* **1996**, *35*, 731–744. [PubMed]
6. Datta, N.R.; Puric, E.; Klingbiel, D.; Gomez, S.; Bodis, S. Hyperthermia and Radiation Therapy in Locoregional Recurrent Breast Cancers: A Systematic Review and Meta-analysis. *Int. J. Radiat. Oncol. Biol. Phys.* **2016**, *94*, 1073–1087. [CrossRef]
7. Datta, N.R.; Rogers, S.; Klingbiel, D.; Gomez, S.; Puric, E.; Bodis, S. Hyperthermia and radiotherapy with or without chemotherapy in locally advanced cervical cancer: A systematic review with conventional and network meta-analyses. *Int. J. Hyperth.* **2016**, *32*, 809–821. [CrossRef] [PubMed]
8. Franckena, M.; Fatehi, D.; de Bruijne, M.; Canters, R.A.; van Norden, Y.; Mens, J.W.; Van Rhoon, G.C.; Van der Zee, J. Hyperthermia dose-effect relationship in 420 patients with cervical cancer treated with combined radiotherapy and hyperthermia. *Eur. J. Cancer* **2009**, *45*, 1969–1978. [CrossRef]
9. Rau, B.; Wust, P.; Tilly, W.; Gellermann, J.; Harder, C.; Riess, H.; Budach, V.; Felix, R.; Schlag, P.M. Preoperative radiochemotherapy in locally advanced or recurrent rectal cancer: Regional radiofrequency hyperthermia correlates with clinical parameters. *Int. J. Radiat. Oncol. Biol. Phys.* **2000**, *48*, 381–391. [CrossRef]
10. Overgaard, J.; Gonzalez, D.G.; Hulshof, M.C.C.H.; Arcangeli, G.; Dahl, O.; Mella, O.; Bentzen, S.M. Hyperthermia as an adjuvant to radiation therapy of recurrent or metastatic malignant melanoma. A multicentre randomized trial by the European Society for Hyperthermic Oncology. *Int. J. Hyperth.* **1996**, *12*, 3–20. [CrossRef]
11. Bakker, A.; Van der Zee, J.; van tienhoven, G.; Kok, H.P.; Rasch, C.R.N.; Crezee, H. Temperature and thermal dose during radiotherapy and hyperthermia for recurrent breast cancer are related to clinical outcome and thermal toxicity: A systematic review. *Int. J. Hyperth.* **2019**, *36*, 1024–1039. [CrossRef] [PubMed]
12. Overgaard, J. Formula to estimate the thermal enhancement ratio of a single simultaneous hyperthermia and radiation treatment. *Acta Radiol. Oncol.* **1984**, *23*, 135–139. [CrossRef]
13. van Rhoon, G.C. Is CEM43 still a relevant thermal dose parameter for hyperthermia treatment monitoring? *Int. J. Hyperth.* **2016**, *32*, 50–62. [CrossRef]
14. Yarmolenko, P.S.; Moon, E.J.; Landon, C.; Manzoor, A.; Hochman, D.W.; Viglianti, B.L.; Dewhirst, M.W. Thresholds for thermal damage to normal tissues: An update. *Int. J. Hyperth.* **2011**, *27*, 320–343. [CrossRef]
15. Stoll, A.M.; Greene, L.C. Relationship between pain and tissue damage due to thermal radiation. *J. Appl. Physiol.* **1959**, *14*, 373–382. [CrossRef] [PubMed]
16. Craciunescu, O.I.; Stauffer, P.R.; Soher, B.J.; Wyatt, C.R.; Arabe, O.; Maccarini, P.; Das, S.K.; Cheng, K.S.; Wong, T.Z.; Jones, E.L.; et al. Accuracy of real time noninvasive temperature measurements using magnetic resonance thermal imaging in patients treated for high grade extremity soft tissue sarcomas. *Med. Phys.* **2009**, *36*, 4848–4858. [CrossRef]
17. Gellermann, J.; Hildebrandt, B.; Issels, R.; Ganter, H.; Wlodarczyk, W.; Budach, V.; Felix, R.; Tunn, P.U.; Reichardt, P.; Wust, P. Noninvasive magnetic resonance thermography of soft tissue sarcomas during regional hyperthermia: Correlation with response and direct thermometry. *Cancer* **2006**, *107*, 1373–1382. [CrossRef] [PubMed]
18. Winter, L.; Oberacker, E.; Paul, K.; Ji, Y.; Oezerdem, C.; Ghadjar, P.; Thieme, A.; Budach, V.; Wust, P.; Niendorf, T. Magnetic resonance thermometry: Methodology, pitfalls and practical solutions. *Int. J. Hyperth.* **2016**, *32*, 63–75. [CrossRef]

19. Bruggmoser, G.; Bauchowitz, S.; Canters, R.; Crezee, H.; Ehmann, M.; Gellermann, J.; Lamprecht, U.; Lomax, N.; Messmer, M.B.; Ott, O.; et al. Quality assurance for clinical studies in regional deep hyperthermia. *Strahlenther. Onkol.* **2011**, *187*, 605–610. [CrossRef] [PubMed]
20. Kok, H.P.; Cressman, E.N.K.; Ceelen, W.; Brace, C.L.; Ivkov, R.; Grull, H.; Ter Haar, G.; Wust, P.; Crezee, J. Heating technology for malignant tumors: A review. *Int. J. Hyperth.* **2020**, *37*, 711–741. [CrossRef]
21. Zweije, R.; Kok, H.P.; Bakker, A.; Bel, A.; Crezee, J. Technical and Clinical Evaluation of the ALBA-4D 70MHz Loco-Regional Hyperthermia System. In Proceedings of the 48th European Microwave Conference, Madrid, Spain, 23–27 September 2018; pp. 328–331.
22. Wust, P.; Beck, R.; Berger, J.; Fahling, H.; Seebass, M.; Wlodarczyk, W.; Hoffmann, W.; Nadobny, J. Electric field distributions in a phased-array applicator with 12 channels: Measurements and numerical simulations. *Med. Phys.* **2000**, *27*, 2565–2579. [CrossRef]
23. Turner, P.F.; Tumeh, A.; Schaefermeyer, T. BSD-2000 approach for deep local and regional hyperthermia: Physics and technology. *Strahlenther. Onkol.* **1989**, *165*, 738–741.
24. Stauffer, P.R. Evolving technology for thermal therapy of cancer. *Int. J. Hyperth.* **2005**, *21*, 731–744. [CrossRef]
25. Kok, H.P.; Van Haaren, P.M.A.; van de Kamer, J.B.; Wiersma, J.; Van Dijk, J.D.P.; Crezee, J. High-resolution temperature-based optimization for hyperthermia treatment planning. *Phys. Med. Biol.* **2005**, *50*, 3127–3141. [CrossRef]
26. Kok, H.P.; Crezee, J. Hyperthermia Treatment Planning: Clinical Application and Ongoing Developments. *IEEE J. Electromagn RF Microw. Med. Biol.* **2021**, *5*, 214–222. [CrossRef]
27. Kok, H.P.; van der Zee, J.; Guirado, F.N.; Bakker, A.; Datta, N.R.; Abdel-Rahman, S.; Schmidt, M.; Wust, P.; Crezee, J. Treatment planning facilitates clinical decision making for hyperthermia treatments. *Int. J. Hyperth.* **2021**, *38*, 532–551. [CrossRef]
28. Das, S.K.; Clegg, S.T.; Samulski, T.V. Electromagnetic thermal therapy power optimization for multiple source applicators. *Int. J. Hyperth.* **1999**, *15*, 291–308.
29. Bardati, F.; Borrani, A.; Gerardino, A.; Lovisolo, G.A. SAR optimization in a phased array radiofrequency hyperthermia system. *IEEE Trans. Biomed. Eng.* **1995**, *42*, 1201–1207. [CrossRef]
30. Wiersma, J.; Van Maarseveen, R.A.M.; van Dijk, J.D.P. A flexible optimization tool for hyperthermia treatments with RF phased array systems. *Int. J. Hyperth.* **2002**, *18*, 73–85. [CrossRef]
31. Wust, P.; Seebass, M.; Nadobny, J.; Deuflhard, P.; Monich, G.; Felix, R. Simulation studies promote technological development of radiofrequency phased array hyperthermia. *Int. J. Hyperth.* **1996**, *12*, 477–494. [CrossRef]
32. Bellizzi, G.G.; Drizdal, T.; van Rhoon, G.C.; Crocco, L.; Isernia, T.; Paulides, M.M. The potential of constrained SAR focusing for hyperthermia treatment planning: Analysis for the head & neck region. *Phys. Med. Biol.* **2019**, *64*, 015013. [CrossRef]
33. Zanoli, M.; Trefna, H.D. Iterative time-reversal for multi-frequency hyperthermia. *Phys. Med. Biol.* **2021**, *66*, 045027. [CrossRef]
34. Das, S.K.; Clegg, S.T.; Samulski, T.V. Computational techniques for fast hyperthermia temperature optimization. *Med. Phys.* **1999**, *26*, 319–328. [CrossRef]
35. Nikita, K.S.; Maratos, N.G.; Uzunoglu, N.K. Optimal steady-state temperature distribution for a phased array hyperthermia system. *IEEE Trans. Biomed. Eng.* **1993**, *40*, 1299–1306. [CrossRef]
36. De Greef, M.; Kok, H.P.; Correia, D.; Bel, A.; Crezee, J. Optimization in hyperthermia treatment planning: The impact of tissue perfusion uncertainty. *Med. Phys.* **2010**, *37*, 4540–4550. [CrossRef]
37. De Greef, M.; Kok, H.P.; Correia, D.; Borsboom, P.P.; Bel, A.; Crezee, J. Uncertainty in hyperthermia treatment planning: The need for robust system design. *Phys. Med. Biol.* **2011**, *56*, 3233–3250. [CrossRef]
38. Kok, H.P.; Ciampa, S.; De Kroon-Oldenhof, R.; Steggerda-Carvalho, E.J.; Van Stam, G.; Zum Vörde Sive Vörding, P.J.; Stalpers, L.J.A.; Geijsen, E.D.; Bardati, F.; Bel, A.; et al. Toward on-line adaptive hyperthermia treatment planning: Correlation between measured and simulated specific absorption rate changes caused by phase steering in patients. *Int. J. Radiat. Oncol. Biol. Phys.* **2014**, *90*, 438–445. [CrossRef]
39. Kok, H.P.; Schooneveldt, G.; Bakker, A.; de Kroon-Oldenhof, R.; Korshuize-van Straten, L.; de Jong, C.E.; Steggerda-Carvalho, E.; Geijsen, E.D.; Stalpers, L.J.A.; Crezee, J. Predictive value of simulated SAR and temperature for changes in measured temperature after phase-amplitude steering during locoregional hyperthermia treatments. *Int. J. Hyperth.* **2018**, *35*, 330–339. [CrossRef]
40. Kok, H.P.; Korshuize-van Straten, L.; Bakker, A.; De Kroon-Oldenhof, R.; Geijsen, E.D.; Stalpers, L.J.A.; Crezee, J. On-line adaptive hyperthermia treatment planning during locoregional heating to suppress treatment limiting hot spots. *Int. J. Radiat. Oncol. Biol. Phys.* **2017**, *99*, 1039–1047. [CrossRef]
41. Kok, H.P.; Korshuize-van Straten, L.; Bakker, A.; de Kroon-Oldenhof, R.; Westerveld, G.H.; Versteijne, E.; Stalpers, L.J.A.; Crezee, J. Feasibility of on-line temperature-based hyperthermia treatment planning to improve tumour temperatures during locoregional hyperthermia. *Int. J. Hyperth.* **2018**, *34*, 1082–1091. [CrossRef]
42. Canters, R.A.; Franckena, M.; Van der Zee, J.; Van Rhoon, G.C. Complaint-adaptive power density optimization as a tool for HTP-guided steering in deep hyperthermia treatment of pelvic tumors. *Phys. Med. Biol.* **2008**, *53*, 6799–6820. [CrossRef]
43. Franckena, M.; Canters, R.; Termorshuizen, F.; Van der Zee, J.; Van Rhoon, G.C. Clinical implementation of hyperthermia treatment planning guided steering: A cross over trial to assess its current contribution to treatment quality. *Int. J. Hyperth.* **2010**, *26*, 145–157. [CrossRef]
44. Kok, H.P.; De Greef, M.; Bel, A.; Crezee, J. Acceleration of high resolution temperature based optimization for hyperthermia treatment planning using element grouping. *Med. Phys.* **2009**, *36*, 3795–3805. [CrossRef]

45. Kok, H.P.; Kotte, A.N.T.J.; Crezee, J. Planning, optimisation and evaluation of hyperthermia treatments. *Int. J. Hyperth.* **2017**, *33*, 593–607. [CrossRef]
46. Hasgall, P.A.; Di Gennaro, F.; Baumgarter, C.; Neufeld, E.; Gosselin, M.C.; Payne, D.; Klingenböck, A.; Kuster, N. IT'IS Database for Thermal and Electromagnetic Parameters of Biological Tissues. Version 4.0. 2018. Available online: www.itis.ethz.ch/database (accessed on 6 September 2021).
47. Rossmann, C.; Haemmerich, D. Review of temperature dependence of thermal properties, dielectric properties, and perfusion of biological tissues at hyperthermic and ablation temperatures. *Crit. Rev. Biomed. Eng.* **2014**, *42*, 467–492. [CrossRef]
48. Song, C.W. Effect of local hyperthermia on blood flow and microenvironment: A review. *Cancer Res.* **1984**, *44*, 4721s–4730s.
49. ESHO Taskgroup Committee. *Treatment Planning and Modelling in Hyperthermia, a Task Group Report of the European Society for Hyperthermic Oncology*; Tor Vergata: Rome, Italy, 1992.
50. Gabriel, C.; Gabriel, S.; Corthout, E. The dielectric properties of biological tissues: I. Literature survey. *Phys. Med. Biol.* **1996**, *41*, 2231–2249. [CrossRef]
51. Cheng, K.S.; Yuan, Y.; Li, Z.; Stauffer, P.R.; Maccarini, P.; Joines, W.T.; Dewhirst, M.W.; Das, S.K. The performance of a reduced-order adaptive controller when used in multi-antenna hyperthermia treatments with nonlinear temperature-dependent perfusion. *Phys. Med. Biol.* **2009**, *54*, 1979–1995. [CrossRef]
52. Pennes, H.H. Analysis of tissue and arterial blood temperatures in the resting human forearm. *J. Appl. Physiol.* **1948**, *1*, 93–122. [CrossRef]
53. Erdmann, B.; Lang, J.; Seebass, M. Optimization of temperature distributions for regional hyperthermia based on a nonlinear heat transfer model. *Ann. N. Y. Acad. Sci.* **1998**, *858*, 36–46. [CrossRef]
54. Van der Wal, E.; Franckena, M.; Wielheesen, D.H.; Van der Zee, J.; Van Rhoon, G.C. Steering in locoregional deep hyperthermia: Evaluation of common practice with 3D-planning. *Int. J. Hyperth.* **2008**, *24*, 682–693. [CrossRef]
55. Canters, R.A.; Franckena, M.; Paulides, M.M.; Van Rhoon, G.C. Patient positioning in deep hyperthermia: Influences of inaccuracies, signal correction possibilities and optimization potential. *Phys. Med. Biol.* **2009**, *54*, 3923–3936. [CrossRef]
56. Kok, H.P.; Beck, M.; Loke, D.R.; Helderman, R.; van Tienhoven, G.; Ghadjar, P.; Wust, P.; Crezee, H. Locoregional peritoneal hyperthermia to enhance the effectiveness of chemotherapy in patients with peritoneal carcinomatosis: A simulation study comparing different locoregional heating systems. *Int. J. Hyperth.* **2020**, *37*, 76–88. [CrossRef]
57. Canters, R.A.; Paulides, M.M.; Franckena, M.; Mens, J.W.; Van Rhoon, G.C. Benefit of replacing the Sigma-60 by the Sigma-Eye applicator. A Monte Carlo-based uncertainty analysis. *Strahlenther. Onkol.* **2013**, *189*, 74–80. [CrossRef]
58. De Greef, M.; Kok, H.P.; Bel, A.; Crezee, J. 3-D versus 2-D steering in patient anatomies: A comparison using hyperthermia treatment planning. *Int. J. Hyperth.* **2011**, *27*, 74–85. [CrossRef]
59. Fatehi, D.; van der Zee, J.; Van Rhoon, G.C. Intra-patient comparison between two annular phased array applicators, Sigma-60 and Sigma-Eye: Applied RF powers and intraluminally measured temperatures. *Int. J. Hyperth.* **2011**, *27*, 214–223. [CrossRef]
60. Crezee, J.; Van Stam, G.; Sijbrands, J.; Oldenborg, S.; Geijsen, E.D.; Hulshof, M.C.C.M.; Kok, H.P. Hyperthermia of deep seated pelvic tumors with a phased array of eight versus four 70 MHz waveguides. In Proceedings of the 47th European Microwave Conference, Nuremberg, Germany, 10–12 October 2017; pp. 876–879.

MDPI
St. Alban-Anlage 66
4052 Basel
Switzerland
Tel. +41 61 683 77 34
Fax +41 61 302 89 18
www.mdpi.com

Cancers Editorial Office
E-mail: cancers@mdpi.com
www.mdpi.com/journal/cancers

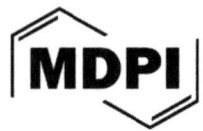

www.ingramcontent.com/pod-product-compliance
Lightning Source LLC
LaVergne TN
LVHW070224100526
838202LV00015B/2087